OPHTHALMOLOGY

Principles and Concepts

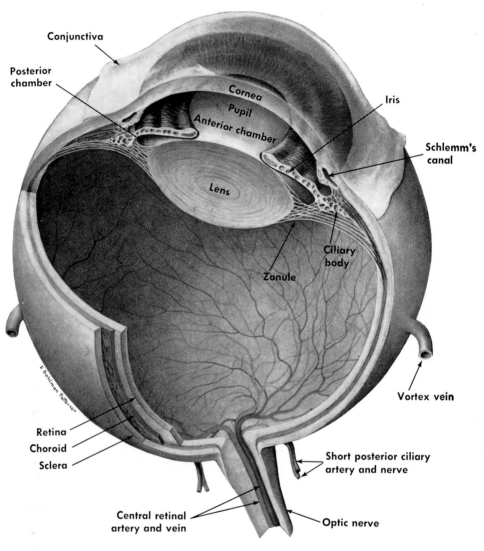

Conjunctiva

Posterior chamber

Cornea

Pupil

Anterior chamber

Iris

Schlemm's canal

Lens

Zonule

Ciliary body

Vortex vein

Retina

Choroid

Sclera

Short posterior ciliary artery and nerve

Central retinal artery and vein

Optic nerve

The human eye

OPHTHALMOLOGY

Principles and Concepts

FRANK W. NEWELL, M.D., M.Sc.(Ophth.)

Professor and Chairman, Section of Ophthalmology,
The University of Chicago

Second edition

With 233 illustrations

Saint Louis

The C. V. Mosby Company

1969

To Marian,
Frank, Mary Susan,
Elizabeth Ann, and David

Preface

The response of students and their instructors to this textbook has been extremely gratifying. Thus the general pattern of the first edition has been retained; however, an attempt has been made to minimize the duplication that arises because of involvement of several different parts of the eye by some systemic diseases. A number of sections have been shortened, particularly that on bacterial diseases, inasmuch as many of these have become curiosities, although the student and practitioner are as responsible for diagnosing curiosities as they are for diagnosing common disorders. In addition, a number of illustrations have been substituted and many sections have been rewritten.

The student's complaint that the study of ophthalmology often consists of learning a particular jargon has been met, hopefully, by the inclusion of a glossary. However, this book is not intended to be used solely within the increasingly limited time assigned to undergraduate instruction. It is meant to correlate diseases of the eye with the anatomy, embryology, biochemistry, optics, pharmacology, and clinical courses the student has studied earlier.

I am particularly grateful to my secretary, Mrs. Karin Cassel, for typing and correcting the typescript. Tibor G. Farkas was extremely helpful in providing photographs of typical histologic sections and reviewing portions of the manuscript. Portions of the manuscript have also been read by Steven G. Kramer, Alex E. Krill, Joel Pokorny, Vivianne Smith Pokorny, and Albert M. Potts. Four classes of medical students have indicated what material was not clear, and friends and readers have suggested changes.

Frank W. Newell

Contents

Part IV

Systemic diseases and the eye

Part I

Basic mechanisms

Chapter 1

Anatomy and embryology

Anatomy

To an unusual extent, the understanding of ocular functions and their modification in disease is dependent upon an appreciation of the anatomy of the eyeball, the surrounding structures, and the central vascular and nervous connections. Dissection of a fresh animal eye readily reveals the interrelationship of the intraocular tissues and the organization of the eyeball as a multichambered, nearly spherical structure. The surface anatomy is easily studied by direct inspection of a living subject, using a small penlight for illumination and a +15 diopter lens for magnification.

Eyeball

The eyeball (frontispiece) rests in the front half of the cavity of the orbit upon a fascial hammock surrounded by fat and connective tissue; only its anterior aspect is exposed. Attached to it and arising within the orbit are four rectus and two oblique muscles. These are innervated by the oculomotor (N III), trochlear (N IV), and abducens (N VI) cranial nerves that enter the orbit at its apex. The optic nerve connects the eye with the brain and leaves the apex of the orbit in the optic foramen, which also transmits the ophthalmic artery and the sympathetic innervation of the eye. The ophthalmic branch of the trigeminal nerve (N V), transmitting sensory impulses from the upper portion of the face and the eye, also enters the cranial cavity through the orbital apex. The exposed anterior one third of the eyeball consists of a central transparent portion, the cornea, and a surrounding opaque portion, the sclera. The sclera is covered with conjunctiva that is reflected onto the inner surface of the protective tissue curtains, the eyelids. Located in the upper outer portion of the bony orbit is the lacrimal gland.

The anterior pole of the eyeball is the center of curvature of the cornea. The posterior pole marks the center of the posterior curvature of the globe, and it is located to the temporal side of the optic nerve. The geometric axis is a line connecting these two poles. The equator encircles the eyeball midway between the two poles (Fig. 1-1).

The anteroposterior diameter of the normal eyeball is about 22 to 27 mm. The circumference is between 69 and 85 mm. In the average eye (24 mm. diameter) the equator is considered to be 16 mm. behind the junction of the cornea and the sclera, and the posterior pole is considered to be 32 mm. behind this junction. The anterior termination of the sensory retina is approximately 8 mm. posterior to the corneoscleral limbus.

The length of the eye cannot be directly measured during life. The normal emmetropic or nearly emmetropic eye, measured by roentgen-ray or ultrasonic methods, is between 22 and 27 mm. long. As in other biologic measurements in man, the length varies about a mean, with a normal (binomial) distribution if refractive

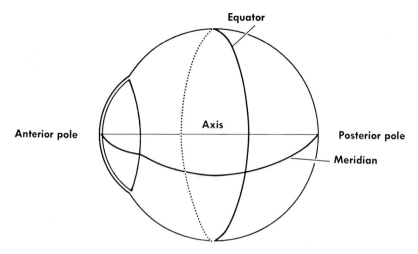

Fig. 1-1. Principal coordinates of the eye. The geometric axis connecting the anterior and posterior poles does not correspond with the visual axis, which is a line connecting an object in space with the fovea.

errors of more than 4 diopters hyperopia and 6 diopters myopia are excluded.

The globe has three main layers, each of which is further divided. The outer supporting coat is composed of the transparent cornea, the opaque sclera, and their junction, the corneoscleral sulcus or limbus. The middle vascular layer, or the uvea, consists of the choroid, the ciliary body, and the iris, which contains a central opening, the pupil. The inner layer consists of the photosensitive retina, which is composed of two parts, a light-sensitive nervous complex and a layer of pigment epithelium.

The lens is a transparent structure located immediately behind the iris and supported in position by a series of fine fibers, the zonule. These are attached to the ciliary body and the capsule of the lens.

Three chambers are described: (1) the vitreous cavity, (2) the posterior chamber, and (3) the anterior chamber. The *vitreous cavity*, by far the largest, is located behind the lens and zonule and is adjacent to the retina throughout. The *posterior chamber* is minute in size and is bounded by the lens and zonule behind and the iris in front. The *anterior chamber* sep-

arates the iris from the posterior surface of the cornea and communicates with the posterior chamber through the pupil. Anterior chamber aqueous humor enters the venous circulation through a filtration area located in the corneoscleral limbus. This is the trabecular meshwork that opens into the canal of Schlemm, an endothelium-lined channel that encircles the anterior chamber.

Outer coat of the eye

The outer coat of the eye consists of relatively tough fibrous tissues shaped as segments of two spheres: the sclera with a radius of curvature of about 13 mm. and the cornea with a radius of curvature of about 7.5+ mm. The white, opaque sclera constitutes the posterior five sixths of the globe, and the transparent cornea is fitted into a beveled opening in the anterior sclera to provide the anterior one sixth of the globe. The junction of the cornea and the sclera, the corneoscleral limbus, is an important functional and anatomic area.

Sclera. The sclera is a dense, fibrous, relatively avascular structure that comprises the posterior five sixths of the eyeball. Anteriorly it comprises the "white"

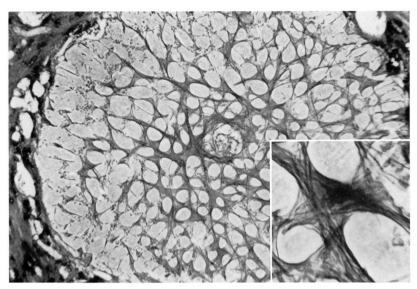

Fig. 1-2. Flat section of lamina cribrosa (posterior scleral foramen) of the cat. Fibers are continuous with the scleral fibers but are lined with microglia. (Wilder stain.) (From Ernest, J. T., and Potts, A. M.: Amer. J. Ophthal. **66:**373, 1968.)

of the eye, and here it is covered with Tenon's capsule and conjunctiva through which fine blood vessels can be seen. Posteriorly it is connected by loose, fine collagen fibers to the dense fascia bulbi (Tenon's capsule, p. 33).

At a point 3 mm. medial to the posterior pole the sclera is perforated by a 3 mm. opening, the posterior scleral foramen, or lamina cribrosa, through which the optic nerve exits from the eye. The scleral foramen is bridged by thin elastic fibers of the inner sclera that form a sievelike structure, the lamina cribrosa (Fig. 1-2). The sclera is thickest in the region surrounding the optic nerve where the dural coverings of the nerve blend into the scleral fibers. The sclera is perforated by the long and short posterior ciliary arteries and nerves in the area surrounding the optic nerve.

The anterior scleral foramen is the beveled opening of the sclera into which the cornea fits. On its inner surface is the scleral spur to which the ciliary muscle is attached. About 4 mm. posterior to the equator, in the region between the recti

muscles, are the openings for the four vortex veins that are the collecting channels for choroidal veins. In the anterior segment, about 4 mm. posterior to the corneoscleral limbus, the anterior ciliary arteries and veins pierce the sclera. Occasionally a long posterior ciliary nerve loops through the sclera and is evident by a small pigmented dot 2 to 4 mm. from the corneoscleral limbus.

Structure. Three ill-defined layers of the sclera (Fig. 1-3) are described: (1) the episclera, (2) the sclera proper, and (3) the lamina fusca.

The *episclera* is the outermost superficial layer. It is composed of loosely intertwined fibrous tissue strands connected to Tenon's capsule. The episclera has a rich blood supply and may become violently congested in inflammation.

The *sclera proper* consists of elastic fibers and typical collagen fibers with cross striations of 640 Å. The collagen fibers vary in diameter from 10 to 15μ and are 100 to 150μ long. They are arranged approximately parallel to the surface of the

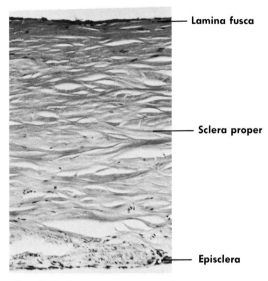

Choroid

— **Lamina fusca**

— **Sclera proper**

— **Episclera**

Fig. 1-3. Transverse section of sclera. (Masson trichrome stain; ×160.)

globe to form an interlacing basketlike weave (Fig. 1-4). Their pattern differs at the area of insertion of the extraocular muscles and at the scleral foramen, apparently in response to mechanical stresses induced by traction of the muscles and the intraocular pressure.

The *lamina fusca* is adjacent to the choroid, from which it derives a large number of melanocytes that give it a brown color. It contains more elastic tissue than the sclera proper. Delicate elastic fibers covered with endothelium with adjacent smooth muscle run between the lamina fusca and the choroid in the potential perichoroidal space.

Blood supply. Posterior to the insertion of the rectus muscles the blood supply of the sclera is sparse. It is provided by the episcleral branches of the short and long posterior ciliary arteries.

Anterior to the insertion of the rectus muscles the anterior ciliary arteries form a dense episcleral plexus. It is these ves-

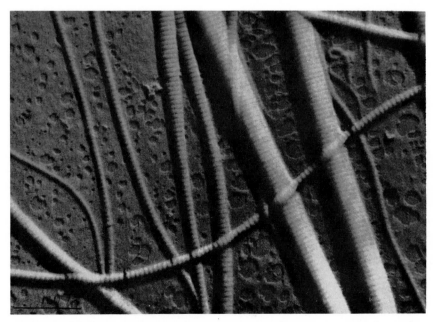

Fig. 1-4. Scleral fibrils mechanically dissociated. The fibrils vary markedly in diameter. (Electron photomicroscopy, ×28,000.) (Courtesy Prof. J. François, Ghent, Belgium.)

sels that become congested in "ciliary injection" (p. 131).

Nerve supply. The sensory nerves supplying the sclera are branches of the short and long posterior ciliary nerves.

Cornea. The cornea is the transparent anterior one sixth of the eyeball. It is approximately circular in shape and fits, as a watch glass, into the beveled edge of the sclera. The corneal diameter is about 11.5 mm. Exact measurement of the diameter is difficult because the peripheral border is covered by conjunctiva at the corneoscleral limbus. The central optical portion of the cornea is only 0.5 to 0.7 mm. thick and has nearly parallel anterior and posterior surfaces. Its peripheral portion thickens to about 1.0 mm. The radius of curvature of the anterior surface is slightly less than 8 mm., and the radius of curvature of the concave posterior surface is slightly

more than 6 mm. The cornea is the chief refracting surface of the eye because it separates media of such different indexes of refraction as air and aqueous humor. Variations in curvature of different corneal meridians cause astigmatism.

Structure. The cornea (Fig. 1-5) is composed of five layers: (1) epithelium, (2) Bowman's membrane (continuous with the stroma), (3) substantia propria (stroma), (4) Descemet's membrane (the basement membrane of the endothelium), and (5) endothelium.

The *epithelium* covers the substantia propria anteriorly and is continuous with the epithelium of the conjunctiva. It consists of stratified squamous cells formed in the deepest basal layer which shed 4 to 8 days later from the superficial layer. The basal cells are columnar in shape and rest upon a delicate basement membrane 100 to 300 Å thick. This consists of a superficial lipid layer adherent to the overlying cells and of a deeper reticular network that merges into the adjacent Bowman's membrane. With maturation, basal cells are pushed forward to form three layers of progressively flatter cells called wing cells. The outermost squamous cells are two layers thick and consist of thin, flat cells that form the outer surface of the cornea and are attached to adjacent cells by desmosomes 500 to 1,500 Å thick. Because of these attachments, sheets of epithelial cells may be mechanically removed from the cornea.

The anterior corneal stroma is condensed into a homogeneous layer, *Bowman's membrane.* It is grossly evident as a brilliant, glistening membrane when epithelial cells are removed or when corneal sections are examined by light microscopy. Electron microscopy indicates Bowman's membrane to be continuous with the substantia propria and not a separate structure. Its abrupt termination at the corneal periphery is the proximal, anterior margin of the corneoscleral limbus (p. 9). The injured

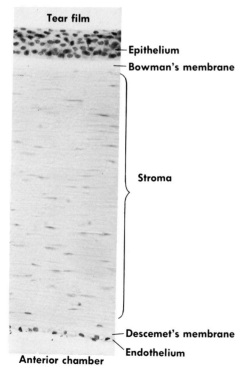

Fig. 1-5. Transverse section of cornea. (Hematoxylin and eosin stain; ×105.)

Tear film — Epithelium — Bowman's membrane — Stroma — Descemet's membrane — Endothelium — Anterior chamber

epithelium quickly regenerates by sliding and proliferation of adjacent cells, and healing occurs without scarring. Damage to the substantia propria results in scar formation.

The *substantia propria*, or stroma, forms 90% of the cornea. It consists of cells and fine fibrils. The cells are long, flattened, compressed keratocytes or corneal corpuscles and correspond to fibroblasts in other tissues. In addition, there are flattened,

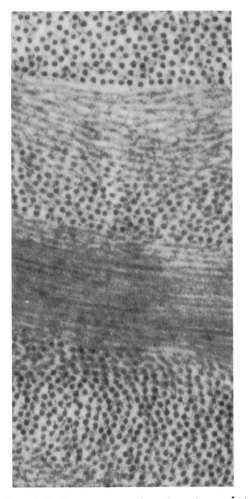

Fig. 1-6. Transverse section through corneal stroma showing several lamellas in which collagen fibers are oriented parallel to each other and perpendicular to those in adjacent layers. (Electron photomicroscopy, ×12,000.)

wandering leukocytes. The fibrils are composed of collagen and are approximately of uniform thickness. The fibrils are covered with a dense layer of a mucopolysaccharide cement substance (p. 445). They are collected into bundles that form some 100 to 200 corneal lamellas. The lamellas are arranged parallel to the corneal surface but crisscross at right angles to each other in alternate layers (Fig. 1-6).

The posterior cornea is lined with endothelium composed of a single layer of flat cells of irregular size arranged on the inner surface of *Descemet's membrane*. This is a glassy membrane loosely attached to the back surface of the stroma and secreted by the endothelial cells. Descemet's membrane is composed of collagen fibrils embedded in a mucopolysaccharide matrix. Both the matrix and the fibrils differ from those found in the substantia propria. Descemet's membrane regenerates readily and, following injury, may form a double layer. At the periphery of the cornea it becomes fenestrated at the openings of the trabecular meshwork and forms the proximal, posterior margin of the corneoscleral limbus. Desmosomes have not been demonstrated in the endothelium lining the substantia propria, but adjacent cells are bound together by extensive interdigitation.

Blood supply. The central cornea is avascular, but the region of the corneoscleral limbus is generously supplied by conjunctival branches of the anterior ciliary arteries. These form a superficial marginal plexus that sends blood vessels at right angles toward the cornea. They give rise to two systems: branches forming terminal vascular loops at the corneoscleral limbus and recurrent branches that anastomose with posterior conjunctival arteries (p. 37).

Nerve supply. The corneal nerves are entirely sensory, subserving the sensation of pain and possibly of touch. The nerve endings are either terminal beadlike thickenings or bare fibers in the epithelium or in the anterior stroma. Near the limbus, Krause's end-bulbs and endings for cold sensation are present. The nerves become medullated as they exit from the corneal periphery and pass to the semilunar ganglion by way of the long and short posterior ciliary nerves, branches of the ophthalmic division of the trigeminal nerve.

Corneoscleral limbus. The corneoscleral limbus, or junction (Fig. 1-7), is a transitional zone 1 to 2 mm. wide between the cornea proper and the sclera and conjunctiva. Its proximal margin is a line extending from the termination of Bowman's membrane to the end of nonfenestrated Descemet's membrane. Its distal margin is the corneoscleral junction through a plane drawn perpendicular to the scleral spur and parallel to the proximal margin. The area is clinically important because it encompasses the trabecular meshwork and the canal of Schlemm, which forms the drainage system of the anterior chamber. In addition, surgical incision into the globe for cataract extraction and glaucoma procedures is usually at the limbus. The trabeculum can be seen clinically by using a gonioscope.

Structure. Basically the corneoscleral limbus is composed of but two layers: (1) the epithelium and (2) the stroma. Buried in its inner aspect is the trabecular meshwork that communicates between the anterior chamber and the canal of Schlemm.

In the limbal area the corneal *epithelium* thickens, and in some areas papillary formation may be seen. The corneal *stroma* loses its regular pattern, and the lamellas do not lie parallel to the corneal surface. Imperceptibly there is a gradual change from the regularly arranged corneal lamellas to the random distribution of the collagen bundles of the sclera.

Trabecular meshwork. Surrounding the entire circumference of the anterior chamber is the trabecular meshwork, a pore-like structure through which aqueous humor percolates to the canal of Schlemm (Fig. 1-8). In cross section the trabeculum forms an obtuse triangle with a short base

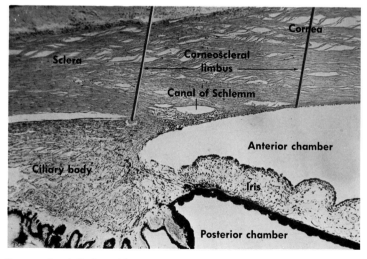

Fig. 1-7. Corneoscleral limbus. The central margin of the corneoscleral limbus is a line drawn between the termination of Bowman's membrane and the point where Descemet's membrane becomes discontinuous. The posterior margin is a line drawn parallel to the central margin and passing through the scleral spur. (Hematoxylin and eosin stain; ×105.)

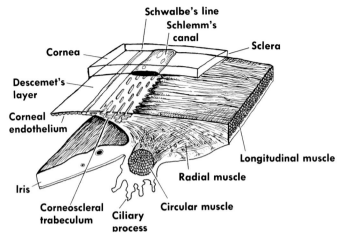

Fig. 1-8. Schematic construction of the ciliary body and angle recess in man. (Redrawn from Rohen, J. W.: In Von Mollendorf, W., editor: Handbuch der mikroskopischen Anatomie des Menschen, Berlin, 1964, Springer-Verlag.)

and two long sides. The base of the triangle is in contact with the scleral spur and the free surface of the ciliary body. One long side is in contact with the cornea and the sclera and in communication with Schlemm's canal—this is described as the corneoscleral portion. The other long side opens directly into the anterior chamber and is described as the uveal portion. The meshwork is arranged in sheets, with round or oval openings between layers. An acid mucopolysaccharide coats the meshwork. The angle formed at the junction of the two long sides is the anterior termination of the trabecular meshwork and forms the border ring of Schwalbe.

The trabecular meshwork is innervated by a plexus of delicate axons that terminate without specialized endings within the endothelium of Schlemm's canal. The nerves arise from both divisions of the autonomic nervous system and from the trigeminal nerve. They may function in controlling the rate of flow of aqueous humor through the system.

Canal of Schlemm. The canal of Schlemm is an endothelium-lined chan-

nel, approximately oval in cross section, that surrounds the entire circumference of the anterior chamber. On its inner surface it communicates with the anterior chamber through the trabecular meshwork. Its outer wall is buried in the stroma of the corneoscleral sulcus. The canal contains numerous pores through which the aqueous humor percolates. The canal of Schlemm connects with the venous system through a system of 25 to 35 collector channels that anastomose to form a deep intrascleral plexus. This intrascleral plexus sends branches to the ciliary body and the anterior ciliary veins. The anterior ciliary veins may appear subconjunctivally as minute vessels containing clear aqueous, the aqueous veins.

Middle coat of the eye

The middle or uveal coat of the eyeball (from *uva* [Latin], meaning grape) consists of the choroid, the ciliary body, and the iris. The choroid is a vascular layer providing the blood supply to the retinal pigment epithelium and the outer one half of the neural retina adjacent to it. The ciliary body secretes aqueous humor and

Neural retina

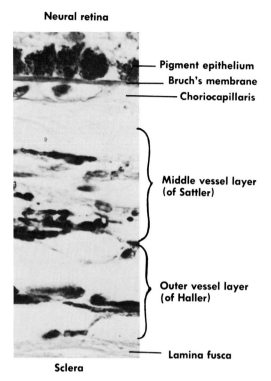

Pigment epithelium

Bruch's membrane

Choriocapillaris

Middle vessel layer (of Sattler)

Outer vessel layer (of Haller)

Lamina fusca

Sclera

Fig. 1-9. Transverse section of choroid. (Hematoxylin and eosin stain; ×625.)

contains the smooth muscle responsible for the change in shape of the lens, causing accommodation (p. 86). The iris surrounds a central opening, the pupil, which controls the amount of light entering the eye.

The choroid is of mesodermal origin, whereas the epithelium of the ciliary body and the iris represents the anterior extremities of the primitive secondary optic vesicle. The dilatator and sphincter muscles of the iris arise from neural ectoderm, and the ciliary muscles arise from mesoderm.

Choroid. The vascular sheet provides the blood supply for that half of the retina adjacent to it. It is composed mainly of an inner layer of capillaries (choriocapillaris) and successively larger collecting veins arranged roughly in layers. The choroid extends from the optic nerve posteriorly to

the ciliary body anteriorly. Perhaps reflecting a variation in nutritional requirements of the different parts of the retina, it is thickest (0.25 mm.) at the posterior pole and gradually thins anteriorly to 0.10 mm. It is attached firmly to the sclera in the region of the optic nerve where the posterior ciliary arteries enter the eye and at the points of exit of the four vortex veins.

Structure. The choroid (Fig. 1-9) consists of three layers of blood vessels with supporting structures on either side: (1) the suprachoroid (lamina fusca), (2) the blood vessel layer, and (3) the basal lamina (membrane of Bruch).

The outermost layer, the *suprachoroid (lamina fusca)*, is made up of delicate lamellas composed of elastic and collagenous fibers to form a synechia that is dense posteriorly and becomes looser anteriorly. Chromatophores are abundant in this layer and decrease in number in the vascular layers. Also found in this area are smooth muscle fibers, fibroblasts and endothelial cells, long and short posterior ciliary arteries, and nerves. The short posterior ciliary arteries have but a short course in the suprachoroid and extend directly to the choriocapillaris layer. Thus the outer and middle coats of vessels consist nearly exclusively of veins, although the middle layer contains some arterioles.

The *blood vessel layer* has three components: (1) the outer (nearest the sclera) vessel layer (of Haller), which consists of large veins that lead to the vortex veins and have no valves; (2) the middle vessel layer (of Sattler), which consists of medium-sized veins and some arterioles and which contains a loose collagenous stroma with numerous elastic fibers and fibroblasts containing pigment (chromatophores); and (3) the choriocapillaris, which consists of widely dilated capillaries that form a dense network extending from the optic disk to the ora serrata.

The *basal lamina (membrane of Bruch)* is about 7 mμ thick and separates the choroidal blood vessels from the retinal pigment epithelium. It has a dual origin from the choroid and the retinal pigment epithelium. The outer layer nearest the choroid is composed of the walls of a single layer of endothelial cells of the choriocapillaris and contains numerous pores. Adjacent to this is a delicate layer of collagen fibers. Centrally there is a layer of elastic tissue fibers that extend outward to form the supporting structure of the choriocapillaris. The inner (cuticular) layer originates from the retinal pigment epithelium and is composed of collagen fibers surrounded by acid mucopolysaccharides. Resting upon this is the delicate basement membrane of the retinal pigment epithelium. At the optic nerve, Bruch's membrane stops abruptly with the pigment epithelium. Anteriorly, at the ciliary body, the two component layers divide.

Blood supply. The blood supply of the choroid is derived from the short posterior ciliary arteries, the long posterior ciliary arteries, and the anterior ciliary arteries, all of which are interconnected through the choriocapillaris and intra-arterial anastomoses (Fig. 1-10). The short posterior ciliary arteries arise as two branches of the ophthalmic artery. These two branches subdivide into 10 to 20 branches that perforate the sclera around the circumference of the optic nerve. The majority pass at once into the choroid and communicate directly with the choriocapillaris layer. The two long posterior ciliary arteries perforate the sclera on either side of the optic nerve and extend anteriorly in the suprachoroidal space on the medial and lateral sides of the globe to the ciliary body. There each divides into two branches to form the major arterial circle of the iris, which is

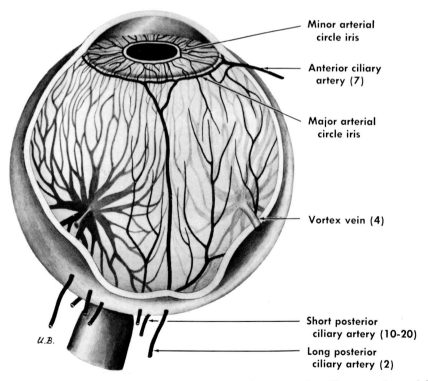

Minor arterial circle iris

Anterior ciliary artery (7)

Major arterial circle iris

Vortex vein (4)

Short posterior ciliary artery (10-20)

Long posterior ciliary artery (2)

U.B.

Fig. 1-10. Blood supply of the uveal tract. The two long posterior ciliary arteries mainly supply the iris, the anterior ciliary arteries the ciliary body, and the short posterior ciliary arteries the choroid. The blood vessels anastomose freely.

located in the ciliary body. Recurrent choroidal branches extend posteriorly to the choriocapillaris.

The anterior ciliary arteries are the terminal branches of the two muscular arteries of each rectus muscle (except the lateral rectus muscle, which has but one muscular artery). The anterior ciliary arteries bifurcate into vessels that penetrate the sclera and nonpenetrating vessels that extend toward the cornea. The penetrating vessels provide the blood supply to the ciliary body and send branches to the anterior extremity of the choriocapillaris of the choroid and the major arterial circle of the iris. The nonpenetrating vessels extend forward in the episclera as anterior conjunctival arteries, anastomose with posterior conjunctival arteries, and terminate in the superficial (conjunctival) and deep (episcleral) pericorneal plexus.

Venous blood is collected from the choroid, ciliary body, and iris by a series of veins of increasingly larger diameter. These lead to four large vortex veins located behind the equator of the globe. In addition to venous blood from the choroid, the vortex vessels contain blood from the iris and from the ciliary body. The vortex veins empty into the superior and inferior ophthalmic veins, each of which drains into the cavernous sinus.

Nerve supply. The choroid is innervated by the short ciliary nerves derived from the ciliary ganglion. As they enter the choroid, they branch repeatedly to form a plexus, losing their myelin sheath. Numerous ganglion cells are present, and nerve endings are in contact with pigmented cells and with smooth muscle in the walls of the arterioles and the arteries.

Ciliary body. The ciliary body (Fig. 1-11) is a ring of tissue about 6 mm. wide intermediate between the base of the iris and the choroid.

In cross section the ciliary body forms approximately a right triangle with a short base and with the right angle attached to the scleral spur. The base faces the anterior chamber and provides insertion for the iris. The hypotenuse faces the vitreous and posterior chambers, and the intermediate side is adjacent to the sclera.

Structure. The ciliary body is divided into the following: the uveal portion adjacent to the sclera, which includes the ciliary muscle, the suprachoroid (lamina fusca), the vessel layer, the lamina vitrea, and the elastic, connective tissue, and cuticular layers, and the epithelial portion adjacent to the posterior chamber, which includes the pars plana (orbiculus ciliaris) and the pars plicata (corona ciliaris).

Uveal portion. The *ciliary muscle* is the most prominent structure in the uveal portion of the ciliary body. It is composed of three groups of smooth muscle: (1) the longitudinal fibers (Brücke's muscle) are the outermost—they parallel the surface of the overlying sclera and constitute the main bulk of the muscle; (2) the radial fibers arise from the anterior portion of the longitudinal fibers and run obliquely to become continuous with circular fibers; and (3) the circular fibers (Müller) are the innermost portion of the ciliary muscle and have a direction approximately parallel to the equator of the lens.

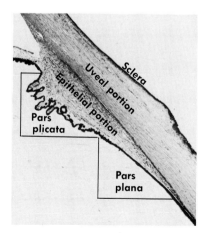

Fig. 1-11. Ciliary body. (Hematoxylin and eosin stain; ×160.)

There is general agreement that in accommodation (p. 86) the ciliary muscle contracts and causes relaxation of the zonule, permitting the lens to become convex. The mechanism of this action is in doubt, particularly in respect to the longitudinal fibers that have an indefinite insertion. The motor innervation is by the short ciliary nerves. The motor fibers arise in the Edinger-Westphal nucleus and reach the ciliary ganglion from the inferior division of the oculomotor nerve (N III). Postganglionic fibers are then distributed with the short posterior ciliary nerves.

The scleral surface of the ciliary body is the *suprachoroid (lamina fusca)*, which is comparable to that of the choroid but contains fewer lamellas. The *vessel layer* is composed mainly of the major arterial circle of the iris, its tributaries, and veins. There is no choriocapillaris. The *lamina vitrea* is the anterior extension of Bruch's membrane, which becomes split by connective tissue. The *elastic layer* (choroid) diminishes and disappears, but the *cuticular layer* (retinal) continues forward to the root of the iris.

Epithelial portion. The epithelial portion of the ciliary body forms the hypotenuse of the triangular ciliary body and faces the vitreous cavity and the posterior chamber. It is divided into (1) the *pars plana* (orbiculus ciliaris), about 4 mm. broad and adjacent to the retina, and (2) the *pars plicata* (corona ciliaris), the anterior 2 mm. The pars plicata is thrown into some 60 to 70 folds, the ciliary processes, each of which is 0.8 mm. high and 1 mm. broad. The junction of the pars plana portion of the ciliary body with the retina presents a toothed or scalloped margin, the ora serrata (Fig. 1-12). Each tooth corresponds with the valley of a ciliary process, and narrow striae extend to them from the ora. In this area the sensory retina is transformed abruptly into a single layer of elongated, columnar, nonpigmented ciliary epithelium.

The epithelial portion of the ciliary body is composed of a layer of nonpigmented epithelium constituting the anterior continuation of the sensory retina and pigmented epithelium constituting the anterior continuation of the outer portion of the optic cup, the retinal pigment epithelium. Each has an adjacent basement membrane. That of the nonpigmented epithelium is the continuation of the internal limiting membrane of the retina and is on the vitreous side of the cell (its base). The basement membrane of the pigmented

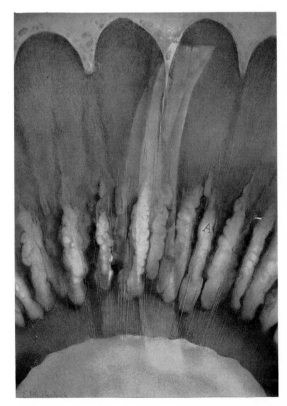

Fig. 1-12. Ciliary body viewed from behind with the ora serrata above and the lens below. Zonular fibers extend toward the lens from the valleys between the ciliary process. The area between the ciliary processes, **A**, and the ora serrata is the pars plana. (From McCulloch, C.: Trans. Amer. Ophthal. Soc. **52:**525, 1954.)

epithelium is the cuticular portion of the lamina vitrea and is on the side of the cell nearest the sclera. The apexes of these cells are thus in apposition, and cell secretion is by extrusion through the apex rather than through the base of the cell in contact with the basement membrane. The material then passes into intercellular spaces to make its way between cells to the vitreous or the posterior chamber. Electron microscopy suggests that the non-pigmented epithelium of the ciliary processes elaborates aqueous humor and hyaluronic acid. The Golgi complex of these cells is prominent, and their structure is closely comparable to mucus-secreting glandular cells.

Each ciliary process consists of a delicate finger of tissue with a covering of nonpigmented epithelium over a layer of pigmented epithelium surrounding a vascular core (Fig. 1-13). Each process has an arteriole extending to the apex, where it breaks into a rich capillary system.

Iris and pupil. The iris is a delicate diaphragm lying in front of the lens and the ciliary body and separating the anterior and posterior chambers. Located slightly to its nasal side is a circular aperture, the pupil, which reflexly controls the amount of light admitted to the eye. The iris inserts into the scleral spur by means of its connection to the middle of the anterior surface of the ciliary body. The pupillary border rests upon the lens. When the lens is absent, the iris is tremulous (iridodonesis) and flat.

The anterior surface is divided into a pupillary zone, in which the anterior leaf of the stroma is absent, and a peripheral ciliary zone. These are divided by a ridge, the collarette, which is concentric with the pupillary margin (Fig. 1-14). The collarette marks the position of the minor vascular circle of the iris from which the pupillary membrane arises in fetal life. Atrophy of the membrane begins in the seventh month and is usually complete by 8½ months, frequently leaving behind a few delicate strands.

The central pupillary zone of the iris is relatively flat, and its width varies with the degree of atrophy of the anterior leaf of the stroma and the degree of pupillary dilation. The anterior leaf of the iris stroma is not strongly attached to the underlying tissue and, with pupillary dilation, the

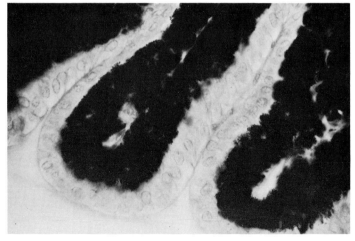

Fig. 1-13. Ciliary processes. The nonpigmented epithelium is on the surface facing the posterior chamber. (Periodic acid–Schiff stain; ×63.)

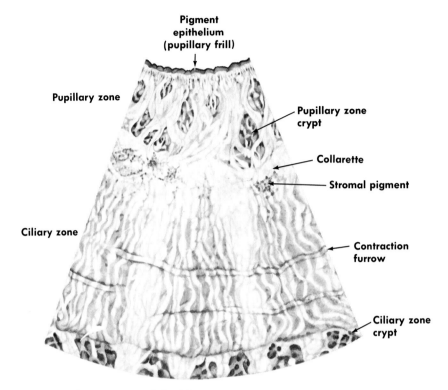

Fig. 1-14. Surface pattern of the iris.

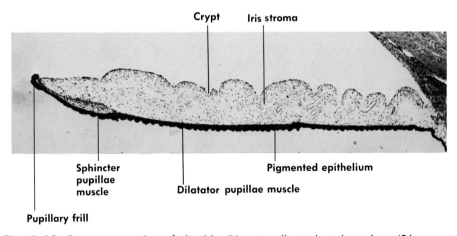

Fig. 1-15. Transverse section of the iris. (Hematoxylin and eosin stain; ×43.)

pupillary zone slides under the anterior leaf of stroma in the ciliary zone.

The ciliary zone of the iris is marked by many radial interlacing ridges, giving a gossamer-like appearance. Additionally, in lightly pigmented eyes, concentric con-traction furrows may be seen. The color of the iris depends upon the amount of melanin in the mesodermal stroma. If very slight, reflection from the pigment of the posterior layer causes scattering and thus a blue appearance. If more marked, the eye is hazel, and if very marked, the eye is brown.

Structure. The iris consists of two layers: (1) stroma, located anteriorly and arising from mesoderm, and (2) pigmented epithelium, located posteriorly and arising from neural ectoderm (Fig. 1-15).

The *stroma* may be divided into an anterior and a posterior leaf. The anterior stroma contains numerous vessels radiating at different levels from the great circle of the iris and crossing each other at different angles. There are fine collagen fibers in which chromatophores that vary in pigment content are enmeshed. The anterior limiting membrane of the iris is a condensation of the anterior stroma, producing a dense matting. The anterior leaf is most highly developed about the seventh month of fetal life. Thereafter it atrophies in the pupillary zone of the iris and in irregular areas in the ciliary zone to form crypts. The posterior leaf is similar to the anterior leaf but contains more elastic fibers, fewer chromatophores, and blood vessels that are less likely to atrophy. It is visible in the pupillary zone and at the depth of iris crypts.

The *pigmented epithelium* consists of two layers of cells, constituting a fusion of the two layers of the primitive optic vesicle. They are densely packed with pigment. The anterior layer of pigment cells is closely identified with the dilatator pupillae muscle. This layer is absent in the area of the sphincter muscle. The posterior layer of epithelium is covered on its lenticular surface with an internal limiting membrane, presumably continuous with that of the retina and the ciliary body. The pupillary margin may have a pigment frill that is continuous with the ectodermal pigment layer. This frill constitutes the anterior extremity of the secondary optic vesicle.

The sphincter pupillae muscle is located in the pupillary zone of the posterior stroma. It is a smooth muscle about 1 mm.

broad that forms a sphincter around the pupillary margin. The dilatator muscle is located between the stroma and the pigmented epithelium, and it extends as a thin sheet of smooth muscle from its origin in the ciliary body to the sphincter pupillae muscle.

Blood supply. The blood supply is provided by radial vessels in the stromal layer that extends from the major arterial circle of the iris (circulus arteriosus iridis major) located in the ciliary body (Fig. 1-12). This is formed by two long posterior ciliary arteries and the seven anterior ciliary arteries. The iris blood vessels pass radially in a corkscrew pattern toward the pupillary margin, giving rise to the meridional striations of the ciliary portion of the iris. At the collarette they anastomose to form the incomplete minor vascular circle of the iris. The vessels have an unusually thick collagen adventitia. The muscularis layer of the arteries is very thin. The veins have a perivascular sheath bordering the endothelium.

Nerve supply. The iris is richly supplied with nerves from the short and long posterior ciliary nerves that carry sensory, motor, and sympathetic fibers. The nerves are partially medullated and have a thick neurilemma. They are distributed to the stroma (sensory, N V), the dilatator muscle (sympathetics), blood vessels (sympathetics), and the sphincter muscle (N III).

Inner coat of the eye

Retina. The retina develops from invagination of the optic cup (discussion on embryology, p. 61) to form an outer layer, the pigment epithelium, and an inner layer, the neurosensory retina. The inner layer becomes stratified into many layers. By custom, the layers of the retina nearest the choroid are designated as the outer layers, and those nearest the center of the eye are designated as the inner layers. The photosensitive neurosensory retina extends from the optic nerve posteriorly to the scalloped margin, the ora serrata, anteriorly.

The pigment epithelium is of fairly uniform structure throughout. The structure of the neurosensory retina varies both histologically and functionally in its central and peripheral portions in the distribution of neural and supporting elements.

Pigment epithelium. The pigment epithelium (Fig. 1-16) extends to the optic nerve margin posteriorly and to the ora serrata anteriorly, where it fuses with the anterior continuation of the neurosensory retina and continues forward as the pigmented ciliary epithelium. The cells of the pigment epithelium contain varying amounts of pigment which, on ophthalmo-

scopic examination, give a grandular appearance to the fundus. The retinal pigment epithelium consists of a single layer of cuboidal cells that are firmly attached to the cuticular portion of the membrane of Bruch.

Individual pigment epithelium cells may have from four to eight sides but are usually hexagonal. They are fitted together like cobblestones in a regular arrangement. They are separated from, but also bound to, each other by a clear cement substance that also binds the entire layer to the cuticular layer of Bruch's membrane. In cross section the pigment epithelium cells are divided into a base, body, and processes or microvilli. The base, which does not contain pigment, contains the cell nucleus and

Neural retina

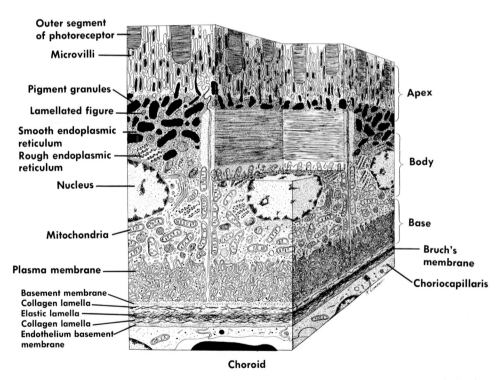

Outer segment of photoreceptor
Microvilli
Pigment granules
Lamellated figure
Smooth endoplasmic reticulum
Rough endoplasmic reticulum
Nucleus
Mitochondria
Plasma membrane
Basement membrane
Collagen lamella
Elastic lamella
Collagen lamella
Endothelium basement membrane

Apex
Body
Base
Bruch's membrane
Choriocapillaris

Choroid

Fig. 1-16. Retinal pigment epithelium and its relationship to the choriocapillaris (below) and the neural retina (above). Sheep pigment epithelium illustrated here has more marked infolding of the plasma membrane than in man. (From Leure-duPree, A.: Amer. J. Ophthal. **65:**383, 1968.)

Layers of sclera, choroid, and retina

I. Sclera
   A. Episclera
   B. Sclera proper
   C. Lamina fusca

II. Choroid
   A. Lamina fusca
   B. Layer of large veins (of Haller)
   C. Layer of smaller-sized veins (of Sattler)
   D. Choriocapillaris (the blood supply of the outer retina)
   E. Bruch's membrane
      1. Elastic portion

III. Retina
   A. Bruch's membrane
      1. Cuticular portion (basement membrane of pigment epithelium)
   B. Pigment epithelium (outer layer of secondary optic vesicle)
   C. Neurosensory retina (inner layer of secondary optic vesicle)
      1. Photoreceptors (outer and inner segments of rods and cones)
      2. External limiting membrane (terminal bars of Müller's cells)
      3. Outer nuclear layer (cell bodies of rods and cones)
      4. Outer plexiform layer (synapse of rod and cone fibers with bipolar cell dendrites)
      5. Inner nuclear layer (nuclei of bipolar, Müller, and association cells)
      6. Inner plexiform layer (synapse of bipolar cell axons with ganglion cell dendrites)
      7. Ganglion cell layer
      8. Nerve fiber layer (axons of ganglion cells)
      9. Inner limiting membrane (Müller's fibers)
         a. Basement membrane of retina

is in contact with the basement membrane. The body contains rod-shaped and elliptic pigment granules that extend into the processes, which in turn surround the outer segments of the rods and cones.

Neurosensory retina. The neurosensory retina (inner layer of primitive optic vesicle, Fig. 1-17) basically consists of a photoreceptor layer of cells and two neurons. A neuron is simply a nervous element consisting of a nucleus with a dendrite and an axon with their terminal arborizations. The photoreceptor cells, the rods and cones, correspond to the sensory endings elsewhere in the nervous system. The first neuron is the bipolar cell whose dendrites synapse with rods and cones and whose axons synapse with the dendrites of ganglion cells. Ganglion cells constitute the second neuron; their axons extend through the optic nerve and radiate to the midbrain. The skeletal support of the retina is provided by fibers from Müller's cells.

The neurosensory retina may thus be divided into the following: a layer of photoreceptor cells, the layer of rods and cones; a layer composed of cell bodies of the rods and cones, the outer nuclear layer; an inner nuclear layer containing the cell bodies of bipolar, Müller, and association cells; and a ganglion cell layer. The region of synapse between rods and cones and dendrites of the cells with nuclei in the inner nuclear layer is the outer plexiform (molecular) layer. The

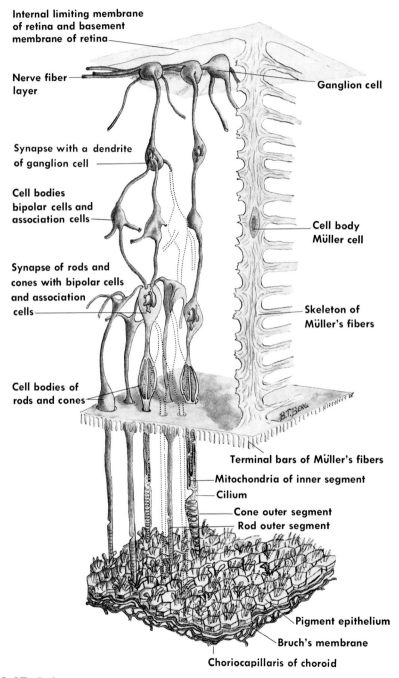

Internal limiting membrane
of retina and basement
membrane of retina

Nerve fiber
layer

Ganglion cell

Synapse with a dendrite
of ganglion cell

Cell bodies
bipolar cells and
association cells

Cell body
Müller cell

Synapse of rods and
cones with bipolar cells
and association
cells

Skeleton of
Müller's fibers

Cell bodies of
rods and cones

Terminal bars of Müller's fibers

Mitochondria of inner segment

Cilium

Cone outer segment

Rod outer segment

Pigment epithelium

Bruch's membrane

Choriocapillaris of choroid

Fig. 1-17. Retina.

region of synapse between axons of cells with nuclei in the inner nuclear layer and dendrites of ganglion cells is the inner plexiform (molecular) layer. The axons of ganglion cells constitute the nerve fiber layer. There are thus three layers of nuclei and three fiber layers.

Photoreceptor layer (rods and cones). Each rod and cone may be divided into (1) an outer segment in close relationship to the pigment epithelium; (2) a cilium, a tubelike structure connecting the outer and inner segments; (3) an inner segment; (4) the outer rod (or cone) fiber connecting the inner segment to the cell body; (5) the cell body that contains the nucleus, and (6) the inner rod (or cone)

fiber that terminates in a specialized synaptic ending (Fig. 1-18).

The *outer segment* is composed of a stack of flattened sacs or disks arising from infoldings of a plasma membrane and consisting of a double layer of membrane connected to a tubelike outer wall. The space included in the double layer is occupied by the visual pigments (p. 78). The disklike structure increases the membrane surface and orients the visual pigments for optimum absorption of light. There are some 700 disks in each outer segment.

The outer segment is connected to the inner segment by a *cilium* that, on electron microscopy, is observed to have nine pairs of linear striations (as does hair) and

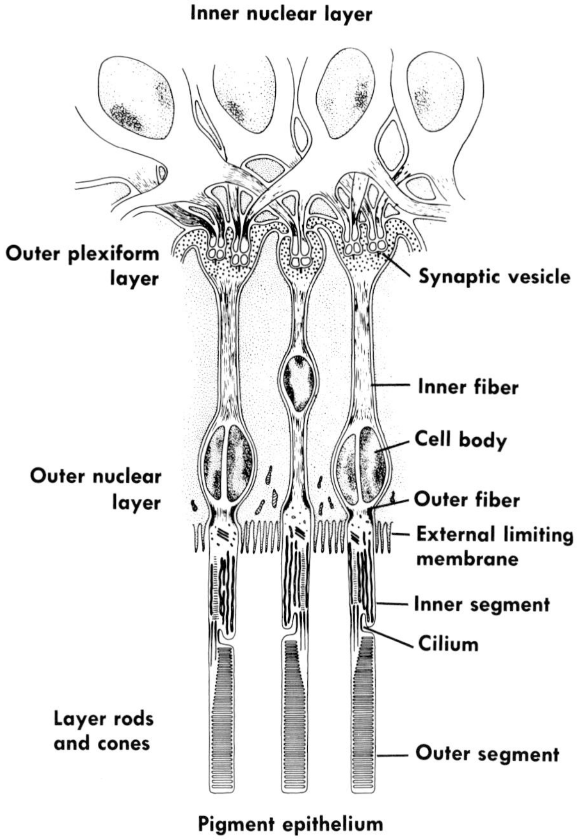

Fig. 1-18. Schematic drawing of retinal receptors in the guinea pig retina. (From Sjöstrand, F. S.: In Smelser, G. K., editor: The structure of the eye, New York, 1961, Academic Press, Inc.)

appears to have a supporting rather than a nervous function.

The *inner segment* is divided into a refractile outer portion or ellipsoid and a nonrefractile basophilic inner portion or myoid. The ellipsoid is filled with mitochondria. The myoid contains the large Golgi complex and associated vesicles and ribosomes. In some amphibian cones the myoid is contractile—hence the name "myoid"; it has no muscle properties in man. The inner segment may synthesize the acid mucopolysaccharide that surrounds the outer segment. The mitochondria are present in great abundance. The nervous signal initiated by the chemical change in the visual pigment of the outer segment may be amplified in this region. The inner segment of a cone is plump—hence the name "cone"; division into ellipsoid and myoid portions is more distinct than in rods. Generally, rods are of similar shape throughout the retina, but cones differ quite markedly both in length and plumpness in different areas of the retina.

The inner segment is connected to the cell body that contains the nucleus by a delicate *outer rod (or cone) fiber,* which may be long or short, depending upon the distance between the structures it is connecting. The outer rod fiber is surrounded by the terminal bars of Müller's fibers. In light microscopy these are seen as the outer limiting membrane and provide the vertical orientation for the photoreceptors.

The *cell body* consists almost entirely of nucleus and is located in the outer nuclear layer. An *inner rod (or cone) fiber* passes to the outer plexiform layer and terminates in a rod spherule, or end-knob, or in a cone pedicle, or cone-foot, which synapses in the outer plexiform layer with cells whose nuclei are in the inner nuclear layer. There are several different types of synaptic endings, and it is possible at this level that there are both inhibition and integration of the nervous impulse. Also

at this level some chemical intermediate is secreted, possibly acetylcholine, which is involved in the transsynaptic transmission of impulse.

In man there are approximately 120 million rods and 5 million cones. The cones are mainly concentrated in the fovea centralis and surrounding area, although a few are scattered throughout the retina (see Fig. 2-5). The optic nerve has but 1 million fibers—thus it is evident that the nerve fibers transmit impulses arising from a number of photoreceptors. The analogy of an eye to a camera, with the retina constituting the film, has been used so frequently that it may be difficult to appreciate that the nervous impulse transmitted to the brain when the retina is stimulated is not a neat miniature scene resembling the colored transparency but instead a complex code of electrical impulses (p. 85).

Inner nuclear layer. The cell bodies of bipolar cells, association cells (the horizontal and the amacrine), and Müller's supporting cells are located in this layer. The layer is composed of densely staining nuclei, and in the usual histologic preparations it is not possible to distinguish different types of cells.

Bipolar cells consist of a cell body located in the inner nuclear layer, an outer dendritic portion, and an inner axis cylinder. The outer dendritic portion synapses with the inner fiber of rods or cones in the outer plexiform layer. The axon synapses with dendrites of ganglion cells in the inner plexiform layer.

Some bipolar cells synapse with a number of photoreceptors (mop and brush bipolars), whereas others synapse with but a single cone. Traditionally, those that synapse with a single cone, the midget bipolars, synapse with but one ganglion cell and characterize the cells transmitting the impulse from the cones in the fovea centralis to the brain. Physiologically this one to one representation of the fovea centralis cones is an oversimplification. Bipolar cells likely synapse with more than one foveal photoreceptor and ganglion cell but with fewer than elsewhere in the retina.

Located in the inner nuclear layer with the cell bodies of bipolar cells are the cell bodies of the *association cells,* the horizontal and the amacrine cells. Horizontal cells have a dendrite that synapses with several closely adjoining cones and an axon that synapses with several rods and cones in a distant part of the retina. Possibly they act as condensers, as in an electric circuit, and collect impulses from a group of cones and, with discharge, trigger a visual impulse. Amacrine cells are oriented in the wrong direction to be explained in terms of the transmission of the light impulse. The amacrine dendrite synapses with ganglion cells, and its thin axons synapse with cone-foot pedicles. They may have an inhibitional function in integration of the visual impulse.

Müller's cells (radial fibers of Müller) form the bulk of the neuroglial supporting framework of the retina. They provide an elaborate arrangement of astroglia that invests the cell bodies, axons, dendrites, and blood vessels of the retina. It so completely invests retinal structures that the retina has no extracellular space. It functions in a manner analogous to the sheath of Schwann about a peripheral nerve. In addition, Müller's cells synthesize and store glycogen and contain many of the enzymes required by the tricarboxylic acid cycle. The cell body is located in the inner nuclear layer. The outer or scleral ends of Müller's cells are terminal bars, interpreted by light microscopy as the external limiting membrane, which closely surround the outer fibers of the photoreceptor cells. The inner ends of Müller's cells form the inner surface of the sensory retina and secrete the basement membrane of the retina.

Ganglion cell layer. The nuclei of ganglion cells are located in the innermost cellular layer of the retina. In the region surrounding the fovea centralis, ganglion cells are five to seven layers thick. In the retinal periphery, ganglion cells are but a single cell thick. Ganglion cell dendrites synapse with the axons of bipolar cells and the dendrites of amacrine cells. The axons of ganglion cells constitute the afferent fibers of the optic nerve and extend to the lateral geniculate body (visual fibers) and to the pretectal nucleus (pupillary fibers).

Fiber layers. The retina contains three fiber layers. Synapse is made in both the inner and the outer plexiform layers. The nerve fiber layer, the innermost, consists of ganglion cell axons.

The *outer plexiform (molecular) layer,* which is located between the cell bodies in the outer and inner nuclear layers, contains the synapses of rods and cones with bipolar and association cells together with Müller's fibers. In the region of the fovea centralis the fibers of the outer plexiform layer parallel the surface of the retina and are called Henle's outer fiber layer.

The *inner plexiform (molecular) layer* contains the synapses between bipolar, association, and ganglion cells plus Müller's fibers. The inner plexiform layer is of uniform thickness throughout, except in the region of the fovea where it is spread apart to expose the cones.

The *nerve fiber layer* is arranged with fibers approximately radial to the optic nerve. The fibers are parted temporally by the mass of axons from the fovea centralis. The major retinal blood vessels are embedded in this layer. The distribution of the nerve fibers in this layer plays an important role in determining the configuration of visual field defects (p. 308).

Regions of the retina. The retina has been divided into regions that differ histologically and functionally: (1) the optic disk is the termination of all retinal layers except the nerve fiber layer; (2) the ora serrata is the scalloped anterior termination of the neurosensory retina; (3) the

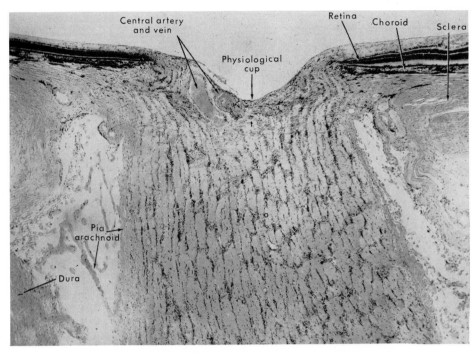

Fig. 1-19. Optic disk and optic nerve. (Hematoxylin and eosin stain; ×43.)

central retina, or macula lutea, surrounds the fovea centralis; and (4) the extra-central peripheral retina includes the other portions of the retina.

Optic disk. The optic disk (Fig. 1-19) is composed of axons of ganglion cells that leave the eyeball through the sieve-like opening, the lamina cribrosa. The choroid and all layers of the retina, except the nerve fiber layer, terminate at the disk margin. Inasmuch as the photosensitive rods and cones are absent, this area is blind and gives rise to the blind spot of Mariotte in visual field testing (p. 148). The central artery and vein of the retina (p. 26) emerge on the surface of the optic disk. Frequently a physiologic cup is present, formed by atrophy of vascular elements that, during fetal life, emerged from the central portion of the optic disk.

Ora serrata. The ora serrata is the anterior termination of the retina and consists of scalloped fringe that parallels the ciliary processes (Fig. 1-20). It is located about 8 mm. from the corneoscleral limbus. In this area the neurosensory retina abruptly loses its laminated structure, and the two layers of the primitive optic vesicle fuse and continue forward as the ciliary epithelium.

Central retina. This is a specialized region about 6 mm. in diameter. It extends from the fovea centralis to the optic disk nasally to about the same distance temporally and above and below to the major temporal blood vessels (Fig. 1-21). In this area the ganglion cell layer is several cell layers thick. The retinal layers from the outer nuclear layer inward have a yellow pigmentation, the macula lutea. The fovea is not pigmented where these layers are absent. The yellow pigment is visible in eyes opened within 15 minutes after death and in red-free ophthalmoscopic light. The

---

*The optic disk is at the same level as the surrounding retina; the term "papilla" is a misnomer.

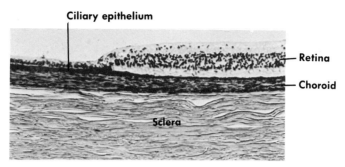

Fig. 1-20. Abrupt termination of the retina to form the ora serrata and the forward continuation as the ciliary epithelium. (Hematoxylin and eosin stain; ×43.)

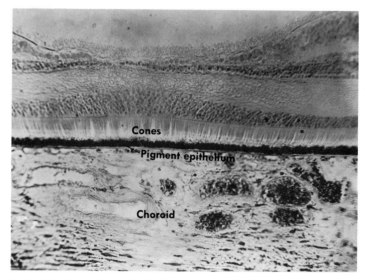

Fig. 1-21. Retina in the region of the fovea centralis. Bruch's membrane is seen as a thin line immediately beneath the pigment epithelium. (Hematoxylin and eosin stain; ×450.)

human retina is thickest (0.4 to 0.5 mm.) just peripheral to the foveal depression because of the great accumulation of nuclear cells in this area.

The central retina surrounds the fovea centralis. The fovea centralis is located about 3 mm. temporal to the optic disk at the posterior pole of the eye and is about 1.5 mm. in diameter. At its center is the *foveola,* an area measuring about 0.4 mm. in diameter, which is characterized by the presence of cones only and

by the absence of the inner layers of the retina with their accompanying vascular and neuroglial elements. The fovea centralis is nurtured solely by the choriocapillaris of the choroid. The vertebrate retina is so constructed that light must pass through the inner transparent retinal layers to stimulate the photoreceptors. In the fovea centralis these inner layers are displaced peripherally so that light falls directly upon cones without passing through intervening inner retinal layers.

Extracentral peripheral retina. The cells in the extracentral peripheral retina are quite regularly arranged. The majority of photoreceptors are rods, but cones are scattered throughout.

Blood supply. The retina is nurtured from two sources: (1) the outer one half is nurtured by the choriocapillaris of the choroid (p. 12) and (2) the inner one half is nurtured by the central retinal artery and its branches. This does not provide a double blood supply—both must be intact to maintain active retinal metabolism.

The *central retinal artery,* the first branch of the ophthalmic artery, enters the inferior medial side of the optic nerve about 12 mm. posterior to the globe. It extends forward to the optic disk where it bifurcates into superior and inferior papillary branches. As the vessel passes through the lamina cribrosa, its wall is reduced to about one half its previous thickness, the internal elastic lamella is lost, and the medial muscle coat becomes incomplete.

The superior and inferior papillary branches of the central retinal artery bifurcate on the surface of the disk to form nasal and temporal branches. The nasal branches follow a relatively direct course to the periphery. The temporal vessels arch above and below the fovea centralis and pass to the periphery.

Capillaries. Traditionally, two closely interconnected capillary networks have been described in the neurosensory retina, one at the level of the nerve fiber layer and the other at the level of the inner nuclear layer (Fig. 1-22). Trypsin digestion of the retina followed by staining of the capillaries indicates that capillaries plunge nearly at right angles to the retinal surface and connect with venular capillaries at all levels from the inner nuclear layer inward to the nerve fiber layer. There is usually a relatively large arteriole connected to a venule by a rich capillary

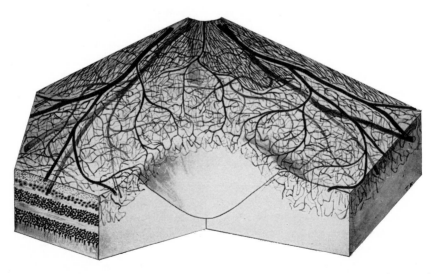

Fig. 1-22. Retinal blood supply of the inner layers of the retina. (The outer layers of the retina are nurtured by the choroid.) The blood vessels are shown with the arteries superficial and the veins deeper. Capillaries are present throughout the inner retina and do not form layers. The fovea is capillary free. There is a capillary-free zone about the arteries and veins, but the zone around the veins has capillaries that course over the veins. (From Toussaint, D., Kuwabara, T., and Cogan, D. G.: Arch. Ophthal. [Chicago] **66:**575, 1961.)

plexus without arteriovenous shunts. The arterioles and veins have a capillary-free zone surrounding them.

The endothelial cells line the retinal capillaries and are regularly arranged with their nuclei parallel to the direction of the vessel. The vessel wall contains mural cells or pericytes that are separated from the endothelium by a homogeneous basement membrane.

Veins. The veins in the retina essentially follow the distribution of the arteries. They consist of an endothelial coat supported by a small amount of connective tissue. At points in the retina where veins and arteries cross the vessels are bound together with a common adventitial sheath. The central retinal vein emerges from the optic nerve at about the same point where the central retinal artery enters, about 12 mm. behind the globe. As the central retinal vein passes through the meninges surrounding the optic nerve, it is considered vulnerable to increases in intracranial pressure, a factor important in the production of papilledema.

Chambers of the eye. The eye contains three main chambers: the anterior chamber, the posterior chamber, and the vitreous cavity.

Anterior chamber. The anterior chamber is bounded anteriorly by the cornea, posteriorly by the front surface of the iris and lens, and peripherally by the angle recess. The anterior chamber is deepest in its central portion (3 mm.) and shallowest at the peripheral insertion of the iris. It has a volume of a little more than 0.1 ml.

Posterior chamber. The posterior chamber is bounded anteriorly by the iris, posteriorly by the front surface of zonular fibers, medially by the lens, and laterally by the ciliary processes. Its volume in adults is about 0.06 ml. The aqueous humor secreted by ciliary processes flows from the posterior chamber through the pupil into the anterior chamber.

Vitreous cavity. The vitreous cavity is surrounded by the retina and the optic nerve posteriorly. Anteriorly it is bounded by the zonule, the ciliary body, and the posterior surface of the lens. Its volume is 4.5 ml.

Vitreous body. The vitreous body is a transparent gel having the shape of a sphere with a segment removed anteriorly to provide a hollowed-out space for the lens. In the healthy eye the vitreous body is in contact with the retina throughout. It has firm attachments to the ciliary body and the retina in the region of the ora serrata and to the margin of the optic disk. Sometimes there is a loose attachment to the posterior lens capsule (Weigert's hyaloid-capsular ligament).

The vitreous body is divided into two parts: (1) a cortical portion adjacent to the retina and (2) a gel proper. The *cortical portion* contains a few cells together with fibrils that attach to the basement membrane of the retina and to the ciliary body and extend fanwise into the vitreous body. The *gel proper* is a true physical and biologic gel, having a collagen-like fibrous network and a mucopolysaccharide, hyaluronic acid, in which is suspended a large amount of water (99%).

Lens. The crystalline lens (Fig. 1-23) is a grossly transparent, biconvex structure located directly behind the iris and the pupillary aperture and in front of the vitreous body. It is held in position by zonular fibers. The lens has a diameter of about 10 mm. and is 4 mm. thick. Its anterior and posterior surfaces meet at the equator. The center of curvature of the anterior surface is the anterior pole; the posterior pole is the corresponding point on the posterior surface. The equator is separated from the free edge of the ciliary body by a distance of about 0.5 mm. The zonular fibers insert into the lens capsule in a zone concentric with the equator and extend further over the anterior than over the posterior surface.

The lens continues to form fibers

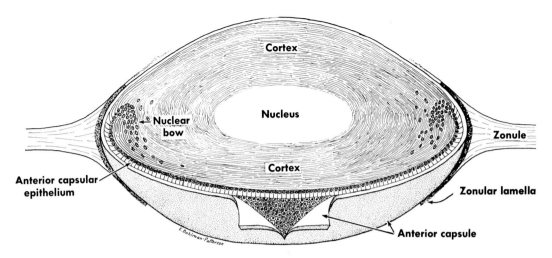

Fig. 1-23. Crystalline lens.

throughout life. Old fibers are not des-quamated, but they become compressed centrally to form an increasingly larger and more inelastic nucleus. Although gross-ly the lens appears brilliantly transparent, by microscopic examination it is seen to contain minute opacities and concentric areas of different indices of refraction.

The lens is composed of (1) a lens cap-sule entirely surrounding it, (2) epithelium beneath the anterior capsule, and (3) a lens substance that consists of the cortex (newly formed soft layers) and the nu-cleus (a dense central area of old fibers).

The *lens capsule* is a typical glassy mem-brane that is homogeneous, acellular, and elastic. It is thickest on either side of the equator just central to the insertion of zonular fibers. It is divided into two layers: (1) a superficial, thin zonular lamella com-posed of acid polymucosaccharides, which constitutes the attachment of the zonule to the lens, and (2) the cuticular capsule or capsule proper, which is probably the basement membrane of the lens epithe-lium. This is a homogeneous structure composed of fine filamentary lamellas em-bedded in cement substance.

The *epithelium* is located directly under the anterior lens capsule. It consists of a single row of cuboidal cells. Electron microscopy indicates that these cells have an irregular shape and numerous inter-digitations.

The *lens substance* consists of fibers embedded in an amorphous cement sub-stance with a concentric construction simi-lar to that of an onion. Each new fiber has its nucleus at the equator, and a long (10 mm.), tapering, six-sided, ribbonlike process extends toward the anterior and posterior poles. The most recently formed fibers have their nuclei closest to the equator. As the fiber ages, the cell and its nucleus are pushed axially into the lens substance. This produces a "nuclear bow" of cell nuclei that approximately parallels the anterior lens surface. With further aging, the fiber nucleus degenerates, the cell fiber shrinks, and the fibers become compressed centrally. The nucleus of the lens, composed of cell membranes, is in-elastic, yellowish, and increases in size with aging.

Zonule. The lens zonule (zonule of Zinn, or suspensory ligament of the lens, Fig. 1-24) supports the lens in position. It is composed of a series of fine fibers that arise from the ciliary body and attach to the zonular lamellar portion of the lens

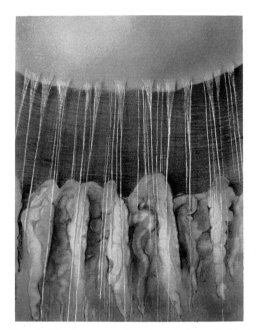

Fig. 1-24. Lens zonule viewed from behind. This specimen is from a man 68 years of age. A child would have many more zonular fibers. (From McCulloch, J. C.: Trans. Amer. Ophthal. Soc. **52:**525, 1954.)

capsule on either side of the equator. The zonular fibers attach to the internal limiting membrane covering the ciliary epithelium. Their point of attachment is in the valley between the ciliary processes and not to their apices. The ciliary attachment is very broad, and fibers may extend to the pars plana of the ciliary body. Other fibers attach to the anterior vitreous face. The insertion is to the equator of the lens in a zone extending from about 2 mm. in front to 1 mm. behind it.

Optic nerve. The optic nerve is a portion of a white fiber tract of the central nervous system consisting of axons of retinal ganglion cells together with nerve fibers that extend from the brain to the eye. The optic nerve extends from the eyeball to the optic chiasm. Thereafter, these fibers constitute the optic tract. The optic nerve leaves the eye about 3 mm. nasal to,

and slightly above, the posterior pole.

The optic nerve is divided into four portions: (1) intraocular, 1 mm.; (2) orbital, 30 mm.; (3) intracanalicular, 0.5 to 0.1 mm.; and (4) intracranial, 10 mm.

The *intraocular portion* of the optic nerve includes the optic disk and that portion of the optic nerve within the posterior scleral foramen. This opening is bridged by a sievelike connective tissue membrane, the lamina cribrosa (p. 5). This is derived from connective tissue of the choroid and the sclera together with astroglia derived from the septal system of the optic nerve. Posterior to the optic disk the nerve fibers are myelinated, whereas anterior to the disk they are unmyelinated. The portion of the optic nerve visible within the eye (optic disk) measures about 1.5 mm. in diameter.

The *orbital portion* of the optic nerve has an S-shaped curve to permit movements of the eyeball. Near the globe the long and short ciliary arteries and nerves are arranged about its circumference. The central retinal artery and vein penetrate the optic nerve 12 mm. behind the globe. At the apex of the orbit the nerve is surrounded by the ligament of Zinn, the tendinous origin of the rectus muscles. It is surrounded by the coverings of the brain, the pia mater, the arachnoid, and the dura mater.

In the *intracanalicular portion* the optic nerve passes through the optic foramen in company with the ophthalmic artery and the sympathetic nerves accompanying this vessel. Within the foramen the nerve acquires the three meningeal coverings of the brain: the pia mater, the dura mater, and the arachnoid. The pia mater extends to the globe. The dura mater lines the optic foramen and splits within the orbit in such a manner that one portion is continuous with the orbital periosteum (periorbita) and the other continues to the globe as the dural sheath of the optic nerve. Within the optic foramen the dura mater is adherent to bone, arachnoid, and pia mater, so that the nerve is firmly fixed in this region. The dura mater and the arachnoid sheaths extend anteriorly and blend with the sclera.

The *intracranial portion* of the optic nerve is located above the diaphragm of the sella covering the pituitary gland. Lateral to each optic nerve is the internal carotid artery, each of which gives off the ophthalmic artery on the inferior side of the nerve. Superior to the nerve is the anterior perforated substance, the medial root of the olfactory tract, and the anterior cerebral artery.

Structure. The optic nerve contains approximately 1 million fibers classified as efferent axons of ganglion cells subserving vision and the pupillary reflex, efferent fibers of unknown function (vasomotor?), autonomic fibers, and photostatic fibers to the superior colliculi.

The nerve is composed of bundles of nerve fibers separated by septa that are continuous with the pial sheath and carry minute blood vessels to the nerve (Fig. 1-25). As in the brain, nerve fibers are supported by astroglia and oligodendroglia derived from the neural ectoderm and by mesenchymal microglia having a phagocytic function. Myelinization of the optic nerve begins at the chiasm at about the twenty-fourth week of fetal life and, at birth, has reached a point just behind the lamina cribrosa. Oligodendrocytes are associated with the synthesis and metabolism of myelin; these cells are more numerous behind the lamina cribrosa. Inasmuch as the optic nerve loses its myelin sheath within the lamina cribrosa (Fig. 1-2), astrocytes are more common in this area. They provide a framework on the intraocular surface of the optic nerve and are probably important in providing mechanical support for nerve fibers that make a right angle turn from the retina.

Blood supply. The blood supply of the optic nerve is derived from several sources.

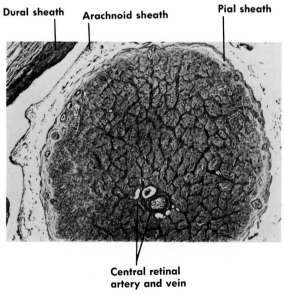

Dural sheath   **Arachnoid sheath**   **Pial sheath**

Central retinal artery and vein

Fig. 1-25. Cross section of optic nerve showing bundles of nerve fibers separated by septa derived from the pial sheath and carrying blood vessels. The nerve is surrounded by the same coverings as the brain. (Hematoxylin and eosin stain; ×160.)

The intraocular portion is supplied by the short posterior ciliary arteries that, as they penetrate the sclera, give off branches to form the anastomotic circle of Haller-Zinn, which in turn anastomoses with the central artery of the optic nerve. The central retinal artery may also contribute to the anastomotic circle before entering the eye. Considerable attention has been focused on the blood supply to this area because of involvement of the optic disk in glaucoma.

The intraorbital portion of the nerve has a peripheral and possibly an axial system. The peripheral vessels arise from the pia mater and are derived from the neighboring blood vessels. The axial vessels are derived from the central optic nerve artery, a branch of the ophthalmic artery. The axial vascular system nurtures the macular fibers.

The intracanalicular and intracranial portions of the optic nerve are nurtured by the pial fibrovascular meshwork

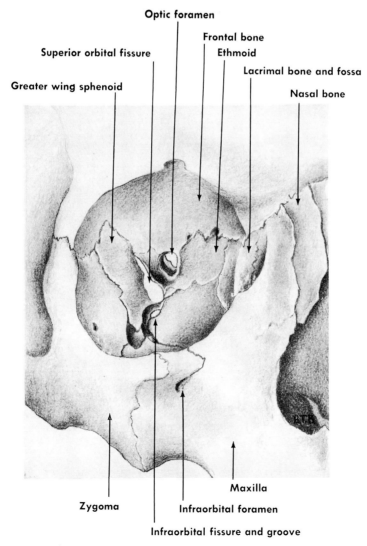

Fig. 1-26. Bony orbit.

from branches of the internal carotid artery.

Bony orbit

The eyes rest in two bony cavities, the orbits, located on either side of the nose. The anterior two thirds of the orbit is roughly the shape of a quadrilateral pyramid. The posterior one third of the orbit narrows to the shape of a triangular pyramid. The lateral walls of the orbit diverge from the medial walls, which are approximately parallel, at an angle of about 45°. The eyeball is located closer to the medial wall than to the lateral wall. Seven bones make up the orbit: the maxilla, the palatine, the frontal, the sphenoid, the zygoma, the ethmoid, and the lacrimal bones.

Structure. The *bony anterior margin* of the orbit is quadrilateral with rounded corners (Fig. 1-26). The bones in this area are relatively heavy and provide protection for the soft parts of the eye. The *lateral margin* is formed by the zygomatic bone and the zygomatic process of the frontal bone. The *superior margin* is formed entirely by the frontal bone. The *medial margin* is poorly defined because of the fossa of the lacrimal sac. It is formed by the medial angular process of the frontal bone and the frontal process of the maxilla. The *inferior margin* is formed by the zygoma and the body of the maxilla.

The walls of the orbit, with the exception of the medial wall, are approximately triangular with the base located anteriorly. The *lateral wall* is formed by two bones: the zygoma anteriorly and the greater wing of the sphenoid posteriorly. The zygomatic portion of the lateral wall is composed of dense bone that separates the orbit from the fossa of the temporalis muscle. The posterior portion of the lateral wall is extremely thin and separates the orbit from the temporal lobe of the brain. On the anterior margin of the lateral wall is located the lateral orbital tubercle to which is attached the suspensory ligament of the globe (ligament of Lockwood), the aponeurosis of the levator palpebrae superioris muscle, and the check ligament of the lateral rectus muscle.

The *medial wall* is quadrilateral in shape. It is formed mainly by the orbital plate of the ethmoid bone. The ethmoid bone is extremely thin (lamina papyracea), and when inflamed this sinus may rupture into the orbit. In the anterior portion of the orbit the fossa of the lacrimal sac is located between the anterior lacrimal crest of the frontal process of the maxilla and the posterior lacrimal crest of the lacrimal bone. The lacrimal sac occupies this fossa and extends inferiorly through the lacrimal canal. The medial canthal ligament divides into two leaves that insert into the anterior and posterior lacrimal crests. The posterior portion of the medial wall of the orbit is formed by the body of the sphenoid bone and contains the optic foramen.

The *roof* of the orbit is formed mainly by the orbital plate of the frontal bone. The lesser wing of the sphenoid contributes slightly to the apex. In the anterior lateral portion of the roof is the fossa for the lacrimal gland. Located medially is the trochlea, which forms the pulley for the tendon of the superior oblique muscle. The bone of the roof is thin and fragile. The frontal sinus and the anterior cranial fossa are located immediately above.

The *floor* of the orbit does not extend to the apex so that the posterior orbit is triangular in shape. The floor is formed mainly by the orbital plate of the maxilla. The orbital surface of the zygoma contributes laterally, and the orbital process of the palatine bone contributes medially. Extending across the floor of the orbit from the inferior orbital fissure is the infraorbital sulcus for the infraorbital artery and the maxillary nerve. About midway this becomes a canal that opens at the infraorbital foramen located about 4 mm. below the inferior orbital margin, through which the artery and the nerve emerge on the face. Inferior to the floor of the orbit is the maxillary sinus.

Optic foramen. The optic foramen is located at the apex of the orbit in the body of the sphenoid bone. Through it passes the optic nerve, the ophthalmic artery, and the sympathetic nerves from the carotid plexus. Just lateral to the optic foramen is the superior orbital fissure that separates the greater and lesser wings of the sphenoid bone (Fig. 1-38). Passing through the superior orbital fissure are the motor nerves to the ocular muscles (N III, IV, and VI) and the ophthalmic branch of the trigeminal nerve (N V). The inferior orbital fissure (sphenomaxillary), located at the junction of the orbital plate of the greater wing of the sphenoid bone and the lateral margin of the floor of the orbit, transmits the infraorbital and the zygomatic nerves and an anastomosis between the inferior ophthalmic vein and the pterygoid plexus. This fissure is covered by the muscle of Müller, a smooth muscle of questionable function in man, which is the analogue of the retractor bulbi muscle of lower animals.

Orbital fascia. The orbital contents are bound together and supported by connective tissues that, although connected, divide the orbit into spaces of clinical importance in limiting the spread of hemorrhage and inflammation. The main orbital fascias are (1) the periorbita (periosteum of the orbit), (2) the orbital septum (palpebral fascia), (3) the bulbar fascia (Tenon's capsule), and (4) the muscular fascia.

The *periorbita (periosteum of the orbit)* is the periosteal lining of the orbit. It is derived from the dura mater, which splits at the optic foramen into two layers, one contributing to the periosteum and the other continuing as the dural sheath of the optic nerve.

The *orbital septum (palpebral fascia)* stretches from the bony margins of the

orbit to the lid in close relationship with the posterior surface of the palpebral portion of the orbicularis oculi muscle (p. 41). The septum prevents orbital fat from entering the lids and limits the spread of inflammation—therefore it has been designated as "the firewall of the orbit."

The *bulbar fascia (Tenon's capsule)* separates the globe from orbital fat and constitutes the socket in which the eyeball moves. It extends forward to the insertion of the deeper layers of the conjunctiva at the corneoscleral limbus. Its lower portion is thickened to form a sling (the ligament of Lockwood), upon which the globe rests. Posteriorly the fascia is very thin and is perforated by the structures passing to or from the globe.

The *muscular fascia* surrounds the ocular muscles, particularly their anterior portions, like the sleeves of a coat surround an arm. The portion that covers the medial and lateral rectus muscles sends expansions to the orbital margin as check ligaments. Other fibers extend to the conjunctiva and hold it taut in ocular rotation.

Extrinsic muscles

The extrinsic muscles of the eye (Fig. 1-27) are the four rectus and the two oblique muscles. (The ciliary muscle and the sphincter and dilatator muscles of the pupil are the intrinsic muscles.)

Origin

The four rectus muscles originate at the apex of the orbit from the ligament of Zinn (annulus tendineus communis), which encircles the optic foramen and the medial portion of the superior orbital fissure. The superior oblique muscle originates at the apex of the orbit from the periosteum of the body of the sphenoid bone medial to and above the optic foramen. The inferior oblique muscle arises from the floor of the orbit from the periosteum covering the anteromedial portion of the maxilla. The four rectus muscles insert into the sclera

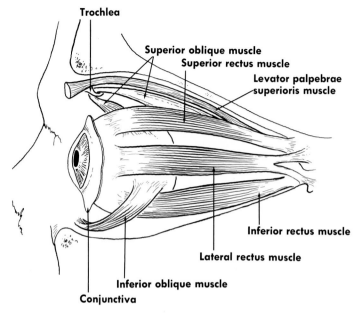

Trochlea

Superior oblique muscle
Superior rectus muscle

Levator palpebrae
superioris muscle

Inferior rectus muscle

Lateral rectus muscle

Inferior oblique muscle

Conjunctiva

Fig. 1-27. Extrinsic muscles of the eye.

anterior to the equator of the globe. The two oblique muscles insert into the sclera posterior to the equator.

The extraocular muscles appear to be the most highly organized of all striated muscles. They contain slow fibers capable of a graded contracture on their exterior surface and fast fibers responsible for rapid movements on the surface adjacent to the globe. The slow fibers correspond to red muscle fibers, which contain a high content of mitochondria and oxidative enzymes. The fast fibers correspond to white muscle fibers and contain greater amounts of glycogen and glycolytic enzymes and less oxidative enzymes than do the slow fibers.

Rectus muscles

The rectus muscles are (1) the medial rectus muscle, (2) the lateral rectus muscle, (3) the superior rectus muscle, and (4) the inferior rectus muscle. They originate from the ligament of Zinn and pass forward in the orbit, gradually diverging to form the ocular muscle cone. Each mus-

cle is about 40 mm. long and 9.5 to 10.5 mm. wide at its point of insertion to the sclera. By means of a tendon, the muscles insert into the sclera between 5 and 7 mm. from the corneoscleral limbus.

The *medial rectus muscle* arises from the medial portion of the ligament of Zinn in close contact with the optic nerve. It is innervated by the inferior division of the third cranial nerve, which enters on the bulbar side. Its sole function is adduction of the globe.

The *lateral rectus muscle* arises by two heads from the upper and lower portions of the ligament of Zinn, where it bridges the superior orbital fissure. It passes forward, crossing the insertion of the inferior oblique muscle, to insert into the sclera. It is innervated by the abducens nerve (N VI), which enters on its bulbar surface at about the middle. The sole function of this muscle is abduction of the eye.

The *superior rectus muscle* arises from the superior portion of the ligament of Zinn in close contact with the meningeal sheaths surrounding the optic nerve.* The muscle passes forward and laterally from the apex, forming an angle of 23° with the sagittal diameter of the globe. Superiorly it is in close contact with the levator palpebrae superioris muscle throughout its course. The superior rectus muscle is innervated by the superior division of the third cranial nerve, which enters its bulbar surface at the junction of the anterior one third with the posterior two thirds. The muscle functions mainly as an elevator, with elevation becoming more efficient as the eye is turned laterally and becoming entirely absent as the eye is turned medially. When the eye is turned medially, the muscle aids in adduction. The muscle intorts (rotates inward) the superior meridian of the cornea.

The *inferior rectus muscle* arises from the inferior portion of the ligament of Zinn and passes forward and laterally, forming an angle of 23° (as does the superior rectus muscle) with the sagittal diameter of the globe. It is innervated by the inferior division of the third cranial nerve, which enters on its superior edge at the junction of the anterior one third with the posterior two thirds. The muscle functions mainly as a depressor, with depression becoming more efficient as the eye is turned laterally and becoming entirely absent as the eye is turned medially. In medial rotation the muscle aids in adduction. Additionally, the muscle extorts (rotates outward) the superior meridian of the cornea.

Oblique muscles

There are two oblique muscles, the superior oblique and the inferior oblique.

The *superior oblique muscle* originates from the periosteal covering of the body of the sphenoid bone above and medial to the optic foramen. It consists of two parts:

a direct portion extending from its insertion to the trochlea and a reflected portion, composed entirely of tendon, from the trochlea to its insertion.

The direct portion passes forward in the angle between the roof and the medial wall of the orbit to the trochlea. The trochlear nerve (N IV) enters its upper surface at 8 to 13 mm. from its origin. The trochlea is a V-shaped fibrocartilage attached to the trochlear spine of the frontal bone located on its medial aspect a few millimeters behind the orbital margin. The tendon of the superior oblique muscle begins about 10 mm. behind the trochlea. It is encased in a synovial sheath through the pulley. From the trochlea the tendon passes downward, laterally, and posteriorly beneath the superior rectus muscle to be inserted on the upper outer quadrant of the eyeball behind the equator. The tendon is shaped as a fibrous cord about 1 by 2 mm. in size, but it becomes flat and wide as it approaches the medial margin of the superior rectus muscle. The main function of the muscle is depression, which increases as the eye is rotated medially and becomes entirely absent as the eye is rotated laterally. In lateral rotation the muscle aids in abduction. The muscle intorts (rotates medially) the 12 o'clock meridian of the cornea.

The *inferior oblique muscle* arises from the periosteum covering the orbital plate of the maxilla a few millimeters behind the orbital margin and near the orifice of the nasolacrimal duct. It passes laterally and posteriorly, and after crossing the inferior rectus muscle on the inferior aspect, it curves upward around the globe to insert into the posterior sclera on the inferior lateral surface of the globe. It has little or no tendon. The muscle is innervated by the inferior division of the oculomotor nerve (N III), which enters the bulbar surface just after the muscle has passed to the lateral side of the inferior rectus muscle. The main function of the inferior oblique

---

*Pain on movement of the eye in retrobulbar neuritis (p. 282) occurs because of close association of the superior and medial rectus muscles with the optic nerve.

muscle is elevation, which increases as the eye is rotated medially and is absent in abduction. The muscle holds the globe steady in abduction and extorts (rotates outward) the 12 o'clock meridian of the cornea.

Blood supply
Arteries

The eyeball and the orbital contents receive their main blood supply from the ophthalmic artery. The lids and conjunctiva have a generous anastomotic supply from branches of both the external carotid and the ophthalmic arteries. There are numer-

ous variations in the pattern of vasculature.

Ophthalmic artery. The ophthalmic artery is the first intracranial branch of the internal carotid artery and arises just as the artery exits from the cavernous sinus. The ophthalmic artery enters the orbit through the optic foramen immediately below and lateral to the optic nerve, turns forward and upward, and passes over the optic nerve to its medial side. It ascends to the medial wall of the orbit and passes forward with the nasociliary nerve between the medial rectus and the superior oblique muscles to terminate by divid-

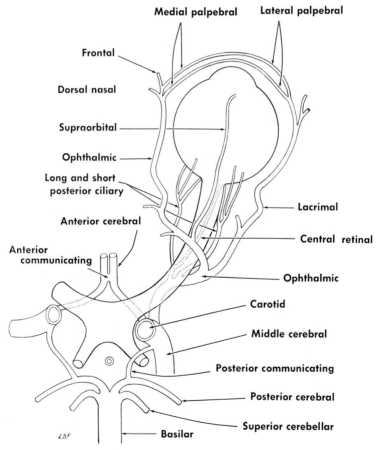

Fig. 1-28. Blood supply to the orbit and the ocular adnexa. There are numerous variations.

ing into dorsonasal and supratrochlear branches (Fig. 1-28).

The majority of branches of the ophthalmic artery are given off while the vessel is lateral to the optic nerve. These branches include the following arteries:

1. The central retinal artery sends nutrient vessels to the optic nerve and to the circle of Haller-Zinn at the lamina cribrosa. It then divides into superior and inferior papillary branches that in turn divide into nasal and temporal branches providing blood to the inner layers of the retina.

2. The posterior ciliary arteries give rise to 6 to 20 short posterior ciliary arteries and to the medial and lateral long posterior ciliary arteries. The short posterior ciliary arteries enter the globe around the optic nerve and rapidly divide to form the choriocapillaris. The long posterior ciliary arteries anastomose with the anterior ciliary arteries to form the circulus arteriosus iridis major.

3. The lacrimal artery gives off a large recurrent meningeal artery that anastomoses with the middle meningeal branch of the maxillary artery. The lacrimal artery terminates in temporal and zygomatic branches that anastomose with the anterior deep temporal and transverse facial arteries. These form lateral palpebral branches that anastomose with medial palpebral branches to form the tarsal and peripheral arterial arcades of the lid. Branches of the peripheral arterial arcade are distributed to the conjunctiva as the posterior conjunctival arteries.

4. A variable number of recurrent arteries anastomose with branches of the internal carotid artery. These may replace major blood vessels, even the ophthalmic artery itself.

5. Muscular branches are distributed to each of the extrinsic muscles in the orbit and have many anastomoses. The anterior ciliary arteries (Fig. 1-35) are forward continuations of the muscular arteries of the rectus muscles. Each rectus muscle has

two muscular arteries except the lateral rectus muscle, which has one. The anterior ciliary vessels extend to the limbus as the anterior conjunctival arteries and form the pericorneal arcade. The superficial conjunctival arteries anastomose with the posterior conjunctival arteries derived from the palpebral arcade. About 4 mm. from the corneoscleral limbus, branches of the anterior ciliary arteries penetrate the sclera to contribute, together with the long posterior ciliary arteries, to the circulus arteriosus iridis major and to provide blood vessels to the ciliary processes.

While superior to the optic nerve, the ophthalmic artery gives off the supraorbital artery, which extends anteriorly to anastomose with the superficial temporal and supratrochlear arteries in the scalp.

When medial to the optic nerve, the ophthalmic artery gives off posterior and anterior ethmoidal arteries. The anterior ethmoidal artery has an anterior meningeal branch. Superior and inferior palpebral branches anastomose through the tarsal and peripheral palpebral arcades with the corresponding branches of the lacrimal artery. The ophthalmic artery terminates in two terminal branches: (1) the dorsonasal artery, which is distributed to the skin of the nose and to the lacrimal sac and anastomoses with angular and nasal branches of the facial artery, and (2) the supratrochlear artery.

External carotid artery. The blood supply to the eye and eyelids from branches of the external carotid artery arises from (1) the external maxillary (facial) artery, (2) the superficial temporal artery, and (3) the internal maxillary artery.

The *external maxillary (facial) artery* gives off a number of branches to the face. Its terminal branch is the angular artery, which anastomoses at the medial canthus with the dorsonasal branch of the opthalmic artery to provide blood for the inferior arterial arcades of the lids. It also anastomoses with the infraorbital artery, a branch of the internal maxillary artery.

The *superficial temporal artery* is the smaller terminal branch of the external carotid artery. The transverse facial artery, the largest branch of the superficial temporal artery, anastomoses with the infraorbital and angular arteries. The zygomatico-orbital artery anastomoses with the lacrimal artery and its palpebral branches to participate in the arterial arcade of the lids. The frontal artery anastomoses with the supraorbital and frontal branches of the ophthalmic artery and the corresponding artery from the opposite side.

The *internal maxillary artery* is the larger of the terminal branches of the external carotid artery. Its largest branch is the middle meningeal artery, which supplies bone and dura mater at the base of the skull. The internal maxillary artery sends an orbital branch through the superior orbital fissure, which anastomoses with a recurrent branch of the ophthalmic artery. The infraorbital artery arises in the pterygopalatine (sphenomaxillary) fossa; it enters the orbit through the infraorbital sulcus and groove canal in the orbital plate of the maxilla and passes forward to emerge on the face from the infraorbital foramen. The infraorbital branch anastomoses with the angular branch of the external maxillary (facial) artery, the transverse facial branch of the superficial temporal artery, and the lacrimal and dorsonasal branches of the ophthalmic artery.

These vessels provide a generous anastomosis for nutrition of the eyelids and the globe. The many anastomoses make it unusually difficult to correct aneurysms involving the circle of Willis.

Veins

Venous drainage of the orbit is mainly through the superior and inferior orbital veins. These are markedly tortuous, have no valves, and empty into the cavernous sinus. The superior orbital vein communicates with the angular vein, which is continuous with the facial vein. The inferior ophthalmic vein communicates with the pterygoid plexus through the inferior orbital fissure. The inferior ophthalmic vein may either communicate directly with the cavernous sinus or may empty into the superior ophthalmic vein. The central vein of the retina usually exits from the optic

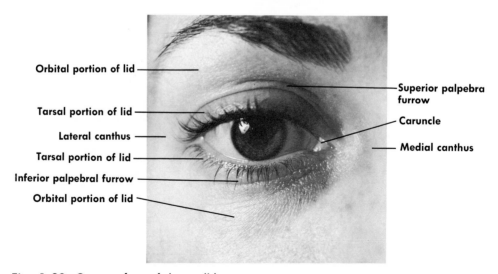

Fig. 1-29. Outer surface of the eyelids.

nerve close to the entrance of the artery. It enters the cavernous sinus separately or empties into the superior ophthalmic vein.

Eyelids

The eyelids are thin curtains of skin, muscle, fibrous tissue, and mucous membrane that protect the eye from external irritation, limit the amount of light entering the eye, and distribute tears over the surface of the globe. The upper lid is limited above by the eyebrow; the lower lid merges with the cheek. Each lid is divided by a horizontal furrow into an orbital and a tarsal portion. The upper furrow is formed by skin insertions of the levator palpebrae superioris muscle (Fig. 1-29). The lower furrow is poorly defined and is formed by a few cutaneous connections from the orbicularis oculi mus-

cle. The corneoscleral limbus is covered above and below by the lids.

When the eyes are open, the lids form an elliptic opening, the palpebral fissure, which measures about 12 by 30 mm. Laterally this fissure forms a 60° angle. It is about 2 mm. higher than the medial portion in Caucasians and 4 to 5 mm. higher than the medial portion in Mongols. Medially the palpebral fissure is rounded. In Mongols it is obscured by a characteristic vertical skin fold (epicanthus) which, when present in Caucasians, may cause the eyes to appear to be crossed.

Located on the free margin of each lid are the opening of the lacrimal canaliculus (the punctum), the eyelashes or cilia, and the openings of glands (Fig. 1-30). Each lid margin is 2 mm. thick and 30 mm. long. At a point 5 mm. from the medial angle is a small eminence, the papilla

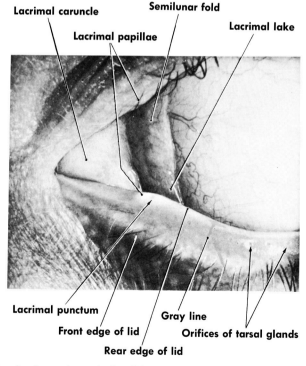

Lacrimal caruncle
Semilunar fold
Lacrimal papillae
Lacrimal lake

Lacrimal punctum
Gray line
Front edge of lid
Orifices of tarsal glands
Rear edge of lid

Fig. 1-30. Lacrimal portion of the lid margin. (From Gibson, H. L.: Med. Radiogr. Photogr. **28:**126, 1952.)

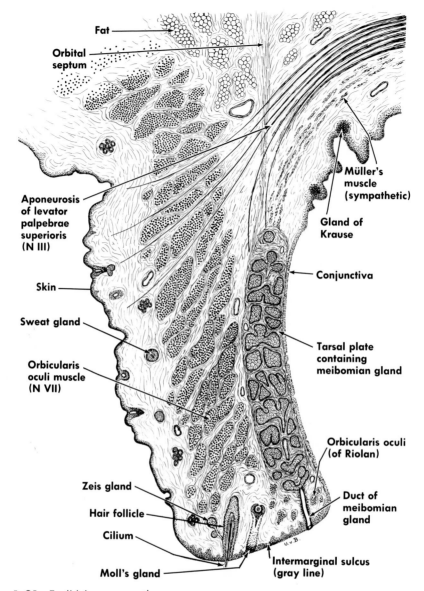

Fat

Orbital
septum

Müller's
muscle
(sympathetic)

Aponeurosis
of levator
palpebrae
superioris
(N III)

Gland of
Krause

Conjunctiva

Skin

Sweat gland

Tarsal plate
containing
meibomian gland

Orbicularis
oculi muscle
(N VII)

Orbicularis oculi
(of Riolan)

Zeis gland

Hair follicle

Duct of
meibomian
gland

Cilium

Moll's gland

Intermarginal sulcus
(gray line)

Fig. 1-31. Eyelid in cross section.

lacrimalis, which contains the minute central opening of the lacrimal canaliculus, the punctum. The medial one sixth of the lid, or the lacrimal portion, has no cilia or gland openings, and the lid margins are rounded. The lateral five sixths of the lid margin has square edges.

The intramarginal sulcus, or gray line, divides the lid margin into anterior and posterior leaves. The eyelashes originate anterior to the gray line, and the orifices of the tarsal glands are posterior to it. The junction of the conjunctiva and the stratified epithelium of the skin is at the level of the orifices of the tarsal glands.

The eyelashes on the upper lid margin curve upward and are more numerous than those on the lower lid margin, which curve downward. Opening into the follicle of each cilium are the ducts of the sebaceous glands of Zeis. Large sweat glands (of Moll) open into these follicles or directly onto the lid margin between the cilia.

Structure. The eyelids contain the following parts (Fig. 1-31):

Skin
Muscles
    Orbicularis oculi (N VII)
        Orbital portion
        Palpebral portion
    Levator palpebrae superioris (N III)
    Palpebral smooth muscles of Müller (sympa-
        thetic nerves)
Fibrous tissue
    Palpebrum fascia or septum orbitale
    Tarsal plates
    Medial and lateral palpebral ligaments

The *skin* of the eyelids is the thinnest in the body. It contains no fat in the subcutaneous areolar area and is thrown into numerous folds. The skin may be markedly distended by blood or fluid and, because of its thinness, underlying blood vessels may appear as dark blue channels.

The *muscles* of the eyelids are the orbicularis oculi (N VII), the levator palpebrae superioris (N III), and the palpebral smooth muscles of Müller (sympathetic nerves).

The orbicularis oculi muscle (N VII) is a thin, oval sheet of striated muscle composed of concentric fibers arranged approximately parallel to the palpebral fissure. There are two main portions: a peripheral orbital part involved in forcible closure of the eyelids and a central palpebral part involved in involuntary blinking. Both portions of the orbicularis oculi muscle originate from the anterior and posterior leaves of the medial palpebral ligament attached to the anterior and posterior lacrimal crests. The muscle inserts into the lateral palpebral ligament attached to the lateral orbital tubercle.

The levator palpebrae superioris muscle (N III) is closely related to the superior rectus muscle in its origin and course. It arises from the periosteal covering of the lesser wing of the sphenoid bone, with its origin blending with that of the superior rectus muscle below and the superior oblique muscle medially. It runs forward beneath the roof of the orbit to a point about 1 cm. behind the septum orbitale, where it expands to the aponeurosis, which passes through the septum to find wide insertion. The aponeurosis inserts into the skin of the lid to form the superior palpebral furrow, into the anterior surface of the tarsal plate, and into the medial and lateral palpebral ligaments. The nerve supply is from the superior division of the oculomotor nerve (N III), which passes through the underlying superior rectus muscle to reach the levator muscle.

The superior and inferior palpebral smooth muscles of Müller (sympathetics) are small sheets of smooth muscle located immediately beneath the orbital portion of the palpebral conjunctiva. The superior palpebral muscle arises from the undersurface of the levator palpebrae superioris muscle. The inferior palpebral muscle has an indefinite origin from the muscular fascia covering the inferior rectus muscle. Each of the palpebral muscles inserts into the tarsal plate. They function in providing "tone" to the lids.

The *fibrous tissue* of the eyelids consists of a peripheral layer, the palpebral fascia or septum orbitale (p. 33), and a thickened central portion, the tarsal plates.

The tarsal plates consist of firm connective tissue (not cartilage) that gives form and density to the free margin of the eyelids. Each tarsal plate is about 1 mm. thick and 25 to 30 mm. long. Medially they extend from the lacrimal puncta to the lateral canthus. The upper tarsus is about 11 mm. wide, and the lower tarsus is about 5 mm. wide. Each tarsus contains sebaceous (meibomian) glands, the ducts of which open onto the lid margin. These glands are arranged in a single row in the tarsal plate, and each consists of 10 to 15 acini placed irregularly around a central canal opening onto the lid margin. The sebaceous secretion prevents the overflow of tears, makes for an airtight closure of the lid, provides the superficial layer of the precorneal tear film, and prevents the rapid evaporation of tears.

The free edge of the tarsal plate extends the length of the ciliary portion of the lid margin. The posterior surface of the tarsus is firmly attached to the tarsal conjunctiva and conforms to the curvature of the globe. The anterior surface of the tarsus is separated from the orbicularis oculi muscle by loose areolar tissue, so that the muscle moves freely over its surface. The deep margin of the tarsus gradually merges into the orbital septum. Medially and laterally the tarsal plates attach to palpebral ligaments.

Blood supply. The blood supply to the eyelid is derived from marginal and peripheral vascular arcades. These are formed by the lateral palpebral branches of the lacrimal artery and the medial palpebral branches of the dorsonasal artery, both of which are derived from the internal carotid artery through the ophthalmic artery (p. 36). There is a wide anastomotic circulation provided by branches of the external carotid artery through the facial, superficial temporal, and infraorbital arteries.

Nerve supply. The ophthalmic (first) division of the trigeminal nerve (N V) provides the afferent sensory innervation to the upper lid and to a small lateral portion of the lower lid. Innervation of the remaining portion of the lower lid is by the maxillary division (second) of the trigeminal nerve through the infraorbital nerve. The facial nerve (N VII) innervates the orbicularis oculi muscle, and the oculomotor nerve (N III) supplies the levator palpebrae superioris muscle. Postganglionic sympathetic fibers from the superior cervical ganglion innervate the palpebral muscles of Müller.

Lymphatic supply. The lids are drained by two groups of lymphatic vessels: (1) a medial group drains the medial two thirds of the lower lid and the medial one third of the upper lid and ends in the maxillary lymph nodes and (2) a lateral group drains the remaining portion of the lids and ends in the parotid (preauricular) nodes (Fig. 1-32).

Lacrimal apparatus

The lacrimal apparatus consists of a secretory and a collecting portion. The secretory portion is composed of the lacrimal gland and the accessory lacrimal glands of Krause and Wolfring. The col-

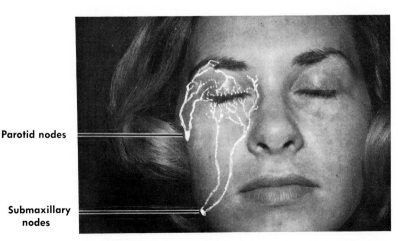

Parotid nodes

Submaxillary nodes

Fig. 1-32. Lymphatics of the eyelids.

lecting portion consists of the canaliculi with their orifices (the puncta), the lacrimal sac, and the lacrimal duct, which has its opening in the inferior nasal meatus.

Secretory portion

Lacrimal gland. The lacrimal gland is lodged in the fossa of the lacrimal gland located in the roof of the orbit on its anterior lateral aspect. It is divided into a large orbital portion and a small palpebral portion by the lateral part of the aponeurosis of the levator palpebrae superioris muscle (Fig. 1-33). The lacrimal gland is of the tubuloalveolar type, with numerous acini composed of a double layer of cells surrounding a central canal. The canals open into the larger ducts that in turn open into excretory ducts. Three to five ducts drain the orbital portion of the gland, and five to seven ducts drain the palpebral portion. The ducts of the orbital portion pass through the palpebral lobe, and each of the ducts opens separately onto the superior temporal fornix.

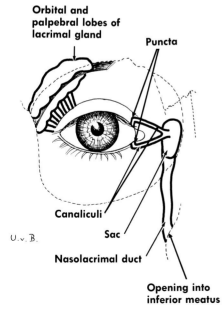

Orbital and palpebral lobes of lacrimal gland

Puncta

Canaliculi

U. v. B.

Sac

Nasolacrimal duct

Opening into inferior meatus

Fig. 1-33. Lacrimal apparatus.

Secretory innervation to the lacrimal gland arises in the lacrimal (salivatory) nucleus in the floor of the fourth ventricle and runs through the facial nerve to the geniculate ganglion. The fibers do not synapse here but leave the facial pathway via the greater superficial petrosal nerve to reach the sphenopalatine (Meckel's) ganglion. From here postganglionic fibers are distributed to the lacrimal gland, passing either directly or with the zygomatic branch of the maxillary branch of the trigeminal nerve. Postganglionic sympathetic fibers from the superior cervical ganglion pass by way of the deep petrosal nerve to the sphenopalatine ganglion, where they are distributed with fibers destined for the lacrimal gland. The sympathetic innervation is mainly to blood vessels of the gland and have no direct effect upon secretion.

The lacrimal gland is drained by the lymphatic vessels ending in the preauricular lymph nodes.

Accessory lacrimal glands of Krause and Wolfring. The accessory lacrimal glands of Krause and Wolfring are isolated lobules of secretory tissue having a structure identical to the lacrimal gland. They are located mainly in the superior fornix.

Collecting portion

The collecting portion of the lacrimal apparatus is composed of the canaliculi, the lacrimal sac, and the nasolacrimal duct.

Canaliculi. Tears enter the canaliculi through the puncta and then pass to the lacrimal sac and through the nasolacrimal canal to an opening in the inferior nasal meatus. The canaliculi extend from the superior and inferior puncta medially to the lacrimal sac. They are lined with stratified columnar epithelium continuous with that of the conjunctiva, and they are surrounded by elastic connective tissue. The canaliculi consist of a vertical portion about 2 mm. long opening directly to the lacrimal puncta and a horizontal portion that begins at a right angle bend and is directed medially.

The puncta, the orifices of the lacrimal canaliculi, are situated upon the surface of the lid margin on a slight elevation, the lacrimal papilla. Upon closing the lids, the puncta are inverted into the lacrimal lake and are prevented from collapsing by a dense surrounding ring of connective tissue.

Lacrimal sac. The lacrimal sac is located in the lacrimal fossa. The sac is closed superiorly and is continuous below with the nasolacrimal duct. The medial palpebral ligament covers the upper end of the sac (the fundus), so that inflammations always point below the ligament. The canaliculi enter the sac about 3 mm. below its apex.

Nasolacrimal duct. The nasolacrimal duct extends 15 mm. from the lacrimal sac above to the inferior nasal meatus below. The duct is surrounded by the bone of the nasolacrimal canal. Its opening into the inferior nasal meatus may not be direct, but the duct may pass for several millimeters beneath the nasal mucous membrane before opening. A variety of constrictions and folds in the sac and the nasolacrimal duct have been described as valves.

Conjunctiva

The conjunctiva is a thin, transparent mucous membrane lining the inner surface of the eyelids and covering the anterior portion of the sclera. Its epithelium is continuous with that of the cornea and the lacrimal drainage system through the puncta. The conjunctiva is divided into

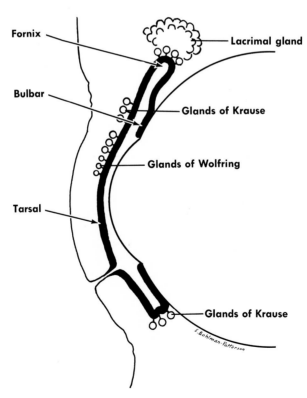

Fig. 1-34. Conjunctiva. Note the lacrimal and accessory lacrimal glands. Epithelium is continuous with that of the cornea.

three areas: (1) the palpebral conjunctiva, (2) the conjunctiva of the superior and inferior fornices, and (3) the bulbar conjunctiva.

The *palpebral conjunctiva* is divided into marginal, tarsal, and orbital portions. That portion on the margin of the eyelid contributes to the mucocutaneous junction at the gray line. The tarsal portion is closely adherent to the tarsal plate, from which it can be removed only with difficulty. The orbital portion is thrown into folds.

The *conjunctiva of the superior and inferior fornices* forms transitional areas between the palpebral and bulbar conjunctivae (Fig. 1-34). It is but loosely applied to the underlying tissue and may become markedly swollen.

The *bulbar conjunctiva* is closely adherent to the sclera, which can be seen as the "white" of the eye through the transparent conjunctival tissue.

At the medial angle of each eye are two specialized structures formed in part by the conjunctiva: the semilunar fold and the lacrimal caruncle (Fig. 1-30). The semilunar fold (plica semilunaris) consists of a delicate vertical crescent of conjunctiva, the free edge of which is concave and concentric with the corneal margin. It is separated from the bulbar conjunctiva by a cul-de-sac 2 mm. deep. The semilunar fold is the homologue of the nictitating membrane in other species, which constitutes the third eyelid innervated by the sympathetic nervous system. The lacrimal caruncle is a minute piece of modified skin located in the lacus lacrimalis medial to the semilunar fold. It is covered by stratified epithelium that is not keratinized. It consists of large sebaceous glands similar to meibomian glands and has fine hairs with sebaceous glands similar to the glands of Zeis. The caruncle is conspicuous when the eye is rotated laterally.

Structure. Like other mucous membranes, the conjunctiva is composed of two layers: (1) stratified columnar epithelium and (2) a lamina propria composed of an adenoid and a fibrous layer.

The *stratified columnar epithelium* varies in thickness from two cell layers in the upper tarsal portion to five to seven layers at the corneoscleral junction. It is never keratinized in health. After the age of 3 months, the development of the adenoid layer makes the surface of the conjunctiva moderately irregular. Goblet cells secreting mucin are numerous in the conjunctival fornices and occur less frequently in the bulbar portion. They secrete the inner layer of the precorneal tear film.

The *lamina propria* is composed of dense connective tissue containing blood vessels, nerves, and conjunctival glands. The bulbar and fornix conjunctiva and the orbital portion of the palpebral conjunctiva contain an adenoid layer with numerous lymphocytes enmeshed in a fine reticular network. True lymphatic follicles are not present. The fibrous layer of the conjunctiva is continuous with the attached margin of the tarsal plates and contains the smooth palpebral muscle of Müller.

Blood supply. The blood supply of the palpebral conjunctiva arises from the peripheral and marginal arterial arcades of the lid. The marginal arcade nourishes the margin and a portion of the tarsal part of the palpebral conjunctiva. The bulbar and fornix conjunctiva is nourished by the peripheral arcade.

The posterior conjunctival branches of the peripheral arterial arcade are the blood supply of the peripheral bulbar conjunctiva. These vessels are superficial, nearly invisible, and extend within 4 mm. of the corneoscleral junction. In this area, anterior conjunctival branches of the seven anterior ciliary arteries pass toward the cornea to form a superficial (conjunctival) and a deep (episcleral) pericorneal plexus. The anterior and posterior conjunctival vessels anastomose (Fig. 1-35).

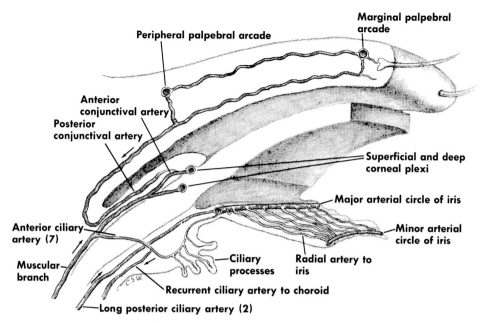

Fig. 1-35. Blood supply of the anterior ocular segment. Only portions of the arteries are illustrated. Two anterior ciliary arteries arise from the muscular branches of each rectus muscle, except for the lateral rectus muscle, which contributes only one. There are two long posterior arteries that enter the globe on either side of the optic nerve and extend anteriorly to the ciliary body on the lateral and medial sides of the eye in the suprachoroidal space. The vascular arcades in the eyelid derived from the lateral palpebral branches of the lacrimal artery and the medial palpebral branches of the dorsonasal artery have generous anastomoses with branches of external carotid artery distributed to the face.

The posterior conjunctival vessels are dilated in inflammations of the bulbar conjunctiva (p. 131). Because of their superficial position, they appear bright red and move with the conjunctiva. They are most evident in the fornices and fade toward the limbus. Because they are superficial, they may be constricted with the instillation of 1:1,000 epinephrine. The superficial (conjunctival) pericorneal plexus, which is derived from the anterior ciliary arteries, is injected in inflammations of the cornea. The deep (episcleral) pericorneal plexus is injected in inflammations of the iris and the ciliary body and in angle-closure glaucoma. Because of their deep position, these vessels appear dull red to purple and do not move with the conjunctiva. They are not affected by topical epinephrine. These vessels are most evident near the corneoscleral limbus and fade toward the fornices. Because of the generous anastomoses between the anterior and posterior conjunctival arteries, severe inflammations always cause injection of both ciliary and conjunctival vessels.

Nerve supply. The bulbar conjunctiva is innervated by sensory and sympathetic nerves from the ciliary nerves. The remaining palpebral and fornix conjunctiva is innervated by the ophthalmic and maxillary branches of the trigeminal nerve, which parallels the innervation of the overlying skin.

Lymphatic supply. The lymphatics of

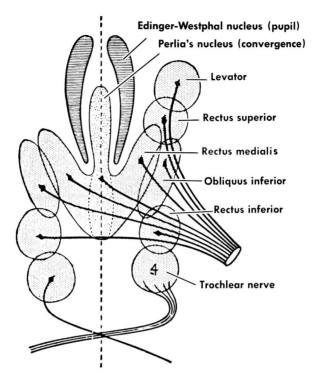

Fig. 1-36. Ventral view of the oculomotor and trochlear nerve nuclei. A variety of arrangements has been suggested. This is Brouwer's modification of Bernheimer's scheme. (From Warwick, R.: In Bender, M. B., editor: The oculomotor system, New York, 1964, Hoeber Medical Division, Harper & Row, Publishers.)

the conjunctiva parallel those of the eyelid (p. 42).

Glands. The conjunctival epithelium, unlike that of the cornea, contains numerous unicellular mucous glands (goblet cells) that secrete the mucoid layer of the precorneal tear film (p. 74). The glands are most numerous in the bulbar conjunctiva and fornices and are absent at the lid margins and corneoscleral limbus. Located deep in the substantia propria in the superior and inferior fornices, particularly laterally, are the accessory lacrimal glands of Krause, which have the histologic structure of the lacrimal gland proper. The accessory lacrimal glands of Wolfring are situated near the upper margin of the superior tarsal plate.

Nerves to the eyes
Cranial nerves

The distribution and function of the cranial nerves to the eyes are as follows:

Motor
  Oculomotor (N III)
    Superior division to superior rectus and levator palpebrae superioris muscles
    Inferior division to medial and inferior rectus and inferior oblique muscles and motor (short) root to ciliary ganglion (ciliary and sphincter pupillae muscles)
  Trochlear (N IV) to superior oblique muscle
  Abducens (N VI) to lateral rectus muscle
Mixed
  Facial (N VII)
    Motor to face
    Secretory to submaxillary, sublingual, and lacrimal glands
    Taste from anterior one third of tongue

Trigeminal (N V)
  Motor to muscles of mastication
  Sensory from face
  Proprioceptive from muscles of mastication
    (mesencephalic nucleus and perhaps
    ocular muscles)

Oculomotor (third cranial) nerve. The oculomotor (third cranial) nerve supplies the superior, medial, and inferior rectus muscles and the levator palpebrae superioris muscle. Its visceral efferent fibers innervate the ciliary muscle and the sphincter pupillate muscle after synapse in the ciliary ganglion.

Nucleus. The nucleus of the oculomotor nerve is an elongated mass of cells located beneath the cerebral aqueduct of Sylvius,

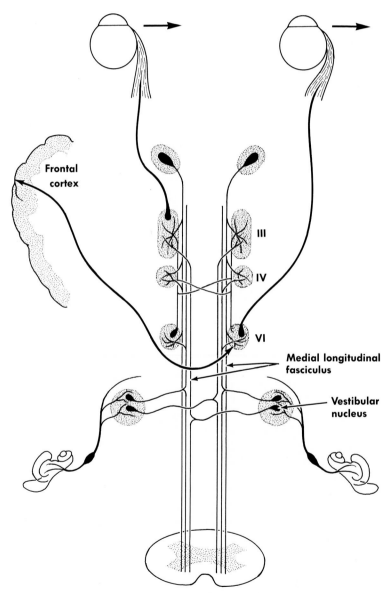

Fig. 1-37. Medial longitudinal fasciculus that coordinates the nuclei of the ocular muscles with each other and with other nuclei in the brain stem.

which connects the third and fourth ventricles. Many different arrangements of its component parts have been described. The nucleus is frequently stated to be composed of two parts: lateral cells that are paired, located posteriorly, which are nearly continuous with the nuclear cells of the trochlear nerve, and medial cells that are unpaired, located at the anterior extremity of the nucleus and related to convergence. The latter group of cells is the nucleus of Perlia (Fig. 1-36).

The lateral paired cells send fibers to all of the extrinsic muscles of the eye except the superior oblique (N IV) and the lateral rectus (N VI) muscles. At their anterior termination on each side is the nucleus of Edinger-Westphal, which innervates the sphincter pupillae and ciliary muscles.

The medial (posterior) longitudinal fasciculus connects the lateral motor cells of the oculomotor nerve to each other and to the nuclei of the fourth and sixth

cranial nerves, the vestibular nuclei, and the sensory nucleus of the trigeminal nerve (Fig. 1-37). This is an important fiber tract that transmits stimuli that coordinate conjugate movements of the eyes (eyes right, eyes left, eyes up, or eyes down). Lesions in this tract produce an internuclear ophthalmoplegia in which convergence is retained with an inability to turn the eyes to the right or to the left.

Intracerebral course. From the third cranial nerve nucleus, efferent fibers run through the tegmentum, red nucleus, and substantia nigra and leave the midbrain in the interpeduncular fossa between the cerebral peduncles.

Intracranial course. In their intracranial course the oculomotor nerves are closely associated with the posterior cerebellar arteries above and the superior cerebral arteries below. From the midbrain they pass down forward, outward, and downward to pierce the dura mater and enter the roof and lateral wall of the cavernous

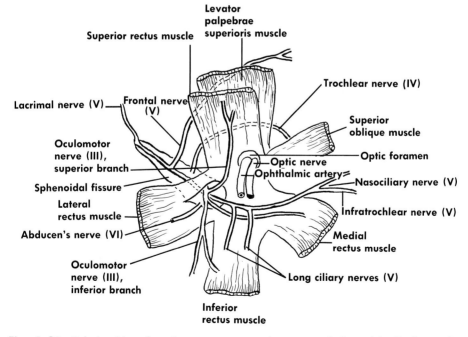

Fig. 1-38. Relationship of major structures at the apex of the orbit. (Redrawn from Labat, G.: Regional anesthesia, Philadelphia, 1924, W. B. Saunders Co.)

sinus about midway between the anterior and posterior clinoid processes. In the cavernous sinus, each nerve is close to the trochlear and ophthalmic division of the trigeminal nerve.

Orbital distribution. The oculomotor nerve leaves the cavernous sinus near the lesser wing of the sphenoid bone and enters the orbit through the superior orbital fissure (Fig. 1-38). Here it divides into a small superior and larger inferior division. The superior division is distributed to the superior rectus muscle on its bulbar surface and passes through this muscle to terminate in the levator palpebrae superioris muscle. The inferior division is distributed to the medial and inferior rectus muscles. Its terminal portion ends in the posterior border of the inferior oblique muscle. The terminal branch to the inferior oblique muscle sends the short, or motor, root branch to the ciliary ganglion.

Ciliary ganglion. The ciliary ganglion is located between the lateral rectus muscle and the optic nerve near the apex of the orbit. Its motor root consists of visceral motor fibers (nucleus of Edinger-Westphal) given off by the terminal branch of the inferior division of the oculomotor nerve, which ends in the inferior oblique muscle. After synapse in the ciliary ganglion, emerging fibers are distributed as cholinergic fibers to the ciliary muscle (accommodation) and the sphincter pupillae muscle (pupillary constriction).

The sensory root (long) is derived from the nasal ciliary branch of the ophthalmic division of the trigeminal nerve. These fibers do not synapse in the ciliary ganglion. The sympathetic root consists of fibers derived from the cavernous and internal carotid plexuses. The sympathetic fibers synapse in the superior cervical ganglion and pass through the ciliary ganglion as postganglionic fibers that do not synapse. The sympathetic fibers mainly provide vasoconstrictor fibers to uveal blood vessels. The sensory root to the ciliary ganglion also carries sympathetic fibers that may entirely replace a separate sympathetic root.

The branches of the ciliary ganglion are three to six short ciliary nerves that divide into some twenty branches and pierce the sclera about the optic nerve. They are distributed mainly to the uveal tract and to the ciliary and sphincter pupillae muscles.

Trochlear (fourth cranial) nerve. The trochlear (fourth cranial) nerve innervates the superior oblique muscle only. Its fibers decussate in the brain, and it is the only cranial nerve to emerge from the dorsal surface of the brain.

Nucleus. The nucleus of the trochlear nerve is a small group of cells located at the posterior end of the lateral (paired) portions of the oculomotor nerve. It is located beneath the cerebral aqueduct of Sylvius, near its connection with the fourth ventricle, at about the level of the inferior colliculus (Fig. 1-36). The cells are connected, by the medial longitudinal fasciculus, to other motor nuclei of the eye, the vestibular nuclei, and the trigeminal sensory nucleus.

Course in the brain stem. The trochlear is the sole cranial nerve to decussate dorsally. The axons pass laterally and then curve around the aqueduct of Sylvius, progressing caudally and passing over the aqueduct, at which point they leave the brain stem.

Intracranial course. After emerging from the brain stem on its dorsal surface, the trochlear nerve passes as a slender filament around the cerebral peduncle to reach the ventral surface of the brain just posterior to the oculomotor nerve. It enters the dura mater posterior to the entrance of the oculomotor nerve at about the level of the posterior clinoid process. It is located in the lateral wall of the cavernous sinus somewhat below the oculomotor nerve. The trochlear nerve emerges from the cavernous sinus and enters the lateral portion of the superior orbital fissure outside the ligament of Zinn. In the orbit it passes anteriorly and medially, crossing above the oculomotor nerve, the levator palpebrae superioris muscle, and the superior rectus muscle. It enters the superior oblique muscle on its orbital surface. This is the only ocular muscle that does not receive its innervation on its bulbar aspect.

Abducens (sixth cranial) nerve. The abducens (sixth cranial) nerve has the longest intracranial course of any of the motor nerves of the eye. It makes a sharp turn over the petrous ridge, which makes it vulnerable to trauma and increased intracranial pressure.

Nucleus. The nucleus of the abducens nerve is located in the gray matter in the floor of the fourth ventricle lateral to the medial longitudinal fasciculus. The genu of the facial nerve curves over the dorsal and lateral surfaces of the abducens nucleus.

Course in the brain stem. The axons of the abducens nerve cells pass anteriorly and ventrally through the pons and between the medially located superior olivary nucleus and the laterally located pyramidal tract. The fibers emerge on the ventral surface of the brain stem in a deep groove between the pons anteriorly and the medulla posteriorly.

Intracranial course. The fibers of the sixth cranial nerve pass anteriorly on the surface of the pons to which they are bound by the anterior inferior cerebellar artery, the first branch of the basilar artery. The nerve then pierces the dura mater and passes vertically over the posterior part of the petrous portion of the temporal bone to enter the cavernous sinus. Just prior to entering this sinus, the nerve passes under the petrosphenoid ligament. In the cavernous sinus it is the most inferiorly located of the motor nerves of the eye. The nerve enters the orbit through the superior orbital fissure between the two heads of the lateral rectus muscle. It passes forward and laterally in the orbit to innervate the lateral rectus muscle from its bulbar surface.

Facial (seventh cranial) nerve. The facial nerve supplies derivatives of the second branchial arch. It is mainly motor to the muscles of the face and scalp, but it has a small sensory component carrying sensations of taste from the anterior one third of the tongue. In addition, it provides motor fibers to the submaxillary, sublingual, and lacrimal glands.

Nuclei. The motor nucleus of the facial nerve is located in the pons medial to the spinal trigeminal tract and lateral to the fibers of the abducens nerve. The gustatory (taste) nucleus receives fibers from cranial nerves VII, IX, and X. The cell bodies are located in the geniculate ganglion, and the axons extend centrally to the gustatory nucleus in the medulla. Fibers that stimulate salivary and lacrimal secretion originate in the salivary nucleus.

Course in the brain stem. The motor axons pass medially and posteriorly to the floor of the fourth ventricle to form a compact genu around the abducens nucleus. The fibers pass laterally to emerge from the ventral surface of the brain stem at the inferior border of the pons considerably lateral to the abducens nerve.

Intracranial course. Upon emerging from the brain stem, the motor fibers of the facial nerve pass in the posterior cranial fossa anterior and lateral to the internal auditory meatus, which it enters in company with the acoustic and vestibular nerves and the intermediate nerve of Wrisberg. The facial nerve makes a sharp backward bend in the temporal bone to enter the facial canal, which curves over the superior and dorsal aspects of the middle ear. It leaves the temporal bone at its lower portion through the stylomastoid foramen.

As soon as the nerve emerges, it turns

anteriorly around the base of the styloid process to enter the parotid gland, where it divides into its terminal divisions, the upper temporofacial and the lower cervicofacial. The temporofacial division gives off temporal and zygomatic branches supplying the orbicularis oculi, the frontalis, the corrugator supercilii, and the anterior and superior auricularis muscles. The cervicofacial division supplies the lower face. These upper and lower branches of the facial nerve have separate areas of origin in the facial nucleus. The upper branches have cortical connections with each hemisphere, but the lower branch has connections only with the opposite motor cortex. Thus, in a unilateral supranuclear lesion, structures innervated by the upper portion of the facial nerve are not affected, but those innervated by the lower portion are affected. The structures are similarly affected in infranuclear lesions.

The taste fibers have a complicated course. Those from the anterior tongue join the chorda tympani nerve, which runs across the middle ear cavity to join the facial nerve. Then the fibers pass with the facial nerve to a point where the internal acoustic meatus joins the facial canal. It is here that the geniculate ganglion is located. Other taste fibers are located in the petrous ganglion (glossopharyngeal nerve) and in the nodose ganglion (vagus nerve).

Motor fibers to the salivary and lacrimal glands are contained in the intermediate nerve of Wrisberg, which passes with the facial nerve into the internal auditory meatus. As the facial nerve turns to enter the facial canal, most of the visceral efferent fibers leave at the apex of the angle as the greater superficial petrosal nerve, which runs forward through the petrous bone to reach the intracranial cavity. The greater superficial petrosal nerve then runs under the semilunar ganglion to emerge from the cranial cavity through the foramen lacerum—it passes through the pterygoid canal to join the sphenopalatine ganglion. Motor fibers to the lacrimal gland join the maxillary branch of the trigeminal nerve, which joins the zygomatic branch to enter the lacrimal gland.

Fibers to the maxillary gland pass with the chorda tympani nerve to emerge from the skull by a fissure between the tympanic and petrous portions of the temporal bone. Fibers join the lingual branch of the mandibular nerve and then synapse with the submaxillary ganglion, with postganglionic fibers distributed almost immediately to the maxillary and sublingual glands. The parotid gland receives its innervation from the lesser petrosal nerve.

Trigeminal (fifth cranial) nerve. The trigeminal nerve has a complicated structure. It is not only the sensory nerve of the face and head, but it also sends motor fibers to the muscles of mastication. It has extensive central connections with reflex arcs associated with cranial nerves III to XII.

Motor nucleus and root. The masticator is the motor portion of the trigeminal nerve. Its nucleus is located cephalad to the facial nerve nucleus near the floor of the cerebral aqueduct of Sylvius. The fibers are distributed with the mandibular nerve and innervate the muscles that move the mandible and the muscles of mastication: the masseter, the temporalis, the internal pterygoid, the mylohyoid, the anterior belly of the digastric, and the external pterygoid. In addition, motor fibers supply the tensor tympani muscle, which tenses the eardrum, and the tensor veli palatine muscle, which stretches out the soft palate.

The mesencephalic root of the trigeminal nerve is situated between the main sensory and the motor nuclei. Fibers of this root are distributed with each of the main divisions of the trigeminal nerve. In the act of biting, impulses pass to the mesencephalic root. It has been postulated that proprioceptive fibers in the extraocular muscles terminate in the mesencephalic nucleus, but this has not been demonstrated.

Sensory nuclei. The principal sensory nucleus of the trigeminal nerve is located near the point of entry of the sensory root into the pons; it lies near the lateral surface of the pons close to the margin of the inferior cerebral peduncle. Functionally, it appears related to tactile impulses.

The nucleus of the spinal trigeminal tract extends down to the second cervical segment of the spinal cord and becomes continuous with the substantia gelatinosa of the dorsal horn. It is functionally associated with the sensation of pain and temperature.

The sensory root is composed of fibers that arise in the semilunar (gasserian) ganglion together with a few fibers from the ciliary ganglion and possibly from other ganglia. The sensory root extends from the posterior border of the semilunar ganglion to the pons. As it leaves this ganglion, it pierces the dura mater under the attached border of the tentorium, which contains the superior petrosal sinus. It then lies on the trochlear nerve and crosses over the facial and auditory nerves as they pass to enter the internal auditory foramen. It is then related to a groove in the medial aspect of the petrous portion of the temporal bone lateral to the abducens nerve.

The sensory root of the trigeminal nerve enters the brain on the lateral surface of the pons about midway between its anterior and posterior margins. Inside the pons it divides into ascending and descending tracts. The thick ascending fibers terminate almost immediately in the principal sensory nucleus. The thin descending fibers are adjacent to the nucleus of the spinal trigeminal tract.

Semilunar ganglion. The semilunar ganglion is a crescent-shaped mass of cells lying in Meckel's cave, which is a cleft located between layers of dura mater in the middle fossa of the skull on a depression on the anterosuperior surface of the petrous bone. At its anterior concave aspect the semilunar ganglion receives three branches: (1) the ophthalmic branch, (2) the maxillary branch, and (3) the mandibular branch.

The *ophthalmic branch* may be outlined as follows:

Frontal nerve
Lacrimal nerve
Nasociliary nerve
    Long (sensory) root of ciliary ganglion
    Long ciliary nerves
    Posterior ethmoidal nerves
    Infratrochlear nerves: superior and inferior palpebral nerves
    Anterior ethmoidal nerves
    Interior nasal nerves: medial and lateral nasal nerves
    External nasal nerves

The ophthalmic is the smallest branch of the semilunar ganglion. It is located in the lateral wall of the cavernous sinus. Just posterior to the sphenoid fissure it divides into the frontal, the lacrimal, and the nasociliary nerves. The frontal and lacrimal nerves enter the orbit above the ligament of Zinn, whereas the nasociliary branch enters through the ligament and accompanies the ophthalmic artery as it passes over the optic nerve and under the superior rectus muscle to the medial wall of the orbit.

The *frontal nerve* is located in the roof of the orbit between the levator palpebrae superioris muscle and the periosteum. It terminates in the supraorbital and supratrochlear nerves. The supraorbital nerve leaves the orbit through the supraorbital notch and supplies the forehead, scalp, and upper lid. Its terminal branches are the medial and lateral frontal nerves. The supratrochlear nerve contains fibers from the medial scalp, lid, and conjunctiva that enter the orbit near the trochlea.

The *lacrimal nerve* follows the upper border of the lateral rectus muscle accompanied by the lacrimal artery. Its superior branch terminates as the lateral palpebral nerve, supplying the skin and conjunctiva of the upper and lower lids. The inferior division receives a twig from the zygomaticotemporal branch of the maxillary division of the trigeminal nerve, which may be secretory to the lacrimal gland.

The *nasociliary nerve* has much the same course as the ophthalmic artery and provides the sensory innervation of the globe. The long (sensory) root of the ciliary ganglion is given off at the superior orbital fissure and runs to the ciliary ganglion. Two long ciliary nerves arise from the nasociliary nerve as it crosses above the optic nerve. They pierce the sclera with the short posterior ciliary nerves and accompany the long posterior ciliary arteries anterior to the ciliary plexus. The fibers are mainly sensory and combined with sympathetic fibers to the dilatator pupillae muscle and the choriocapillaris. The other branches of the nasociliary nerve have the regional distribution anticipated from their nomenclature.

Autonomic nervous system

The autonomic nervous system is a subdivision of the motor portion of the nervous system that carries impulses to smooth muscles, cardiac muscle, and glands. These structures receive a double innervation, so that stimulation of one will cause excitation and stimulation of the other will cause inhibition. In contrast to innervation of skeletal muscle in which a single neuron extends from the central nervous system to the muscle fiber, the autonomic nervous system is composed of a two-neuron chain. The first, or preganglionic, neuron has its cell body in the central nervous system and synapses in a ganglion with postganglionic neurons. The second, or postganglionic, neuron has its cell body in an autonomic ganglion and terminates in smooth muscle, cardiac muscle, or glands.

The autonomic nervous system is composed of two parts: visceral efferent fibers in cranial nerves III, VII, IX, X, and XI and sacral nerves II, III, and IV, which comprise the parasympathetic portion (craniosacral division), and visceral efferent fibers of thoracic and lumbar nerves, which comprise the sympathetic system (thoracolumbar division).

A nerve impulse at an autonomic ganglion initiates an impulse in the postganglionic fibers through the liberation of acetylcoline, which is rapidly destroyed by cholinesterase (p. 95). A postganglionic impulse results in stimulation of the innervated structure. In the case of parasympathetic nerves, stimulation is through release of acetylcholine, and in the case of most sympathetic nerves, stimulation is through release of norepinephrine (see discussion on pharmacology, p. 100).

Parasympathetic nervous system. The visceral efferent branch of the oculomotor nerve arises from cell bodies located in the Edinger-Westphal nucleus. The axons pass, with the inferior division of the oculomotor nerve, with the branch to the inferior oblique muscle and form the preganglionic motor root (short) of the ciliary ganglion. Here synapse is made with the cells of postganglionic fibers, which pass with the short ciliary nerves to innervate the ciliary and sphincter pupillae muscles.

Sympathetic nervous system. The sympathetic nervous system (Fig. 1-39) has centers located in the hypothalamus and the medulla: (1) the superior ciliospinal center and (2) the inferior ciliospinal center (of Budge). The *superior ciliospinal center* is located near the nucleus of the hypoglossal nerve. The *inferior ciliospinal center* (of Budge) is located in the upper portion of the spinal cord. Sympathetic efferent fibers arise in the anterior lateral columns of the spinal cord that leave the spinal cord in the ventral roots of thoracic I to lumbar II spinal nerves. These fibers pass with the anterior rami lateral to the vertebral column when they leave the anterior rami in the white ramus communi-

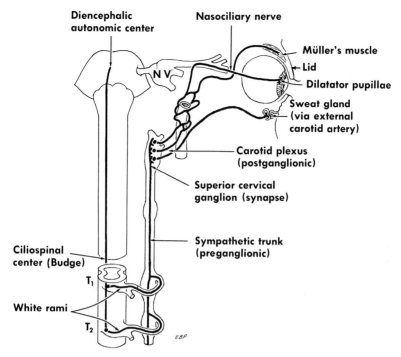

Fig. 1-39. Sympathetic nervous system.

cans. The white rami turn at right angles at the vertebral column to form the sympathetic nerve trunk, which extends from the base of the skull to the tip of the coccyx. Within the trunk are ganglia in which synapse is made with peripheral postganglionic sympathetic nerves.

The ganglia at the level of cervical I, II, and III spinal nerves fuse to form a superior cervical ganglion. Most of the preganglionic fibers making synapse in the superior cervical ganglion have left the spinal cord at the level of the first two thoracic nerves and have coursed upward in the sympathetic nerve trunk.

Postganglionic fibers from the superior cervical ganglion are widely distributed. The internal carotid branch extends intracranially with fibers distributed to the internal carotid artery and the cavernous plexus. These fibers provide nearly all of the sympathetic nerve branches to the eye and the orbit. Fibers for sweating of the face, however, are distributed with the external carotid artery.

Sympathetic nerve fibers are mainly vasomotor and are distributed by the short posterior ciliary nerves from the ciliary ganglion. Fibers to the dilatator muscle are mainly carried to the globe by the long ciliary nerves that do not pass through the ciliary ganglion.

Supranuclear centers

The supranuclear centers of the cranial nerve nuclei to the eye are complicated structures and are the subject of considerable present-day research. In general, these centers control both reflex and voluntary ocular movements, and they are concerned with conjugate movements of the two eyes, such as eyes right, eyes left, eyes up, and eyes down.

Voluntary control and regulation of ocular movements that are not dependent upon visual stimuli are functions of the frontal motor cortex in areas designated as 8 alpha, 8 beta, and 8 gamma, located at the posterior end of the second frontal convolution. Stimulation of these areas causes both eyes to turn to the side opposite the area stimulated. Extirpation of the frontal lobe causes the eyes to turn to the same side. Fibers from the frontal cortex reach the cranial nerves of the brain stem through the corticobulbar pathway that courses through the internal capsule. The fibers either enter the appropriate nuclei directly or course in the medial longitudinal fasciculus.

In movements in which the eyes follow a moving object (pursuit movement, p. 89) the supranuclear centers are in the occipital lobe. Stimulation of the occipital lobe causes conjugate deviation to the opposite side. The connections of visual centers in the occipital lobe with cranial nuclei are by corticotectal fibers to the superior

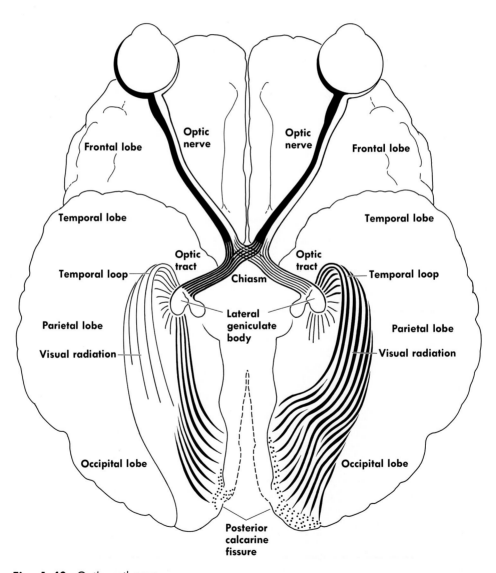

Fig. 1-40. Optic pathways.

colliculi, by corticotegmental fibers to centers for lateral gaze, and by corticotectal fibers that are involved in vertical gaze. The corticotegmental fibers, which end in the abducens nuclei of the opposite side, are involved in lateral gaze. Midbrain lesions tend to cause vertical defects of gaze (Parinaud's syndrome), and pontine lesions produce horizontal defects.

The frontal motor cortex and the occipital lobe on the same side are connected to each other. The frontal area is dominant, but if both frontal lobes are lost, the lack of voluntary eye movements is compensated by voluntary head movements in response to stimuli arising from the occipital area (oculomotor apraxia).

In addition to the supranuclear centers noted, there are others in the cerebellum, basal ganglion, and extrapyramidal systems.

Optic pathways

The retina, as discussed previously, may be divided into a macular portion (mainly cones), used in central vision and color vision, and a peripheral portion (mainly rods), used in dark adaptation and in the detection of peripheral movements. Insofar as the visual pathways are concerned, the retina may be divided into four quadrants by horizontal and vertical lines that intersect at the fovea centralis. (Note that the fovea and not the optic nerve is the point of division.) Thus each eye may be divided into superior, inferior, temporal, and nasal portions, which in turn may be divided into peripheral and central portions.

All fibers arising from the nasal half of each retina decussate to the opposite side at the chiasm to join uncrossed temporal fibers to form the optic tract. Visual fibers synapse in the lateral geniculate body and then pass to the optic radiation as the optic tract (Fig. 1-40).

Optic chiasm. The optic chiasm (Fig. 1-41) is about 13 mm. wide. It is attached by the pia mater and the arachnoid to the dorsal surface of the diencephalon, and it forms a portion of the floor of the third ventricle. Its posterior surface is in close contact with the tuber cinereum from which extends the infundibulum or stalk

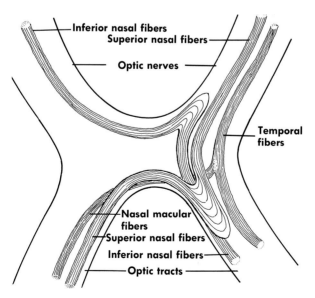

Fig. 1-41. Decussation of nasal fibers in the optic chiasm. Decussating fibers of the fovea are located most posteriorly.

of the pituitary gland (hypophysis cerebri). The chiasm is superior to the tuberculum sellae turcicae and the diaphragma sellae and is usually posterior to the optic groove of the sphenoid bone. It is closely related to the internal carotid arteries laterally and to the anterior cerebral arteries and anterior communicating artery anteriorly.

Optic tract. Crossed nasoretinal fibers and uncrossed tempororetinal fibers sweep laterally and posteriorly to form the optic tracts. These encircle the hypothalamus (in the ventral wall of the third ventricle) and wind around the ventrolateral aspect of the pes pedunculi (the ventral portion of the midbrain). The majority of visual fibers terminate in the lateral geniculate body. A smaller number continue as the superior quadrigeminal brachium to the superior colliculi (reflex ocular movements) and to the pretectal area (pupillary reflexes). Other fibers enter the hypothalamus and terminate in the supraoptic nucleus and the medial nuclei of the tuber cinereum. The significance of these endings in man is unknown—in some species they may govern the distribution of skin pigment in response to different light intensities.

Lateral geniculate body. The lateral geniculate body is the area of synapse of axons of ganglion cells of the retina carrying visual impulses. It is located in the diencephalon lateral to the medial geniculate body, and it consists of a dorsal and an inconspicuous (in man) ventral nucleus. The dorsal nucleus is composed of six concentrically arranged cell layers separated by fiber bands: fibers from the temporal retina terminate in three alternate layers, and crossed fibers from the contralateral nasal retina terminate in the other three layers. Synapse is made in the lateral geniculate body so that corresponding nasal and temporal retinal fibers have the same representation in the optic radiation (geniculocalcarine tract).

Optic radiation. The geniculocalcarine tract passes through the internal capsule to form the optic radiation that terminates in the striate area (Brodmann's area 17) of the occipital lobe. Upon emerging from the internal capsule, the fibers flare around the lateral ventricles. Fibers from the lower retina (lower temporal on the same side and lower nasal on the contralateral side) turn downward into the temporal lobe and loop around the lateral ventricle to form the Flechsig-Archambault-Meyer loop.

Visual cortex. The fibers of the optic radiation terminate in the calcarine cortex of the occipital lobe, which is located in the walls of the calcarine fissure and the adjacent portion of the lingual and cuneus gyri. The macular fibers terminate in an extensive posterior area, whereas the peripheral retinal representation is located anteriorly along the lips of the calcarine fissure. The visual cortex is exceedingly thin, being only 1.5 mm. thick in the floor of the calcarine fissure. Six cell layers typical of the cortex are present but are modified by the occurrence of numerous granule (stellate) cells that form a grossly visible band of Gennari.

Localization in the visual pathways. The visual field (p. 147) is composed of the total perception arising from retinal stimulation at one moment. Its orientation is directly opposite that of the distribution of retinal elements. Objects located on the temporal side stimulate the nasal retina; objects located below stimulate the retina above, and so on (Fig. 1-42).

As fibers enter the optic nerve, central macular fibers occupy the lateral portion nearest the fovea. Thereafter the various sectors have the same distribution in the optic nerve as in the retina. The macular fibers are central, surrounded by the peripheral fibers; fibers from the inferior retina are below, and those from the superior retina are above.

In the optic chiasm the temporal fibers retain their temporal position, with the

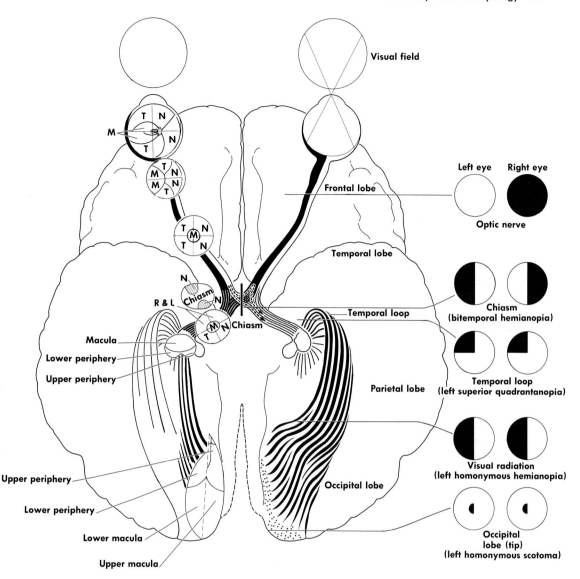

Fig. 1-42. Typical visual field defects that follow damage to different regions of the optic pathways. Note that the visual fields are diagrammed to reflect the source of the light that stimulates the retina. Thus light from the temporal side stimulates the nasal portion of the retina, light from above the lower portion, and so on. Thus the visual field defect arising from a lesion in the nasal retina is diagrammed as a temporal field defect.

nasal fibers from the macula located more posterior than the peripheral fibers. Both peripheral and macular nasal fibers decussate in the chiasm (Fig. 1-41). Fibers from the inferior nasal sector lie on the anterior and inferior surfaces of the chiasm (closest to the pituitary gland). After decussating, they loop forward in the optic nerve of the opposite side to pass back to the optic tract. (The inferior position of these fibers in the chiasm makes them the most vulnerable in pituitary enlargements, so that the earliest visual sign of pituitary disease is involvement of the superior temporal visual field. The anterior loop in the contralateral optic nerve is responsible for the occasional involvement of the visual field of each eye in disease involving the opposite optic nerve.)

The superior nasal fibers cross in the superior portion of the chiasm in its posterior aspect. They first pass posteriorly in the optic tract on the same side and then loop forward to decussate.

In the anterior portion of the optic tract the distribution of nerve fibers is similar to that in the optic nerve, except that the nasal fibers are those that have crossed from the opposite side. The fibers are rapidly redistributed so that those from corresponding parts of each retina become associated. Thus crossed (nasal) lower fibers become related to uncrossed (temporal) lower fibers, and crossed superior fibers become related to uncrossed superior fibers. In the optic tracts, defects produce homonymous field defects as fibers from corresponding parts of each retina are involved in a single lesion (hemianopsia is half-blindness; the reference is to the blind portion of the field).

The distribution of fibers in the lateral geniculate body is complicated. Macular fibers have conspicuous representation. Visual field defects here are similar to those in the optic tract.

The fibers emerging from the lateral geniculate body in the optic radiation have exact correspondence in each eye so that a defect causes exactly similar visual field defects in each eye.

In the striate area of the visual cortex of the occipital lobe (area 17), superior retinal fibers are located anteriorly, and inferior retinal fibers are located posteriorly. There is no anatomic evidence that the nasal fibers in the macular area do not decussate completely. The "sparing of the macula," in which defects involving the occipital area seem not to affect all macular fibers, apparently arises from minute changes in fixation and not from any anatomic exception.

Embryology

The development of the eye is evident at the eight-somite state, and thereafter any adverse environmental influence can cause ocular developmental abnormalities. In general, genetic or exogenous factors that influence development early in embryonic life cause such severe defects that the fetus seldom survives. Ocular defects seen clinically thus arise relatively late in ocular development.

The eye arises from neural and surface ectoderm and from mesoderm. Both the neural and pigment layers of the retina develop from neural ectoderm, and both layers continue anteriorly to give rise to the ciliary epithelium and the pigmented epithelium of the iris and its sphincter and dilatator muscles. The neuroglial and neural portions of the optic nerve arise from neural ectoderm.

The surface ectoderm gives rise to the lens, the epithelium of the cornea, the conjunctiva, and the lid together with the epithelium of their glandular structures. The mesoderm gives rise to the corneal endothelium and stroma, the sclera, the iris stroma, the extrinsic muscles of the eye, and the blood vessels and bones of the orbit (Table 1-1).

Following fertilization of the ovum, a solid cluster of cells is formed, the morula. This then develops in a hollow sphere, the blastula or blastocyst, containing a central cavity, the blastocele. Cells multiply on one section within the blastocyst to form an inner cell mass destined to form the embryo, amnion, and primitive gut (the yolk sac or archenteron). The outer wall of the blastocyst is destined to form the placenta.

The cells adjacent to the wall of the blastocyst give rise to the primitive ectoderm and line the amniotic cavity. The

Table 1-1. Primordia of ocular structures

Neural ectoderm	Surface ectoderm	Mesoderm
Pigment and sensory retina	Lens	
Ciliary epithelium	Corneal epithelium	Corneal stroma,† endothelium, and Descemet's membrane
Pigmented epithelium of iris	Conjunctival epithelium	Blood vessels
Sphincter and dilatator iridis	Lid	Sclera
Neuroglial and neural portions of optic nerve	Cilia Epithelium, tarsal glands Epithelium, Zeis and Moll glands Epithelium, lacrimal and accessory lacrimal glands	Iris stroma Extrinsic eye muscles Ciliary muscle Bones of orbit
	Vitreous body* Zonule*	Corneal stroma†

*From neural ectoderm and surface ectoderm.
†From surface ectoderm and mesoderm.

inner cell mass grows freely within the blastocyst, and the initial primitive layer of cells, the entoderm, multiplies to form the yolk sac (Fig. 1-43).

The embryo, developing as the embryonic disk or plate at the area of contact between the amnion and the yolk sac, consists of two layers: a dorsal ectoderm and a ventral entoderm connected to the wall of the blastocyst by a body stalk. A primitive streak, then a groove, develops on the dorsal or ectodermal surface and provides an axial symmetry to the embryonic disk. From the area of the groove, intraembryonic mesoderm or mesenchyme appears and divides the disk into three layers.

In the dorsal ectoderm anterior to the primitive streak there first develops a longitudinal (neural) groove and then, by cell proliferation, the neural or medial plate. At the anterior extremity of the neural plate the ectoderm develops markedly to form two parallel (the neural) folds. From this area grows the primary brain vesicles, the hindbrain or rhombencephalon, which divides into the metencephalon and mye-

lencephalon, the midbrain or mesencephalon, and the forebrain or prosencephalon, which divides into the telencephalon (the frontal, parietal, and temporal cerebral hemispheres) and the diencephalon (the thalamus).

The first indications of ocular development are two barely noticeable dents, the beginnings of the optic grooves or sulci. These deepen into optic foveolae or pits. Simultaneously the neural folds merge to transform the neural groove into a primitive neural tube with the cerebral vesicle located at the anterior end. Along each neural fold at the line of closure, ectodermal cells (neural crests) appear, which are destined to form ganglia of cranial, spinal, and sympathetic nerves, the neurilemmal sheaths of peripheral nerves, the pia mater and the arachnoid, the chromaffin organs, and the melanoblasts. The ectoderm covering the now closed nervous system gives rise to the surface ectoderm.

With further development of the cerebral vesicle, the optic primordia come to lie far apart and then expand to form vesicular protrusions, so that the entire

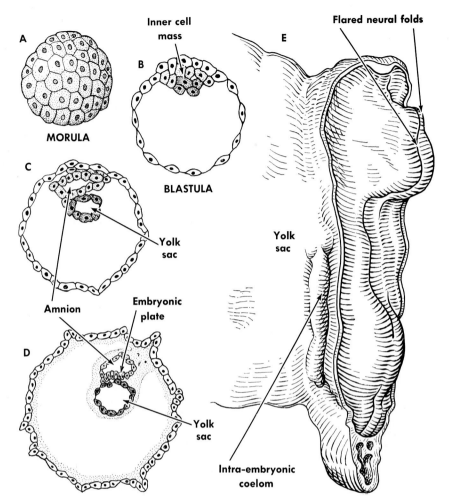

Fig. 1-43. A, Morula. **B,** Blastula containing the inner cell mass. **C,** Outer wall of the blastula is destined to form the placenta; the inner cell mass adjacent to the wall of the blastula gives rise to the amnion; the remaining cells form the yolk sac. **D,** Embryo develops at the area of contact between the amnion and the yolk sac. **E,** Amnion is cut away to show the neural folds at the anterior extremity of the neural plate.

anterior portion of the primitive brain consists of a cerebral vesicle separating two lateral optic vesicles.

The lateral optic vesicles become invaginated at their centers, forming double-walled secondary optic vesicles or cups. The thicker inner layer of the wall, by a complex process of differentiation, develops into the nervous layer of the retina, whereas the single-celled outer wall be-

comes the pigment epithelium. The space that separates these layers is reduced to a cleft communicating with the cerebral vesicle through a hollow, tubelike stalk (the optic stalk), the future optic nerve (Fig. 1-44). Failure of the optic cup to invaginate causes a congenital cystic eyeball in which the orbit contains a large cyst with traces of nervous elements.

Invagination of the optic vesicle in-

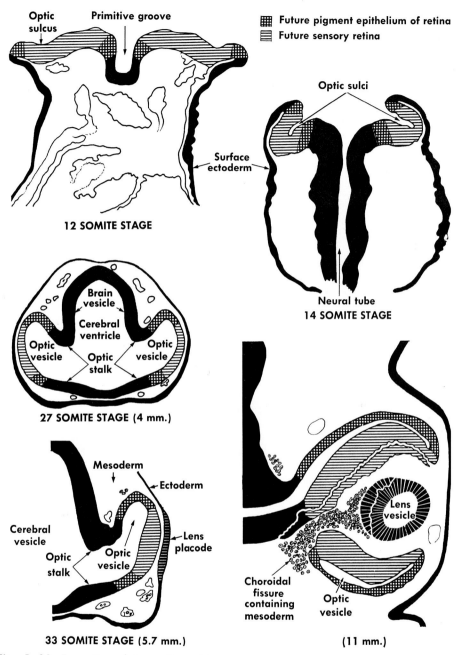

Fig. 1-44. Formation of the optic vesicle.

volves not only the superficial lateral surface but also its inferior surface and the distal end of the optic stalk, so that a linear cleft or fissure forms on its undersurface. This cleft is called the embryonic or fetal fissure, although the fetal stage has not been attained. It is also called the choroidal fissure but has nothing to do with the choroid of the brain. The embryonic fissure provides a shortcut for blood vessels and optic nerve fibers to enter and leave the optic vesicle—otherwise they would have to pass around its lateral margin. Defects in the region of the choroidal fissure result in colobomas that may involve the choroid, the retina, the ciliary body, the iris, or the optic nerve.

Eyeball

Sclera. The sclera arises as a condensation of the mesoderm surrounding the optic cup. Its anterior portion forms first concomitant with the insertion of the rectus muscle.

Cornea. The cornea is derived from both surface ectoderm and mesoderm. The surface ectoderm, from which the lens vesicle detaches itself, forms the epithelium, and the mesodermal fibers give rise to the remainder of the cornea and the endothelium lining the anterior chamber. Descemet's membrane is secreted by the endothelial layer, whereas Bowman's layer is a condensation of the anterior surface of the stroma.

Choroid. The choroid arises from the mesoderm surrounding the primary optic vesicle. All of its layers can be recognized by the fifth month. Pigment develops relatively late, first in the neighborhood of the entrance of the posterior ciliary arteries and then extending forward.

Ciliary body. The ciliary body is formed on the back surface of the iris by a fusion of the optic cup and the growth of blood vessels to form the major circle of the iris. The base of the ciliary body gives rise to the numerous ciliary processes. The *ciliary muscle* grows in from mesoderm between the sclera and the ciliary ectoderm, with the longitudinal fibers being formed at about the fourth month and the circular portion being formed at the end of the sixth month. A cleavage of the structures in the angle of the anterior chamber gives rise to the *trabecular meshwork*.

Iris and pupil. The pattern of the iris in life closely reflects its embryologic origin. The most anterior extremity of the optic cup is evident at the pigmented margin of the pupil. Both the sphincter pupillae and dilatator muscles of the pupil are derived from neural ectoderm and, with the arrectores pili muscles, are the sole muscles of ectodermal origin. Mesoderm grows over the surface of the optic cup, forming the anterior stromal layers of the iris. Up to the third month of embryonic life the margin of the optic cup extends only a short distance beyond the equator of the lens. The mesoderm is continuous with that of the ciliary body, and there is no pupil as such. About the fourth month the optic cup grows forward with an attachment to the mesoderm. The mesoderm in the pupillary area then atrophies as far back as this attachment, which forms the collarette.

Retina. The inner neural or sensory layer of the retina develops, as does the neural tube, into ependymal, mantle, and marginal layers. Because of invagination of the optic cup, the distribution is the reverse of that in the neural tube, so that the marginal layer is closest to the developing vitreous cavity. Differentiation of the retina is a complex process. The ependymal layer forms the external limiting membrane, and rods and cones may originate from cilia on its surface projecting into the vesicle between the neural and the pigmented epithelium. The inner marginal layer gives rise to the nerve fiber layer. The mantle layer gives rise to other neural and glial retinal elements. Development proceeds from the posterior pole toward the periphery. The specialized area of the macula lutea begins in the third month, but its development proceeds slowly. It is not until the sixth month that there is a thinning of ganglion cells, and its anatomic differentiation continues after birth. Inasmuch as central vision does not fully develop until the third to the fifth year, it is evident that functional differentiation lags behind anatomic differentiation.

At the anterior edge of the secondary optic cup the inner sensory and outer pigmentary layers fuse together to form the following structures: (1) the ciliary epithelium (pars ciliaris retinae), the inner layer of which is a continuation of the neural layer and a pigmentary layer, which is the continuation of pigmented epithelium, and (2) the iris epithelium (pars iridica retinae) together with the sphincter and dilatator pupillae muscles.

The optic stalk provides the neuroglial supporting structures of the optic nerve. The nerve fibers consist of axons of ganglion cells located in the inner layer of the retina together with fibers extending from the brain to the retina. The sheaths and septa of the optic nerve develop from mesoderm.

Vitreous body. The vitreous body has a complex development, presumably arising from both neural ectoderm and mesoderm. It is described as consisting of primary and secondary vitreous; the zonule of the lens is termed tertiary vitreous. Primary vitreous is formed by fibers that bridge the area between the surface of the lens vesicle and the inner wall of the optic cup. Thus it seems to be evolved from both lenticular and retinal ectoderm. Secondary vitreous appears to arise from mesoderm that gives rise to the hyaloid system of blood vessels.

Lens. The optic vesicle, as it extends laterally, is covered by surface ectoderm that becomes thickened into several layers, the lens placode. A groove or pit appears in this placode, forming a vesicle that becomes cut off from the surface ectoderm and forms the lens. Lens fibers are laid down concentrically and their ends meet to form suture lines. The nuclei form the nuclear bow, and new lens fibers develop throughout life from the peripheral equator.

Recent studies suggest that the surface ectoderm is cytolyzed and that this causes the stimulation of neural tissue to form the lens. Death of the surface ectoderm cells and their subsequent autolysis are necessary stimulants to the neural cells and will even cause the formation of new lenses in adult rabbits and mice in which the lens has been removed.

Zonule. The zonule arises from the vitreous body, filling the gap between the rim of the optic cup and the lens.

Blood supply

The fetal fissure extends to about the anterior one third of the optic stalk. About the end of the first month (7 to 8 mm.) an arterial plexus below the optic cup consolidates into (1) a hyaloid artery that enters the optic nerve and cup through the fissure and (2) a small annular vessel that ramifies on the rim of the cup and that eventually becomes the choroid.

The hyaloid artery forms a network of vessels covering the back of the lens (tunica vasculosa lentis) and filling the vitreous body (vasa hyaloidea propria). The hyaloid system disappears about the fifth month, but a small branch is retained, the central retinal artery, which ultimately provides the blood supply for the inner layers of the retina. The ophthalmic artery and its branches to the eye and the orbit are defined during the second month and take their final form during the third month.

The vascular return of the entire hyaloid system is by the capsulopupillary membrane that covers the lens from the equator to the edge of the pupil. As the hyaloid system atrophies, the pupillary membrane is supplied by the long posterior arteries and thus continues to develop until early in the sixth month, when they begin to atrophy and disappear.

A wide variation in orbital blood vessels occurs, mainly because of failure of early branches to disappear. Portions of the pupillary membrane commonly persist over the pupillary aperture, and persistence of the hyaloid artery is quite common. It appears to arise from the optic disk and extends a variable distance into the vitreous cavity, sometimes as far as the lens. It may form a small opacity (the Mittendorf dot) on the posterior lens capsule.

Eyelids

The eyelids are derived from both mesoderm and surface ectoderm. The upper lid develops in medial and lateral parts from the frontonasal process. The mesodermal portion of the lower lid arises from an upgrowth of the maxillary process. The covering ectoderm gives rise to the skin on the outside and the conjunctiva on the inside. The tarsal plate and muscular tissues of the lid are derived from mesoderm; their glands and cilia arise from ectoderm. The *lacrimal puncta* do not open onto the lid margins until just before the lids separate during the seventh month. The lower ends of the ducts frequently do not open until birth or shortly thereafter.

Lacrimal apparatus

The lacrimal passages develop in a cleft between the lateral nasal and maxillary processes. This cleft is converted into a tube by canalization of a solid rod of ectodermal tissue cells found beneath the surface, and these epithelial cells form the lacrimal passages. The *lacrimal gland* arises from the ectoderm forming the conjunctival surface of the eyeball. Once formed, it receives connective tissue septa and supporting structures from the mesoderm.

Chapter 2

Physiology of the eye

The human eye is by no means the best of all possible eyes. Its central visual acuity is exceeded in birds, some of which have two maculas. Phenomena caused by polarized light may be appreciated by man under special conditions, but he is unable to utilize the polarized light of the sky for orientation, as do bees. Although the human eye becomes markedly sensitive with dark adaptation, undoubtedly some nocturnal animals have a lower threshold to light. Some creatures are able to utilize ultraviolet light that is invisible to man.

Despite this inferiority of particular functions, the human eye is so organized that it provides vision in a wide variety of conditions. Man has fairly good visual acuity for both far and near. In spite of his inability to detect ultraviolet radiation, his color vision is well developed, and he can adapt to light and dark. The decussation of the fibers from the nasal half of each retina and the nondecussation of fibers from the temporal half of each retina lead to a retinal correspondence so that an object in space may be viewed with stereopsis.

A number of physiology texts deal solely with the eye; a practical volume by Adler; a four-volume monograph edited by Davson well epitomized in a single-volume text; *Biochemistry of the Eye* by Pirie and Van Heyningen; and a number of special monographs. Many of the topics in ocular physiology are, of necessity, complicated, involving as they do interrelationships be-tween quantum mechanics, biophysics, biochemistry, psychology, and electrical phenomena in the nervous system. It is thus possible to emphasize in this section only the highlights.

Cornea

As already noted, the cornea is a transparent structure composed mainly of stroma and having a regularly arranged epithelium on its outer surface and a single layer of endothelial cells lining its inner or posterior surface. Its anterior surface is bathed with tears, whereas the endothelium is immersed in the anterior aqueous humor.

The corneal stroma consists of collagen fibers of unusually uniform diameter that are gathered together in bundles of corneal lamellas. These are arranged regularly at right angles to each other, and they are immersed in a cement substance consisting of three mucopolysaccharides: keratin sulfate, chondroitin sulfate, and chondroitin. The metabolism of the stroma is intimately related to the metabolism of the epithelium and the endothelium, both of which must be intact to prevent stromal edema.

Inasmuch as the cornea is avascular, it must derive the materials and oxygen required for metabolism either by diffusion from the pericorneal capillaries or from the aqueous humor and tears. It seems likely that only the peripheral cornea receives adequate nutrients from the bloodstream, and that the central cornea must depend for its nutrition upon exchange of metabolites from the aqueous humor and tears together with atmospheric oxygen.

Metabolism. It will be recalled that glucose becomes phosphorylated to form glucose 6-phosphate, which may follow one of several metabolic pathways:

1. It may form glucose 1-phosphate that in turn may form uridine diphosphoglucose that may play a role in the synthesis of glycogen, mucopolysaccharides, or glucuronic acid.
2. It may be metabolized by a series of reactions, each of which involves a specific dehydrogenase.
3. The chief metabolic pathway is glycolysis (Embden-Meyerof), which does not require oxygen and in which lactic acid is the end product.
4. The phosphogluconate ("shunt") pathway requires oxygen, and its end products are carbon dioxide and a triose.

Neither of these last two pathways provides as much energy as does the tricarboxylic acid cycle (Krebs or citric acid) in which the trioses formed by the glycolytic and phosphogluconate pathways are degraded in a stepwise manner to carbon dioxide and water. If there is an imbalance so that an excess of lactate is produced, the excess is excreted and does not enter the tricarboxylic acid pathway.

The metabolism of glucose constitutes the chief source of energy for the cornea. The glucose is utilized by the glycolytic (anaerobic) and the phosphogluconate (aerobic) pathways. About 65% of the metabolism proceeds by way of glycolysis, and the remainder proceeds by way of the phosphogluconate pathway. The tricarboxylic acid cycle is present in the epithelium but absent in the stroma, so that lactic acid from the stroma is not further metabolized and diffuses into the aqueous humor and the epithelium. The lactic acid that is not utilized by the epithelium diffuses into the tears.

The oxygen required for the phosphogluconate pathway is derived mainly from atmospheric oxygen. If the entire corneal surface is deprived of ready access to oxygen by means of a contact lens, corneal edema results. This suggests the inability of glycolysis alone to support metabolism and the inadequacy of the oxygen supply from the limbus vasculature.

Transparency. The cornea transmits electromagnetic radiation having a wavelength* of between 300 nm. in the ultraviolet to 2,500 nm. in the infrared. Transmission is about 80% at 400 nm. and nearly 100% at 500 to 1,200 nm. There are two absorption bands of water beyond 1,200 nm., but transmission between the bands is high. Wavelengths of more than 700 nm. are not absorbed by the retinal photoreceptors and do not cause sensory stimulation. Wavelengths between 300 and 400 nm. in the ultraviolet range are partially absorbed by the cornea, and those transmitted are entirely absorbed by the lens and do not reach the retina. Transmission of light by the cornea with this high efficiency indicates that (1) the cornea does not contain pigment that would absorb and reflect light; (2) the number of opaque particles within the cornea that would absorb light must be minimal; and (3) the structure of the cornea is such that light is not scattered, that is, reflected from a number of minute particles.

The transparency of the cornea arises from two factors: (1) the anatomic arrangement of its structure and (2) the deturgescence mechanism of the stroma that maintains a partial dehydration.

The *anatomic factors* concerned are the absence of blood vessels and pigment in the cornea, the regular arrangement of the epithelial and endothelial cells, and the paucity of cells in the stroma. Addi-

---

*The wavelength of electromagnetic energy may be designated as nanometers (nm. = m. $\times 10^{-9}$), Angstrom units (Å = mm. $\times 10^{-7}$), or millimicrons (mμ = $\mu \times 10^{-3}$ = m. $\times 10^{-9}$).

tionally, the epithelial cells are not cornified and are covered with tears to form a regularly refracting surface. The epithelial and endothelial cells and Descemet's membrane are transparent because they all have the same index of refraction.

The collagen fibrils of the corneal stroma have an index of refraction of 1.4; that of the surrounding mucopolysaccharide tissue juice is about 1.34. This difference should produce considerable scattering of light, causing the cornea to be more translucent than transparent. Maurice proposed that the collagen fibers are oriented regularly and precisely in a two-dimensional lattice (Fig. 2-1). The components of this lattice have a diameter of much less than one wavelength of light, so that the lattice is transparent in the direction of the incident beam. That portion of the light striking the lattice itself is eliminated by destructive interference. This mechanism of transparency in the eye is unique. In other transparent tissues such

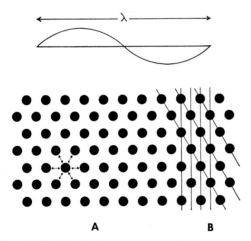

Fig. 2-1. A, Lattice structure of the cornea explains its transparency. Arrows between the fibrils indicate the system of forces that are supposed to maintain the regularity of the structure. The wavelength of light is drawn above for comparison. **B,** The lines are two sets of lattice planes. (From Maurice, D. M.: J. Physiol. [London] **136:**263, 1957.)

as the lens, vitreous body, and inner layers of the retina, the transparency arises because of the uniform index of refraction of the cellular components.

Hydration. Each corneal lamella contains about 65% of the water it is capable of binding. If a button of cornea is placed in isotonic saline solution, it will swell to three times its normal thickness and lose the property of transmitting light. A similar swelling of the stroma occurs if the epithelium or the endothelium is removed, or if the carbohydrate metabolism is inhibited by metabolic poisons.

The mechanisms involved in the maintenance of this deturgescence of the corneal stroma are not clearly understood. It has been postulated that an active transport mechanism is involved, most likely involving the endothelium. Because of the role of the sodium ion in water binding by tissues, it has been suggested that this postulated active transport system should constantly remove sodium from the stroma. Such a transport mechanism is present, but it transports sodium into, rather than out of, the corneal stroma and is in the wrong direction to support the hypothesis. The endothelium provides an additional confusing factor in being freely permeable to water. However, after disease or injury to the endothelium, edema of the cornea stroma occurs.

Epithelial defects cause subepithelial edema, and endothelial defects cause stromal edema. The anterior condensation of the corneal stroma (Bowman's layer) apparently limits the extent of the edema. When a contact lens is worn for a long period, preventing access of oxygen to the cornea, subepithelial corneal edema occurs. This condition is known clinically as Sattler's veil. It is presumably the result of inadequacy of the glycolytic pathway alone to maintain corneal function when oxygen is not available for the phosphogluconate pathway. The edema disappears spontaneously over a period of time when the cornea is in contact with the atmossphere.

Permeability. The peripheral cornea may maintain its metabolism by means of the capillary network at the corneoscleral limbus. The central cornea, however, depends for its nutrition upon substances penetrating either the endothelium or the epithelium. Any substance reaching the epithelium must be water soluble so as to penetrate the film of tears covering the cornea. The epithelium constitutes the principal

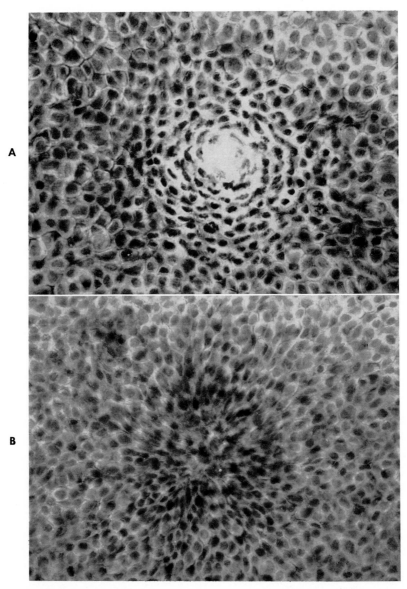

Fig. 2-2. A, Pinprick injury of corneal epithelium of rat. **B,** Healing of pinprick injury by the sliding of adjacent epithelium to form typical rosette. (Flat preparation, hematoxylin stain; ×550.) (From Alexander, A. M., and Newell, F. W.: Amer. J. Ophthal. **48:**22, 210, 1959.)

barrier of the cornea. It is extremely impermeable to ions and other lipid-insoluble substances but is readily permeable to fat-soluble substances, presumably because the cell membranes are composed of a lipoprotein. Thus fat-soluble material passes through the epithelial walls, whereas fat-insoluble substances must either go through pores in the cells or around cells.

Wound healing. Wound healing of the cornea has been widely studied because of the avascularity, the distinct cellular and chemical lamination, and the clinical significance of corneal grafting. Minute epithelial wounds heal by a sliding of adjacent epithelium (Fig. 2-2). Larger epithelial wounds heal by both sliding and mitosis of surrounding epithelium. The sliding is influenced only by severe injury of the epithelium, but epithelial mitosis is inhibited by many compounds commonly used in the treatment of eye disease and injury: sulfonamides, anesthetics, antibiotics, and lanolin ointments.

If Bowman's layer in injured, scar formation results. Wound repair is similar in both Bowman's layer and the stroma: there is stimulation of corneal cells (keratocytes) together with migration of fibrocytes from the blood in the vessels at the corneoscleral limbus. Intact epithelium is required for initiation of stromal healing. The endothelial cell layer regenerates rapidly. Descemet's membrane may be reduplicated and form a double-glass membrane either in the anterior chamber or adjacent to the cornea.

In corneal grafting the donor cornea becomes hydrated, and the swelling causes a watertight wound, permitting the anterior chamber to re-form. Corneal grafts always "take." A hypersensitivity reaction manifests itself not by rejection of the donor graft but by loss of transparency and vascularization of the graft. Presumably because of its avascularity, the normal cornea participates minimally in the immune processes of the body.

Lens

It will be recalled that the lens is derived either from surface ectoderm or from stimulation of the optic vesicle by cytolysis of the surface ectoderm. The lens is covered by a homogeneous capsule and has epithelium only beneath the anterior capsule. The lens contains a central "nucleus" that is surrounded by cortex. Throughout life, new cells are formed at the equator and migrate inward toward the nucleus where ultimately the cell fibers become compressed and the nuclei lost. The lens is held in position behind the pupil by means of zonular fibers. These fibers transmit contractions of the ciliary muscle that result in the change of shape of the lens known as accommodation.

Transparency. The lens transmits nearly 100% of electromagnetic energy between 400 and 1,000 nm. Its transparency arises because of its acellularity and because all of its parts have nearly the same index of refraction. The single layer of epithelial cells beneath the anterior capsule is not thick enough to interfere with transparency, and these are the sole nuclei in the visual axis.

Despite the homogeneity of the lens structure, its total index of refraction is greater than any single portion. This results from a concentric, onionlike structure in which older central layers have a greater index of refraction than the surrounding younger layers. Total refractive power of the lens is thus much greater than one would anticipate from its external curvature, thickness, and the index of refraction of individual layers. In a simplifying assumption in physiologic optics the lens is considered as being composed of a central core with a high index of refraction that has a layer with a lower index of refraction on either side.

Metabolism. The lens is composed almost entirely of protein. For many years these have been termed alpha and beta crystalline and an insoluble portion, albuminoid, which remains after extraction of the two crystallines. Electrophoresis indicates a number of different types of protein with different electrophoretic motility, antigenicity, and structure. Alpha crystalline, composed of a single protein, is formed before birth, remains in the lens throughout life, and has been called embryonic lens protein. With denaturation and dehydration of alpha crystalline, the insoluble protein fraction, albuminoid, is formed. Beta crystalline is composed of a number of fractions and is formed throughout life.

The nature of protein synthesis in the lens is of considerable interest. The amino acids required for protein synthesis must be transported through the ciliary body and then through the posterior aqueous humor and the lens capsule to the lens. The mode of synthesis is unknown, but it involves mainly cells whose nuclei are located at the equator.

In many respects the lens behaves like a large cell. Thus it maintains a large intracellular potassium content, although bathed in a solution with a relatively high sodium content. The epithelium of the anterior capsule is necessary for the maintenance of this gradient and to transport sodium out of the lens. When there is interference with the metabolism of the lens, sodium and water accumulate and there is loss of potassium.

Glycolysis (Embden-Meyerof pathway) accounts for about 85% of the glucose metabolism of the lens. It will be recalled that this pathway yields lactic acid. The lactic acid is further metabolized by the tricarboxylic acid cycle. The lactic acid not metabolized diffuses into the aqueous humor.

The remaining glucose of the lens is metabolized by the phosphogluconate pathway ("shunt"), which accounts for all of the carbon dioxide production by the lens. Inasmuch as the amount of oxygen that can be dissolved in the aqueous humor is extremely small, the rate of this pathway is markedly limited. In addition to these pathways, sorbitol and fructose are found in the lens. It has been suggested that glucose may be converted to sorbitol and then to fructose. The significance of this pathway is not known—it does not appear to contribute to the metabolic economy of the lens.

Considerable attention has been directed to the large amount of gluthione present in the lenses of all species. The concentration of glutathione is reduced in cataract formation, and it disappears prior to the loss of transparency of the lens. It is evident that glutathione plays some role in lens metabolism, but its nature has not been defined. Ascorbic acid is also present in high concentration in the lens and is derived from the aqueous humor. It has been suggested that dihydroascorbic acid oxidizes glutathione, and that the hydrogen thus released reduces triphosphopyridine nucleotide (TPN).

Cataract. Any loss of transparency of the lens is designated as cataract. The mechanisms involved include hydration of the lens and denaturation of lens protein. Cataracts may follow perforating injuries of the lens capsule or any interference with mitosis of the cells at the equator. In experimental animals the administration of galactose, 5-carbon sugars, or metabolic poisons may cause cataract. Cataract always develops in alloxan diabetes, with its time of onset directly proportionate to the blood sugar concentration.

A variety of chemical changes occur in cataract: decrease of potassium, increase of sodium and water, and decrease of glutathione, free amino acids, adenosine triphosphate, and beta crystalline. The hydration is in part reversible, but the protein denaturation is not.

Aqueous humor

The aqueous humor contributes to the maintenance of intraocular pressure and supports the metabolism of the lens, which does not have a blood supply and thus has mainly an anaerobic metabolism. Additionally, it contributes to the nutrition of the cornea. The aqueous humor is formed by both secretion and diffusion by the epithelium of the ciliary processes. The fluid thus formed is elaborated by the non-pigmented epithelial cells of the ciliary body that are closest to the posterior chamber. Once compounds are secreted, their concentration is modified by water and chloride diffusion into the posterior chamber. Sodium is the chief cation of the aqueous humor and enters the eye mainly by secretion. Water is believed to follow the sodium mainly by diffusion. The aqueous humor formed in the posterior chamber flows through the pupil into the anterior chamber, with a minimal amount flowing posteriorly through the zonule to the vitreous cavity. The composition of the aqueous humor in the anterior chamber is modified by diffusion of water from blood vessels in the iris stroma. The aqueous humor leaves the eye through the trabecular meshwork, passing to Schlemm's canal and then to veins in the deep scleral plexus (Fig. 2-3).

The aqueous humor of the posterior chamber differs in composition from the aqueous humor of the anterior chamber. In man, posterior chamber aqueous humor contains chloride and ascorbate in excess of that of plasma and the anterior chamber aqueous humor. There is a deficiency of bicarbonate. In animals having large lenses, chloride is deficient, and there is an excess of bicarbonate, which is presumably required to buffer the lactic acid produced in glycolytic metabolism of the large lens.

In vitro the ciliary body, like the kidney

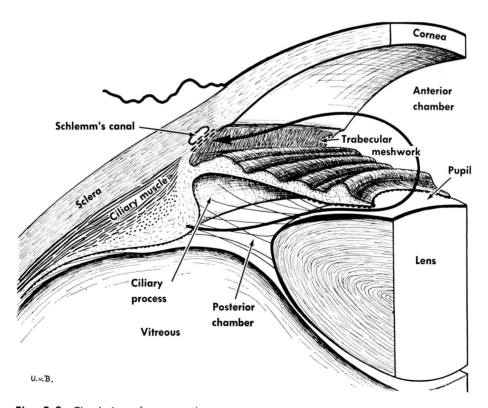

Fig. 2-3. Circulation of aqueous humor.

tubule, can concentrate organic acids such as phenolsulfonphthalein, para-aminohippurate, and iodopyracet (Diodrast). This activity results in the transport of these organic anions out of the eye.

The composition of the aqueous humor depends upon the integrity of the walls of the intraocular blood vessels. If these are damaged through injury or if the aqueous humor is removed by paracentesis, a plasmoid aqueous humor or aqueous humor of secondary formation results. Such an aqueous humor has the same composition as plasma, and there is no difference between anterior and posterior chamber fluids.

Inhibition of carbonic anhydrase decreases the secretory activity of the epithelium by about two thirds. The carbonic anhydrase inhibitors have become important compounds in the management of glaucoma (p. 315). Sodium- and potassium-activated adenosine triphosphatase (ATPase) are involved in electrolyte secretion into the posterior chamber. The cardiac glycosides, which inhibit ATPase, thus decrease the secretion of aqueous humor and have been used experimentally in the management of glaucoma. Interference with the sodium transport mechanism, metabolic poisoning of the ciliary epithelium, and reduction of the temperature of the ciliary body to 19° C. also decrease secretory activity.

Tears

The anterior surface of the eye is kept moist by tears formed by the lacrimal gland and by the accessory lacrimal glands of Krause and Wolfring. The major flow of tears is along the lid margin and in the conjunctival fornices. Periodic involuntary blinking distributes the tears over the surface of the globe and causes a pumping action of the lacrimal drainage system.

The corneal epithelium is covered by a relatively stagnant layer, the precorneal tear film. This is composed of a superficial oily layer derived from the meibomian glands, a middle fluid layer arising from the lacrimal glands, and a deep mucoid layer derived from the goblet cells of the conjunctiva. The oily layer is important in retarding evaporation of the tears and providing a smooth and regular anterior optical surface of the eye. The mucoid layer is in intimate contact with the outermost layer of corneal epithelium (p. 7), which must be intact to retain the precorneal film.

The average normal secretion of tears is between 0.5 and 2.2 μl/min.$^{-1}$. The maximum capacity of the cul-de-sac is about 30 μl, so that tears would overflow if the rate of drainage did not increase with increasing rate of secretion. However, once the rate of tear secretion exceeds 100 μl/min.$^{-1}$, overflow occurs.

With the eyes open and the precorneal oily film intact, a maximum of 0.85 μl of tears are evaporated each minute and the remainder pass through the lacrimal passages. The evaporation causes the tears to become slightly hypertonic, so that there is an osmotic flow of water from the anterior chamber, through the cornea, to the tear film. When the eye is closed, the precorneal tear film is in osmotic equilibrium with the aqueous humor, no osmotic flow occurs, and the corneal stroma thickens.

Determination of the composition of tears is complicated either by evaporation or by the dilution resulting from stimulation. The concentration of chloride, sodium, urea, and phosphate is approximately the same as in plasma, whereas the sugar content is markedly less.

There is a relatively large amount of protein, averaging about 1 to 2 Gm./100 ml. The concentration is lower in the aged than in the young. The protein is composed of 30% albumin, 40% globulins, and 30% lysozyme, an enzyme. The albumin and globulin differ from the albumin and globulin of plasma.

Lysozyme is an antibacterial enzyme widely distributed in nature—egg white is the commercial source. It is mainly effective against nonpathogenic bacteria by dissolving their mucopolysaccharide coating. In keratoconjunctivitis sicca (p. 210) the concentration of the enzyme is reduced, and the pH of tears is decreased from the normal of 7.2.

Tears are secreted in response to (1) psychic stimuli and (2) reflex stimuli. Reflex stimuli involve uncomfortable retinal stimulation by bright lights, irritation of the cornea, conjunctiva, and nasal mucous membrane, and application of heat to the tongue and mouth. Normal moisture of the eye may be entirely maintained by the accessory lacrimal glands, and secretion of tears may constitute a purely emergency response.

Clinically, tear formation is measured by hooking a piece of filter paper 5 mm. wide over the middle portion of the lower lid and determining how much wetting occurs in 4 minutes (p. 183). The filter paper, however, irritates the conjunctiva and the response is more likely to be indicative of reflex tearing rather than normal secretion. A more accurate method is measurement of the dilution of a dye, usually fluorescein, which also causes some reflex tearing. These tests indicate less tear formation after the age of 50 years, but the results may be interpreted as decreased reflex sensitivity rather than decreased tear formation.

Vitreous body

The vitreous body is a transparent gel that fills the vitreous cavity. It is firmly attached to the ciliary body and the retina in the region of the ora serrata and to the periphery of the optic disk. It is composed of (1) a cortical tissue layer adjacent to the retina and forming the hyaloid membrane behind the lens and (2) a vitreous body proper.

The *cortical tissue* is approximately 100μ thick and covers the entire vitreous body. It contains fine fibrils composed of collagen fibrils, an accumulation of proteins and a high concentration of hyaluronic acid, and a few cells. The collagen fibrils run approximately parallel to the surface of the vitreous body, and up to the age of

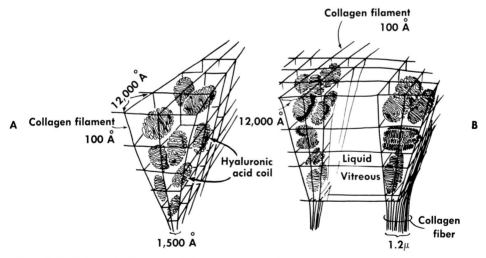

Fig. 2-4. Schematic drawing of fine structure of the vitreous gel showing fibrous network reinforced with hyaluronic acid molecules. **A,** Structural units are distributed randomly. **B,** There has been partial collapse of the network and the formation of a liquid pool. (From Balazs, E. A.: In Smelser, G. K., editor: Structure of the eye, New York, 1961, Academic Press, Inc.)

20 years they attach to the basement membrane of the retina and the ciliary body. Thereafter such attachments are found only in the anterior one third of the eye.

The *vitreous body proper* is a true biologic and chemical gel. Its framework is composed of fine collagen fibrils (Fig. 2-4). The spaces between the fibrils (the interfibrillar spaces) are filled with hyaluronic acid. This is a polysaccharide acid that occupies in water some 1,000 times the volume it would with close packing. It is considered to be a random coil with overlapping and entanglement of the polysaccharide chains. The hyaluronic acid forms a continuous molecular network with definite chain interspacing.

Intraocular pressure

Inasmuch as the eye is a hollow sphere, its interior pressure must exceed that of the surrounding atmosphere to prevent collapse. Two factors are mainly concerned with the maintenance of intraocular pressure: (1) the rate of secretion of the aqueous humor, which is approximately 1.0 to 2.0 μl/min.$^{-1}$, and (2) the ease with which the aqueous humor passes through the trabecular meshwork to the canal of Schlemm and into the veins that collect fluid from the canal. The ease with which the fluid exits is usually indicated as the facility of outflow and in normal eyes is about 0.28 μl/min.$^{-1}$/mm. Hg pressure within the eye.

A number of additional factors contribute to the intraocular pressure. Variations are usually quickly compensated, so that the intraocular pressure is affected but momentarily. The pressure in the episcleral veins connecting to Schlemm's canal is somewhat less than 10 mm. Hg. If this pressure is markedly increased, there is a reflux of blood into Schlemm's canal and increased resistance to outflow. The intraocular arterial and venous pressure and the volume of the arteries usually remain quite constant. Markedly increased

venous pressure, as occurs in the Valsalva maneuver, is accompanied by a marked increase in intraocular pressure because of intraocular venous dilation. The intraocular pressure rapidly returns to normal, presumably because of increased arteriolar resistance that decreases the volume of arteries and permits the veins to empty. Marked variation in the osmotic pressure of the blood affects intraocular pressure and is used in the treatment and diagnosis of glaucoma. Increased osmotic pressure brought about by rapid intravenous administration of mannitol or urea decreases the intraocular pressure. Decreased osmotic pressure induced by intravenous saline solution or drinking a large quantity of water with the stomach empty causes a modest increase in intraocular pressure. The elasticity of the cornea and the sclera remains relatively constant but is an important factor in the measurement of the intraocular pressure by tonometry.

The normal intraocular pressure fluctuates 2 to 5 mm. Hg daily. In glaucoma this fluctuation may exceed 10 mm. Hg. There is a 1 to 2 mm. Hg variation in intraocular pressure with each heartbeat, but this may be observed only with special recording equipment.

The intraocular pressure is measured exactly only by means of a sensitive transducer connected to the interior of the eye in a manner that avoids disturbance of the flow of aqueous humor and the vasculature. This is done mainly in experimental animals and in man only before enucleation of the eye for disease. Clinically the intraocular pressure is measured by means of a tonometer that determines the resistance of the surface of the globe to a change in shape. There are two main types of tonometers: (1) the indentation type and (2) the applanation type. The applanation type is more accurate, but it requires a biomicroscope and greater clinical skill than the indentation type.

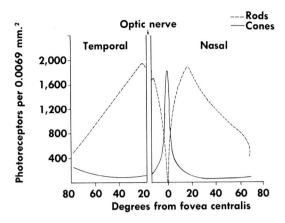

Fig. 2-5. Distribution of rods and cones in the human eye. (Redrawn from Østerberg, G.: Acta Ophthal. [Kobenhavn] supp. **6:**1, 1935.)

Retina

As has been noted (p. 61), the optic cup consists of two layers: (1) the outer layer, which forms the pigment epithelium of the retina and is one cell layer thick, and (2) the inner layer, which gives rise to the complicated sensory layer consisting of the photoreceptor cells, the rods and cones, their nervous connections, the bipolar and ganglion cells, and the supporting glia. The rods serve vision at low levels of illumination (scotopic vision), whereas the cones are effective at high levels of illumination (photopic vision) and in color vision. The cones are concentrated in the fovea centralis where rods are absent but are also scattered in the peripheral retina. The rods are the main photoreceptor of the periphery (Fig. 2-5).

Man's retina contains about 120 million rods and 5 million cones. The optic nerve contains approximately 1 million fibers. However, the distribution of optic nerve fibers to receptors is not uniform. In the center of the fovea the approximately 200,000 cones are connected to at least that many optic nerve fibers. In the far periphery, however, there may be as many as 10,000 rods connected in clusters to a single nerve fiber with considerable overlapping, so that a point of light may stimulate several clusters at once. The resultant perception of a point of light may not constitute the firing of an elementary neural unit—rather it may be an abstraction derived from the particular pattern of impulses transmitted by several nerve fibers, similar to a pinprick on the skin or a pure tone sound in the ear. It is likely that many optic nerve fibers are shared by both rods and cones. However, inasmuch as the sensation arising from cone stimulation is quite different from that arising from rod stimulation, it is likely that different combinations of optic nerve fibers are involved.

The outer segment (nearest the choroid) of each rod and cone is composed of about 700 protein-lipid disks containing light-sensitive pigments. The inner segment contains a dense concentration of mitochondria. The axons of the rods and cones synapse with dendrites of bipolar cells to form a portion of the outer plexiform layer. The axons of the bipolar cells synapse with dendrites of the ganglion cells in the inner plexiform layer. The axons of the ganglion cells join to form the optic nerve and extend to the brain.

The cell bodies and neurons of the retina are closely invested with astroglia and the glia of Müller's cells. These form an elaborate plexus so that the retina has no true extracellular space.

Metabolism of the retina is intimately related to its special function and may be divided into two parts: (1) general metabolism required for the maintenance of cell integrity and (2) specialized reactions related to photoreception and nerve impulse transmission.

General metabolism. Retinal function is dependent upon a continuous supply of glucose from the bloodstream. In man the blood supply from the choriocapillaris nurtures the outer one half of the retina and branches of the central retinal artery, the inner one half. Both systems must be intact for normal function. The retinal glia contains glycogen that is easily available to the neuron. However, in experimental animals, interruption of the blood supply for as short a period as 6 minutes causes irreversible retinal degeneration.

It is believed that glucose diffuses from the choriocapillaris of the choroid, is then converted into glucose 6-phosphate, possibly by the pigment epithelium, and finally diffuses down the neuron. The enzymes of the phosphogluconate pathway are concentrated in the rod and cone nuclei and may be involved in some specific activity of these receptor cells. Possibly this pathway supplies the reduced TPN required in some specific reaction of photoreception by the outer segments of the rods and cones.

The enzymes of the glycolytic pathway are mainly concentrated in the inner layers of the retina. Those of the tricarboxylic acid cycle are localized in the inner segments of rods and cones where mitochondria are concentrated. This pathway is not active enough to utilize all the lactic acid produced, which must either diffuse to the pigment epithelium and then the choriocapillaris or be metabolized by Müller's cells.

Müller's cells contain the enzymes required for glycogen synthesis and degradation. Additionally, these cells contain the enzymes required for the tricarboxylic acid cycle.

Attention has been focused on glutamic acid and glutamine in the retina because these constitute a connecting link between carbohydrate and protein metabolism. The administration of glutamic acid to newborn mice and rats interferes with the development of the inner nuclear layer containing the cell bodies of bipolar cells, association cells, and Müller's fibers, and as a result the animals are sightless. These compounds are also involved in maintenance of a high intracellular potassium concentration against a gradient. Carbonic anhydrase also participates in this reaction.

Photochemistry of vision. Electromagnetic energy (and all other energy) must first be absorbed to exert an effect. To initiate a chemical change, that portion of the electromagnetic spectrum known as light must first be absorbed by the pigment molecules of the disks in the outer segments of the rods and cones. This causes a chemical change, which then gives rise to a nervous impulse that is amplified in the retina and is propagated to the brain where perception occurs. In common with other types of nervous stimulation the sensitive material must be continuously restored so that continued stimulation is possible. Similarly, the sensitive material must be rapidly removed so that stimulation ceases after removal of the stimulus.

The human eye contains at least four photosensitive pigments. Rhodopsin, the pigment of rods, has been best characterized. Its maximum absorption spectrum is about 500 nm. The cones contain three different photosensitive pigments that have maximum absorption at about 445 (blue-sensitive), 535 (green-sensitive), and 570 nm. (red-sensitive) (Fig. 2-6). Rhodopsin and presumably the cone pigments are composed of two parts: (1) a colorless protein called opsin and (2) a pigment carrying a prosthetic group or chromo-

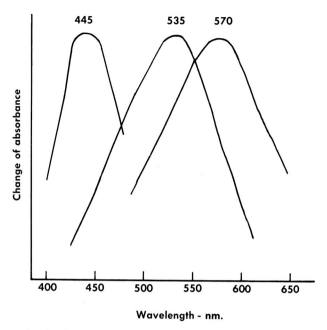

Fig. 2-6. Absorption by blue-, green-, and red-type cones. (Redrawn from Marks, W. B., Dobelle, W. H., and MacNichol, E. F.: Science **143:**1181, 1964.)

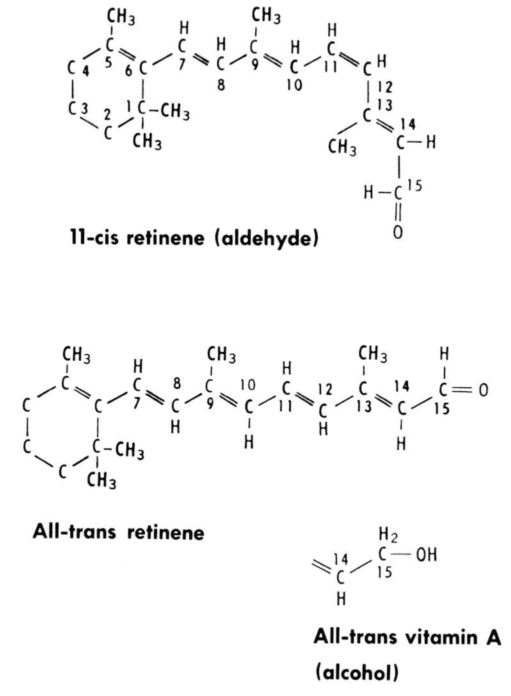

11-cis retinene (aldehyde)

All-trans retinene

All-trans vitamin A

(alcohol)

Fig. 2-7. The 11-cis isomer of retinene and the all-trans isomer.

phore called retinene. Each of the opsins differs, whereas the retinene is the same in human rhodopsin and in the green-sensitive and red-sensitive pigments of cones. Retinene has not yet been demonstrated in the blue-sensitive pigment.

Retinene, the aldehyde of vitamin A, which is an alcohol, occurs in five different molecular shapes called cis-trans isomers of each other. Only the 11-cis isomer conjugates with opsin to form the pigment of rods and cones. Steric hindrance prevents conjugation of any other cis or trans isomer. When the pigment absorbs light, retinene undergoes a change in molecular shape and becomes all-trans (Fig. 2-7). For additional photosensitive pigment to be synthesized, the all-trans retinene must first be isomerized to the 11-cis configuration. The isomerized molecule then couples with opsin to form a retinal pigment. The 11-cis retinene is derived from two sources: (1) all-trans retinene that is isomerized by simple exposure to light or by a specific

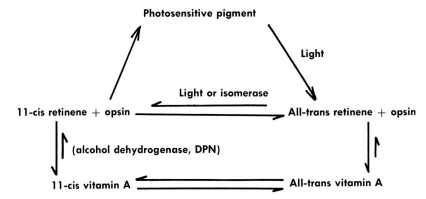

Fig. 2-8. Visual cycle.

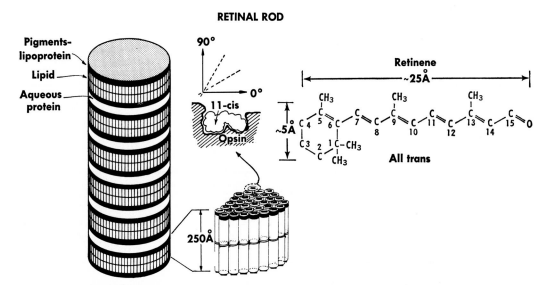

Fig. 2-9. Protein lipid disks of the photoreceptor outer segment, which number about 600, are shown to the left. Each disk contains 1 molecule of photosensitive pigment. The inset shows the photosensitive pigment of opsin coupled with 11-cis retinene. When stimulated by light, the 11-cis retinene becomes all-trans and is uncoupled from the opsin. (From Wolken, J. J.: J. Opt. Soc. Amer. 53:1, 1963.)

enzyme, retinene isomerase, and (2) 11-cis vitamin A (alcohol) that is oxidized to 11-cis retinene (aldehyde) in a reaction requiring alcohol dehydrogenase and DPN (cozymase). Vitamin A is derived from the circulating blood or is stored in the choroid or retinal pigment epithelium (Fig. 2-8).

It is postulated that the absorption of

1 photon of electromagnetic energy by 1 molecule of retinal pigment causes a steric change in retinene from 11-cis to all-trans. This in turn causes an unstable isomeric configuration so that retinene and opsin are uncoupled. The uncoupling of opsin and retinene exposes two sulfhydryl groups and one hydrogen ion–binding group on the opsin molecule (Fig. 2-9). This chemi-

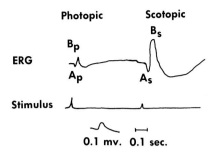

Photopic   Scotopic

ERG

Stimulus

0.1 mv.   0.1 sec.

Fig. 2-10. Components of normal ERG with high-intensity stimuli. A_p, Photopic a-wave; A_s, scotopic a-wave; B_p, photopic b-wave; B_s, scotopic b-wave. (Redrawn from Krill, A. E.: In Hughes, W. F., editor: Year book of ophthalmology, Chicago, 1960, Year Book Medical Publishers, Inc.)

cal change triggers and electrical charge, but the nature of the events is entirely speculative.

Electroretinography. When the retina is stimulated with light, an action potential is produced known as the electroretinogram (ERG). The record is obtained by placing an active electrode on the cornea, usually one embedded in a corneal contact lens, with saline solution bridging the gap between the electrode and the cornea, and an indifferent electrode upon the forehead. The small voltage is amplified and usually photographed from the face of an oscilloscope. The retina is stimulated with light when either dark adapted or light adapted. After the stimulus there is a latent period and then an initial negative deflection known as the a-wave, followed by a positive deflection designated as the b-wave (Fig. 2-10). The a-waves are thought to originate at the distal ends of the rod and cone layer and the b-waves somewhere between the distal end of the inner sector of photoreceptor cells and the beginning of the bipolar cell layer.

The positive deflection usually exceeds the largest amplitude of the negative wave by a factor of at least 1.5. The duration of the entire response is usually less than 250 milliseconds. The value for the positive waves is generally between 75 and 200 microvolts for photopic b-waves and between 250 and 450 microvolts for scotopic b-waves. The ERG is a mass response of the entire external layer of the retina. The record varies with the state of adaptation of the retina, the color of the light used in adaptation, and the intensity and color of the light used for stimulation.

Pathologic responses are described as supernormal, subnormal, negative, or extinguished. When a large area of the retina is damaged or diseased, the ERG is subnormal. When the entire retina is involved, an extinguished ERG is recorded.

Visual mechanisms

Electromagnetic spectrum. Electromagnetic radiation consists of energy having rhythmic oscillation and a velocity of 186,-000 miles a second (3×10^{10} cm./sec.) in a vacuum. The wavelength (distance from crest to crest) of electromagnetic radiation varies from thousands of meters for radio and electric waves to a minute fraction of a micron for cosmic rays. Electromagnetic waves may be reflected, absorbed, or transmitted. Only the energy that is absorbed causes a reaction. Most wavelengths pass through the body without eliciting physiologic change or awareness. Thus the atmosphere is filled with radio waves from all of the stations in the world, but they are not absorbed and do not cause sensation. However, that portion of the electromagnetic spectrum with a wavelength between 400 and 700 nm. passes through the cornea and the lens, is absorbed by the photosensitive pigment in the rods and cones, and initiates the chemical change triggering the visual impulse. This small segment of the electromagnetic spectrum differs from the remainder solely in being absorbed by the photosensitive pigment in the outer segments of rods and cones. Energy with wavelengths of greater or lesser frequency are either absorbed by the cornea and the lens or are entirely transmitted by the eye. They give rise to no photochemical reaction in the retina and hence to no subjective sensation. (When transmitted through the dark-adapted eye, however, x-rays cause a sensation of greenish light, a property that has been used in measurements of the length of the eye.)

Concepts of optics such as reflection, diffraction, polarization, and interference are most easily explained if one regards the electromagnetic spectrum as a series of waves having velocity, wavelength, and frequency. The absorption and scattering by matter are explained if one regards electromagnetic radiation as being composed of small bundles of energy—quanta or photons. The energy of these quanta varies inversely with the wavelengths of the radiation and thus increases as the wavelength becomes shorter. (Cosmic waves have more energy per quantum than radio waves.) The energy of a quantum is found by the formula $E = h\dfrac{c}{\lambda}$ where:

E = Energy
h = Planck's constant $(6.6253 \times 10^{-27}$ ergs/sec.$)$
c = Velocity in cm./sec. $(3 \times 10^{10}$ cm./sec.$)$
λ = Wavelength in centimeters

Action of light upon the eye. When that portion of the electromagnetic spectrum known as visible light (400 to 700 nm.) is absorbed by the visual pigment in the rods and cones, a nervous impulse arises that is transmitted to the brain and causes a subjective sensation.

It has been found experimentally that equal amounts of radiant energy of different wavelengths do not produce visual sensations of equal brightness. Thus 1/1,000 watt of green light appears bright to an observer, whereas 1/1,000 watt of blue light appears dim. Luminous units express the amount of radiant light energy in terms of the production of the sensation of brightness in the observer. Luminous energy is thus radiant energy corrected for the sensitivity of the retina to different wavelengths. Since individuals show slight differences in this sensitivity, luminous units are expressed in terms of the average of many observers (the standard observer). Photopic or cone luminosity function is the sensitivity of a light-adapted human eye and has a maximum sensitivity at 555 nm. The scotopic luminosity function is the sensitivity of the dark-adapted human eye and has a maximum sensitivity at 507 nm. (rhodopsin). When viewed in dim illumination, a colored object appears to have no color. As illumination is increased, the object appears colored. This change from achromatic to chromatic vision reflects the change from scotopic (rod) vision to photopic (cone) vision. This is called the Purkinje shift and reflects a change in the luminosity function of the eye.

Dark adaptation. When a subject is placed in a dark room, the sensitivity of the visual mechanism increases. The luminous energy required to see a light decreases about 100-fold, at first rapidly and then leveling at 5 to 9 minutes. This portion of dark adaptation is attributed to regeneration of the photosensitive pigment in the cones.* The luminous energy required to detect a light decreases some 1,000- to 10,000-fold between 10 and 15 minutes and finally levels at 30 to 45 minutes. This increased dark adaptation is attributed to regeneration of rhodopsin in the rods. The rapidity of full dark adaptation depends upon the amount of light to which the eye was exposed prior to being placed in the dark. Long exposure to bright lights delays dark adaptation (thus the increased danger of driving at night after a day in bright sunshine).

When fully dark adapted, the retina is about 10,000 times more sensitive to light

---

*This is an oversimplification inasmuch as there is both photochemical and neural adaptation.

than when light adapted. Additionally, the dilation of the pupil in decreased light makes the total increase in sensitivity about 100,000 times greater than in the light-adapted eye. (Notice that there has to be some light to stimulate the retina.) This sensitivity is related to detection of light and not to detection of form.

The dark-adapted retina is not uniformly sensitive to light. The most sensitive region is 15° to 20° from the fovea, where the rods are most dense. In the fully dark-adapted eye a visual sensation can be evoked by the activity of only seven rods, each being stimulated by the absorption of a single quantum. Since a retinal rod (or cone) is capable of being stimulated by the absorption of a single quantum, the variation in sensitivity in different parts of the retina probably re-reflects differences in receptor density and the neural summation mechanism rather than differences in receptor sensitivity per se.

Light adaptation. Exposure of the dark-adapted eye to bright light results in a marked decrease in sensitivity involving two changes: (1) a neural process that is completed in about 0.05 second and (2) a slower process, apparently involving the uncoupling of retinene and rhodopsin, occurring in about 1 minute. The neural mechanism occurs regardless of the area of the retina stimulated, whereas the photochemical mechanism involves only the region of stimulation. In the light-adapted eye the rhodopsin is bleached, the pupil is constricted, there is a shift of luminosity to the yellow-red end of the spectrum, and hydrogen ion concentration (pH) of the retina shifts from 7.3 to 7.0.

Color vision. The radiant energy of visible light is not colored; the sensation of color arises solely from absorption of the energy by photosensitive visual pigments in the retina. Thus the absorption of electromagnetic energy with a wavelength of 450 nm. initiates perception of blue, 540

nm. leads to green, 570 nm. to yellow, and 650 nm. to red.

There are two theories to explain the color vision mechanism. The trichromatic theory (Thomas Young, 1801) in its modern form postulates three classes of cone photoreceptors. Each class of receptors is sensitive to a range of wavelengths in the visible spectrum, and their maximal sensitivities are in different parts of the spectrum. It is customary, although inaccurate, to describe receptor classes with maximal sensitivity somewhere in the blue, green, and red regions of the spectrum as "blue," "green," and "red" receptors.

The main evidence for this theory for many years was based upon the matching of any hue by a mixture of three monochromatic lights such as a blue, a green, and a red. Recently two independent laboratories made microspectrophotometric measurements in intact individual primate cones. The absorption spectrum of a single cone was measured before and after bleaching of its photosensitive pigment, and three classes of cones were isolated having maximal absorptions at about 445, 535, and 570 nm. (Fig. 2-6).

Color perceptions are based upon the differential stimulation of these three types of photoreceptor. The sensation of white arises when all three types of photoreceptors are stimulated simultaneously, each to a specific degree, and yellow is produced by stimulation of the red and green types.

The opponent-process theory (Karl E. K. Hering, 1872) is based upon the quality of color sensation. Additive mixtures of certain pairs of colors do not produce an intermediate hue but give a sensation of gray (achromatic). Thus when red and blue-green or yellow and blue are mixed, a perception of gray occurs. Such pairs of colors are called complementary colors.

In its modern form the opponent-process theory postulates neural elements central to the retina that respond to stimu-

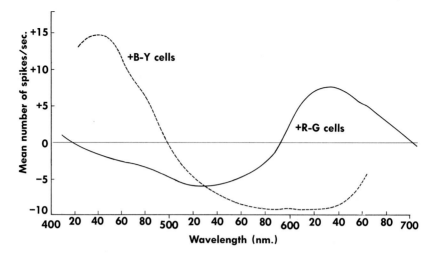

Fig. 2-11. Mean spectral response curves for an equal energy spectrum for +B-Y and +R-G cells. In addition, there are +Y-B and +G-R cells. The curves have been corrected for a spontaneous rate. (Redrawn from DeValois, R. L., Abramov, I., and Jacobs, G. H.: J. Opt. Soc. Amer. **56:**966, 1966.)

lation with different wavelengths with either an increase or decrease in their spontaneous base line activity. DeValois has recently demonstrated the existence of such cells in the lateral geniculate body of the macaque monkey, which either increase or decrease in firing rate when the retina is stimulated with light (Fig. 2-11). Four characteristic types of opponent-process cells are labeled according to the region of the spectrum in which they show peak activity. A cell that shows an increase in firing to stimulation by long wavelengths and a decrease in firing to wavelengths in the middle of the spectrum is thus designated as +R-G. A cell that increases activity to wavelengths in the middle of the spectrum and decreases activity at long wavelengths is called +G-R. The other two types of cells are +B-Y and +Y-B, designating the blue and yellow portions of the spectrum. Spectrally opponent cells have been reported in fish and the spider and squirrel monkey.

The currently accepted theory as to how we perceive color includes elements of both the trichromatic and opponent-process theories. The initial events at the cone photoreceptor level appear to be trichromatic. This information is then recoded into the opponent-process scheme for neural transmission.

Color blindness is believed to arise from a deficiency or abnormality in one or more of the three cone photosensitive pigments. A person with normal color vision is a trichromat and has all three cone pigments in a normal proportion. A dichromat has but two cone pigments.

An anomalous trichromat has abnormal color vision because of a deficiency or an abnormality but not a complete absence of one of the cone pigments. In protanomaly (*protos*, meaning first) there is a deficiency of the "first" color, the red-sensitive pigment. There is poor red-green discrimination and the red end of the spectrum appears dimmer than it does in normal individuals.

In deuteranomaly (*deuteros*, meaning second) there is a deficiency of the "second" color, the green-sensitive pigment. Again, red-green discrimination is poor, but the luminous efficiency is very close to normal.

In tritanomaly (*tritos,* meaning third) there is a deficiency in the "third" color, the blue-sensitive pigment. There is blue-green and blue-yellow insensitivity present.

A dichromat has but two cone pigments and is differentiated from the anomalous trichromat by tests involving color and brightness matching. Dichromats are classed as protanopes (absence of red-sensitive pigment), deuteranopes (absence of green-sensitive pigment), and tritanopes (absence of blue-sensitive pigment).

Probably both protanopes and deuteranopes see red and green as yellow. Some form of protan or deutan defect occurs in about 8% of American and European males. Less than 1% of females show either defect. The defect is inherited as a sex-linked abnormality. The tritan defect is extremely rare and appears to be inherited as an autosomal dominant.

Neural activity. Formation of a minute image upon the retinal rods and cones tempts one to consider the optic nerve as conveying a neat colored photo to the brain. However, each ganglion cell receives its input from a number of receptors, and there are many more rods and cones than there are ganglion cells or axons. Furthermore, if all retinal connections were excitatory, such an arrangement would lead to blurring of information. However, all connections do not excite. When light is flashed upon the retina, the rate of firing of a ganglion cell may decrease. The signal sent to the brain thus consists of a complex code of increased and decreased rates of firing.

Kuffler, in 1953, indicated that in the cat the same ganglion cell could be stimulated or inhibited, depending upon the part of the stimulated photoreceptor field to which it was connected. He found two types of photoreceptor fields: (1) a cen-ter, causing ganglion cell stimulation, surrounded by a periphery, causing ganglion cell inhibition (an "on"-center field), and (2) the reverse type in which the center caused ganglion cell inhibition and the periphery caused stimulation (an "off"-center field). When both the center and the periphery of such fields were stimulated, their effects tended to cancel each other. The size of the center of these receptor fields varied widely, although the total field seemed relatively constant.

Other studies in the frog have indicated an integrative function of the retina highly adapted to its biologic needs. Some optic nerve fibers seem to signal small, dark, moving objects ("bug detectors") but not large or stationary objects. On-off fibers, responding to the general level of illumination, may be present but do not affect other functions.

The nature of the integrative neural activity of man's retina is not known. With such known complexity in lower species, it seems likely that the retina carries out a highly complex process of filtering information before sending it to the brain. It is also evident that not all of the information received by the eye is perceived, as witnessed by one's unawareness of his surroundings unless particular attention is directed to it either by thinking or by an abrupt change in the surroundings.

The perceptual processes of vision are not understood. It is known that the lateral geniculate body contains cells that receive impulses from many optic nerve fibers and others that are related to only one fiber. The theory is advanced that both inhibitory and excitatory cells are present and that not every impulse reaching a cell in the geniculate body is relayed. However, it is believed that, in general, there is little reorganization of incoming messages.

Likewise, the exact function of the visual cortex is unknown. It is questioned whether messages are modified there or are passed to still higher centers for further elaboration. Areas of "on" and "off" centers like the retina are not separated by circles but by straight lines. Thus a field may be a long, narrow excitatory area with inhibitory areas on either side. This implies that stimuli shaped like a rectangle with light on one side and dark on the other ("edges") are likely to be the most potent for cortical cells. A moving stimulus also evokes a potent response in cortical cells. In lower mammals the visual cortex is essential for form perception but not for simple light-dark discrimination.

Image-forming mechanisms

Refraction. When a ray of light passes from one transparent medium to another, its velocity is either decreased in a more dense medium or increased in a less dense medium. If the medium is bounded by surfaces that are not perpendicular to the ray of light, then, in addition to the change in velocity, the emerging ray has a different direction than the entering ray. This change in direction of light is called refraction. It is proportionate to the sine of the angle formed by the light ray and the surface of the refracting medium and the velocity of light in this medium. (The index of refraction is the ratio of the velocity of light in a vacuum to the velocity of light in the medium.) Usually, rather than stating this angle and the index of refraction, the refractive power of a lens is stated as the distance from the surface that the rays come to a focus (the focal length) or as the reciprocal of this distance in meters (diopters). Thus, if the focal length of a lens is 20 cm., its dioptric power is 5 (1.0 m. divided by 0.2 m.).

Refractive surfaces. A ray of light entering the eye is refracted by the cornea and then, after passing through the aqueous humor, by the lens. The anterior surface of the cornea is the chief refractive surface of the eye by virtue of separating media of such different optical density as air and corneal substance. The total refractive power is approximately 43 diopters. The anterior and posterior surfaces of the lens are convex, but inasmuch as it is immersed on either side in fluid, it has less refractive power than the cornea. Optically the lens behaves as though it were composed of a series of concentric lenses, so that its total index of refraction is greater than any individual portion of the lens. With accommodation, in a youthful eye the refractive power of the lens increases from about 19 to 33 diopters.

Refractive error. A refractive error is determined by two factors: (1) the refractive power of the cornea and the lens and (2) the length of the eye. Usually there is a remarkable correlation between the refractive power and the length of the eyeball. Most individuals have a refractive power nearly exactly appropriate to cause parallel rays of light to fall upon the retina. The normal eye varies in length from about 22 to 27 mm., and the total refractive power of the normal eye at rest thus varies from about 52 to 63 diopters. Failure of the refractive power of the anterior segment to be correlated with the length of the eye results in an error of refraction.

Accommodation. Accommodation is the process by which the refractive power of the anterior segment increases so that both distant and near objects may be distinctly imaged upon the retina. Accommodation arises from an increase in thickness and curvature of the lens in response to contraction of the ciliary muscle.

The stimulus to accommodation is a blurred image upon the retina that causes active contraction of the ciliary muscle. The contraction of the ciliary muscle causes *relaxation* of the zonule. When the ciliary muscle is at rest, tension of the zonule causes compression of the lens. With relaxation of the zonule, the lens is freed from the compressing force and, by virtue of the elasticity of its capsule, it tends to assume the shape of a sphere. The anterior suface of the lens, particularly its central portion, becomes markedly more curved. Additionally, the anterior pole of the lens moves forward so that the lens increases in thickness in its center (Fig. 2-12).

With aging, the lens nucleus becomes harder and less compressible and the lens capsule less elastic, so that progressively less change in shape of the lens occurs with zonular relaxation. This results in gradual loss of accommodation. It is a process that begins shortly after birth and continues thereafter until about the age of 50 years, when only about 1 diopter of accommodation remains. The process is mainly the result of lens changes, but increased weakness of the ciliary body musculature with age may also be of some importance.

Extraocular muscular mechanisms

Each eye is moved by six extraocular muscles. Normally their action is so sensitively adjusted that each eye is directed to the same object in space.

The medial rectus muscle (N III) has the single function of adduction, or turning the eye medially. The lateral rectus muscle (N VI) has the single function of abduction, or turning the eye temporally. The four vertical muscles steady the eye in abduction or adduction, elevate or depress the eye, or rotate it around an anteroposterior plane (extorsion or intorsion) (Table 2-1).

When the eye is directed straight ahead, it is said to be in the primary position. If it is directed upward, downward, laterally, or medially, it is said to be in a secondary position. If it is directed in an oblique position (up and in or down and in), it is said to be in a tertiary position.

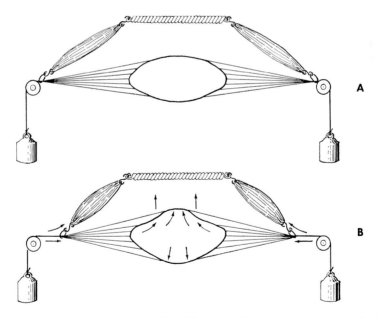

Fig. 2-12. Accommodation. **A,** When the ciliary muscle is at rest, the zonule is contracted, and the power of refraction of the lens is minimal. **B,** When the ciliary muscle contracts, the zonule is relaxed, and the inherent elasticity of the lens causes it to increase in thickness and power of refraction. (Redrawn from Krieg, W. J. S.: Functional neuroanatomy, New York, 1953, The Blakiston Co.)

Table 2-1. Actions of ocular muscles

Muscle	Action
Medial rectus	Adduction only
Lateral rectus	Abduction only
Superior oblique:	
If eye is adducted	Depression
If eye is abducted	Aids abduction
Inferior oblique:	
If eye is adducted	Elevation
If eye is abducted	Aids abduction
Superior rectus:	
If eye is abducted	Elevation
If eye is adducted	Aids adduction
Inferior rectus	
If eye is abducted	Depression
If eye is adducted	Aids adduction
Muscles originating superiorly: Superior oblique and superior rectus	Intorsion
Muscles originating inferiorly: Inferior oblique and inferior rectus	Extorsion

The movement of one eye from one position to another is called duction.

The movement of two eyes from the primary position to a secondary position is called version: (1) eyes right, dextroversion; (2) eyes left, levoversion; (3) eyes up, sursumversion; and (4) eyes down, deorsumversion. In tertiary positions, one usually states the position as up and right, up and left, and so on.

The muscles of one eye that work together to perform duction are called synergists in that function. In adduction the medial rectus muscle is aided by the superior and inferior rectus muscles, whereas in abduction the lateral rectus muscle is synergistic with the superior and inferior oblique muscles. In elevation the superior rectus and the inferior oblique muscles are synergistic, and in depression the inferior rectus and the superior oblique muscles are synergistic (Table 2-1).

Each extraocular muscle is opposed by an antagonist that has the opposite action in a particular position. Thus the antagonist of the medial rectus muscle is the lateral rectus muscle, and when the eye is elevated by the superior rectus muscle, its antagonist is the inferior rectus muscle.

The muscles of the two eyes primarily responsible for directing the eyes in version movements are yoke muscles. Thus in moving the eyes to the right the right lateral rectus muscle is yoked to the left medial rectus muscle. Each superior rectus muscle is yoked with the contralateral inferior oblique muscle, and each inferior rectus muscle is yoked with the contralateral superior oblique muscle.

Version. Version is the term applied to simultaneous movements of the eyes to the right or the left, up or down, and the like. In version an equal innervational impulse flows from the cerebral oculogyric centers to each muscle involved in rotating each eye (Hering's law). This equal innervation is important in the diagnosis of a paretic muscle. Thus, if the paretic muscle is on the right side and the right eye is used for fixing (as might be accomplished by covering the left eye), the nerve impulse required to hold the right eye in position is greater than it would be if the muscles were normal. Inasmuch as the impulse is directed equally to the left eye, then the left yoke muscle of the paretic right muscle will receive an excessive innervational impulse. The deviation of the left eye will thus be greater when the paretic right eye is used for fixation. If the nonparetic left eye fixes, a normal innervational impulse is relayed, and the deviation of the paretic right eye is minimal.

Vergence. Vergence is the term applied to simultaneous ocular movements in which the eyes are directed to an object in the midbody plane, that is, somewhere in front of the nose. The term is applied to convergence, in which the eyes rotate inward toward each other, or to divergence, in which they rotate outward simultaneously. Vertical (sursumvergence) and torsional vergences are uncommon.

The locations of convergence and divergence centers are not known, although many assume them to be present, inasmuch as convergence and divergence paresis is observed clinically. The nucleus of Perlia has long been considered the center for convergence. Convergence palsy occurs in midbrain disease, and the convergence center is assumed to be located in this region. Divergence paresis may occur following head injury associated with perceptual deafness, and the center is considered to be located in the midbrain near the acoustic nerve nucleus.

Duction. Duction is the term applied to the movements of one eye only.

Ocular movements. The two basic types of eye movements are saccadic and vergence. *Saccadic movements* are involved in version or duction, and they may reach an angular velocity of 500° of arc/ sec. They are also called following reflexes and are involved in movements of an eye when the fovea follows a moving target. They also constitute the fast phase of opticokinetic and vestibular nystagmus. Saccadic movements are typically found during reading. *Vergence movements* are designed to maintain the fovea of each eye fixed upon an object of attention located approximately directly in front of the eyes. Their average velocity is about 8° to 20° of arc/sec. On the basis of the difference in velocity in saccadic and vergence movements, it has been suggested that saccadic movements involve large muscle fibers innervated by coarse myelinated nerves and that vergence movements involve small specific muscle fibers innervated by thin, nonmedullated autonomic nerve fibers. Saccadic and vergence movements play a part in a variety of movements related basically to (1) maintaining the eyes in a forward position despite movements of the head and body and (2) bringing an image from the peripheral retina to the fovea or maintaining it on the fovea of either one or both eyes.

The eyes maintain a horizontal position, despite movements of the head, by means of postural reflexes originating in the neck muscles and in each labyrinth. Thus, when the chin is depressed on the chest, an innervational impulse stimulates the elevators of the two eyes, inhibits the depressors, and the eyes remain directed ahead. Elevation of the chin causes the opposite reaction, the depressors stimulated and the elevators inhibited. If the head is tilted to either shoulder, torsion occurs so that the 12 o'clock meridian rotates and the vertical meridian of the cornea remains vertical, providing the tilting of the head is less than 20°.

If the fovea is fixed on a *steady target,* three types of movement occur: (1) those with a frequency of 30 to 70/sec. and an amplitude of 20 seconds; (2) those with irregular frequency of about 1 every second and an amplitude of 3 minutes (saccade or flick movements); and (3) irregular drifts of about 6 minutes. The fine high-frequency movements permit new retinal receptors to be stimulated during the latent period so that the image does not disappear. The saccadic or flick movements tend to correct either drift or previous saccade.

If the fovea is fixed on a *moving target* with an angular velocity of less than 30°/ sec., the eye follows the target almost exactly (pursuit or tracking movement). With greater velocity, an irregular type of saccadic movements results, with overcorrection and correction involving a feedback mechanism from the visual system and, more importantly, a parametric feedback arising from muscle receptors.

Fusional movements are vergence movements directed toward the maintenance of a single perception by maintenance of the retinal image on receptors having the same visual direction.

The *near reflex* is related to vergence movements involving the visual response to the awareness of the nearness of an object. It may occur without visual response when an individual converges for the distance he believes the object to be, basing his judgment on sound or touch.

Electrical phenomena. There is continuous electrical activity in the extraocular mucles during a waking state. Moving the eye into the major field of action of a muscle causes a marked increase in the number and frequency of electrical discharges of the muscle involved. Accompanying this is a reduction in activity of the antagonistic muscle. The ocular muscles demonstrate *Sherrington's principle* of reciprocal innervation. Thus, if the superior rectus muscle elevates the eye, the inferior rectus muscle is inhibited.

The ocular muscles do not exhibit the electrical phenomena of fatigue. Sleep, however, reduces the electrical activity of the extraocular muscles to zero. It should be noted that during dreaming there are bursts of electrical activity and ocular movements. During sleep the eyes are usually directed upward and outward in *Bell's phenomenon*. During general anesthesia, anatomic-mechanical factors position the eyes in the anatomic position of rest in which there is no muscle tone, so that the eyes are somewhat divergent.

Iris and pupil

The iris is a delicate diaphragm originating from the anterior extremity of the optic vesicle and the adjacent mesoderm. The iris surrounds a central aperture, the pupil, and contains the sphincter pupillae muscle (N III) and the dilatator pupillae muscle (sympathetics), which are smooth muscles arising from the ectoderm of the primitive optic vesicle.

The pupil functions to regulate the amount of light entering the eye, increases the depth of focus of the eye, and minimizes spherical and chromatic aberrations of the eye and the astigmatism caused by oblique pencils of light.

Pupillary reflexes. When the amount of light falling upon the eye is increased, the pupil constricts. This is called the *direct light reflex*. The latent period is 0.18 second, and maximum contraction occurs about 1 second after the beginning of the stimulus. There is considerable variability in the state of the pupil thereafter unless the stimulus is maintained. The pupil may dilate again and then constrict, or it may remain constricted.

Light falling upon one eye and causing pupillary constriction also causes the pupil of the fellow eye to constrict—the *indirect* or *consensual light reflex*.

The pupillary reflex to light is a true reflex. The receptors for the pupillary response are the rods and cones of the retina. The afferent fibers responsible for conducting pupillary impulses from the retina to the brain do not synapse in the lateral geniculate body but pass through its medial border by way of the brachium of the superior colliculus into the pretectal nucleus, which is located at the junction of the diencephalon and the tectum of the midbrain. Fibers synapse here and pass to the Edinger-Westphal nucleus on both the same and opposite sides. From the Edinger-Westphal nucleus, pupillary constrictor fibers pass with the inferior division of the oculomotor nerve to the ciliary ganglion. Here they synapse with the postganglionic fibers, which pass by the short posterior ciliary nerves to the sphincter muscle (Fig. 2-13).

Accommodative reflex. When an individual directs his eyes to, and focuses upon, a nearby object, there is pupillary constriction. This miosis involves two mechanisms that ordinarily work together but may be disassociated experimentally. With convergence at near, the reaction is likely one of synkinesis, or an associated movement involving the common innervation of the medial rectus muscles and

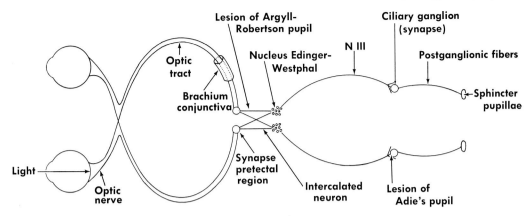

Fig. 2-13. Pathway of reflex for pupillary constriction when retina is stimulated with light.

the sphincter pupillae muscle by the same branch of the oculomotor nerve.

The accommodation reflex is activated in the retina, and the afferent fibers extend to the calcarine cortex and then to areas 19 and 22. The efferent paths travel down the corticotectal tract to the Edinger-Westphal nucleus and thence to the sphincter pupillae muscle.

Lid closure reaction (orbicularis muscle reflex). The lid closure reaction does not occur consistently. When effort is made to close the eyes by contraction of the orbicularis muscle (N VII), there may be constriction of the pupil on the side of closure. This reaction indicates the close association between the third and the seventh cranial nerves.

Trigeminal reflex. Continued stimulation of the trigeminal nerve from irritation of the cornea, conjunctiva, or skin of the face results in constriction of the pupil. Reflex dilatation of the blood vessels of the iris also causes pupillary constriction.

Chapter 3

Pharmacology

A wide variety of drug actions may be observed within the eye. The intraocular musculature provides an excellent area to observe the effects of cholinergic or adrenergic stimulation or blockade. The hypersensitivity of denervation can be observed easily in the pupillary response to drugs. A large variety of anti-inflammatory and anti-infective agents has been developed for ophthalmic use, and unusually high tissue concentrations may follow local instillation. Toxic reactions are commonly observed. These range in seriousness from dermatitis medicamentosa of the eyelids to glaucoma induced by local instillation of corticosteroids or mydriatics to permanent pigmentary changes of the fundi and visual disturbances induced by the phenothiazines.

Routes of drug administration
Systemic route

The intraocular concentration of drugs administered systemically varies considerably. The blood-aqueous barrier is comparable in many respects to the blood-brain barrier, and many compounds enter the eye only in extremely small concentration, if at all. Binding of drugs to plasma proteins may also limit their penetration into the eye. In activity comparable to that of the choroid plexus the ciliary epithelium may also actively remove certain compounds from the eye. When severe inflammation occurs, the blood-aqueous barrier breaks down, and compounds that do not normally enter the eye in high concentration become distributed as in other tissues.

Penicillin and the tetracyclines penetrate the noninflamed eye very poorly. Chloramphenicol enters the eye in high concentration following systemic administration. Iodides, bromides, and organic acids, which are found in low concentration in the ocular fluids, are actively transported out of the posterior chamber by the nonpigmented ciliary epithelium. The uveal pigment of the uvea and retinal pigment epithelium, like melanin-containing cells elsewhere, absorb and retain phenothiazine derivatives, so that there may be 50 times the mean tissue distribution for many days after administration.

Local route

Drugs may be applied to the eyelids or the anterior globe in solution, suspension, ointment, or as a fine powder to be dissolved in the tears. Drugs applied to the anterior segment of the globe penetrate the posterior segment in very low concentration unless there is systemic absorption. Occasionally drugs are injected into the anterior chamber, into the vitreous body, or into the subconjunctival or retrobulbar spaces. Such injections are usually reserved for intraocular infections in which the eye is threatened with destruction because the drugs themselves may cause violent inflammation. Placing a drug under a contact lens or applying saturated cotton pledgets to the conjunctiva ensures prolonged contact and enhances penetration. In iontophoresis, a method not widely used, the drug is placed beneath a contact lens, and an electrical charge is used to enhance intraocular penetration of ionized compounds through the cornea.

Corneal penetration. Compounds enter the anterior chamber mainly through the cornea. The epithelium is the chief barrier to intraocular penetration—if it is diseased or damaged, relatively high drug concentrations may be obtained in the anterior segment. Local anesthetics, wetting agents, massage, and abrasion damage the epithelium and enhance penetration.

The medication must have a greater affinity for the cornea than for the vehicle. If the medication has a greater affinity for the vehicle, it will not be released and will remain in the vehicle rather than be absorbed into the eye. Theoretically, compounds are administered in vehicles in which they have low solubilities.

The quantity of a drug penetrating the cornea is proportionate to the area of cornea in contact with the medication and the duration of contact. A maximal effect is obtained by having the individual look downward. Then the drug is instilled so that it flows over the entire cornea, bathing it in a pool of the medication that collects in the inferior fornix. Gentle closure of the eyelids to eliminate rapid blinking will prevent dilution of the drug by tears. Increased viscosity of the vehicle minimizes dilution and prolongs contact. Thus medications may be prescribed in oils, ointments, methyl cellulose, and other viscous vehicles.

Topical preparations. A number of factors relate to the effectiveness, safety, and comfort of topically applied eye medications: sterility, hydrogen ion concentration, tonicity, physiologic activity, stability, toxicity, surface tension, and compatibility. It is unusually difficult to prepare sterile eye medications, and in recent years nearly all commonly used medications are prepared commercially for interstate commerce.

Sterility. To prevent inactivation by heating, many compounds intended for ocular use are filtered through a Berkefeld-type filter. This ensures the initial sterility required in interstate commerce, but the solution is easily contaminated once the container is opened. The physician should regard a solution in an unsealed container as contaminated.

Epidemic keratoconjunctivitis, which is caused by APC virus type 8 (p. 175), may be transmitted by means of contaminated eye anesthetic solutions. Fluorescein solution is notoriously liable to contamination by *Pseudomonas aeruginosa*, and it may introduce the the organism when used in the diagnosis of corneal abrasions. To avoid infection, fluorescein should be instilled only from a sterile individual container or should be applied by means of a filter paper strip that has been saturated with fluorescein and then sterilized. It must never be used from a stock bottle.

Eyecups are usually contaminated and constitute a common method of recurrent infections in self-treatment. Ointments are often contaminated and should be prescribed sparingly. Eyedroppers are easily contaminated by touching the eyelids or the conjunctiva, and they may then contaminate a stock bottle. Eyedroppers or glass rods that are resterilized after each use may be used if more than one patient is treated with medication from the same container. Plastic "squeeze" bottles in which many commercially available medications are now distributed are far more difficult to contaminate than those with eyedroppers.

Autonomic drugs

The sphincter pupillae and ciliary muscles are mainly innervated by postganglionic parasympathetic efferent fibers of the oculomotor nerve (N III) that have synapsed in the ciliary ganglion. The dilata-

Drugs acting predominantly on cholinergic nervous system

I. Cholinergic stimulating drugs

    A. Direct-acting drugs

        1. Choline esters: acetylcholine; bethanechol (Urecholine); methacholine (Mecholyl); carbachol (carbamylcholine, Carcholin, Doryl)

        2. Pilocarpine

    B. Cholinesterase inhibiting drugs (anticholinesterases)

        1. Physostigmine (eserine)

        2. Neostigmine (Prostigmin)

            a. Edrophonium chloride (Tensilon)

            b. Demecarium bromide (Humorsol)

            c. Pyridostigmine (Mestinon)

            d. Benzpyrinium (Stigmonene)

            e. Ambenonium (Mytelase)

        3. Alkyl phosphates

            a. Echothiophate iodide (Phospholine I)

            b. Diisopropyl fluorophosphate (DFP)

            c. Tetraethylpyrophosphate (TEPP)

            d. Hexaethyltetraphosphate (HETP)

            e. Octamethylpyrophosphoramide (OMPA)

II. Cholinergic blocking drugs

    A. Atropine group (blocks muscarine actions of acetylcholine)

        1. Atropine (1-hyoscyamine)

        2. Scopolamine (1-hyoscine)

        3. Homatropine

        4. Eucatropine (Euphthalmine)

        5. Cyclopentolate (Cyclogyl)

        6. Tropicamide (Mydriacyl)

        7. Banthine

        8. Pamine

        9. Artane

    B. Ganglionic blocking drugs (block nicotine stimulating actions)

        1. Tetraethylammonium chloride

        2. Hexamethonium chloride

        3. Pentolinium tartrate (Ansolysen)

        4. Chlorisondamine chloride (Ecolid)

    C. Neuromuscular blocking drugs

        1. Complete with acetylcholine for motor end plate, preventing its depolarization

            a. *d*-Tubocurarine

            b. Dimethyl tubocurarine

        2. Depolarize end plate

            a. Decamethonium bromide (Syncurine)

            b. Succinylcholine chloride (Anectine)

        3. Central nervous system skeletal muscle depressants

            a. Mephenesin (Tolserol)

            b. Meprobamate (Miltown)

tor pupillae muscle is mainly innervated by postganglionic fibers of the sympathetic nervous system that have synapsed in the superior cervical ganglion.

The autonomic nervous system may be divided into parasympathetic cholinergic and sympathetic adrenergic systems. Drugs affecting these systems may be divided into cholinergic stimulating and cholinergic blocking agents and adrenergic stimulating and adrenergic blocking agents. Acetylcholine is the cholinergic effector substance, and norepinephrine is the main adrenergic effector substance. Acetylcholine is inactivated by the enzyme cholinesterase, whereas norepinephrine is largely inactivated by diffusion and uptake by tissue. Two enzymes, catechol-O-methyl transferase and monoamine oxidase, are involved in norepinephrine metabolism, but they have little or no role in inactivation after release.

The sphincter pupillae and ciliary muscles belong mainly to the cholinergic group, whereas the dilatator pupillae muscle belongs to the adrenergic group. Stimulation of the sphincter pupillae muscle causes constriction of the pupil (miosis). Stimulation of the ciliary muscle causes an increase in accommodation. When the cholinergic system is blocked, the pupil dilates (mydriasis) and the ciliary muscle relaxes, causing a decrease of accommodation (cycloplegia).

Adrenergic stimulation causes dilation of the pupil, whereas adrenergic blockade causes pupillary constriction. The ciliary muscle may have some sympathetic fibers that, when stimulated, cause decreased accommodation. Adrenergic effects frequently are obscured by the more prominent cholinergic effects.

Cholinergic stimulating drugs

The neurohumoral theory of nerve transmission postulates that acetylcholine is the effector substance responsible for (1) synaptic transmission at all autonomic ganglia (including the sympathetic ganglia and the adrenal medulla); (2) some synaptic transmission in the central nervous system; (3) activation of skeletal muscles innervated by spinal nerves; (4) activation of smooth and cardiac muscles innervated by postganglionic parasympathetic nerves; and (5) activation of sweat glands and arrectores pilorum muscles, which are innervated by postganglionic sympathetic nerves (Fig. 3-1).

Acetylcholine has two distinct types of action that have been named after drugs that exhibit mainly only one of these types of action as their principal effect. The "muscarinic" effect is the effect on autonomic effector sites; the "nicotinic" effect is the effect on autonomic ganglia and skeletal muscle.

Acetylcholine is synthesized by the neuron and stored at the site of activity in small synaptic vesicles. When released, it causes depolarization of the postsynaptic membrane and transmission of the nervous impulse. The released acetylcholine is quickly inactivated by the enzyme cholinesterase to permit repolarization of the membrane and transmission of the next impulse.

There are two types of cholinesterase: (1) specific acetylcholinesterase, which is present in nerve, muscle tissue, and erythrocytes, and (2) nonspecific cholinesterase or pseudocholinesterase, which is found in plasma and many tissues and is likely synthesized by the liver. Nonspecific cholinesterase inactivates long-chain choline esters as well as acetylcholine. Specific acetylcholinesterase inactivates acetylcholine only. It is the main cholinesterase of the iris.

Cholinergic drugs are compounds that mimic the action of acetylcholine on effector cells or at synapses. The action may be brought about directly by compounds related to acetylcholine or those such as pilocarpine that act directly upon smooth muscle. Indirect stimulation occurs when the activity of acetylcholine is prolonged

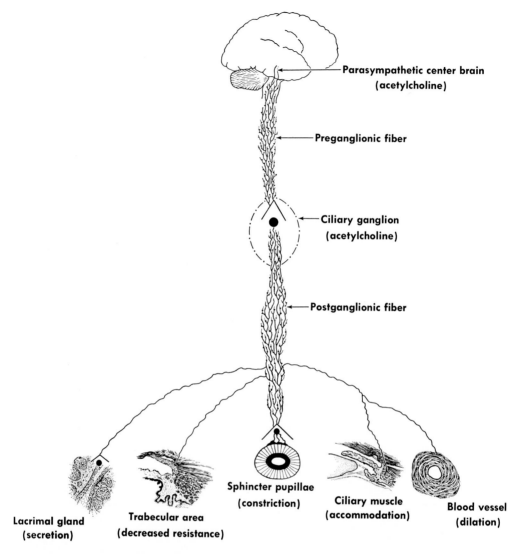

Parasympathetic center brain
(acetylcholine)

Preganglionic fiber

Ciliary ganglion
(acetylcholine)

Postganglionic fiber

Lacrimal gland
(secretion)

Trabecular area
(decreased resistance)

Sphincter pupillae
(constriction)

Ciliary muscle
(accommodation)

Blood vessel
(dilation)

Fig. 3-1. Effects of cholinergic nervous system stimulation. Acetylcholine, the active principle, is inactivated by cholinesterase.

by inactivating the cholinesterase that normally hydrolyzes it. Such compounds are called anticholinesterases and are commonly classified as reversible if their action is relatively short or irreversible if it is long.

Direct-acting cholinergic drugs. Most direct-acting cholinergic drugs are chemically related to acetylcholine and are so potent and have such marked effects when systemically administered that their therapeutic uses are limited. They cause vasodilation, decreased blood pressure and heart rate, stimulation of the salivary, lacrimal, sweat, and gastric secretions, and increased tone of the gastrointestinal, urinary, and bronchiolar musculature.

When instilled in the conjunctival sac, choline esters cause dilatation of the conjunctival and uveal arterioles, constriction of the pupil, and increased permeability of the blood-aqueous barrier. Most of the compounds penetrate the intact cornea poorly; therefore their application is mainly limited to the treatment of simple glaucoma.

The direct-acting cholinergic drugs used in ophthalmology include the following compounds.

Acetylcholine. Acetylcholine (1:5,000) may be injected into the anterior chamber to contrict the pupil following cataract extraction.

Methacholine (Mecholyl). Methacholine (Mecholyl) is instilled in the conjunctival sac in a 10 to 25% aqueous solution in the treatment of glaucoma. It is used in conjunction with an anticholinesterase compound. It is used in a 2.5% solution to demonstrate the supersensitivity (p. 105) of the pupil in Adie's syndrome (p. 221).

Carbachol (Carcholin, Doryl). Carbachol (Carcholin, Doryl), 0.75 to 1.5%, must be combined with a wetting agent so as to penetrate the cornea. It is not hydrolyzed by cholinesterases and is so potent that it is not used systemically. Frequently this drug is substituted for pilocarpine in patients who have developed a tolerance to pilocarpine.

Pilocarpine. Like acetylcholine, pilocarpine acts directly upon glandular and smooth muscle receptors, that is, structures innervated by postganglionic cholinergic nerves. It is effective even though the ciliary ganglion has been blocked. It causes pupillary constriction, stimulates the ciliary muscle so as to increase accommodation, and increases the permeability of the trabecular meshwork. In some patients it decreases aqueous secretion. Its chief value is in the treatment of glaucoma, where it is used topically in a 0.5 to 4.0% solution. It is stable, penetrates the cornea well, is well tolerated, and is rarely toxic. It is prescribed in the minimum concentration that will prevent progression of the glaucoma and is seldom instilled more frequently

than once every 4 hours. In open-angle glaucoma the increased permeability of the trabecular meshwork is its most useful function, while in angle-closure glaucoma the pupillary constriction is most important.

Anticholinesterase drugs. Anticholinesterase drugs permit the accumulation of acetylcholine by inactivating cholinesterase. There are three main types of anticholinesterase compounds: physostigmine (eserine), a tertiary amine with a urethane group; neostigmine (Prostigmin), a quaternary ammonium compound; and alkyl phosphates. The first two are classified as reversible cholinesterase inhibitors. Neostigmine has an additional direct blocking effect on acetylcholine receptors at skeletal muscle sites. The alkyl phosphates produce irreversible inactivation of cholinesterase.

Administration of anticholinesterase compounds causes widespread cholinergic stimulation. There is constriction of gastrointestinal, urinary, and bronchiole muscles. The skeletal muscle is weak and fibrillates. There is increased salivation, lacrimation, and sweating together with increased pulmonary secretions. Central nervous system symptoms range from giddiness to coma and convulsions.

The sphincter pupillae and ciliary muscles are contracted so that the pupil is miotic and accommodation is increased. The alkyl phosphates cause more marked dilation of the conjunctival and ciliary blood vessels with increased permeability of the blood-aqueous barrier than do physostigmine or neostigmine.

The anticholinesterases of ophthalmic interest are discussed in the following paragraphs.

Physostigmine (eserine). This drug was the first miotic used in the treatment of glaucoma (1875). It is used in an aqueous solution of the salicylate salt in a concentration of 0.25 to 1% or as a 0.25% ointment. Usually it is given only at bedtime to supplement the instillation of pilocarpine. Prolonged use causes conjunctival irritation.

Neostigmine (Prostigmin). Neostigmine (Prostigmin) was synthesized as an analogue of physostigmine. It is used in the treatment of glaucoma as a 5% solution every 4 to 6 hours and systemically in the treatment of myasthenia gravis. It penetrates the cornea poorly. Edrophonium chloride (Tensilon), an analogue of neostigmine, has a systemic action of very short duration. It is injected intravenously in doses of 2 to 5 mg. in the diagnosis of myasthenia gravis.

Alkyl phosphates. Echothiophate iodide (Phospholine I) is an alkyl phosphate in which a quaternary ammonium compound has been substituted. It is extremely active against nonspecific cholinesterases. Echothiophate iodide is used locally every 12 hours in a 0.06 to 0.25% solution. It causes intense miosis and a spasm of the ciliary muscle, which causes a dull, aching pain in the eye.

All alkyl phosphates are contraindicated in angle-closure glaucoma (p. 315), bronchial asthma, gastrointestinal spasm, vascular hypertension, myocardial infarction, and Parkinson's disease.

Despite the long list of contraindications, echothiophate iodide has proved particularly useful in controlling open-angle glaucoma in eyes not responsive to other medications. Prolonged use may be followed by a marked improvement in the flow of aqueous humor through the trabecular meshwork of the chamber angle.

The muscle relaxant succinylcholine is rapidly destroyed by the pseudocholinesterases in the normal patient. The reduction of these enzymes by the local use of anticholinesterase drugs may cause a dangerously prolonged apnea when the compound is used in conjunction with general anesthetics.

Reactivators of cholinesterase. Severe toxicity from administration of anticholinesterase compounds arises because of the accumulation of acetylcholine. Atropine is the classical antidote. In recent years attention has been directed to compounds that reactivate cholinesterase and permit it to hydrolyze the accumulated acetylcholine. The most widely studied cholinesterase reactivator is pyridine-2-aldoxime methiodide (PAM). This compound is effective because it displaces the phosphoryl group of anticholinesterase compounds from the esteratic site of the enzyme cholinesterase. These compounds have proved useful in the study of enzyme structure and in the treatment of poisoning by anticholinesterase compounds, particularly insecticides.

Cholinergic blocking drugs

The action of acetylcholine in nerve transmission may be blocked at (1) the motor end plate of postganglionic parasympathetic nerve fibers in smooth and cardiac muscle—these structures are stimulated by muscarine and blocked by the atropine group of drugs; (2) the autonomic ganglia of both the parasympathetic and the sympathetic nervous system—nicotine in small doses stimulates ganglionic transmission, the action being opposed by ganglionic blocking agents, whereas nicotine in large doses is a ganglionic blocking agent; (3) both the central nervous system and the motor end plate of skeletal muscle.

Atropine group. In general, these drugs prevent the action of acetylcholine at postganglionic nerve endings in smooth muscle, cardiac muscle, and glands. Systemic administration increases the heart rate and decreases sweating, lacrimation, salivary secretion, gastric secretion, gastrointestinal motility, and tone. Many of the compounds have a depressant effect on the central nervous system and have been used in the treatment of parkinsonism and as sedatives (scopolamine).

The ocular effects of the atropine-like drugs are mainly dilation of the pupil through paralysis of the sphincter pupillae and decrease of accommodation through paralysis of the ciliary muscle. The duration of these effects varies with different compounds. Systemic administration has less effect than local administration because of decreased concentration of the compounds at the effector sites in the eye. Systemically administered atropine has a greater pupillary effect than the newer atropine-like compounds used for their antispasmodic action on the gastrointestinal tract.

Atropine and related compounds are regarded as reducing the permeability of blood vessels of the iris and the ciliary body. This action, which is well documented, is quite opposite to the vasodilation observed in flushing of the face when large doses of atropine are administered systemically. Peripheral vasodilation cannot be explained by any known neural transmission to blood vessels.

The atropine-like compounds developed as gastrointestinal antispasmodics have varying degrees of mydriatic and cycloplegic activity upon local instillation. Systemic administration in younger persons may cause an annoying decrease in accommodation. A surprising number of patients with ill-defined gastrointestinal complaints for whom atropine-like antispasmodics are prescribed also have unsuspected glaucoma (p. 302).

Members of the atropine group of drugs used in ophthalmology include atropine, scopolamine, homatropine, eucatropine (Euphthalmine), cyclopentolate (Cyclogyl), and tropicamide (Mydriacyl).

Atropine. Atropine is the principal alkaloid of belladonna, the deadly nightshade plant. It is used in a 0.5 to 4% aqueous solution, in an ointment, or in a castor oil base to minimize the possibility of systemic absorption. It causes pupillary dilation that begins in about 15 minutes and persists 10 to 12 days. Paralysis of accommodation begins at 20 to 30 minutes after instillation and persists 3 to 5 days. Atropine is widely used in the treatment of anterior uveitis and keratitis and in the refraction of children, particularly those with strabismus. In inflammatory conditions it may be used every 1 to 6 hours. For refraction it is commonly instilled three times daily for 3 days, and examination is carried out on the fourth day.

Scopolamine. This drug is closely related to atropine but has a shorter duration of action (2 to 3 days) on both pupillary dilation and accommodative paralysis. It is frequently substituted for atropine, which may cause conjunctival irritation or contact allergy when prolonged mydriasis and cycloplegia are used in conditions such as retinal detachment or uveitis.

Homatropine. This synthetic atropine-like compound is used mainly to paralyze accommodation for refraction. It is used in a 1 to 5% aqueous solution and produces mydriasis and cycloplegia lasting 12 to 36 hours.

Eucatropine (Euphthalmine). This synthetic compound has mainly a mydriatic action without cycloplegic effects. It is used almost exclusively to dilate the pupil in a provocative test in patients suspected of having angle-closure glaucoma.

Cyclopentolate (Cyclogyl). Cyclopentolate (Cyclogyl) is a relatively new atropine-like compound that causes mydriasis and cycloplegia, with a return to normal within (usually) 6 hours. It is used almost exclusively in refraction.

Tropicamide (Mydriacyl). This cholinergic blocking drug causes a more rapid paralysis of accommodation and quicker recovery than any other such compound. It is commonly used in a 1% concentration instilled at least two times at 5-minute intervals to produce effective cycloplegia. Its effect usually disappears within 2 to 4 hours. It causes more pupillary dilation than other cholinergic compounds and is often combined with phenylephrine for ophthalmoscopy.

Ganglionic blocking drugs. These compounds affect the transmission of impulses across both sympathetic and parasympathetic autonomic ganglia. They are used mainly in the treatment of hypertensive cardiovascular disease to reduce peripheral resistance by decreasing sympathetic tone to vascular beds. They have additional utility in the therapy of vasospasm and in producing a controlled hypotension in general anesthesia.

The ocular side effects of ganglionic blockade constitute their main ophthalmic interest. The conjunctival blood vessels and pupil are dilated. The tears and accommodation are decreased. The intraocular pressure is slightly decreased, apparently because of a decreased secretion of aqueous humor. The decrease is accompanied by an increased resistance to the exit of aqueous humor through the trabecular meshwork. Increased intraocular pressure does not occur because of the reduced aqueous secretion.

Neuromuscular blocking drugs. These compounds may be effective in the spinal cord and subcortical centers or at the motor end plates of skeletal musculature. Curare is the typical agent affecting skeletal musculature. These agents block transmission of nerve impulses at neuromuscular junctions and selectively involve the extraocular muscles first and then the pharyngeal muscles, skeletal muscles, and the diaphragm in that order.

The main ophthalmic application of this group of drugs arises in general anesthesia in which the administration of *d*-tubocurarine chloride causes relaxation of the extraocular musculature desirable in cataract extraction. Succinylcholine produces a short period of muscular relaxation but also muscular contraction before paralysis develops. Its use is therefore contraindicated in intraocular surgery inasmuch as an increased intraocular pressure occurs.

The compounds that depress skeletal muscle activity because of central nervous system activity do so without affecting consciousness in the usual doses. Mephensin (Tolserol, Myanesin) has some use in muscle spasm. Study of this group of drugs led to the compounds meprobamate (Miltown, Equanil) and chlordiazepoxide (Librium), whose muscle-relaxing qualities are overshadowed by their tranquilizing effects.

Adrenergic stimulating drugs

The effector substances responsible for the stimulation of the majority of structures innervated by postganglionic sympathetic nerves are the catecholamines. (The arrectores pilorum muscles and sweat glands are exceptional in having acetylcholine as the postganglionic effector substance.) Four catecholamines have been identified in the body: epinephrine, the major secretion of the adrenal medulla, which acts mainly as a hormone and has considerably less effect than catecholamines released locally; norepinephrine, which is the major adrenergic neuroeffector substance and a precursor of epinephrine; dopamine, which is a precursor of norepinephrine and epinephrine; and *N*-methylepinephrine, the role of which has not been established (Fig. 3-2).

The cells that form catecholamines convert tyrosine from the blood to dopa, which is changed to dopamine by dopa decarboxylase in the cytoplasm. Dopamine is stored in cytoplasmic granules or converted into norepinephrine by the enzyme dopamine β-oxidase. The norepinephrine is either stored in the cell or in the adrenal medulla and may be converted to epinephrine by a methylating enzyme.

It is postulated that there are two major types of adrenergic receptors: (1) alpha receptors, which are mainly excitatory to smooth muscle and gland cells but cause relaxation of intestinal smooth muscle, and (2) beta receptors, which are mainly inhibitory and cause relaxation of smooth muscle, including that of the intestine, but

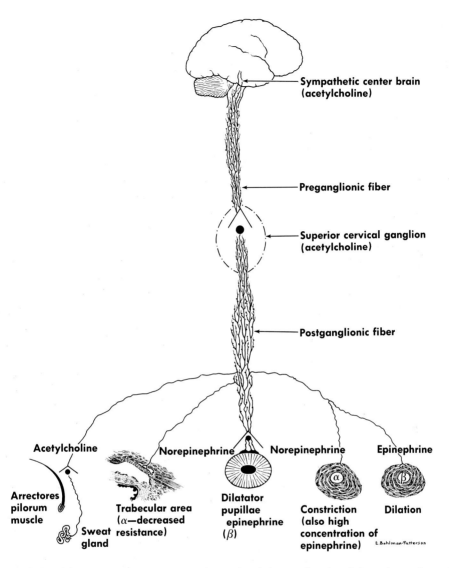

Fig. 3-2. Adrenergic nervous system. Norepinephrine and epinephrine, the active principles, are inactivated by catechol-O-methyl transferase. The effects of stimulation are illustrated.

also cause myocardial stimulation. Vasoconstriction mediated by alpha receptors is the most important physiologic response to adrenergic stimulation, but activation of beta receptors by epinephrine (after alpha receptors are blocked) or isoproterenol produces marked vasodilation.

Both norepinephrine and epinephrine

activate both major types of receptors, but the ratio of the two actions can vary widely. Norepinephrine is most effective at alpha receptor sites. Epinephrine affects beta receptors in low concentration and alpha receptors in high concentration. Their action differs when the compounds are administered in large or small doses or when given systemically or locally.

Norepinephrine and epinephrine both cause a decrease in intraocular pressure when administered intravenously. Norepinephrine causes an increase in the facility of outflow, whereas epinephrine both decreases the secretion of aqueous humor and increases the facility of outflow.

The receptors in the human intraocular musculature have not been determined. In the monkey the dilatator pupillae and sphincter muscles contain mainly alpha receptors. Thus stimulation of alpha receptors in the iris musculature would provide antagonistic actions, although the greater number of receptors in the dilatator muscles causes pupillary dilation. The ciliary muscle of the monkey contains only beta receptors; therefore stimulation should cause relaxation of the muscle.

The released catecholamines at the neuroeffector site are inactivated by reuptake by axonal terminations and by diffusion into the circulation. Slower inactivation is mediated by the enzymes catechol-O-methyl transferase and monoamine oxidase.

Direct-acting adrenergic drugs. The major use of adrenergic drugs in ophthalmology is by local administration. They have three main effects: (1) dilation of the pupil, (2) enhancement of the flow of aqueous humor through the outflow channels of the eye, and (3) decreased secretion of aqueous humor by the ciliary epithelium. In addition, they are widely used to cause vasoconstriction of conjunctival vessels and thus "whiten" the eye. They minimize discomfort in hypersensitivity reactions of the conjunctiva.

A large number of compounds have actions similar to those of epinephrine and norepinephrine. Many are used by inhalation or systemically because of their effect in dilating bronchiole musculature. Amphetamines are widely used to stimulate the central nervous system. Systemic administration of adrenergic drugs may cause some stimulation of the dilatator pupillae muscle with mydriasis. Usually, however, pupillary dilation is not conspicuous, and the pupil reacts readily to light.

Epinephrine. Epinephrine penetrates the cornea poorly, and pupillary dilation requires instillation of a 1% or stronger solution. In denervation hypersensitivity when the sympathetic fibers to the dilatator muscle have been interrupted, a 0.1% solution will dilate the pupil. Two percent epinephrine is used in the treatment of glaucoma to increase the outflow of aqueous humor through the trabecular meshwork and to decrease aqueous humor production. The action on outflow is presumably a direct one and may be mediated by adrenergic nerve endings in the endothelium of the trabecular meshwork. In the therapy of glaucoma, epinephrine is usually combined with a cholinergic stimulating drug such as pilocarpine to maintain pupillary constriction. In some individuals the epinephrine produces black, localized, isolated subconjunctival deposits of melanin in the conjunctiva of the lower lid (p. 179).

Phenylephrine hydrochloride (Neo-Synephrine). Phenylephrine hydrochloride (Neo-Synephrine) is an effective agent for pupillary dilation and stimulates the motor end plates of the dilatator pupillae muscle. It penetrates the cornea well and is commonly used to dilate the pupil for examination of the ocular fundus. It is available in 1, 2.5, and 10% solutions. It is a powerful vasoconstrictor—it constricts the arterioles of the conjunctiva and, if systemically absorbed, may increase the systemic blood pressure. It is sometimes used in combination with cholinergic blocking agents to enhance pupillary dilation in the treatment of uveitis.

Phenylephrine is the agent of choice for dilating the pupil to study the ocular fundus because it can be easily neutralized with cholinergic drugs. It is used to prevent the formation of cysts of the pupillary pigment epithelium in children in whom anticholinesterase preparations are instilled to interfere with peripheral accommodation in accommodative esotropia.

Other direct-acting adrenergic drugs. Adrenergic drugs such as norepinephrine, hydroxyamphetamine hydrobromide (Paredrine), and other amphetamines cause a variable degree of pupillary dilation when instilled into the conjunctival sac. With the exception of Paredrine, which is a less effective dilating agent than phenylephrine, they are not used in clinical ophthalmology. Isoproterenol acts almost exclusively on beta receptors. Its use in ophthalmology is limited to pharmacologic investigation and its clinical uses are as a bronchodilator and cardiac stimulant.

Indirect-acting adrenergic drugs. Nor-

epinephrine and epinephrine are partially inactivated by the enzyme catechol-O-methyl transferase. This enzyme is inhibited by pyrogallol and by quercetin, which therefore permit the accumulation of norepinephrine and epinephrine and prolong their physiologic effects. Pyrogallol and quercetin do not have identical pharmacologic effects on the adrenal medulla or on the central nervous system. These compounds are of pharmacologic interest mainly; they do not have activities comparable to those of the anticholinesterase compounds in the cholinergic nervous system.

Monoamine oxidase was previously considered the enzyme responsible for inactivation of intracellular epinephrine and norepinephrine. At present it seems likely

---

Compounds acting predominantly on adrenergic nervous system

I. Adrenergic stimulating compounds
  A. Direct-acting drugs
    1. Catecholamines: norepinephrine; epinephrine
    2. Isoproterenol
    3. Noncatecholamines: amphetamine; methamphetamine; hydroxyamphetamine (Paredrine); ephedrine; phenylephrine HCl (Neo-Synephrine)
  B. Inhibition of enzyme inactivators of catecholamines
    1. Catechol-O-methyl transferase inhibitors: pyrogallol; quercetin
    2. Amine oxidase inhibitors: iproniazid; ephedrine (?)
  C. Potentiation of catechol action by preventing uptake by adrenergic nerve terminals: cocaine (?)
  D. Increased release of catecholamines: guanethidine (Ismelin); rauwolfia alkaloids (early effect)
  E. Increased sensitivity of receptors to catecholamines: guanethidine; rauwolfia alkaloids

II. Adrenergic blocking compounds
  A. Prevent catecholamine synthesis: alpha-methyldopa (Aldomet)
  B. Decreased binding of catecholamines: guanethidine; bretylium; rauwolfia alkaloids (late effect)
  C. Alpha receptor blockade: dibenamine; ergot alkaloids; phenoxybenzamine (Dibenzyline); tolazoline (Priscoline); phenothiazines; yohimbines; phentolamine (Regitine)
  D. Beta receptor blockade: dichloroisoproterenol (DCI); isoproterenol

III. Secondary adrenergic blocking agents
  A. Ganglionic blocking agents acting on sympathetic ganglia such as superior cervical ganglion
  B. Central nervous system depressants

that the action of monoamine oxidase is concerned with the metabolites of epinephrine and norepinephrine resulting from the action of catechol-O-methyl transferase. If monoamine oxidase is inhibited, there is an accumulation of norepinephrine in the brain and elsewhere. This may occur because there is an accumulation of end products of metabolism inhibiting the inactivation of norepinephrine. This mechanism is not known.

Ephedrine is active as a sympathomimetic compound both through stimulation of sympathetic receptor sites and through inhibition of the effects of monoamine oxidase, which permits accumulation of catecholamines, particularly epinephrine. Monoamine oxidase inhibitors are antidepressants. In most persons they cause a vascular hypotension but may cause a hypertension in some individuals.

Adrenergic blocking agents

The adrenergic nervous system may be blocked at several levels. In many instances the pharmacologic actions are obscured by side effects, and the adrenergic blockade is not conspicuous. The outline on p. 103 shows the levels at which adrenergic blockade may occur: (1) interference with catecholamine synthesis; (2) blocking the effect of catecholamines upon effector cells —there may thus be alpha and beta blocking agents; and (3) prevention of the initial storage and subsequent release of norepinephrine.

In addition to these primary agents, there are a number of secondary adrenergic blocking compounds. Interference with acetylcholine activity at the level of autonomic ganglia, of course, acts upon sympathetic ganglia. Central nervous system depressants also block adrenergic actions.

Compounds that inhibit postganglionic sympathetic nerves at effector sites produce an orthostatic hypotension and nasal stuffiness and some cause a pupillary constriction. They cause reduction of intra-

ocular pressure, presumably through reduced secretion by the ciliary body, and they have been used in the past in the management of angle-closure glaucoma. Many of the compounds have actions in addition to adrenergic blockade and are not widely used clinically.

Interference with catecholamine synthesis. As mentioned previously (p. 100), dopa is changed to dopamine by dopa decarboxylase. The synthesis of dopamine and thence norepinephrine can be blocked by compounds that inhibit decarboxylase.

Alpha-methyldopa (Aldomet) is a decarboxylase inhibitor that interferes with the synthesis of norepinephrine from tyrosine and with serotonin from tryptophan. Topical administration does not affect the intraocular pressure in experimental animals. Systemic administration reduces the arterial blood pressure with a parallel but transient reduction in intraocular pressure.

Interference with catecholamine storage. Several compounds interfere with the storage of catecholamines in the synaptic cytoplasmic vesicles. Generally these compounds cause an initial release of stored norepinephrine and thereafter diminish the amounts of norepinephrine available for endogenous release into the tissues.

Reserpine. Reserpine is one of the alkaloids of *Rauwolfia serpentina*. It causes the release and inhibits the binding of norepinephrine in synaptic vesicles and thus mimics the systemic effects of a sympathectomy. This is perhaps the cause of blood pressure reduction with this compound. The tranquilizing effects are due to a similar effect on serotonin binding. It causes a slight decrease in intraocular pressure, but the mechanism is unknown.

Guanethidine (Ismelin). Guanethidine (Ismelin) prevents the release of norepinephrine by postganglionic sympathetic nerves. Instillation in the eye of a 10% solution causes miosis, narrowing of the palpebral fissure, dilation of conjunctival blood vessels, and a decrease in intraocular pressure. It has been used mainly in the treatment of retraction of the upper eyelid in thyroid disease (p. 394).

Blockade of receptor sites. Compounds that block the receptor response to catecholamines have a high specificity for either alpha or beta sites. A variety of compounds that block alpha sites are available for clinical study, but those causing beta blockade are not as specific and are used solely in pharmacologic studies. The main members of the group are phenoxybenzamine (Dibenzyline), ergot alkaloids, tolazoline (Priscoline), and phentolamine mesylate (Regitine mesylate). Dibenamine, which is similar to but less potent than phenoxybenzamine, has been used effectively in the treatment of angle-closure glaucoma but is not available for clinical use. Tolazoline is used on occasion for retrobulbar injection to cause vasodilation, particularly of the central retinal artery.

The ophthalmic interest in these compounds arises primarily from the alpha receptor blockage produced in the eye: ptosis, miosis, vasodilation, and in glaucoma reduced intraocular pressure.

Beta receptor blockade is produced by dichloroisoproterenol (DCI) and isoproterenol. Neither are available for clinical use but are potent agents for studying the adrenergic nervous system. The ocular response to both alpha and beta receptors has not been studied at any length and is complicated by species differences and nonspecific effects of the drugs.

Denervation hypersensitivity

When a structure innervated by postganglionic autonomic nerves loses its nerve supply, there is a marked decrease in cholinesterase or catechol-O-methyl transferase at the synaptic junction. The denervated structure is thus far more sensitive to exogenous acetylcholine or catecholamines than when normally innervated. Thus in Adie's pupil (p. 221), an abnormality that likely involves the ciliary gan-

glion, the pupil is constricted by the instillation of 2.5% Mecholyl, which does not affect the normal sphincter pupillae muscle —it normally constricts only with instillation of a 15 to 20% concentration. Similarly, if there is interference with the sympathetic pathway between the superior cervical ganglion and the dilatator pupillae muscle, as occurs in Horner's syndrome (p. 221), the pupil dilates with instillation of 1:1,000 epinephrine, which has no effect on the normally innervated pupil.

Relation of autonomic drugs to pupillary dilation and glaucoma

The relation of glaucoma to pupillary dilation is a confusing topic because different mechanisms may be involved in the increase in intraocular pressure in different types of glaucoma (p. 302). Dilation of the pupil in patients who have shallow anterior chambers may cause the iris to interfere mechanically with drainage of aqueous humor through the trabecular meshwork. Once the intraocular pressure exceeds 50 mm. Hg and the diameter of the pupil is greater than 5 mm., the sphincter pupillae muscle no longer responds to miotic drugs—the excessive pressure must be decreased by means of agents that either inhibit carbonic anhydrase (p. 106) or those that increase the osmotic pressure of the blood. Angle-closure glaucoma may be induced in predisposed persons by pupillary dilation with either adrenergic compounds that stimulate the dilatator pupillae muscle or cholinergic blocking drugs that inhibit the sphincter pupillae muscle. Angle-closure glaucoma may be induced in susceptible persons even by minute concentrations of adrenergic drugs used to constrict conjunctival blood vessels. The alkyl phosphates, although they cause miosis, also produce marked dilation and increased permeability of blood vessels of the ciliary body. The extreme miosis may decrease the volume of aqueous humor that can pass through the pupil, and this, combined with ciliary body vascular dilation, may produce angle-closure glaucoma in predisposed individuals.

In open-angle glaucoma, cholinergic blocking drugs may induce a moderate increase in intraocular pressure through an effect either on the ciliary muscle, the trabecular meshwork, or the secretion of aqueous humor.

Caution is indicated in prescribing cholinergic blocking agents systemically in patients who may have glaucoma. These compounds are commonly prescribed for patients in the age group in which glaucoma is most prevalent. Evidence suggests that over 15% of the patients with gastrointestinal symptoms for which antispasmodics are prescribed have open-angle glaucoma. The administration of cholinergic blocking agents prior to surgery in patients with glaucoma is not contraindicated, and any increase in intraocular pressure may be anticipated and controlled with local miotics.

Carbonic anhydrase inhibitors

Carbonic anhydrase catalyzes the equilibrium between carbonic acid and carbon dioxide. The enzyme is widely distributed in (1) erythrocytes, where it functions in the exchange of carbon dioxide in pulmonary capillaries, (2) the renal tubule cell, where it functions in the exchange of intracellular hydrogen for tubular sodium with acidification of the urine and return of glomerulus-filtered carbon dioxide to the blood, (3) the choroid plexus, where it functions in the secretion of cerebrospinal fluid, (4) the gastric mucosa and the pancreas, and (5) the epithelium of the ciliary body, where it functions in the secretion of aqueous humor.

Potent inhibitors of carbonic anhydrase were synthesized after it was observed that the systemic administration of sulfonamides caused an acidosis because of loss of sodium bicarbonate to the urine and failure of the exchange of cellular hydrogen for

tubular sodium. Despite the widespread distribution of carbonic anhydrase in the tissues of the body, the effects of enzyme inhibition are mainly renal. With certain of the agents, however, there is a decreased secretion of aqueous humor and cerebrospinal fluid. Decreased secretion of aqueous humor occurs even in the absence of renal effects and is apparently due to interference with secretory activity of the ciliary body in an as yet unknown manner.

Effective drugs in this group reduce the secretion of aqueous humor from 50 to 60%. There is a concomitant reduction in intraocular pressure. The most commonly used agent is acetazolamide (Diamox). Because of side effects, a number of other compounds have been substituted for acetazolamide.

Acetazolamide (Diamox). This drug is the most widely used carbonic anhydrase inhibitor in ophthalmology. In patients with open-angle glaucoma the usual dosage is 250 mg. orally every 6 hours. It may be used intravenously in patients with angle-closure glaucoma. The ocular effect is observed 1 to 2 hours following oral administration and persists for 3 to 5 hours. The secretion of aqueous humor is reduced, but never stopped, and it is evident that only mechanisms of secretory activity involving carbonic anhydrase are concerned (p. 72). A variety of side effects may occur. Myopia, aplastic anemia, exfoliative dermatitis, and other reactions observed with sulfonamide derivatives occur rarely. Nearly all patients have paresthesia with numbness and tingling in the extremities. Anorexia is common. There is a slight tendency to renal lithiasis. Side effects may necessitate the substitution of another carbonic anhydrase inhibitor.

Ethoxzolamide (Cardrase), dichlorphenamide (Daranide), and methazolamide (Neptazane) are more recently synthesized carbonic anhydrase inhibitors that may be substituted for acetazolamide. It is not unusual for one of them to be effective in reducing intraocular pressure when another fails.

Cardiac glycosides

The production of aqueous humor involves active secretion of sodium, and water follows passively. The ciliary processes contain sodium- and potassium-activated ATPase (adenosine triphosphatase) sensitive to digitalis. This enzyme may be inhibited in man by digoxin and in cats by intravenous ouabain. Inhibition is followed by a moderate reduction in intraocular pressure due to decreased secretion of aqueous humor by the ciliary processes. The effect is potentiated by the simultaneous administration of acetazolamide, which suggests that a different site of action is involved.

There is little change in the ocular pressure of man until digitalization has taken place. A maintenance dose of digitalis may produce gradually falling levels of intraocular pressure for 2 to 3 months. The use of cardiac glycosides in a 0.5 to 5% ointment produces a moderate reduction in intraocular pressure but may also produce corneal opacities. These compounds are mainly of theoretic interest and are not used in the management of glaucoma.

Osmotic agents

If the osmotic pressure of the blood is increased, water is withdrawn from the eye, and the intraocular pressure is decreased. The increased osmotic pressure of the blood is usually maintained for only a short time, and within 5 hours the intraocular pressure is restored to its previous level. Treatment by increasing the osmotic pressure of the blood is used in ophthalmic practice when it is desirable to decrease the intraocular pressure and volume for a relatively short period. Thus it is used in the following instances: (1) in angle-closure glaucoma to reduce the intraocular pressure to less than 50 mm. Hg so that the sphincter pupillae muscle will respond

to miotics; (2) to reduce intraocular pressure immediately prior to surgery, particularly in uncontrollable glaucoma; (3) to reduce intraocular volume to assist scleral wound closure in retinal detachment surgery; and (4) to reduce orbital volume in orbital surgery.

Urea. Urea is used intravenously in a 30% solution in 10% invert sugar in a dosage of 1.0 to 1.5 Gm./kg. body weight. The intraocular pressure falls within 30 minutes after intravenous infusion is started and may fall to levels of less than 10 mm. Hg. The intraocular pressure returns to pretreatment levels about 5 hours after the medication is discontinued.

The increased osmolarity of the blood causes marked reduction of intracranial pressure with severe headache, which is aggravated by elevation of the head. There is marked diuresis, and there may be associated nausea and vomiting. The blood urea nitrogen is markedly increased for 24 to 48 hours, except when there is impaired renal function that causes the levels to remain elevated for as long as a week. Vascular hypertension and acute pulmonary edema may occur.

Mannitol. Mannitol is a 6-carbon alcohol that is not significantly metabolized. It is excreted by filtration through the renal glomeruli and is not reabsorbed by the tubules. Mannitol is administered intravenously in a 20% solution, usually in a 500 ml. volume, irrespective of body weight. The maximum fall in intraocular pressure occurs within 60 minutes, and it returns to pretreatment levels after about 4 hours. The maximum increase in the blood osmolarity precedes the maximum decrease of intraocular pressure by a few minutes.

The complications of mannitol therapy are less severe than those observed with urea. Headache of the same type and severity occurs, as does diuresis. Local infiltration of tissues does not produce induration.

Glycerol. Glycerol is a trivalent alcohol that forms a part of the molecule of glycerides and phosphatides. It is metabolized in the body through the tricarboxylic acid cycle. (Insulin is not required in its metabolism.) It is administered orally in a 50% solution in lemon juice in doses of 1.0 to 1.5 Gm./kg. body weight. The maximum decrease in intraocular pressure is observed within 30 to 60 minutes and returns to pretreatment levels within 4 or 5 hours.

Side effects are few. Usually headache does not occur, and diuresis is not marked. Nausea and vomiting may prevent its long-term use.

Isosorbide (Hydronol). This compound is a dihydric alcohol formed by the removal of two molecules of water from sorbitol. It may be given orally in a 50% ginger-flavored solution without gastrointestinal irritation. In a dosage of 1 to 2 Gm./kg. of body weight the intraocular pressure reaches a minimal value 1 to 2 hours after administration and remains depressed for 5 to 6 hours. Side effects are uncommon, but the drug has not been thoroughly studied.

Dyes

A variety of dyes are used in ophthalmology to stain breaks in the continuity of the epithelium of the cornea or conjunctiva and for a variety of diagnostic tests. The most commonly used are sodium fluorescein and rose bengal.

Sodium fluorescein is used in 2% alkaline solution. Because of the ease of contamination, particularly with *Pseudomonas aeruginosa*, it should be instilled either from a single-dose container or by means of a strip of sterile filter paper saturated with dye. The dye is instilled in the conjunctival sac and after 1 minute the excess dye is washed away. In areas in which the corneal epithelium is diseased or absent, the stroma stains a bright green color. Foreign bodies embedded in the cornea are surrounded by a bright green ring. The intensity of staining is accentuated if 2% cocaine ophthalmic solution is instilled in the eye or if the eye is illuminated with a mercury lamp with a wavelength of 3,600 nm. to stimulate fluorescence.

Fluorescein is also instilled in the eye to demonstrate dilution that occurs when anterior aqueous humor escapes from a postoperative fistula, a penetrating wound, or a conjunctival bleb following glaucoma filtration surgery. It is used to demonstrate areas of pressure on the globe in the fitting of contact lenses. Applanation tonometry is based upon the appearance of the fluorescein pattern when pressure is applied to the eye.

In recent years intravenous sodium fluorescein has been combined with fundus photography to study the dynamics of the retinal circulation. Five to 10 milliliters of a 10 to 20% solution is injected rapidly into the brachial vein and fundus photographs are taken with a cobalt blue glass in the illuminating system and using a fast black and white film. Nausea occurs fairly commonly with the injection and fluorescein is excreted in the urine for the following 24 to 48 hours. Anaphylactic reactions have recently been described.

Intravenous administration is followed by the appearance of fluorescein in the aqueous humor, a method of measuring aqueous flow. Similarly, if fluorescein is allowed to remain in contact with the surface of the globe, it enters the anterior chamber and its disappearance rate can be used to gauge the outflow of aqueous humor.

Rose bengal is used similar to fluorescein in a 1% solution, but in most clinical situations it is inferior to fluorescein. However, it stains devitalized cells better, and staining areas of the conjunctiva are more evident than with fluorescein. Its chief use is in the diagnosis of keratoconjunctivitis sicca (p. 210).

Local anesthetics

The small size of the eye and the accessibility of the nerve supply have made it possible to perform most ocular procedures under local anesthesia. The conjunctiva and cornea are readily anesthetized by means of topically instilled agents, of which cocaine, the prototype, has been succeeded by tetracaine (Pontocaine, 0.5%), benoxinate (Dorsacaine, 0.4%), and proparacaine (Ophthaine, 0.5%). Infiltration or block anesthesia is readily achieved with procaine (Novocain) or lidocaine (Xylocaine) skillfully administered.

Topical anesthetics are used for superficial procedures such as tonometry or removal of corneal foreign bodies. The exquisite pain of corneal abrasions, ultraviolet keratitis, and corneal foreign bodies is quickly relieved. Inasmuch as these agents are potent sensitizers and delay corneal epithelization they should not be prescribed for analgesia.

Infiltration anesthesia is used mainly in the region of the lids for the excision of local lesions. Simultaneous motor and sensory block is obtained by injecting the anesthetic agent in the region of the orbital portion of the orbicularis oculi muscle (Van Lint technique) to prevent eyelid closure in intraocular surgery.

Motor block of the lids is sometimes obtained by infiltrating fibers of the temporal branch of the seventh nerve as they pass anterior to the temporomandibular articulation (O'Brien technique). Motor block of the nerve supply to the extraocular muscles and sensory block of the nerve supply to the globe is obtained by retrobulbar injection of anesthetic solution posterior to the globe in the region between the lateral rectus muscle and optic nerve. This blocks all of the extraocular muscles except the superior rectus muscle, blocks the ciliary ganglion so the pupil dilates, and anesthetizes the entire globe with the exception of the cornea.

Other sensory blocks follow injections of anesthetic agents in the region of the supra- and infratrochlear nerves at the superior medial angle of the orbit, the infraorbital nerve, either in its orbital course or as it emerges through the infraorbital foramen to the face, and the lacrimal and zygomaticofacial nerves as they exit from their respective foramina.

Anti-infective agents

There are several factors that modify the use of anti-infective agents in ophthalmology. When systemically administered, many do not pass the blood-aqueous barrier, and effective intraocular concentrations are not obtained. Conversely, in many infections requiring a high intraocular concentration, the inflammation has impaired the blood-aqueous barrier so that adequate concentrations may be obtained with drugs that ordinarily do not enter the eye.

When anti-infective agents are used locally, unusually high local tissue concentrations may be obtained. Many of the compounds do not penetrate the epithelial barrier of the cornea, but when this is removed or diseased, relatively high concentrations may be obtained in the anterior ocular segment. The use of radioactive isotopes indicates that some drugs instilled in the conjunctival sac diffuse to the posterior pole, but it is unlikely that any useful concentration occurs. Systemic administration is therefore indicated for posterior lesions.

Many of the compounds instilled in the conjunctival sac give rise to a contact dermatoconjunctivitis either of an allergic or an irritative type. Prolonged local use of antibiotics and steroids predisposes to fungus infections, and the possibility of a secondary fungal invader must be considered in any persistent conjunctival or corneal inflammation. Anti-infective agents used locally are diluted rapidly by the tears, and they must be instilled frequently to assure adequate local tissue concentration.

Antibiotics

Antibiotics are chemical substances that inhibit growth or destroy microorganisms in a dilute solution. They may be effective through one of several mechanisms. They may prevent the synthesis of protein either of the cell nucleus or of the cell wall. The agents may primarily inhibit bacterial multiplication or destroy microorganisms. Some agents are both bacteriostatic and bactericidal.

The use of antibiotics is complicated by the occurrence of strains of microorganisms resistant to their action and by a variety of side effects. Side effects range from hypersensitivity reactions, observed particularly with the penicillins, to fatal aplastic anemia, rarely resulting from the administration of chloramphenicol. Suppression of the normal flora of the gastrointestinal tract may give rise to serious staphylococcal or monilial enteritis. Other side effects of antibiotics include toxic effects such as peripheral neuritis, deafness, vertigo, nausea, and vomiting.

Some antibiotics that are too toxic for routine systemic use have been used locally in ophthalmology. These include the following: polymyxin B, effective against *Pseudomonas aeruginosa;* neomycin, which is bactericidal against both rods and cocci; and bacitracin, which is bactericidal against cocci.

Antibiotics may be divided into four main groups: (1) agents that impede replication of genetic information (nalidixic acid and griseofulvin); (2) agents that impair translation of genetic information into protein synthesis (chloramphenicol, tetracyclines, erythromycin, lincomycin, kanamycin, neomycin, and streptomycin); (3) agents that alter the structure and function of the cell wall (penicillins, bacitracin, cephalothin, vancomycin, cycloserine, and ristocetin); and (4) agents that restrict

the function of the cell membrane (gramicidin, tyrocidine, polymyxin B, colistin, amphotericin B, and nystatin). The sulfonamides (p. 112) impair the intermediate metabolism of bacteria.

Penicillins. These drugs are both bacteriostatic and bactericidal and are effective against a wide range of microorganisms, although they are used primarily in the therapy of streptococcal and pneumococcal infections and for gonorrhea and syphilis. The penicillins may be divided into those prepared by fermentation and those formed by isolation of the 6-aminopenicillanic acid from penicillin fermentation media and then conjugated with various side chains to produce a semisynthetic product.

Hypersensitivity to the penicillins is one of the commonest forms of allergy and has virtually eliminated their topical use in ophthalmology. Systemic administration may be followed by hypersensitivity reactions ranging in severity from urticaria to anaphylaxis. The penicillins are all cross-reactive and a patient sensitive to one will be sensitive to other penicillins, though not always to the same extent. Anaphylactic reactions occur most commonly with the natural penicillins and much less frequently with the semisynthetic derivatives which, however, may cause delayed hypersensitivity reactions.

Treatment with the penicillins has become highly individualized and varies from community to community, depending mainly upon the emergence of penicillinase-producing staphylococci. The semisynthetic penicillins administered orally do not provide the high blood level required for ocular penetration. However, ampicillin has a wide antibacterial range and enters the eye well; it is not, however, effective against penicillinase-producing staphylococci.

Neomycin. This deoxystreptomine antimicrobial is effective against most gram-negative bacilli with the exception of

Pseudomonas species. Staphylococci are the only gram-positive organisms inhibited by the compound. It is widely used by topical administration in ophthalmology, usually combined with polymyxin B. Cutaneous hypersensitivity occurs in 5 to 15% of the patients treated topically. Combinations of adrenocorticosteroids in proprietary preparations may mask the cutaneous reaction, but then it may appear after cessation of therapy. Application of heat to the affected area can reactivate these reactions for as long as 5 months following exposure to the drug.

Polymyxins. Polymyxin B belongs to a group of polymyxins that are effective against gram-negative rods including *Pseudomonas aeruginosa*. It is often combined with neomycin. Polymyxin E (colistin) has similar activities and toxicities. At times the polymyxins exert a synergistic action when combined with tetracyclines or chloramphenicol.

Gentamicin. Gentamicin is a unique antibiotic effective against *Pseudomonas* and *Proteus* as well as other gram-negative bacteria and the *Staphylococcus* species. It is active against some bacteria resistant to antibiotics such as neomycin. Toxic reactions following systemic administration include vestibular damage, which is more common in patients with impaired renal function. However, the drug appears to be of use in ocular inflammations not responding to combinations of polymyxin B with neomycin or as a substitute following the development of hypersensitivity.

Tetracyclines. Tetracycline (Achromycin) and the substituted tetracyclines, chlortetracycline (Aureomycin), oxytetracycline (Terramycin), and demethylchlortetracycline (Declomycin), are essentially bacteriostatic and inhibit a broad range of gram-positive and gram-negative bacteria in addition to *Mycobacterium tuberculosis*, *Rickettsia*, Bedsoniae (psittacosis–lymphogranuloma venereum group of agents), and the agent (Eaton) of primary atypical pneumonia, *Mycoplasma pneumoniae*. The compounds penetrate the intact blood-aqueous barrier poorly. In recent years resistant strains have developed during the course of therapy, and after suppression of susceptible microflora the superimposition of resistant strains has developed. Tetracyclines are usually administered orally and may give rise to nausea, vomiting, and diarrhea. Outdated tetracycline may cause nephrotoxicity. Discoloration of developing teeth and fatal hepatic necrosis in pregnant women have been reported. Demethylchlortetracycline causes photosensitivity in some individuals.

The tetracyclines concentrate in the mitochondria of fast-growing tissues, liver, tumors, and areas of new bone formation. The fluorescence of the tetracyclines has thus been used as a diagnostic test of areas where tumor cells are easily available such as the lung or stomach. Most orbital neoplasms fluoresce well following administration of 1 Gm. of oxytetracycline three times daily for 3 days. However, malignant melanomas of the uveal tract do not fluoresce. A number of tetracyclines are available for local use. The compounds have a low antigenicity, and sensitivity reactions are uncommon.

Chloramphenicol (Chloromycetin). Chloramphenicol (Chloromycetin) is a potent inhibitor of microbial protein synthesis and is effective against approximately the same organisms as the tetracyclines. The drug is well absorbed from the gastrointestinal tract and penetrates the blood-aqueous barrier well. High intraocular concentrations are possible following systemic use. Chloramphenicol may cause a reversible anemia as well as fatal aplastic anemia in rare instances. This has limited its systemic use to those diseases for which no other effective antibiotic is available. Optic and retrobulbar neuritis (p. 282) and peripheral neuritis have been described in patients with cystic fibrosis who have received systemic chloramphenicol for at least 12 weeks.

Chloramphenicol is particularly valuable for local instillation. The likelihood of inducing aplastic anemia by this route is extremely remote. It has a low antigenicity and a broad spectrum and is probably the most widely used local antibiotic in ophthalmology that is also used systemically. It is particularly useful topically in combination with systemic administration of other antibiotics in the treatment of infectious endophthalmitis.

Lincomycin (Lincocin). Lincomycin (Lincocin) is effective against most gram-positive bacteria including some strains of *Staphylococcus* that are penicillin resistant. It is primarily bacteriostatic but may be bactericidal in a dosage range up to 30 times that required to produce bacteriostasis. It inhibits bacterial growth by interfering with protein synthesis. It may be administered orally, intravenously, and intramuscularly. High intraocular levels are obtained. Diarrhea is the major toxic manifestation of oral administration. Experience with this compound is limited, but its chief value would appear to be as an alternative drug in penicillin-sensitive individuals.

Erythromycin. Erythromycin is active against gram-positive microorganisms and some strains of gram-negative bacteria. *Staphylococcus* rapidly develops resistance. When administered systemically, the compound penetrates the eye poorly. The topical administration is fairly well limited to instances of specific bacterial sensitivity and would be the second or third choice.

Corticosteroid combinations. A variety of antibiotics for topical use have been combined with corticosteroids for the treatment of conjunctival and lid inflammations. For the most part, such combinations are not indicated. The corticosteroids reduce local tissue immunity and induce increased resistance to the outflow of aqueous and to the development of glaucoma in susceptible eyes. The combination of a cortico-

steroid and an antibiotic may facilitate the development of a fungal keratoconjunctivitis. Additionally, the combination is expensive and does not permit the administration of the two drugs at different time intervals. The effects of the antibiotic on the microorganism may also be obscured by the anti-inflammatory action of the corticosteroid.

Antifungal antibiotics. There are only three useful antifungal antibiotics: amphotericin B, griseofulvin, and nystatin.

Amphotericin B. Amphotericin B inhibits a wide variety of fungi as well as protozoa, flatworms, snails, and higher algae, but not bacteria. The drug is administered intravenously and causes mild renal damage in total dosages between 5 and 10 Gm. and severe damage in total dosages of more than 10 Gm. If the blood urea nitrogen level exceeds 40 mg./100 ml., the drug should be discontinued until the level falls to normal.

Nystatin. Nystatin is administered topically in a concentration of 100,000 units/ml. of commercial diluent in demonstrated fungus infections of the anterior ocular segment. Its main value is in the treatment of superficial *Candida* infection and it is ineffective in cutaneous dermatophyte infections. It does, however, inhibit a wide range of fungi. It is not absorbed from the gastrointestinal tract, but its toxicity is such that it cannot be used intravenously.

Griseofulvin. Griseofulvin is effective in the treatment of infections of the hair, skin, and nails caused by dermatophytes. Infection of the eye or ocular adnexa by fungi sensitive to the antibiotic is extremely uncommon.

Sulfonamides. The sulfonamides are effective because they compete with para-aminobenzoic acids required by microorganisms for the synthesis of folic acid. Sulfonamides have a definite but limited usefulness in the treatment of infections and the management of certain other diseases.

They have a wide antibacterial spectrum, but if resistance develops to one sulfonamide, then cross-resistance to all derivatives is observed. Similarly, cross-sensitivity occurs and therefore no sulfonamide is safe once a patient demonstrates a hypersensitivity reaction to any derivative.

For the most part, the sulfonamides are fairly insoluble, and therapeutic concentrations are not obtained with most compounds when used locally. Two compounds are used locally in ophthalmology, sulfacetamide (Sulamyd) and sulfisoxazole (Gantrisin).

Sulfacetamide (Sulamyd). Sulfacetamide (Sulamyd) is used in a 30% solution and 10% ointment. It is probably the most useful of the sulfonamide compounds for local use. It is minimally antigenetic, and hypersensitivity reactions are rarely observed.

Sulfisoxazole (Gantrisin). Sulfisoxazole (Gantrisin) is used locally in a 4% solution. A white precipitate of the drug may gather at the canthus. Other sulfonamides should not be used for local therapy.

• • •

Short-acting sulfonamides such as sulfadiazine are used in the treatment of toxoplasmosis in conjunction with pyrimethamine and in conjunction with tetracycline in the management of *Bedsoniae* infections.

Virus chemotherapy

Virus chemotherapy dates from 1962 when idoxyuridine was shown to be effective against herpes simplex keratitis. Thus far herpes simplex keratitis has been most effectively treated, although medications are available for the treatment of vaccinia and smallpox.

Idoxyuridine (IDU, 5-iodo-2-deoxyuridine). This antimetabolite has its widest application in herpes simplex keratitis, where a high local tissue concentration may be obtained with no systemic toxicity. IDU inhibits DNA synthesis of the cell at the stage of the final phosphorylation of thymidine and its polymerization into DNA. It is used locally in 0.1% concentration every hour, day and night, in the acute phase of herpes simplex keratitis. Following clinical improvement, the frequency of administration is gradually reduced. Corticosteroids, which are contraindicated in herpes simplex infections, may be employed on occasion for stromal involvement if IDU is used.

A variety of antimetabolites are effective against the herpes simplex virus, but many cause corneal clouding and other toxic reactions. A search thus continues for compounds with a higher therapeutic index than IDU.

Heavy metals. Mercuric chloride is used locally, mainly in an ointment base. Metaphen is used in a 1:2,500 ointment in the conjunctival sac.

Silver nitrate is used as a 1% solution in Credé's prophylaxis of ophthalmia neonatorum (p. 174). It is effective through precipitation of protein, including that of bacteria, and reacts with the sodium chloride of tissues to form insoluble silver chloride. The silver proteinate salts have largely been abandoned in ophthalmic therapeutics. Zinc sulfate is a specific for the diplobacillus of Morax-Axenfeld (p. 171), but antibiotics are superior for this purpose. Zinc sulfate is used as an astringent in many collyria and nonspecific eye preparations for nonspecific eye disabilities.

Corticosteroids and ACTH

The adrenal gland consists of the medulla and the cortex. The medulla secretes epinephrine mainly and possibly a small amount of norepinephrine. The adrenal cortex produces three groups of hormones: (1) the androgenic steroids, concerned with the development of secondary sex characteristics; (2) the mineralocorticoids, mainly aldosterone and desoxycorticosterone, which are concerned with fluid and electrolyte metabolism; and (3) the glucocorticoids, mainly corticosterone and hydrocortisone, which act on the metabolism of carbohydrates, proteins, fats, electrolytes, and water. The glucocorticoids are of main ophthalmic interest.

Corticotropin (ACTH). One of the secretory products of the anterior lobe of the pituitary gland stimulates the cortex of the adrenal gland to synthesize corticosteroids from cholesterol. This adrenocorticotropic hormone (ACTH) is released from the pituitary gland in response to stimulation by the hypothalamus. The release of corticotropins is inhibited by elevated blood levels of adrenal steroids and enhanced by low blood levels of adrenal steroids. Administration of ACTH causes hypertrophy of the adrenal glands. Administration of adrenal steroids may cause atrophy of the adrenal glands inasmuch as the exogenous corticosteroids inhibit release of ACTH by the pituitary gland and remove the normal adrenal cortex stimulation.

Corticosteroids. A large variety of corticosteroids has been proposed for systemic and local anti-inflammatory activity in ophthalmic disease. The synthetic compounds have more marked pharmacologic action than the naturally occurring hydrocortisone and corticosterone, which must be converted to hydrocortisone to have anti-inflammatory activity. The anti-inflammatory actions parallel the facilitation of gluconeogenesis.

Corticosteroids are mainly effective in suppressing the manifestation of inflammation without affecting the actual cause of inflammatory action. Thus the drugs are most useful in self-limited or intermittent disease processes, permitting decrease of acute inflammatory disease until a remission occurs. Inflammations involving the posterior ocular segment require systemic administration of the compounds. Inflammation of the eyelids, cornea, conjunctiva, and anterior segment of the eye usually respond to topical administration in adequate dosage. In inflammations of the anterior segment it may be desirable to supplement topical administration by systemic administration. Subconjunctival injections are occasionally used, but the vehicle may remain beneath the conjunctiva for long periods.

Fungus infections of the cornea are particularly prone to develop in eyes in which there has been long-term treatment with local corticosteroid preparations or antibiotics. A fungus infection must be suspected in any persistent corneal ulceration that has been treated for a long period with these compounds.

Local tissue immunity confines most herpes simplex (p. 205) inflammations of the cornea to the epithelium. If corticosteroid preparations are used locally, this tissue immunity is destroyed, and the virus not only involves additional epithelium but may also cause necrotic lesions of the stroma. This necrosis can cause so much tissue destruction that the cornea ruptures. Frequently when corticosteroids are used there is relief of symptoms and a decrease of ciliary injection so that the patient is unaware of the aggravation of the disease, although the disease continues to progress.

Frequent local instillation of corticosteroids may delay fibroblastic regeneration. For the most part, it is difficult by means of systemic administration to obtain a concentration adequate to interfere with wound healing. However, the abdominal striae seen in Cushing's disease are ample evidence that systemic corticosteroids may interfere with wound healing. Despite the demonstration of interference with stromal regeneration by these drugs, their use postoperatively, particularly in corneal transplants and sometimes in other surgical procedures, does not appear to affect wound healing adversely. Attempts to enhance the effects of glaucoma filtering operations or to prevent neovascularization of corneal transplants by the use of steroids have not been successful.

In recent years it has been demonstrated

that repeated instillation of some cortico-steroid preparations into the conjunctival sac will cause a marked decrease in the coefficient of outflow within 1 to 3 weeks (p. 306). This condition in all respects re-sembles open-angle glaucoma, and if the drug is continued, optic atrophy, excava-tion of the optic disk, and typical glau-comatous field defects will occur. The sus-ceptibility of eyes to the local instillation of steroids is an inherited characteristic and suggests that a single enzymatic defect occurring at the level of the trabecular meshwork is responsible for this type of glaucoma. Instillation of steroids may be used as a provocative test in open-angle glaucoma. However, not all patients who have positive test results develop overt glaucoma (p. 306).

Patients with rheumatoid arthritis who receive systemic corticosteroids in high doses for a long period may develop pos-terior subcapsular cataract. The cataract reduces vision and may require removal. Patients receiving steroids for rheumatoid arthritis are particularly prone to cataract formation—it does not occur as commonly in patients with ulcerative colitis or asthma. This difference in incidence may reflect genetic variations. Local administra-tion of corticosteroids may also be asso-ciated with cataract formation.

Retinal microaneurysms occur rarely in patients receiving corticosteroids over a long period. Papilledema has been ob-served in children receiving triamcinolone or prednisone for a long period.

Systemic administration of the com-pounds may be associated with a number of the following side effects:

Increased gluconeo-genesis	Decreased eosinophils
Inhibition of peripheral glucose utilization	Decreased lymphocytes
	Euphoria
Increased liver glyco-gen	Increased uric acid excretion
Hyperglycemia	Cushing's disease
Glycosuria	Moonface
Inhibited protein anabolism	Hirsutism
	Acne
	Amenorrhea

Inhibition of antibody production	Osteoporosis
Fat mobilization	Muscle wasting
Sodium retention	Hypertension
Potassium excretion	Psychotic manifesta-tions
Inhibition of inflamma-tion	Aggravation of peptic ulcer

It is desirable to use the minimal amount of corticosteroid for as short a period of time as possible. If the compound has been systemically administered for several weeks, it is desirable to reduce the medica-tion gradually because abrupt termination of the treatment may result in an adrenal crisis.

Complications of topical administration of drugs

A surprising number of ocular conditions are either induced, persist, or are aggra-vated because of overtreatment with drugs used locally. Inasmuch as many eye dis-eases are self-limiting, in the absence of exact diagnosis there is no indication for the local instillation of medication.

Mechanical injury

Physicians, nurses, and patients instilling medications into the eye by means of an eyedropper should be instructed to place the eyedropper so that its long axis par-allels the lid margin. If the patient lunges forward, then he is not struck by the end of the eyedropper but by its side. Patients should be reassured that the conjunctival sac holds but a single drop and that exact measurement of a single drop is not neces-sary because the excess medication over-flows.

Pigmentation

Prolonged instillation of various com-pounds may cause pigmentation of the conjunctiva and the lids. For the most part, these are now curiosities and are observed only in patients who used silver and mer-cury preparations in years past. Persistent use of silver preparations causes a condi-tion of argyrosis. Metallic silver is deposited in the conjunctival area—it is particularly evident in the fornices where it causes a slate-gray color. On microscopic examination it is seen to arise from minute, closely packed dots of gray-black matter that have been shown to be metallic silver. There is no effective treatment.

Mercury preparations such as ammoniated mercury or yellow oxide of mercury may cause a similar type of pigmentation from mercury deposition if used for a long period.

Epinephrine used locally over a long period may cause an unusual pigmentation of the lid margins that gives rise to an appearance not unlike that which follows the use of eye makeup. More common is a sharply defined, rounded black area of melanin pigmentation arising from the conversion of epinephrine to adrenochrome in conjunctival cysts, followed by melanin deposition. Dense black corneal pigmentation has also been described.

Ocular injury

A number of compounds may cause direct ocular injury upon instillation. Silver nitrate in concentrations of more than 5% may cause necrosis of the cornea. In the use of 1% silver nitrate in Credé's prophylaxis, one may be assured of a proper concentration by using the wax ampules distributed for this purpose. Physicians who cauterize umbilical cords with silver nitrate find silver nitrate sticks safer to use than strong solutions.

A variety of compounds may cause minute epithelial defects of the cornea, which produce a foreign body sensation. Compounds that denature the protein of the corneal epithelium, such as alcohol and Zephiran, are common offenders. These may be brought to the eye on instruments used for minor ocular surgery. Strong solutions of local anesthetics may cause a white precipitate in the superficial corneal epithelium, which usually disappears when irrigated with distilled water. Compounds

prepared for use on other mucous membranes may injure the corneal epithelium.

Cocaine solutions are markedly hypotonic to the tears and cause desiccation of the corneal epithelium, which may then be removed easily. Cocaine is an excellent local anesthetic, and its use in surgery is sometimes desirable because it produces local vasoconstriction and moderate dilation of the pupil. Many believe that the ease with which epithelium is removed following its use constitutes an overwhelming disadvantage.

Sensitivity reactions

Nearly any compound that is applied frequently to the lids and the conjunctiva may be responsible for causing a contact dermatitis and conjunctivitis. Repeated instillation of drugs such as pilocarpine, which is required in the treatment of glaucoma, may give rise to conjunctival irritation or to a hypersensitivity with many follicles evident in the lower lid.

Contact dermatitis of the skin characterized by an erythematous, desquamating, irritable lesion localized to the lid may be caused by a number of compounds. Adhesive tape, nail polish, and cosmetics are particular offenders. Of the compounds used in local therapy, the sulfonamides, particularly sulfathiazole, and the antibiotics, particularly penicillin and streptomycin, are common offenders. Locally applied antihistamines may cause reactions that may be unrecognized inasmuch as the compounds have been prescribed for a preexisting reaction. Local anesthetics are also a common cause of dermatitis medicamentosa.

Delay of corneal epithelization

Small defects in the cornea heal by sliding of adjacent epithelium; large defects heal by mitosis and sliding of adjacent epithelium (p. 71). Many of the compounds used in ocular therapeutics delay mitosis but have no effect upon epithelial sliding.

Particular offenders are anesthetic solutions and ointments containing lanolin.

Pupillary constriction

Compounds used to produce miosis may give rise to a surprising number of minor and major complaints. The extreme miosis produced by the alkyl phosphates combined with swelling of the ciliary body may cause a physiologic iris bombé with the production of angle-closure glaucoma in susceptible individuals. Marked miosis has been considered a cause of retinal detachment, with traction of the zonular fibers extending back to the anterior retina.

In patients with minor lens opacities, constriction of the pupil may cause a severe diminution in vision that is not present when the pupil is of normal size. The reduction in vision presents a difficult problem in the management of glaucoma in patients with cataract and may necessitate a sector iridectomy, although the patient's glaucoma is adequately controlled with medication and the cataract is not sufficiently opaque to require surgery. In children in whom miotics are used in the treatment of accommodative strabismus, cysts may form at the pupillary margin involving the pigment epithelium. The use of phenylephrine immediately following the instillation of the miotic prevents the development of cysts.

Cataracts occur commonly in patients with glaucoma and are thought to be a part of the glaucomatous process. In recent years it has been demonstrated that the local instillation of compounds used to induce miosis such as pilocarpine and especially strong anticholinesterase drugs such as echothiophate iodide are associated with progressive lens opacities. The opacities consist of minute vacuoles beneath the anterior lens capsule and progressive nuclear sclerosis.

Systemic reactions

The eye may be involved in a variety of reactions following the systemic administration of drugs. Occasionally ocular reactions do not occur in experimental animals, and severe eye lesions may be produced before the relationship between the eye abnormality and the drug is suspected.

Systemic reactions to local instillation

Absorption of atropine, pilocarpine, sympathetic amines, or cholinesterase inhibitors through the mucous membranes of the nose or the lacrimal passages may give rise to characteristic systemic pharmacologic responses. Such reactions are more common with these drugs than with others inasmuch as 1 drop of the ophthalmic preparation (0.15 ml.) may be comparable to, or exceed, the therapeutic systemic dose (Table 3-1).

Drugs should be prevented from entering the nasolacrimal duct by maintaining pressure over the inner corner of the closed eyelids for 2 minutes after instillation. Atropine and scopolamine are often administered either in an oily solution or in ointment to minimize absorption.

Atropine poisoning develops quickly, with dryness and burning of the mouth

Table 3-1. Therapeutic dose of eye medications

	Dosage	
	1 drop	*Therapeutic*
1% atropine	0.75 mg.	0.6 mg.
4% pilocarpine	3.0 mg.	5.0 mg.
0.25% echothiophate iodide	0.16 mg.	Too toxic for systemic therapy
10% phenylephrine	7.5 mg.	5.0 mg.

and difficulty in talking and swallowing. There is intense thirst. The pupils are dilated, and accommodation is paralyzed. The skin becomes flushed, hot, and dry, and a high fever develops. Treatment is symptomatic—reduce the fever with ice packs or sponging and, if necessary, maintain respiration with a respirator.

Pilocarpine poisoning occurs most commonly in the management of angle-closure glaucoma in which a high concentration of the drug is instilled frequently. Sweating and the flow of saliva are stimulated, and vomiting may occur. These are all effects commonly attributed to angle-closure glaucoma.

The anticholinesterase agents, particularly the alkyl phosphates, significantly depress the erythrocyte cholinesterase levels. Systemic absorption may cause diarrhea, abdominal cramps, and the signs and symptoms of an acute abdominal or other gastrointestinal disturbance. Laparatomy has been performed in patients with a poor history.

Phenylephrine (Neo-Synephrine), when absorbed, may cause a marked increase in systolic and diastolic blood pressure. This has been reported as causing a cerebrovascular accident.

Alcohol

Ethyl alcohol, a central nervous system depressant, in large doses causes an esophoria with an accompanying diplopia that the intoxicated individual may not recognize. The condition known as alcohol amblyopia is solely a nutritional deficiency with an accompanying optic neuropathy that causes reduced central visual acuity with a central scotoma. It arises because of reduced food intake and a lack of vitamins, particularly the B complex group. It may be corrected in its early stages by an adequate diet and the administration of large doses of vitamin B, even though excessive use of alcohol continues.

The ingestion of methyl alcohol may cause a fatal acidosis accompanied by abdominal pain, vomiting, and signs of severe intoxication. In patients who survive, severe primary optic atrophy and blindness may occur. The acidosis must be combated by the administration of alkali. Ethyl alcohol in large doses competes successfully with methyl alcohol for metabolic sites and may prevent blindness.

Most central nervous system depressants may give rise to muscle weakness with diplopia and, on occasion, blurred vision. In some instances these compounds aggravate preexisting muscular defects or cause nystagmus. The eye signs are usually reversible with reduced intake of the medication.

Chloroquine

Chloroquine is an antimalarial agent in common use for the treatment of lupus erythematosus, arthritis, and other connective tissue disorders. Prolonged administration of high doses may give rise to a keratopathy, myopathy, or retinopathy. Generally the total chloroquine dosage must exceed 100 Gm. and the drug must be used for more than a year before a retinopathy develops. The drug may be retained in the body for years after administration has been stopped, and the retinopathy may develop several years after it has been discontinued.

Chloroquine keratopathy is a reversible deposition of chloroquine in the cornea. With the slit lamp, minute whitish dots distributed in a whorl pattern can be observed. Patients complain of "glare," ill-defined blurring of vision, and iridescent vision, the halo surrounding lights being identical to that in glaucoma. The condition is entirely reversible upon discontinuing the drug, and it may disappear spontaneously even if the drug is continued.

Chloroquine retinopathy is a serious pigmentary degeneration of the retina that may progress to complete loss of vision. Initially there is a minute degree of pigment clumping in the macular area. A characteristic "bull's-eye" or "doughnut" retinal lesion develops, which may be incomplete. This is followed by a stippled or hyperpigmentation of the fovea centralis, surrounded by a clear zone of depigmentation, which in turn is circled by another ring of pigment. In the end stages there is widespread retinal atrophy, pigment clumping, and threadlike retinal vessels.

Patients requiring chloroquine therapy should be followed up with repeated ophthalmoscopy and careful study of the central visual field for the development of paracentral scotomas.

Quinine

Quinine has long been known as a compound causing damage to the retinal ganglion cells with associated constriction of the retinal arterioles in susceptible individuals. In such persons the administration of even a small amount of quinine (as little as that contained in quinine water) may be followed by constriction of the visual field to a central area 5° or 10° in diameter. There may be associated deafness and other signs of central nervous system damage. The abnormality is usually reversible, but continued ingestion of quinine may cause irreversible constriction of the visual fields, impaired dark adaptation, and loss of central visual acuity.

In rare instances severe atrophy of the pigment epithelium of the iris may follow the quinine amblyopia. The pupils do not react to light in the area of iris atrophy (p. 227). The condition is presumably caused by ischemia of the anterior portion of the eye.

Digitalis

Digitalis toxicity may be associated with disturbed vision in which objects may appear to be covered with frost or have a pale yellow color, or flashing lights may be present. Usually visual symptoms are associated with nausea, vomiting, and bradycardia at high dosage levels, but they may occur in patients using the drug in a therapeutic range. A similar xanthanopsia has been attributed to systemic effects of chlorothiazide and also to aspidium (male fern).

Oral contraceptives

The agents most commonly employed for oral contraceptive therapy are progestin and estrogen in combination or in sequence. These potent drugs are widely used and have been suggested as playing a causative role in occlusive vascular disease in certain patients. Women with vascular hypertension, migraine, or vascular disease are thought to be especially vulnerable. Brain infarction may be associated with ocular signs, depending upon the area of the brain involved. Papilledema and optic neuritis (papillitis or retrobulbar neuritis) appear to occur more commonly in women using contraceptive therapy than in others. However, the role of these agents is not definitely known. It is believed that the indications for using oral contraceptives should be carefully weighed in each case and that the patient should not receive them for long periods without medical supervision. They should be discontinued in the event of thromboembolic disease, neurologic disease, or suggestion of liver damage.

Some wearers of contact lenses develop an intolerance to the lenses while receiving oral contraceptives. Often this is characterized by photophobia, increased irritation caused by the lenses, and prolonged recovery from corneal edema associated with the wearing of the lenses.

Induced refractive errors

A large variety of compounds may cause a spasm of a ciliary muscle or increased refractive power of the lens. The sulfonamides and related compounds, particularly Diamox, may increase the refractive power of the lens. All of the anticholinesterase compounds may cause ciliary spasm and miosis. Many insecticides are anticholinesterases, and spasm of accommodation combined with pupillary constriction has been described as a cause of the crash of a crop-dusting airplane. Increased refractive power or sustained accommodation reduces hyperopia or increases myopia.

The ganglionic blocking agents used in the treatment of vascular hypertension cause a decrease in accommodation that many patients in the younger age groups find extremely annoying. This may be associated with the dilation of the conjunctival blood vessels, giving the appearance of conjunctivitis. The loss of accommodation may have to be corrected by means of bifocal lenses. The conjunctival injection may be alleviated slightly by the local instillation of a vasoconstrictor such as 1:1,000 epinephrine.

Optic atrophy

A large variety of compounds have been reported as causing optic atrophy. These include chloramphenicol, streptomycin, sulfonamides, and isoniazid. Tryparsamide, a pentavalent arsenical previously used in the therapy of central nervous system syphilis, has a direct toxic effect upon the optic nerve.

Erythema multiforme

Sulfonamides are particularly associated with the development of erythema multiforme exudativum. When the eyes are involved, this is usually called Stevens-Johnson syndrome. Many other compounds in common use have been considered as precipitating factors, such as the penicillins, thiouracil, salicylates, codeine, and anticonvulsant medications. The condition is characterized by the occurrence of severe bullous skin lesions, mucous membrane vesiculation and erosion, and involvement of the conjunctiva. It gives rise to severe scarring, symblepharon formation, decreased tears, and lid deformities. The condition is frequently preceded by a systemic disease for which the offending drug is prescribed, and the ocular disease may not be recognized.

Hypercalcemia

Markedly increased blood calcium may give rise to the deposition of calcium salts in the conjunctiva and the cornea (p. 201). The interpalpebral conjunctiva is injected, and biomicroscopic examination indicates crystals in the cornea and in the conjunctiva. The condition is associated with the administration of calcium carbonate and milk (milk-alkali syndrome), an excess of the parathyroid hormone, or excessive ingestion of vitamin D.

Hypercarotenemia

Carotenoids are pigments, the molecule of which usually contains 40 carbon atoms. They are of ophthalmic interest because of the combination of vitamin A and a carotenoid prosthetic group to form visual pigments. Carotenoids contribute the yellow-colored xanthomas and atheromas associated with hyperlipidemia. Excessive ingestion of plants containing carotenoids (2 or more quarts of carrot juice daily for 1½ years) may give rise to a yellow-orange pigmentation of the skin, which starts in the nasolabial folds and palms of the hands and gradually spreads over the entire body. The conjunctiva is diffusely pigmented and has a yellowish color similar to that seen in jaundice.

Vitamin A

Prolonged high doses of vitamin A may give rise to a deposition of the vitamin A pigment (carotenosis) in the skin and in the conjunctiva, which simulates the appearance of jaundice. Papilledema and retinal hemorrhages have also been reported.

Part II

History taking
and examination
of the eye

Chapter 4

History and interpretation

The provisional diagnosis of disease, the clinical examination, and the selection of the most appropriate laboratory studies must be based upon an analysis of the most probable cause of the symptoms. Clinical skill in large measure reflects the ability of the physician to make a correct diagnosis by correlating the relationship of symptoms and signs, the association of which is frequently obscured by a mass of irrelevant details.

The main symptoms of ocular abnormality include the following: (1) disturbances of vision; (2) pain in one or both eyes or in the head; (3) abnormal secretion from the eyes; and (4) physical signs described by the patient as symptoms.

Disturbances of vision

A visual abnormality may arise because of (1) a defect in image formation, (2) an interference with impulse transmission in the visual pathways, and (3) an abnormality in the visual perceptual centers. A defect in image formation is due to an abnormality within the eye itself. Both eyes may be involved, but often one eye is more severely affected. If the defect is eliminated by lenses, it is likely due to a refractive error and not organic disease. If there is interference in nervous impulse transmission anterior to the chiasm, only one eye is involved. If there is interference at the chiasm or posterior to this, both eyes are involved. Visual perceptual defects often produce bizarre patterns of inability to recognize objects. The physician must

learn, therefore, whether the defect involves one or both eyes, if it disappears when correcting lenses are worn, if it is transient or permanent, if it is for distance or near vision or both, if it involves central or peripheral vision, and if the vision itself is normal with visual phenomena such as floaters superimposed. If the visual defect disappears when the patient wears correcting lenses, it should be evident that a refractive error is the most likely cause of symptoms. There are a number of individuals who require lenses and do not wish to wear them. They describe a variety of unusual, apparently inexplicable ocular symptoms that confuse the unwary. A detailed inquiry into such symptoms is seldom rewarding. Many individuals with psychologic disorders with ocular manifestations have accumulated many spectacles, all of which have failed to relieve their complaints. These patients may be anxious to acquire another pair of lenses and are most reluctant to recognize the psychologic basis of their complaints. Symptoms that involve near vision when the distance vision is normal or vice versa are most suggestive of a refractive error. One or both eyes may be involved.

A history of sudden, persistent unilateral decrease of vision is suggestive of a number of serious ocular disorders: angle-closure glaucoma, iridocyclitis, vitreous hemorrhage, retinal artery or vein closure, or optic neuritis. Decrease in vision in which there are episodes of visual loss varying from slight haziness to no light

123

Symptoms of eye disease

I. Disturbances of vision
  A. Decreased central visual acuity
    1. Near
    2. Distance
  B. Abnormal color vision
    1. Hereditary: bilateral
    2. Acquired: often unilateral
  C. Abnormal visual field
    1. Unilateral asymmetric defects in retinal and optic nerve diseases
    2. Bilateral symmetric defects in diseases at or posterior to chiasm
  D. Defective dark adaptation
  E. Iridescent vision ("halos")
  F. Floaters
  G. Photopsia
    1. Unilateral: retinal stimulus other than light
    2. Bilateral: visual hallucination
      a. Unformed: occipital lobe origin
      b. Formed: temporal lobe origin
  H. Micropsia and macropsia
    1. Fovea centralis abnormality
  I. Cortical blindness: bilateral lesions of occipital cortex
  J. Perceptual blindness: lesions of angular gyrus of parieto-occipital fissure
  K. Diplopia
    1. Physiologic
    2. Monocular: local disturbance of one eye
    3. Near only: convergence abnormality
    4. Distance only: divergence abnormality
    5. Varying with eye or head movements: ocular muscle weakness

II. Pain in one or both eyes or in the head
  A. Superficial foreign body sensation
  B. Deep pain within the eye
  C. Headache
  D. Burning, itching, "tired" eyes
  E. Photophobia

III. Abnormal secretion from eyes
  A. Lacrimation (excessive tear production)
  B. Epiphora (defective tear drainage)
  C. Mucus
  D. Pus
  E. Dry eyes

IV. Physical signs described by the patient as symptoms
  A. Red eye
    1. Conjunctival injection
    2. Ciliary injection
    3. Subconjunctival hemorrhage
  B. New growths
  C. Abnormal position of eyes or eyelids
  D. Protrusion of globe
  E. Widened palpebral fissure
  F. Narrowed palpebral fissure
  G. Pupillary abnormality

perception and lasting for a few seconds to minutes may arise from spasm of the ophthalmic artery in occlusive disease of the internal carotid artery or from abnormalities of the aortic arch (p. 422). Gradual unilateral loss of vision may occur with corneal disease, glaucoma, cataract, vitreous opacities, retinal detachment, macular degeneration, or intraocular inflammation.

Sudden loss of vision involving both eyes occurs uncommonly. Inquiry usually indicates that vision failed first in one eye and that the sudden loss described was noted by the patient when vision in the fellow eye became involved. Both eyes may be involved in the diseases that cause sudden unilateral loss of vision, but this occurs rarely. A sudden bilateral decrease of vision is most suggestive of hysteria, the toxic effects of drugs, or poor observation.

Gradual loss of vision in both eyes may arise from nearly any ophthalmic disorder. In the main, if central vision is involved and peripheral vision is intact, the disorder must be anterior to the chiasm. If peripheral vision is involved in both eyes, the disorder may be at the chiasm or posterior to it.

Color vision. Color vision is solely a cone function. A deficiency in color perception is inherited in approximately 7% of males and 0.5% of females. Central vision in these individuals is normal, but color perception is depressed. Acquired unilateral depression of color sense occurs in diseases affecting the cone function of one eye, mainly macular degeneration and optic nerve disease. Loss of central visual acuity parallels the loss of color discrimination. Bilateral acquired depression in color vision may occur in malnutrition and following the ingestion of toxic drugs. Color vision may be uniformly depressed, but not lost, by opacities of the ocular media, particularly those involving the cornea (leukoma) or lens (cataract).

Peripheral vision. The retinal periphery contains rods mainly, but a few cones are scattered throughout. A defect in the visual field may occur in many abnormalities of the retina, optic nerve, and optic pathways. If the abnormality is anterior to the chiasm, the defect is unilateral. Diseases involving the chiasm or visual pathways involve both eyes. When one eye is involved in retinal or optic nerve disease, the patient frequently describes the sensation of a curtain falling over a portion of the visual field. When both eyes are involved, the patient may be unaware of the defect. Cortical blindness is characterized by unawareness of visual loss.

Defects in the visual fields are usually described as central or peripheral. Central field defects are usually measured on a tangent screen (see Fig. 6-4, *B*) and peripheral field defects on a perimeter (see Fig. 6-4, *A*). Localized areas of defective vision surrounded by areas of normal vision are called scotomas. These have been described as islands of blindness in a sea of vision. Central scotomas involve the fixation point, and paracentral scotomas involve an area adjacent to the fixation point (Fig. 4-1). Central scotomas characterize diseases involving the fovea centralis and the papillomacular bundle of nerve fibers in the optic nerve. Centrocecal scotomas (Fig. 4-2) involve both the physiologic blind spot and the fixation point and are characteristic of toxic diseases of the optic nerve. Annular scotomas form a circular defect around the fixation point and are particularly common in diseases that first manifest themselves at the equator of the eye, particularly retinal degenerations such as retinitis pigmentosa. Arcuate scotomas involve a bundle of nerve fibers and characterize the field defect of glaucoma.

Peripheral defects are described as temporal, nasal, superior, and inferior. It should be recalled that the visual field is a projection of visual function opposite to the areas of the retina involved. Thus a temporal defect in the visual field involves fibers of the nasal retina that decussate.

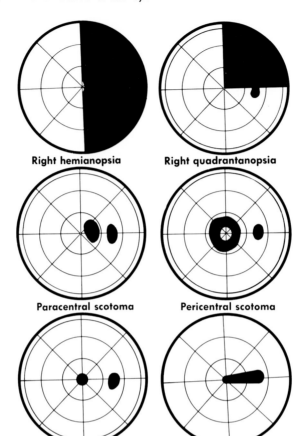

Fig. 4-1. Various types of central field defects. The blind spot is temporal to the point of fixation, and its location to the right of the fixation point indicates that all of these field defects involve the right eye.

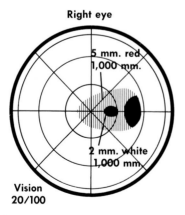

Fig. 4-2. Centrocecal scotoma with an absolute scotoma (in black) surrounded by a relative scotoma (in lines).

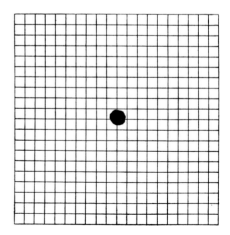

Fig. 4-3. Central scotoma projected onto the grid of an Amsler chart.

A superior field defect involves inferior retinal fibers.

Reference is always to the blind portion of the visual field. Hemianopsia means half-blindness. A right hemianopsia indicates a right half-blindness (Fig. 4-1) and must involve the fibers of the left half of the retina. Homonymous hemianopsia indicates involvement of the right or left portion of each visual field and thus interference with visual transmission posterior to the optic chiasm. (The term "heteronymous" is not used; a bitemporal hemianopsia that occurs in chiasmal disease is, however, heteronymous.)

Dark adaptation. Patients with organic disease with defective dark adaptation frequently do not complain of this defect. Conversely, patients without organic ocular disease not infrequently have numerous complaints of poor vision in reduced illumination. Optic nerve disease, glaucoma, tapetoretinal degenerations such as retinitis pigmentosa, and vitamin A deficiency occurring in cirrhosis of the liver or inadequate nutrition all cause defective dark adaptation. The defect commonly involves slow recovery of vision during night driving after the headlights of an oncoming car shine in the patient's eyes. Defective vision in bright illumination is mainly a sign of toxic involvement of the optic nerve.

Iridescent vision. This term is applied to the halos or rainbows seen surrounding bright lights when there is diffraction by the ocular media. The most common cause is edema of the cornea that may follow a rapid increase in intraocular pressure. Prolonged wearing of contact lenses and swimming in fresh water with the eyes open also cause corneal edema. Pus floating across the cornea in conjunctivitis may cause iridescence that disappears with rapid blinking. Corneal degeneration (dystrophy) and cataract may cause diffraction of light with the iridescent vision identical to that of corneal edema.

Floaters. Floaters are translucent specks of various shapes and sizes that float across the visual field. They can be seen only when the eye is open. Commonly the patient can observe them only when looking at a bright blue sky or a brilliantly illuminated pastel-colored wall. All individuals have small fixed flecks of protein in the vitreous body (muscae volitantes) seen as small dots that dart away as one tries to fix them. Lens opacities may cause fixed floaters. Leukocytes from inflammation of the retina or uvea may cause floaters, but usually such large numbers are present that vision is generally depressed. A sudden shower of floaters may occur in the periphery of the visual field with a vitreous hemorrhage. This may be the initial symptom of hole formation preceding retinal separation. The location of the floaters may be helpful in locating the retinal hole. The sudden appearance of a moderately large floater is an outstanding symptom of vitreous detachment. Rarely a patient learns inadvertently to observe entoptically the erythrocytes in his own capillaries and becomes concerned about the flecks that disturb his reading.

Photopsia. This term is applied to such visual phenomena as specks, rings, lightning flashes, and luminous bodies that are observed with the eyes closed. When unilateral, the condition is caused by an inadequate retinal stimulus, that is, a retinal stimulus other than light. It may occur in vitreous detachment, traction upon the retina, or pressure upon the closed eye.

In bilateral photopsia there are visual hallucinations. They are divided into formed and unformed. Formed visual hallucinations consist mainly of landscapes, prairie fires, seascapes, and similar scenes, usually with minimal detail and with repetitive activity. They are most characteristic of involvement of the visual tract in the temporal lobe. If a homonymous hemianopsia is present, the hallucinations are commonly on the side of the blindness.

Unformed visual hallucinations consist of lightning flashes and expanding circles of light called scintillating scotoma. They originate in the occipital lobe and are a cardinal sign of the aura of migraine.

Micropsia. Micropsia is an abnormality of image formation at the fovea in visual perception. Edema, tumors, and hemorrhages in the foveal region cause the cones to become spread farther apart and give rise to the perception that objects are smaller than they actually are.

Macropsia. Macropsia is an abnormality in which objects appear larger than they actually are. It arises from edema, tumors, and hemorrhages in the foveal region, causing the cones to be closer together.

Cortical blindness. Cortical blindness is an abnormality in perception arising from bilateral impairment of the visual centers of the occipital cortex (area 17). It is characterized by a loss of the visual sensation with retention of the pupillary reaction to light. The patient may not be aware of his loss of vision.

Perceptual blindness. Perceptual blindness is an abnormality caused by lesions in the angular gyrus of the parieto-occipital fissure in which individuals are unable to recognize objects visually (agnosia) but are able to recognize objects by touch or other sensory portals. An individual so afflicted will be unable to recognize a key when looking at it but will readily recognize it when touching it. Defects related to this condition include alexia (inability to read), agraphia (inability to write), and dyslexia (disturbance in the ability to read). These abnormalities may be highly selective and involve the reading of numbers and not the reading of letters and vice versa or involve written script but not printed matter.

Blindness. There are approximately 450,000 blind persons in the United States, and it is estimated that more than one half are 65 years old or over. The exact definition of blindness differs, but generally a person is considered legally blind when his best visual acuity with lenses in the better eye is 20/200 or less or when the peripheral visual field is contracted to within

Table 4-1. Central visual acuity in visually handicapped persons (better eye with best possible correction)*

Common definition	Snellen index	Practical test	Legal significance
Total blindness or light perception only	Less than 2/200	Unable to see hand movement at 3 feet	Satisfies all criteria for legal blindness†
Form and motion	Less than 5/200	Hand movement visible, but unable to count fingers at 3 feet	Total disability for Social Security Administration
Travel vision	Less than 10/200	Unable to read newspaper headlines	Legal blindness
Minimal reading	Less than 20/200	Reads headlines, but not 14-point (4.7 mm.) type	Maximum acuity for legal blindness for Internal Revenue Service and most state industrial commissions
Partially seeing (borderline)	More than 20/200, but less than 20/70	Cannot read 10-point (3.4 mm.) type without marked difficulty	Not legally blind, but eligible for some services

*From Wheeler, J. M.: Missouri Med. **64:**315, 1967.
†Legal blindness also present if visual field is contracted to 20° or less (tunnel vision).

20° (Table 4-1). The chief causes of blindness in the United States are glaucoma, cataract, and retinal disorders, mainly diabetic retinopathy.

The physician managing a blind patient must avoid the slightest hint of condescension and learn that the patient's interpretation of his voice and actions are the major factors in reassurance. A person talking to a blinded individual should identify himself by name, should not shout, should always give detailed verbal directions and not signals, and should always warn the patient before touching him.

A surprising number of blinded individuals are not aware of the agencies and services available to promote their adjustment and independence. Information may be obtained from the American Foundation for the Blind, 15 West 16th Street, New York, N. Y.

Diplopia. Diplopia, or double vision, occurs whenever the visual axes are not directed simultaneously to the same object. Unilateral diplopia is a curiosity in which light rays are split by an opacity in the cornea or lens so that a single object is imaged twice upon the retina. Frequently the images are so blurred that the patient notices the defect only under exceptional optical conditions.

Physiologic diplopia is a normal phenomenon in which objects not within the area of fixation are seen double. Usually it does not impinge upon the consciousness. It is easily demonstrated by looking at a near object with attention directed to a distant object that then appears doubled. Such physiologic diplopia contributes to parallax, which enables one to judge the distance of objects.

Diplopia is a cardinal sign of weakness of an extraocular muscle, and characteristically the separation of images increases in the field of action of the extraocular muscle involved. It must be recalled that diplopia can occur only if binocular vision has developed. The absence of diplopia thus does not indicate that a paresis of an extraocular muscle is not present. Diplopia may also occur without paresis if there is displacement of the globe so that the visual axes cannot be directed simultaneously to the same object.

Pain

Pain and aches in the region of the eye or in the head may be difficult to interpret and require considerable clinical skill in their evaluation. Some patients are phlegmatic about pain, the severity of which would be disabling to others. Moreover, pain is a subjective sensation, and considerable insight into a patient's usual response is required for evaluation.

A superficial foreign body sensation may be caused by a lesion in the lid, a foreign body on the cornea or the conjunctiva, inflammation of the cornea or the conjunctiva, or loss of conjunctival or corneal epithelium. A local anesthetic instilled in the conjunctival sac usually eliminates the sensation of a superficial foreign body but not that due to inflammation of the conjunctiva and the cornea. If the eyelid is drawn away from the globe, the sensation caused by a foreign body on the tarsal conjunctiva will be eliminated, whereas the sensation due to a foreign body on the cornea will continue. Patients invariably localize a foreign body sensation to the outer portion of the upper lid irrespective of its location.

A large number of relatively minor ocular abnormalities manifest themselves by burning, itching, and uncomfortable eyes. These symptoms may arise from an inadequately corrected refractive error, lack of sleep and fatigue, conjunctival irritation, and chronic conjunctivitis (p. 172). Extremely mild and nonspecific inflammation of the lid or the conjunctiva without obvious signs may cause ocular discomfort, particularly when the eyes are used intensively. Minor ocular irritation arising from prolonged use of the eyes is mainly without significance. Often the afflicted individual is unable to do essential reading without early fatigue but is able to read a novel or do other unnecessary light reading without discomfort.

The interpretation of headache as a symptom of ocular disease requires familiarity with its causes. Headaches that are relieved by salicylates are usually not caused by serious organic disease. Severe incapacitating headaches do not arise from uncorrected errors of refraction or from wearing the wrong lenses. Headaches that are present on awakening in the morning are not caused by excessive use of the eyes the previous night.

One should determine whether a headache is intermittent or continuous, its location in the head, and other associated signs. An aura followed by hemicrania, nausea, and vomiting is suggestive of migraine. A headache aggravated by straining and associated with vomiting without nausea is suggestive of an internal hydrocephalus. A severe frontal headache associated with paralysis of all of the ocular muscles is suggestive of an infraclinoid aneurysm of the internal carotid artery. If only the oculomotor nerve is involved, a supraclinoid aneurysm, possibly associated with subarachnoid bleeding, must be considered.

Deep severe pain within the eye may be present in a variety of disorders. The most important causes, inasmuch as they require immediate attention, are inflammations of the ciliary body and rapid increase in the intraocular pressure such as that occurring in angle-closure glaucoma. In each of these instances the eye is red, and vision is decreased.

Tic douloureux gives rise to a characteristic excruciating pain in the region of distribution of the sensory branches of the trigeminal nerve. Usually the history of episodic pain of a similar type alerts one to the nature of the disorder. Herpes zoster ophthalmicus may give rise to severe retrobulbar pain, which may precede the eruption by several days. Often the cause of the pain is not recognized until the typical eruption occurs in the area of distribution of the ophthalmic nerve. Postherpes zoster neuralgia may be extremely disabling in the elderly.

Photophobia is a reflex in which light stimulating the retina causes constriction of the pupil and pain. The term is widely used to indicate any discomfort arising from bright light, such as the reflection of a great amount of light from the sky or an unpleasant contrast between light and dark areas. Glare is the term given to excessive light directed into the eyes from a reflecting surface. A common sign of ocular neurosis is excessive sensitivity of the eye to light.

Abnormal secretion

It is frequently possible to make the diagnosis of an ocular disease by learning the nature of an abnormal secretion from the eyes (p. 172). Pus is found in the conjunctival sac in mucopurulent conjunctivitis. The lashes are frequently agglutinated to each other by drying pus, and it may be difficult to open the eyes in the morning. A foamy secretion at the inner canthus is produced by *Corynebacterium xerose*, which lives solely on desquamated epithelium. A stringy secretion with excoriation of the canthus characterizes the inflammation caused by the diplobacillus of Morax-Axenfeld. A tenacious, stringy secretion occurs in allergic inflammation of the conjunctiva.

A distinction is made between lacrimation (excessive production of tears) and tearing (epiphora), in which there is overflow of a normal amount of tears secondary to closure of some portion of the lacrimal drainage system. Generally the distinction is semantic only, but lacrimation arises from those diseases that cause reflex secretion of tears, whereas epiphora may be recognized by the abnormality of the drainage system. Persistent tearing of one or both eyes of an infant is a cardinal sign of congenital glaucoma. There is an associated corneal edema. Tearing in infancy may occur because of failure of the nasolacrimal duct to open as it normally does about the third week of life. Tearing also occurs in photophobia, in inflammations of the cornea and conjunctiva, and reflexly in inflammations of the ciliary body.

A decrease in tear formation occurs most commonly in Sjögren's syndrome, which is associated with arthritis, dry eyes (keratoconjunctivitis sicca), and decrease in saliva formation, in association with the laboratory signs of a widespread systemic infection. Dry eyes also occur in vitamin A deficiency and in cicatrizing lesions of the conjunctiva that close the orifices of the lacrimal glands. A juvenile form of erythema multiforme (Stevens-Johnson disease), trachoma, and chemical burns are the chief cause of such scarring.

Physical signs described by patient

Red eye. Red eye is a cardinal sign of ocular inflammation. It is customarily divided into ciliary and conjunctival injection (Table 4-2).

Ciliary injection involves branches of the anterior ciliary artery that become dilated in inflammations of the cornea, iris, and ciliary body and in angle-closure glaucoma. Each of these conditions is associated with loss of vision and very frequently with pain deep within the eye.

Conjunctival injection involves mainly the posterior conjunctival blood vessels that extend from the peripheral marginal arcade in the lid to anastomose with the anterior ciliary arteries at the corneoscleral limbus. The posterior conjunctival vessels are most numerous in the conjunctival fornix and are injected in conjunctival inflammations. There is never a loss of vision, and there is ocular discomfort rather than frank pain. Because the posterior conjunctival blood vessels are superficial, they are redder in color than the ciliary arteries, which are violet colored. The posterior conjunctival blood vessels move with the conjunctiva and are bleached with the local instillation of 1:1,000 epinephrine.

Subconjunctival hemorrhage occurs with the rupture of a small blood vessel beneath the conjunctiva and causes a bright red blotch of blood beneath the conjunctiva that frequently alarms the patient. The condition is nearly always unilateral, and

Table 4-2. Red eye

	Conjunctival injection	Ciliary injection
Blood vessels	Posterior conjunctival	Anterior ciliary
Location	Superficial conjunctiva, arise from marginal arcade in lids	Deep conjunctiva, extend anterior from rectus muscle insertion to superficial and deep corneal plexus
Appearance	Vessels superficial, red, movable with conjunctiva, most numerous in fornix, fade toward limbus	Vessels deep, violet, immovable, most numerous at limbus, fade toward fornix
1:1,000 epinephrine	Constricts vessels, "whitens" conjunctiva	No effect
Diseases	Conjunctivitis	Keratitis, iridocyclitis, angle-closure glaucoma
Associated signs	Cornea clear, pupil and iris normal, vision undisturbed, eye uncomfortable	Cornea cloudy, pupil distorted, iris pattern muddy, vision reduced, eye painful

the hemorrhage absorbs spontaneously. It is caused for the most part by the same mechanisms that cause the black-and-blue spots elsewhere. A subconjunctival hemorrhage that involves the entire bulbar conjunctiva following head injury is a serious sign and suggests either rupture of the posterior globe or a fracture of one of the bones of the orbit.

Other signs described by the patient as symptoms are discussed in the following chapter on ocular examination.

Chapter 5

Physical examination of the eyes

A skilled physician, consciously or unconsciously, is constantly and unobtrusively studying his patients for the physical basis of their symptoms. In the hope that eventually such observation will become second nature, students are often given a long list of physical signs to tick off. Rather than memorize such a list for each organ, it is far simpler to begin at the outer anatomic layer and progress inward, first considering anomalies of size, shape, and position of structures, then inflammations and degenerations, and finally the effects of systemic disease.

It is fairly simple in the initial meeting with the patient to note the diameter and shape of the head and the position of the eyes. Gross variations in the insertion of the canthal ligaments are observed easily and the obliquity of the palpebral fissure is readily evident. Simple observation reveals wrinkling of the forehead due to photophobia or an attempt to elevate a paralyzed upper lid in blepharoptosis. Close inspection is not necessary to reveal jaundice or injection of the conjunctival vessels. The position of the lid margins in relation to the eyeball should be evident, and it should be obvious if the individual is having considerable discomfort in holding the eyes open.

The presence or absence of entropion or ectropion is usually evident without formally inspecting the lid margins. In the course of visiting with the patient it should become evident whether the eyes move in unison and whether the movements seem entirely full.

More careful inspection may be carried out by means of a small penlight that will provide a concentrated beam of light upon the eye (Fig. 5-1). Better visualization of details may be obtained if good illumination is combined with inspection through a +10 or +15 diopter convex lens. Such a lens may also be used for indirect ophthalmoscopy and for inspection of dermatologic lesions. Better magnification may be obtained by means of a binocular loupe that provides magnification of three to five times.

External examination

Examination is carried out in a systematic manner beginning with the skin of the lids and continuing inward. First, the examiner notices the symmetry and width of the palpebral fissures and the position of the eyes. The lids usually conceal the corneoscleral limbus in the 12 and 6 o'clock meridians. Proptosis or retraction of the upper lid in thyroid disorders is often first manifest by exposure of a narrow rim of sclera in these meridians. Subtle proptosis and keratoconus are most easily appreciated by viewing from above and behind the contact of the cornea with the lower lid. The examiner stands behind the seated patient and looks over his brow (Fig. 5-2). By drawing the upper lids upward, any difference in prominence of the two eyes is easily noted. In keratoconus

133

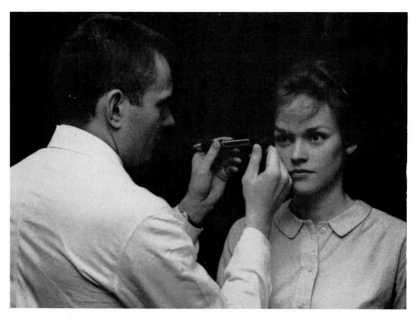

Fig. 5-1. Use of a penlight and a magnifying lens to study anterior segment details.

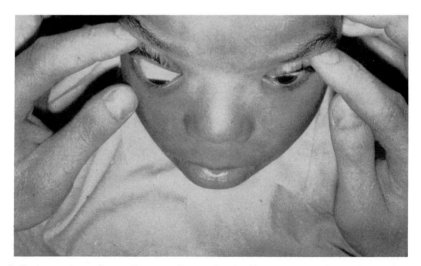

Fig. 5-2. Inspection of prominence of eyes by looking over the brow from above and behind.

the cornea distorts the lower lid outward (Munson's sign).

Lid margin. The cilia and the lid margin are inspected for the characteristic scaling of squamous blepharitis. Abnormalities in position of the lid margin are also noted at this time. Intermittent en-

tropion may be demonstrated if the patient squeezes his eyelids closed and then opens them. Particular attention is directed to the position of the puncta in relation to the lacrimal lake at the inner canthus. The inferior punctum should not be visible when the eyes are rotated up-

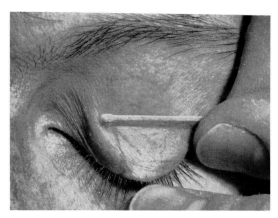

Fig. 5-3. Eversion of the upper lid. The patient must look downward; the eyelashes are grasped, and the lid is drawn outward and everted over an applicator placed at the superior palpebral fold.

ward. A frequent cause of tearing is slight eversion of the puncta. Sties involve the lid margin, whereas chalazia usually appear in the deeper substance of the lid.

Eversion of the upper lid. Inspection of the upper tarsal conjunctiva requires eversion of the upper lid that can be done only with the patient looking downward. It is nearly impossible to evert the upper lid if the patient looks in any other direction. With the patient looking downward, the lashes of the upper lid are grasped by the examiner between the thumb and the index finger. The lid is drawn gently outward to break the suction between the lid and the globe. The lid is then everted on a toothpick or applicator placed on the palpebral sulcus (Fig. 5-3). The tarsal conjunctiva is exposed, and the course of meibomian glands perpendicular to the lid margin can frequently be seen through the transparent tarsal conjunctiva. Frequently a small portion of the lacrimal gland may be seen at the outer canthus.

To inspect the superior fornix, it is first necessary to evert the upper lid and then expose the fornix by means of an instrument placed on the orbital portion of the lid. The conjunctiva here may contain follicles, and frequently several large blood vessels are evident.

Eversion of the lower lid. Inspection of the lower lid is performed easily. The patient looks upward, and the lid is drawn downward by the examiner's index finger applied to its orbital portion (Fig. 5-4). The lower tarsus is not nearly as wide as the upper tarsus. With the exception of trachoma and vernal catarrh, nearly all conjunctival inflammations are more marked in the inferior fornix than in the superior fornix.

Conjunctiva and cornea. The bulbar conjunctiva may be inspected directly. The caruncle is evident as a minute pink mass of tissue at the inner canthus. The semilunar fold is not markedly evident unless the conjunctiva is inflamed. The superior and inferior portions of the bulbar conjunctiva are inspected easily by having the patient look upward and downward while the lids are held apart.

Attention is directed to the diameter and the clarity of the cornea. A cornea measuring more than 10 mm. in diameter may indicate congenital glaucoma or megalocornea. Extremely small corneas in an adult are suggestive of microcornea, with which hyperopia and angle-closure glaucoma occur.

The evaluation of corneal clarity involves several factors. The anterior surface of the cornea should be smooth, regular, and mirrorlike. The iris pattern should be distinctly seen in all areas. Corneal blood vessels should not be present. In corneal edema the cornea has a subtle ground-glass appearance. Marked opacities are usually quite evident, but magnification is required for less severe defects. Corneal vascularization may be superficial or deep and may involve the entire cornea or merely a segment of it. Deep vascularization may be appreciated solely as a loss of corneal clarity, with magnification required to see the individ-

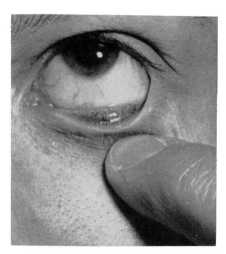

Fig. 5-4. Eversion of the lower lid by drawing the margin downward.

ual blood vessels. The corneoscleral limbus may be involved in arcus senilis, particularly in elderly individuals or in those with lipid disturbances. Corneal staining (p. 139) may be required to demonstrate areas where epithelium is deficient.

Anterior chamber. The normal aqueous humor is acellular and transparent. Even in severe uveal inflammations, good magnification is required to see cells and a Tyndall reaction (flare) in the anterior chamber. Rarely blood in the anterior chamber (hyphema) obscures the view of the iris. A severe leukocytic reaction may cause pus to collect in the inferior portion of the anterior chamber (hypopyon).

The depth of the anterior chamber is estimated. Normally the distance between the posterior surface of the cornea and the front surface of the iris is 3 mm. If the iris appears to parallel the concave surface of the posterior corneal surface and the depth of the anterior chamber is less than 2 mm., there is danger of angle-closure glaucoma (p. 309). If a shallow anterior chamber is present, attention should be directed particularly (1) to episodes of blurring or fogging of vision or severe pain in an eye following movies, tele-

vision, or prolonged darkness and (2) to occasional halos around lights (iridescent vision). An erroneous diagnosis of migraine, impending cerebral aneurysm rupture, or other diseases causing hemicrania may be made in patients with periodic acute episodes of angle-closure glaucoma.

Iris and pupil. The iris pattern should be clearly visible. Normally it is possible to see the iris crypts and the collarette. Inability to visualize the iris pattern suggests a corneal opacity, cells in the aqueous humor, or an iris inflammation. A difference in color of the irides of the two eyes suggests the possibility of uveal inflammation, tumor, or an anomaly in the sympathetic innervation of the dilatator pupillae muscle, as occurs in Horner's syndrome. A retained intraocular foreign body containing iron causes the iris to become brown. A coloboma of the iris, indicating absence of some portion of the iris, may be surgical or congenital. Absence of the crystalline lens removes support from the iris and it becomes tremulous, a condition known as iridodonesis.

Attention is directed to the shape, size, reaction, and equality of the pupils. If the pupil is adherent to the cornea (adherent leukoma) or to the lens (posterior synechiae), it will not be circular. Minor inequalities in pupillary diameter, as occur in Horner's and Adie's syndromes and in Argyll Robertson pupils (p. 220), are often not diagnosed because of inadequate observation.

The direct pupillary response to light is measured by directing the light of a penlight into the eye and observing the pupillary constriction (p. 218). Each eye is measured separately. The pupillary response to accommodation is of diagnostic importance only if there is a defect in the response to light.

Lens. The normal lens can be seen only by observing the image reflected from its anterior surface. An advanced cataract may cause a gray, opaque appearance in the

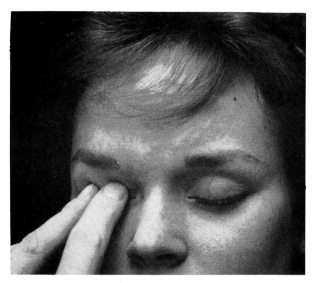

Fig. 5-5. Estimation of intraocular tension by palpation.

pupillary aperture. The lens is usually evaluated by means of the biomicroscope; opacities are evident upon ophthalmoscopic examination.

Ocular movements. The patient is instructed to look to the right, left, up, and down. Full movements indicate integrity of the third, fourth, and sixth cranial nerves. The patient is then directed to look at a penlight held about 13 inches in front of his eyes. Normally the image reflected from the cornea is approximately in the center of the pupil. The presence or absence of a phoria or tropia is determined by the alternate cover test (p. 322).

Corneal sensitivity

The sensory innervation of the cornea is derived from the nasociliary branch of the ophthalmic division of the trigeminal nerve through the long posterior ciliary nerves. Corneal sensitivity is tested clinically by means of a cotton-tipped applicator with a wisp of cotton drawn to a point. The patient is instructed to look directly ahead, and the cornea is touched with the cotton wisp. With normal inner-

vation, a lid closure reflex follows almost immediately. Care must be taken not to touch the eyelashes or the lid margins with the cotton wisp and not to stimulate lid closure by allowing the patient to see the wisp.

Corneal sensitivity is reduced in herpes simplex inflammations of the cornea, following herpes zoster involving the nasociliary branch of the ophthalmic division of the trigeminal nerve, and in APC virus disease of the cornea. Corneal sensitivity is also reduced in lesions at the apex of the orbit, which are also associated with involvement of motor nerves to the eye. Corneal anesthesia is an important sign in cerebellopontine angle tumors.

Measurement of intraocular pressure

By means of palpation of the eyeball through the closed lids, the examiner estimates whether the eye is extremely hard or unusually soft. Accurate pressures cannot be estimated in the intermediate ranges, and palpation is not an accurate or recommended method of determining intraocular pressure. In practice the patient is directed to look downward. The examiner then rests the fingers of both hands on the forehead and gently exerts alternate pressure on the globe through the upper eyelids with each index finger (Fig. 5-5). The pressure should be directed to the globe and not to the orbit. The pressure is estimated by the resistance

encountered. An extremely soft eyeball characterizes diabetic acidosis and penetrating injuries of the eye (a condition in which the measurement of the tactile tension is contraindicated in that it may cause extrusion of intraocular contents). Extremely high pressures of the eyeball occur

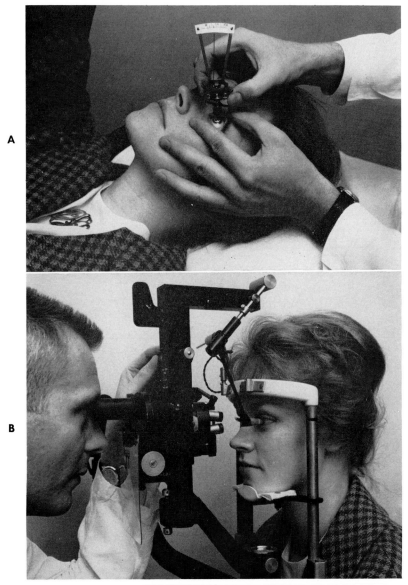

A

B

Fig. 5-6. A, Measurement of the ocular tension with the Schiøtz tonometer. **B,** Measurement of the ocular tension with the Goldmann applanation tonometer.

most commonly in angle-closure and secondary glaucoma. In such conditions there is usually marked reduction of vision.

Intraocular pressure is most accurately measured by means of a cannula within the eye, connected to a suitable transducer and amplifier. Such testing has been carried out in man only immediately prior to removal of an eye for disease, usually tumor. It must be done carefully so as not to disturb the normal pressure equilibrium of the eye by the loss of aqueous humor around the cannula or by excessive manipulation of the eye.

Clinical testing of the intraocular pressure is carried out by means of indentation tonometry, as is done with a Schiøtz tonometer, or by applanation tonometry that requires a biomicroscope (Fig. 5-6).

Corneal staining

Epithelial defects of the cornea may be demonstrated by instillation of a 2% fluo-

rescein solution (p. 108). Areas in which the epithelium is absent stain a brilliant green color. Fluorescein is an unusually valuable agent in the diagnosis of foreign bodies, abrasions, and inflammations of the cornea. As stated in the discussion on pharmacology (p. 108), it should be used solely as a sterile solution.

Bengal rose, 2%, is unusually valuable as a dye for demonstrating loss of conjunctival and corneal epithelium in keratoconjunctivitis sicca, but it causes considerable discomfort. A local anesthetic used prior to its instillation causes minute epithelial defects that may be evaluated incorrectly.

Ophthalmoscopy

Inspection of the interior of the eye through an ophthalmoscope is fundamental to diagnosis and permits visualization of the arteries, veins, optic disk, retina, choroid, and media. There are three methods

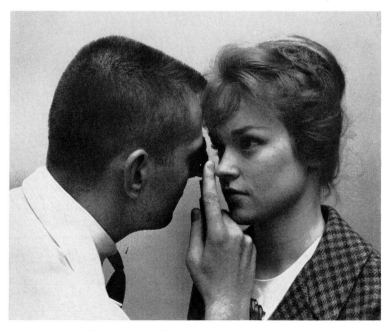

Fig. 5-7. Direct ophthalmoscopy of the patient's right eye. The examiner uses his right eye for observation and holds the ophthalmoscope in his right hand with his index finger on the lens dial.

of viewing the ocular fundus: (1) direct ophthalmoscopy, by which a magnification of about 15 diameters is obtained; (2) indirect ophthalmoscopy, by which a larger field is obtained, but with magnification of 4 to 5 diameters; and (3) biomicroscopy combined with a –40 diopter lens to neutralize corneal refracting power.

Direct ophthalmoscopy. Direct ophthalmoscopy (Fig. 5-7) provides an upright image of the retinal structures that are magnified about 15 times. With maximal pupillary dilation, it is possible to study the ocular fundus as far as an area slightly anterior to the equator—the area between the equator and the ora serrata cannot be seen. The maximum resolving power is about 70μ, and objects smaller than this, such as hemorrhages or microaneurysms, are not seen. The illumination by the modern direct ophthalmoscope is so bright that some translucent structures, particularly opacities in the media, may not be seen, and other features such as copper-wire arteries do not have the color described in original classical reports.

Technique. Only suggestions for ophthalmoscopy are possible by narration. As is true of golf, microscopy, and other individual occupations, there is no substitute for actual participation, but the following suggestions may be helpful.

Adequate pupillary dilation is necessary. This can usually be produced by a single instillation of 10% phenylephrine (Neo-Synephrine) in individuals up to 50 years of age and 2.5% concentration thereafter. Pilocarpine, 1%, is instilled at the conclusion of the eye examination, and the examiner must be assured that the pupils are either normal or beginning to constrict before he discharges the patient. Extreme caution is indicated in dilating the pupils of patients with shallow anterior chambers to avoid precipitating an attack of angle-closure glaucoma. There is more danger, however, of missing significant ocular or systemic disease by failing to dilate the pupils than there is of precipitating glaucoma by dilation.

The patient is examined in a dimly illuminated or dark room. A fixation point should be provided so that the patient does not look at the ophthalmoscope light. If it is possible for the patient to be examined while seated, he should not be examined in the supine position or in bed. If the examiner wears correcting lenses constantly, he should become accustomed to wearing them when learning the technique of ophthalmoscopy. It is frequently easier to examine patients who have a refractive error of more than 5 diopters if these patients wear their lenses during ophthalmoscopy.

The examiner examines the patient's right eye with his own right eye and the patient's left eye with his own left eye. The ophthalmoscope is held in the corresponding hand. The examiner sits or stands to the side of the eye to be examined. The head of the ophthalmoscope is steadied in the mediosuperior margin of the examiner's bony orbit. His index finger is used to change lenses. The examiner's free hand rests at his side. Usually it is not necessary to elevate the patient's lid for an adequate view.

The texture and detail of the retina and the blood vessels are better appreciated by constantly focusing the ophthalmoscope lens for superficial and deep views, much as one adjusts a microscope when studying a tissue section.

Accessories such as slits, special filters, colored lenses, and reticules are seldom useful to the novice ophthalmoscopist, and when used by the experienced examiner, they are usually combined with special attachments.

With the patient looking at a fixation light, the examiner directs the ophthalmoscope light into the eye from a distance of about 15 inches. A red fundus reflex will be observed. Any opacities in the ocular media will stand out as black silhouettes against a red background. Keeping his attention directed to the red reflex, the examiner gradually approaches the patient's eye, and the retinal details should become apparent. If not, a +10 lens is rotated into position in the ophthalmoscope, and the red reflex is focused from a distance of about 10 cm. Then the lens power is decreased as the patient's eye is approached. Once fundus details are seen, a blood vessel is followed to its origin at the optic papilla, and the systematic examination usually begins there.

Indirect ophthalmoscopy. Indirect ophthalmoscopy (Fig. 5-8) is carried out by means of a mirror having a central perforation. Light is directed into the eye, and the emerging rays are observed through the opening in the mirror. The image formed by the emerging rays is observed by means of a convex lens of +10 to +20 diopter power. A binocular indirect ophthalmoscope worn on the examiner's head permits use of his hands to depress the sclera near the ora serrata in order to observe the extreme retinal periphery. The indirect ophthalmoscope provides an inverted image that is magnified about five times. The field of observation is much larger than that seen with the direct ophthalmoscope, and a stereoscopic image may be seen with the binocular instrument. By means of the indirect ophthalmoscope, the entire retina from the disk to the ora serrata may be inspected. The maximum resolving power is about 200μ, but the stereoscopic image of the binocular instrument combined with parallax permits detection and appreciation of details not evident with the direct ophthalmoscope. This method of ophthalmoscopy is particularly useful when there are opacities in the media.

Biomicroscopy. The biomicroscope may be combined with a –40 diopter concave contact lens that neutralizes the corneal refractive power for study of the retina. Its

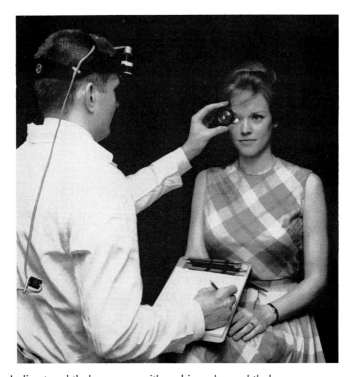

Fig. 5-8. Indirect ophthalmoscopy with a binocular ophthalmoscope.

particular value is increased magnification combined with oblique illumination for more accurate estimation of the depth of lesions. The concave contact lens may be fitted with mirrors so that, with adequate pupillary dilation, it is possible to study the retinal periphery.

The fundus

The red background of the fundus arises from the blood in the choriocapillaris of the choroid, the visibility of which varies with the amount of pigment in the pigment layer of the retina. The pigment usually parallels the complexion of the individual. In lightly pigmented persons, choroidal veins can be seen. The arteries supplying the choroid go almost directly to the choriocapillaris, and the major portion of the choroid is composed of freely anastomosing veins (p. 12) that are the ophthalmoscopically visible choroidal vessels. In some patients the contrast between choroidal pigment and blood viewed through a moderately pigmented retinal epithelium gives rise to a tessellated or tigroid fundus.

The optic disk is about 1.5 mm. in diameter. The diameter of the disk is the standard unit of measurement in the fundus. The disk appears to be approximately the same size in most patients. Marked enlargement in the size of the disk suggests a conus or a posterior staphyloma. If the disk appears smaller than normal, a pseudopapillitis may be present. The disk appears much smaller than normal in aphakia in which the lens is absent. The equator of the globe is about 16 mm., and the ora serrata is about 24 mm. from the optic disk.

The disk has a pale pink color, except for the physiologic cup, which is nearly white. The edges of the disk are usually flat and sharp, but not uncommonly the nasal margin is not as distinct as the temporal margin. Pigment may be visible, particularly on the temporal side, sometimes as a continuous arc and at other times as linear streaks concentric with the disk. This is called the choroidal ring and is of no pathologic significance. Slightly more uncommon is an arc of stark white tissue on the temporal side of the disk, a scleral ring, which may occur in degenerative myopia. It is often combined with a choroidal ring.

The physiologic cup of the optic disk is a funnel-shaped depression of varying size and shape. In some cases it is located nearly at the center of the disk, with grayish areas of the lamina cribrosa evident. In other eyes it has a more oblique course. Irrespective of its position, there is always a rim of nerve tissue between the physiologic cup and the edge of the disk in the healthy eye. Occasionally the area usually occupied by the physiologic cup is filled with glial tissue that may extend for a short distance over the arteries and the veins. This glial tissue should not be mistaken for vascular sheathing. Papilledema is never present if the physiologic cup can be seen.

The bifurcation of the central retinal artery into its superior and inferior papillary branches can usually be observed on the surface of the optic disk or slightly within the optic cup. The central vein usually bifurcates a little deeper within the optic nerve and has a pulsation nearly synchronous with the heart. When this physiologic pulsation is not present, it may be elicited by a very slight increase in intraocular pressure induced by pressing the globe with the index finger through the lids. In the healthy eye the central retinal artery does not pulsate, and the occurrence of pulsation indicates either an extremely high pulse pressure, as occurs in aortic regurgitation, or an increased intraocular pressure. Each of the papillary branches divides into a nasal and a temporal branch. These vessels do not have a continuous muscle coat or an internal elastic lamella and thus are arterioles (p. 26). In the healthy eye the walls of the vessels are never visible. Instead, a column of blood is observed through a transparent tube.

The retinal arterioles have a smaller diameter than venules, the usual ratio of arteriole to venule being 3:4 or 2:3. A broad, bright streak is reflected from the convex surface of arterioles. The reflection from venules is much narrower and not nearly as bright. The oxygenated blood is much brighter red in the arterioles than in the veins. In a complete examination of the fundus the superior and inferior temporal and nasal arteries are followed as far to the periphery as they can be seen.

In the usual ophthalmoscopic examination, final attention is directed to the fovea centralis. This is situated about 2 disk diameters (3 mm.) temporal to the optic disk. Usually pupillary dilation is required for careful examination of this area inasmuch as pupillary constriction is marked when the fovea is illuminated. The pit of the fovea presents a bright dotlike reflex arising from the "central bouquet of cones" that arises slightly above the surrounding foveal depression. The area surrounding the foveal centralis for a distance of about 1 disk diameter (1.5 mm.) appears to be a slightly deeper red than the surrounding fundus, and a very faint, discrete pigmentation may be evident. The temporal blood vessels arch over and under the fovea. The superior temporal artery in particular sends branches toward the fovea centralis, but there are no blood vessels in the fovea centralis.

The area surrounding the fovea extending to the temporal vessels above and below and about 3 mm. on either side has a yellowish pigmentation in primates. This is best observed in a sectioned eye, and it persists for about 15 minutes after the eye has been deprived of its blood supply. This pigmentation can be seen only with the ophthalmoscope when red-free light is used. It is called the macula lutea (yellow spot), and the region is frequently called the "macula," a term loosely interchanged with the term "fovea."

Chapter 6

Functional examination of the eyes

The function of the eye may be evaluated by a number of tests. The cone function of the fovea centralis is assessed mainly by measurement of the form sense, the ability to distinguish the shape of objects. This is designated as central visual acuity. It is measured for both near and far, with and without the best possible correction of any ametropia present. Because only cones are effective in color vision and because they are concentrated in the fovea, the measurement of the ability to recognize colors is also a measurement of foveal function. The function of the peripheral retina, which contains mainly rods, may be assessed by measurement of dark adaptation, which is seldom done in clinical situations, or by estimation of the peripheral visual field.

Any reasonably complete physical examination should indicate (1) that vision is approximately normal for near and far, each eye being measured separately, (2) that the visual field is intact upon gross testing, (3) that the ocular movements are normal, (4) that the pupils constrict with direct stimulation of the retina by light, and (5) that the optic disks are flat and of normal color.

Such an examination cannot be construed as a complete eye examination, but it will exclude a large variety of serious organic disease.

Central visual acuity

Measurement of the central visual acuity is essentially an assessment of the function of the fovea centralis. An object must be presented so that each portion of it is separated by a definite interval. By custom, this interval has become 1 minute of an arc, and the test object is one that subtends an angle of 5 minutes of an arc. A variety of test objects has been constructed on this principle, so that an angle of 5 minutes is subtended at distances varying from a few inches to many feet.

Central visual acuity is designated by two numbers. The first indicates the distance between the test object and the patient; the second indicates the distance at which the test object subtends an angle of 5 minutes. In the United States these numbers are usually given in inches or feet, whereas in Europe the designation is in meters.

The most familiar test objects are letters or numbers (Figs. 6-1 and 6-2). Such tests

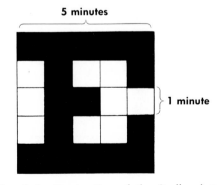

Fig. 6-1. Construction of the Snellen letter to subtend an angle of 5 minutes, with each part subtending an angle of 1 minute.

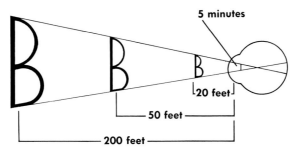

Fig. 6-2. Test letters subtending an angle of 5 minutes at varying distances from the eye. (Not to scale.)

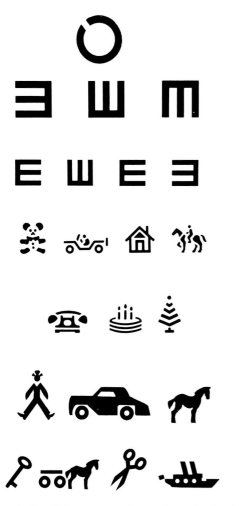

Fig. 6-3. Objects used in testing of visual acuity. The broken ring, the illiterate E, the Allen preschool vision test, and the Østerberg chart are illustrated.

have the disadvantage of requiring some literacy on the part of the patient. Additionally, there is a variation in their recognizability. Thus L is considered the easiest letter in the alphabet to read, and B is considered the most difficult. To obviate this difficulty, a broken ring (Fig. 6-3) has been devised in which the break in the ring subtends a 1-minute angle, and the entire ring subtends a 5-minute angle. Similarly, the letter E may be arranged so that it faces in different directions (Fig. 6-3). These test objects are easier to see than letters, eliminate some of the difficulties inherent in reading, and can be used in the testing of illiterates and persons not familiar with the Western alphabet. A variety of pictures have been designed for testing children.

The measurement of central visual acuity involves a variety of complex factors necessitating, first, that an object be imaged upon the retina and give rise to a photochemical response and in turn a nervous impulse that must result in conscious perception. Visual acuity can vary with motivation, attention, intelligence, and purely physical variants. The testing situation in many physicians' offices varies considerably (as does the patience of the examiner), and exact standards for the measurement of visual acuity have never been adopted.

There is a variety of devices that project letters upon a test screen, and in many testing situations the testing distance is more than 10 feet long but less than 20 feet. Letters are proportionately reduced for the testing situation used, but visual acuity appears to be better when the test distance is less than 20 feet. When a mirror is used, vision may be poorer than when measured in a 20-foot lane.

It is easier to recognize an isolated letter than a series of letters. This is particularly true in individuals with strabismic amblyopia (p. 330), who may have vision as good as 20/40 or 20/50 when measured with isolated letters and as poor as 20/200 when the letters are placed in a series. Visual acuity improves if the individual is given an unlimited time to recognize the test object, and it similarly decreases if the test objects are presented rapidly.

The accurate measurement of central visual acuity in a manner that may be consistently reproduced involves attention to a number of complex physical and psychic details. These are controlled only in experimental situations. The maximum visual acuity should be that in which the individual correctly recognizes 51% of the test objects when they are presented at a definite time interval. If a portion of the test objects is not recognized, it is customary to indicate the best vision minus the number of letters missed, such as 20/30-2. Inasmuch as the number of letters on the 20/30 line is not indicated, this is not particularly meaningful.

Despite the variations that may arise in the measurement of central visual acuity, it constitutes a relatively accurate clinical test of function and, when normal, indicates the following: (1) that myopia is not present or, if present, is of minor degree or has been compensated by partially closing the eyelids; (2) that any hyperopia present has been compensated by accommodation; (3) that the cornea and lens and ocular media are relatively clear in the visual axis, permitting an image to be formed on the retina; (4) that the fovea centralis is relatively intact, as are its nervous connections to the brain; and (5) that perception by the higher visual centers is intact.

The test chart commonly used in the United States has as its largest test object one that subtends an angle of 5 minutes at a distance of 200 feet. Then there are test objects subtending 5-minute angles for distances of 100, 70, 50, 40, 30, 20, and 15 feet. If the individual is unable to recognize the largest test object, he should be brought closer to it, and the distance at which he recognizes it should be recorded. Thus, if he recognizes the test object that subtends a 5-minute angle at 200 feet when he is 12 feet distant, the visual acuity is recorded as 12/200. This is not a fraction but indicates two physical measurements, the test distance and the size of the test object.

Special test objects that subtend a 5-minute angle at distances as great as 1,500 feet are available for measuring markedly decreased vision. If the individual is unable to recognize any test object, then one determines the distance at which he is able to count fingers, and this is recorded as counting fingers at 18 inches, 24 inches, etc. If unable to count fingers, the distance at which he can recognize hand movements is recorded. If unable to recognize hand movements, a small penlight is used to indicate whether he can project the direction from which light is entering the eye. This is recorded as light projection. If unable to project the direction of light, it is determined whether or not he can perceive light. Only in the absence of perception of light is the eye recorded as blind. Because blindness has a variety of legal and sociologic definitions, many institutions record the eye as having no light perception rather than blind. Tests for central visual acuity are carried out in each eye separately and then with both eyes open.

Discussions such as this are unfortunate

in suggesting that the measurement of visual acuity is a complicated, time-consuming, difficult-to-interpret maneuver. In the course of a physical examination it seems adequate to direct the patient's attention to nearly any object and to ask if he sees it equally clearly with each eye. This should be done with the patient wearing any glasses he has to correct distance vision. The variation between vision with and without glasses involves refractive errors solely.

Measurement of near vision is by no means as accurate as that of distance vision. For the most part, the distance at which near vision is tested is not recorded, and one records the smallest type that can be recognized irrespective of the distance. The standard test distance is considered to be 14 inches (33 cm.), and test objects conforming to the 5-minute angle have been designed for measuring near vision. These are used primarily in industrial testing situations.

A surprisingly large number of people have never been tested for visual acuity in each eye separately. Sometimes the first indication that vision is decreased in one eye is a trifling eye injury. If the physician has not measured the vision in an eye before inspecting or manipulating it, he may be wrongfully accused of responsibility for the decreased vision. In an emergency situation it is not necessary to have specific testing equipment available. One may gauge the visual acuity by using such material as a telephone book or a newspaper and recording the smallest-sized print that can be recognized with each eye.

It is desirable to measure central visual acuity of children sometime during their third year so as to prevent the development of amblyopia ex anopsia or to recognize the presence of severe degrees of ametropia. Picture charts may be used for this or illiterate charts with the letter E or broken ring. Objective tests of vision may be made using a rotating drum on which there are painted alternating strips of black and white that induce an opticokinetic nystagmus. This is the common method of measuring visual acuity in experimental animals. A strip of cloth 24 by 3 inches may have a series of 2-inch circles of a different color sewed upon it. Movement of the strip in front of the eyes induces an opticokinetic nystagmus in infants who have vision adequate for subsequent normal schooling.

Visual fields

The visual function of the retinal periphery may be assessed by measurement of the peripheral field of vision. This may be determined accurately by means of one of several instruments, or it may be determined approximately by means of the confrontation test. The confrontation test is so gross that it is significant only when abnormal. If the patient's peripheral vision appears normal with confrontation, a defect still may be detected by more sensitive methods of examination. The confrontation test is carried out as follows:

The examiner sits facing the patient at a distance of 1 m. in an area with good illumination. The patient is asked to close one eye, usually holding the lids closed with his fingers. The examiner closes his own eye, which is directly opposite the closed eye of the patient. Thus, if the patient is occluding his right eye, the examiner closes his left eye. The examiner then places his hand midway between the subject and himself, bringing his hand slowly in from the periphery with one, two, or three fingers extended. The subject is instructed to tell the examiner as soon as he can count the number of fingers visible in his field of vision. When the patient and the examiner have normal vision, each should recognize the number of fingers at the same time. Usually one tests the temporal and nasal fields and the fields above and below each eye in turn. Confrontation testing may also be carried out by substituting a hat pin with a 3 or 5 mm. white tip for fingers. In children the examiner may stand behind the child, who has one eye occluded, and bring his hand into the nasal and temporal fields from behind the child's head.

Two main groups of test equipment have been developed for measurement of the visual field: perimeters and tangent screens.

Perimeters. Perimeters are constructed in such a manner that the eye is at the center of rotation of a hemisphere that has a radius of curvature of 33 cm. Some consist of an arc of a circle that is rotated, whereas others are constructed as a hemisphere (Fig. 6-4, A). In the crudest devices the test object is moved on the end of a wand into the field of view. With all instruments, the testing distance of 33 cm. remains constant. However, the size and color of the test object may be varied, and the contrast of the test object with the surrounding field may be varied with projection types of perimetry. A line connecting the points at which a test object may be just recognized is called the peripheral isopter. It is recorded as (1) the size, 1, 2, 3, 10 mm., etc.; (2) the test distance, 330 mm.; the color; and (4) the contrast. The accurate determination of visual fields may be time-consuming; frequently it is superficially and inaccurately carried out. Quite often the disease process necessitating examination of the visual field disturbs the patient's attention and consciousness, and only the grossest responses are obtained.

Tangent screens. Determination of the retinal function within 30° of the fovea centralis is best performed by use of a tangent screen (tangent because it is a plane tangent to the arc of a perimeter). A tangent screen is usually covered with black felt, and usually the test is con-

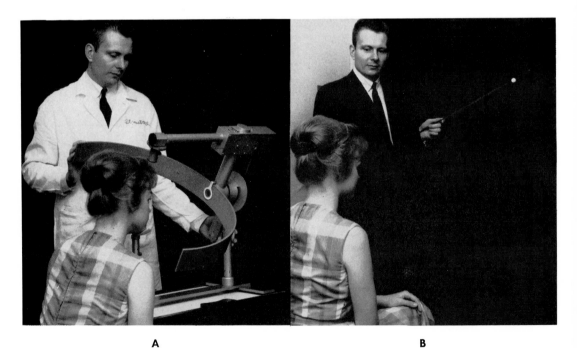

A   B

Fig. 6-4. A, Measurement of the peripheral visual field using a perimeter that projects the test object. **B,** Measurement of the central visual field using the tangent screen. Each eye is tested separately.

ducted 1 or 2 m. from the eye. Test objects varying in size from 1 to 50 mm. are used. For the most part, testing with the tangent screen presents a smaller stimulus to the patient, and the results are more accurate than when the perimeter is used. Similarly, a greater degree of cooperation on the part of the patient is required with tangent screen testing. Defects of the retinal periphery will also be reflected on the tangent screen, and this constitutes the main method of visual field examination by ophthalmologists in the United States (Fig. 6-4, *B*).

The Amsler test is one that involves the use of a pattern consisting of a 20 cm. square divided into 1 cm. squares. The patient looks at the center of the square and projects any defect in the visual field onto the square. It is a sensitive method of assessing abnormalities of the fovea centralis that are so slight as not to be detected by the usual methods of perimetry.

Visual field screening. Visual field screening may be done conveniently by means of a Harrington-Flocks visual field screener. This consists of a screen on which are projected, for one tenth of a second, dots of various sizes in various parts of the visual field. The test involves a mesoscopic recognition of the test objects. The device is of particular value in excluding visual defects and those defects arising from glaucoma and from neurologic involvement of the optic nerve and visual pathways.

Color vision

Color vision testing is seldom routinely carried out. The tests used clinically are often relatively gross and too insensitive to detect small changes. This failure to measure color vision probably arises because color vision defects occur as a hereditary defect in about 7% of males and 0.5% of females, and its value in detection of disease is not appreciated. The severity of the defect varies considerably in different individuals. The grossest test for detecting color deficiency involves the matching of yarns (Holmgren's test) or recognizing red and green lanterns. Color plates are available in which numbers are outlined in the primary colors and surrounded by confusion colors. The color-deficient individual is unable to see the figure that is recognized quickly by a person with normal color appreciation. More sensitive tests of color vision involve the use of the Nagel anomaloscope in which the hue and saturation of a color are matched by mixtures of two other colors. Usually this instrument is employed only in clinical investigation. The Farnsworth-Munsell test of hue discrimination consists of 100 chips of color that are matched in terms of increasing hue.

Color perception is disturbed in a variety of diseases of the optic nerve and fovea as well as in nutritional disturbances. Testing may play an important role in the recognition of total color blindness as a cause of bilateral decrease in vision, the etiology of which is not obvious. The occurrence of glucose 6-phosphate dehydrogenase deficiencies associated with hemolytic anemia and red-green color blindness in the inhabitants of Sardinia has excited geneticists and hematologists, and it seems likely that in years to come the tests will move from the laboratory for clinical investigation to routine clinical use.

Part III

Diseases and injuries
of the eye

Chapter 7

The eyelids

The eyelids are thin curtains of skin, conjunctiva, and striated and smooth muscle that contain a plate of fibrous tissue, the tarsus. They function in distributing tears over the anterior surface of the eye and in limiting the amount of light entering the eye. The eyelids are divided into two portions: (1) the tarsal portion, adjacent to the lid margin, ending at the peripheral margin of the tarsus and involved in reflex blinking, and (2) the orbital portion, the peripheral portion of which merges into the cheek below and the brow above. The lid margins contain a mucocutaneous junction of skin and conjunctiva, the gray line, a triple line of eyelashes or cilia, the orifices of the meibomian glands, and the superior and inferior puncta, which are the openings of the superior and inferior canaliculus. The lid margin is divided into two parts: (1) a lateral five sixths, the ciliary portion containing eyelashes, and (2) a medial one sixth, without eyelashes, that contains the puncta. The lateral junction of the lid margins, the lateral canthus, forms a 60° angle located about 2 mm. above the rounded medial margin, the medial canthus (p. 39). The orbicularis oculi muscle (N VII) originates from two leaves of the medial palpebral ligament and inserts in the lateral canthal ligament.

The eyelids are covered by a thin elastic and easily distensible skin that contains no subcutaneous fat. The skin is, of course, subject to the same diseases as skin elsewhere, but secondary involvement of the globe may overshadow the cutaneous disorder. The eyelids are separated from orbital structures by the palpebral fascia (orbital septum, p. 33), which limits the extension of inflammation, effusions, and fat between the orbit and the eyelids.

The upper eyelid is elevated by the levator palpebrae superioris muscle (N III). Müller's smooth muscle (sympathetics) provides tone to the elevated lid. The eyelids are closed by the orbicularis oculi muscle (N VII). Only the tarsal portion is involved in reflex blinking, whereas both the orbital and the tarsal portions are involved in forcible closure of the eyelids.

The eyelids contain numerous glands: sebaceous (Zeis) and sudoriferous (Moll) glands associated with the cilia, meibomian glands in the tarsal plates, and accessory lacrimal glands of Krause and Wolfring located in the conjunctival fornices (see discussion on lacrimal apparatus and conjunctiva, pp. 42 and 44). Additionally, the skin of the eyelids contains sweat and sebaceous glands subject to the same diseases as elsewhere.

Symptoms and signs of eyelid disease

The variety of structures forming the eyelids, their importance in facial expression and appearance, and their essential function in protection and health of the eye provide the basis for a wide variety of abnormalities.

153

The palpebral apertures are normally similar in size, shape, position, and movement, and the eyelids just conceal the corneoscleral limbus in the 12 and 6 o'clock meridians. The shape of the aperture varies in different races, and it is more slanted and almond shaped in Orientals. The upper lid is highest at the junction of the medial one third with the lateral two thirds, while the lower lid is lowest at the lateral one third. Retraction of the eyelids or forward protrusion of the globe exposes the sclera (scleral rim) above or below the corneoscleral limbus. When the eyelids are closed, the palpebral aperture becomes a fissure and the eye turns up and out (Bell's phenomenon, p. 90), providing protection to the cornea.

The lid margins are normally in close apposition to the globe, with the lashes directed outward. The lashes are more rigid than body hair, darker, and do not gray with aging. The inferior punctum turns slightly inward to dip into the lacrimal lake at the inner canthus. The lacrimal papillae, a small prominence surrounding the punctum, becomes more obvious with aging.

The skin of the eyelids is thin and often translucent, so that a delicate tracery of blood vessels gives a slightly bluish cast to the lids. The skin is thrown into fine folds, and the superior and inferior palpebral sulci (p. 41) provide characteristic folds.

Periodic contraction of the tarsal portion of the orbicularis oculi muscle causes involuntary blinking. With attempts to squeeze both eyes closed, there is normally an equal contracture on both sides. The levator palpebrae superioris and Müller's muscles elevate the eyelids to a similar height on the two sides.

The symptoms caused by abnormalities of the eyelids vary widely. Inturning of the lid margins (entropion, p. 156) causes the lashes to irritate the cornea and bulbar conjunctiva. Failure of the eyelids to cover the globe, as occurs in lagophthalmos (p. 159) or ectropion (p. 156), may cause an inflammation of the conjunctiva and cornea due to exposure. If the lids cover one or both pupils, there may be interference with vision. If one pupil is covered early in life, central visual acuity may fail to develop normally in this eye. If both lids cover the pupils, the patient often compensates by throwing his head back so as to expose the visual axis.

Pain, swelling, and redness of the lids occur with a variety of inflammations. Inflammatory or neoplastic disease may extend from the eyelids to involve the eye. Infection of the upper lid or the outer one third of the lower lid may cause enlargement of the preauricular (parotid) lymph node. Involvement of the medial two thirds of the lower lid may cause a submaxillary lymphadenopathy.

Tearing may arise because of irritation of the eye or because the lids are not in apposition with the globe. Constant tearing may cause excoriation of the skin at the lateral and medial canthi.

Congenital abnormalities

The eyelids are subject to a large number of congenital abnormalities. Failure of an eyeball to develop may result in the absence of the lid, called ablepharon. The lids may be imperfectly separated in ankyloblepharon. There may be failure of a portion of the lid to develop, causing a notching defect of the lid margin, a coloboma of the eyelid. Development of a supernumerary row of lashes, which are frequently directed backward so as to irritate the cornea, is known as distichiasis (p. 162).

Epicanthus is by far the most common congenital variation. A vertical skin fold occurs in the medial canthal region that conceals the medial angle and the caruncle. Such an epicanthal fold occurs normally in the Oriental races (Fig. 7-1). It is present in many Caucasian infants

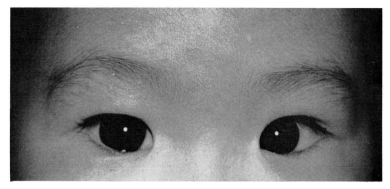

Fig. 7-1. Epicanthal fold in a Japanese child. Concealment of the sclera may simulate the appearance of esotropia.

until growth of the nose and face causes it to be obliterated. An epicanthal fold may conceal the medial sclera and may simulate the appearance of esotropia. The presence or absence of esotropia is quickly determined by means of the alternate cover test (p. 322).

Abnormalities of size, shape, and position

In entropion the lid margin is turned inward, and the eyelashes irritate the eyeball. In ectropion the lid margin is turned outward so that the conjunctival surface is exposed and becomes keratinized. In blepharoptosis the upper lid is not elevated properly so that the palpebral fissure is narrowed. In blepharophimosis the interpalpebral fissure is congenitally short. Blepharoptosis and epicanthal folds may be associated. In lagophthalmos the eyelids fail to cover the globe.

Entropion

Entropion is a condition in which the lid margin is turned inward so that the lashes irritate the eye, causing irritation of the cornea and the conjunctiva, conjunctival injection, tearing, and sometimes secondary infection of the cornea or the conjunctiva. It occurs in three forms: (1) spastic, (2) atonic, and (3) cicatricial. The spastic and the atonic types affect only the lower lid, whereas the cicatricial form may affect either the upper or the lower lid.

The spastic form arises from excessive contraction of the orbicularis oculi muscle (blepharospasm) and may complicate chronic conjunctivitis, keratitis, and ocular surgery. Primary treatment is directed toward removal of the cause. Surgery involves resection of a strip of skin and orbicularis oculi muscle parallel to the palpebral fissure in order to evert the lid margin.

The atonic type of entropion follows a loss of tone of the orbicularis oculi muscle combined with loss of elasticity of the skin. It occurs in the elderly. In the early stages the entropion is often intermittent but may be induced by having the patient forcibly squeeze the eyes closed. The irritation of the globe by the lashes causes a blepharospasm; therefore both a spastic and an atonic entropion may be present (Fig. 7-2). Surgery is usually required. Temporary relief may be obtained by drawing the skin of the outer canthus down and out by means of an adhesive tape strip. Ordinarily this is effective only in the mildest of cases. The usual surgical procedure involves a resection or shortening of the orbicularis oculi muscle fibers adjacent to the lid margin.

Cicatricial entropion follows scarring of

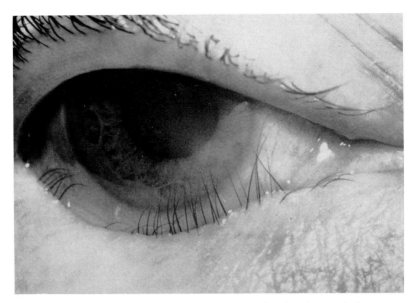

Fig. 7-2. Spastic entropion with irritation of the globe by the eyelashes.

the palpebral conjunctiva, which may be caused by chemical injuries, lacerations, surgical procedures, radiant energy, trachoma, and erythema multiforme. Frequently the tarsus is deformed. A number of surgical procedures have been devised to evert the lid margin and the lashes. It may be necessary to transplant mucous membrane from the mouth to replace scarred conjunctiva.

Ectropion

Ectropion is a condition in which the lid margin is turned away from the eye so that the bulbar and the palpebral conjunctivae are exposed. Symptoms arise from exposure of the conjunctiva and the cornea. When the lower lid is involved, the inferior punctum is not adjacent to the lacrimal lake, and tearing may occur. Ectropion occurs in three main forms: (1) spastic, (2) atonic, and (3) cicatricial. Only the lower lid is involved in the spastic and atonic types, but the cicatricial type may affect either the upper or the lower lid.

Atonic ectropion (Fig. 7-3) is the most common type. It follows paralysis of the orbicularis oculi muscle (N VII). The lower lid sags outward, and there is marked tearing. Usually there is an associated paralysis of other facial muscles. Medical measures are ineffective. A wide variety of surgical procedures is described to correct the condition. In diseases of the facial nerve, nerve grafting is the preferred procedure. If this is not practicable, a shortening operation on the lid is indicated. Surgery is not indicated if spontaneous recovery from the paralysis occurs.

Spastic ectropion usually follows conditions in which the eyeball is proptosed or the conjunctiva chronically thickened. In youth the skin and muscle provide firm support of the lid, and the spasm of the orbicularis oculi muscle causes the lid margin to turn outward. Treatment is directed toward the cause.

Cicatricial ectropion follows burns, lacerations, and infections of the skin of the eyelids. With most thermal burns, the eyelids close tightly, and the lid margins are uninvolved, there being an intact 1 or 2 mm. margin present. Subsequent plastic

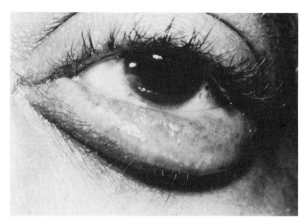

Fig. 7-3. Ectropion with conjunctival hyperplasia and keratinization.

surgery to correct contracture may be unnecessary if the lids are sutured together as early as possible. Early skin transplant is desirable in most instances of cicatricial ectropion. Skin of the opposite upper lid is ideal for this purpose, or skin may be obtained from over the mastoid region. The plastic surgery required for established cicatricial ectropion may be difficult and may necessitate skilled and prolonged care. Symptomatic treatment is usually not helpful.

Blepharoptosis

Blepharoptosis is an abnormality in which there is drooping of the upper lid so that the palpebral aperture is narrowed. It arises either because of an abnormality of the musculature of the lid or its innervation or because of mechanical interference with elevation of the lid. Muscular causes include myasthenia gravis and various muscular dystrophies. Oculomotor nerve interference, either in its nucleus or in its course to the levator palpebrae superioris muscle, gives rise to a marked defect. Interference with the sympathetic innervation of the smooth muscle of Müller, which provides tone to the upper lid, causes 1 to 2 mm. of drooping, as is seen in Horner's syndrome (p. 221). Blepharoptosis may be secondary to increased

weight of a tumor involving the upper lid, which causes a mechanical interference with elevation. With aging, the palpebral fissure becomes narrower due to loss of tone of the levator palpebrae superioris muscle.

Blepharoptosis is often divided into congenital and acquired types. The congenital type, which is present at birth, is almost invariably due to interference with the innervation of the levator palpebrae superioris muscle. There may also be involvement of muscles innervated by the oculomotor nerve. The acquired type may be distinguished from the congenital type by the presence of the superior palpebrae sulcus, which arises at the point of insertion of the levator palpebrae superioris tendon into the skin of the upper lid. In instances in which the levator palpebrae superioris muscle has never functioned, the sulcus is absent.

Congenital blepharoptosis. Blepharoptosis (Fig. 7-4), which is present at birth, is usually due to an abnormality of the oculomotor nerve. There may be an associated paralysis of the superior rectus muscle, which is also innervated by the superior division of the oculomotor nerve. In addition, strabismus is common. The condition is noticed at birth or shortly thereafter when it is evident that the palpebral

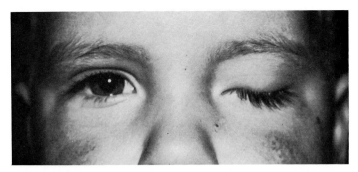

Fig. 7-4. Bilateral blepharoptosis. The absence of a superior palpebral furrow indicates paralysis of the levator palpebrae superioris muscle.

fissure on one or both sides is narrower than normal and that the upper lid does not move upward with the eye. There may be all degrees of severity. If both pupils are covered by the drooping eyelids, the child acquires a characteristic posture with his head thrown back and his forehead furrowed in a perpetual frown as he uses his frontalis muscle to elevate the eyelids. If the pupil of only one eye is covered, the child may develop defective vision from disuse of this eye (amblyopia, p. 330). Because of this visual involvement, a monocular ptosis requires earlier treatment than a bilateral blepharoptosis. The treatment of congenital blepharoptosis is based on the degree of severity. If the pupils are not covered by the lids, treatment may be deferred for a long period. If the pupil of only one eye is covered, surgery is usually carried out between the ages of 1 and 2 years and major attention is directed toward the development of normal visual acuity in the affected eye. When the condition is bilateral, surgery, if indicated, is done between the ages of 3 and 5 years. Although it is exceptional, myasthenia gravis may involve the eyelids of young children, and it is customary to carry out a Tensilon test to be certain that the condition is due to an oculomotor nerve abnormality and not muscle disease.

Acquired blepharoptosis. Acquired blepharoptosis may arise from any affec-tion of the nerve supply of the upper eyelid musculature, from a disease of the muscles themselves, or from mechanical interference in elevating the lid by the weight of a tumor. The most common causes of oculomotor nerve involvement are ruptured intracranial aneurysms, head injuries, diabetes mellitus (p. 385), and toxic and inflammatory disease. Aneu-rysms of the internal carotid artery with-in the cavernous sinus may cause a complete ophthalmoplegia and anesthesia of the cornea from involvement of cranial nerves III, IV, V, and VI. Aneurysms involving the circle of Willis above the cavernous sinus may cause an isolated oculomotor nerve palsy. Medical diseases most often do not involve the pupillary fibers.

The blepharoptosis caused by interfer-ence with the sympathetic nerve supply to Müller's smooth muscle is seldom marked and does not require treatment. There is usually an associated miosis and anhidrosis on the same side (see discussion of Hor-ner's syndrome, p. 221).

Paresis of the levator palpebrae supe-rioris muscle may be the initial sign of myasthenia gravis. Frequently the disease is limited to the upper lid and does not become more generalized. Most commonly only one side is affected. Inasmuch as the disease may be treated medically it is most important to exclude myasthenia

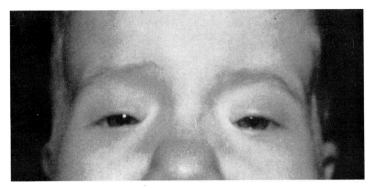

Fig. 7-5. Blepharophimosis. The palpebral fissures are neither wide enough nor long enough. The medial canthi are separated widely. An inverse epicanthal fold is present.

gravis prior to surgical correction of an acquired blepharoptosis. Myotonic dystrophy may cause a bilateral blepharoptosis, but ordinarily the ocular involvement is only incidental to the systemic disease.

• • •

There are three surgical procedures used in the correction of blepharoptosis:

1. Resection of the levator palpebrae superioris muscle through either a skin or a conjunctival incision is the procedure of choice when levator function is present.

2. Suspension of the upper lid from the frontalis muscle by means of fascia lata or other material provides mechanical elevation, but the cosmetic result may not be as pleasing as with a levator resection. This procedure is used more frequently now than previously, and the tendency among some surgeons is to use it solely except when levator function is present.

3. If the superior rectus muscle has normal action, a small slip of muscle may be transplanted to the upper lid. This often causes a vertical muscle imbalance, and the procedure has fallen into disuse in recent years.

Several ingenious devices known as ptosis crutches have been developed that attach to the frame of spectacles and elevate the lid. For the most part, they are not particularly well tolerated. It must also be recalled that a unilateral ptosis may be effective in preventing double vision when ocular muscles are involved.

Blepharophimosis

Blepharophimosis (Fig. 7-5) is a rare condition in which the eyelids are neither wide enough nor long enough. It causes the palpebral fissure to be reduced in length from about 30 to less than 20 mm. and to be reduced in width from some 10 to 5 to 7 mm. It may be associated with microphthalmia, ptosis, and epicanthus. The distance between the medial canthus and the midfacial plane is often very great. Skilled surgery is required to lengthen the palpebral fissure, to shorten the canthal ligaments, and to correct the associated defects.

Lagophthalmos

Lagophthalmos is an abnormality in which inadequate closure of the eyelids results in exposure of the eyeball. It may occur because of seventh cranial nerve weakness, proptosis, lid retraction, or enlargement of the globe. Exposure of the cornea occurs with drying and secondary infection (p. 209). Treatment is directed toward the cause. Surgery to prevent exposure keratitis should be carried out as soon as it is evident that the cornea is threatened. Permanent or temporary adhesions may be created between the upper and the lower lids (tarsorrhaphy). These may be either lateral, medial, or central. In mild lagophthalmos only the central portion of the cornea may be exposed, and the instillation of an ointment base at bedtime may be all that is required to prevent corneal drying during sleep. Saran wrap held in position with gummed cellophane tape may be used to cover the exposed eye and create a moist chamber. Alternatively, a corneoscleral contact lens may prevent corneal drying in a cosmetically more acceptable manner.

Disorders of the orbicularis oculi muscle

Blinking

Blinking spreads tears over the surface of the eyeball and limits the amount of light entering the eye. It may be involuntary or voluntary. Involuntary blinking occurs as a periodic contraction of the tarsal portion of the orbicularis oculi muscle at a rate peculiar to each individual. It is absent in infants and is of low frequency in Parkinson's disease and hyperthyroidism (Stellwag's sign). Periodic blinking normally occurs once every 5 seconds and lasts about 0.3 second.

Reflex blinking may follow peripheral stimulation of the trigeminal, optic, or auditory nerves. Irritation of the cornea, conjunctiva, or eyelashes is followed by lid closure. Bright lights or dazzling in the visual field may initiate reflex blinking through an arc that begins in the retina. A sudden loud noise may cause reflex closure of the eyelids.

Blepharoclonus

Blepharoclonus is an exaggerated form of reflex blinking in which either the rate of blinking is increased or the phase of closure is excessively long. There is often marked contraction of the orbital portion of the lids. Blepharoclonus may be initiated by irritation or inflammation of the conjunctiva or the cornea. Even after removal of the cause, blepharoclonus may continue as a tic, and other muscles of the face may be involved. When the stimulus cannot be found, effective treatment is difficult. A variety of surgical procedures have been described that aim at interrupting the facial nerve supply to the orbicularis oculi muscle or disturbing the muscle fibers themselves.

Children 5 to 10 years of age may develop episodes of rapid blinking. Apparently the child is unaware of the blinking, but the parents may be greatly distressed. Almost invariably, examination of the eyes indicates no ocular abnormality. Reassurance of the parent usually causes the blinking to disappear or the parent to stop noticing it.

Adults may develop a habit of exaggerated blinking that at times involves other muscles of the face. Inasmuch as the disease is not organic in origin, surgical correction is unsatisfactory and may direct the patient's neurosis to an area less accessible to diagnosis.

Orbicularis oculi muscle tremor

Involuntary contraction of a few fibers of the orbicularis oculi muscle causes the patient to sense an annoying twitching that feels very conspicuous. Examination indicates a barely perceptible contraction of a few fibers of the orbicularis oculi muscle. The condition occurs most frequently with fatigue, but often no cause is found. Local instillation or systemic administration of anticholinesterase compounds, particularly the alkyl phosphates, may be a cause. Reassurance and adequate rest are prescribed. Quinine sulfate in doses of 200 to 400 mg. increases the latent period of skeletal muscle contraction with relief of symptoms. If the entire muscle is involved, a search must be made for organic causes, particularly multiple sclerosis, Parkinson's disease, tabes dorsalis, and hyperthyroidism.

Blepharospasm

In this abnormality there is forcible closure of the lids that persist for a few seconds to many days. There may be involvement of other facial muscles, causing the whole face to be in almost incessant motion. Commonly, the opposite side becomes involved, and the patient becomes severely handicapped by inability to see because the eyes are closed. The condition may be caused by painful stimulation of the trigeminal nerve or by stimulation of the facial nerve. In most instances there appears to be a psychosomatic basis, although superficially the patients seem well adjusted. Psychiatric therapy is not particularly helpful. Parkinsonism may also be a cause in some instances. Resection of the lateral insertion of the orbicularis oculi muscle, injection of the seventh cranial nerve with alcohol, and similar procedures have been described as useful.

Miscellaneous conditions
Blepharochalasis

Blepharochalasis is an abnormality in which there is atrophy and loss of elasticity of the skin of the eyelids. It occurs most commonly in aged persons. There is a loss of skin turgor, and a large fold of skin may hang down over the lid margin. Treatment is usually not indicated. If the fold of skin interferes with vision by covering the pupillary area, the excess skin may be excised.

Baggy eyelids

Puffiness or swelling of the eyelids arises from localized edema or protrusion of orbital fat through the orbital fascia. Systemic causes include hyperthyroidism, nephrosis, and angioneurotic edema. In premenstrual edema, fluid retention may be conspicuous in this area, as may be vaso-

dilation with the abundant vasculature of the lid evident through the nearly translucent skin.

Herniation of orbital fat through a dehiscence in the orbital fascia gives rise to a localized swelling in the lid that can sometimes be palpated as a small tumor. The inner portion of the upper lid and the middle portion of the lower lid are partially involved. Successful treatment requires surgical closure of the fascial defect because mere excision of the fat will be followed by replacement of more fat from the orbit.

Symblepharon

Symblepharon is a condition in which there are adhesions between the palpebral and bulbar conjunctiva. It may obliterate conjunctival cul-de-sacs or form bands of scar tissue. Scarring follows conditions in which apposed areas of the conjunctiva lose their epithelial coverings. The chief causes are chemical burns (particularly caustics), trachoma, erythema multiforme (Stevens-Johnson disease), and benign mucous membrane pemphigus. The adhesions cause a mechanical defect since the lids are adherent to the eyeball, and desiccation of the cornea and keratitis occur because of exposure. Treatment frequently is ineffective and disappointing. It is directed toward replacement of the scarred conjunctiva with a buccal mucous membrane graft.

Trichiasis

In this condition the lashes are directed toward the globe and irritate the cornea and the conjunctiva, causing secondary infection. The condition usually follows diseases that cause scarring of the lid margin. Treatment must be directed toward destruction of the irritating lashes. Generally, removal is ineffective because the lashes tend to regrow. Destruction of the hair follicle by electrolysis is indicated when only a few lashes are involved. If many are involved, reconstruction of the margin of the eyelid may be necessary.

Distichiasis

Distichiasis is a congenital abnormality in which the meibomian glands atavistically revert to hair follicles to form an accessory line of lashes. Other congenital malformations may be present. If the lashes are numerous and cause irritation of the globe, the area must be excised and a graft substituted.

Hypertrophy of the eyelids

Immense overgrowth of the eyelids may occur in neurofibromatosis, hemangiomas (particularly in infancy), lymphangioma, and a variety of infections. Treatment is directed toward the cause.

Inflammation

The glands in the lids may be involved in acute suppurative infections such as those occurring with sties that involve the glands of Zeis and Moll associated with the lashes. The meibomian glands may be involved in an acute or chronic inflammation called chalazion.

The lid margins may be involved in inflammations (blepharitis) caused by bacteria, seborrheic dermatitis, or localized hypersensitivity reactions. The skin of the eyelids may be involved in a large variety of inflammations that may be more conspicuous than similar lesions elsewhere in the body because of the looseness of the skin, its exposed position, and secondary involvement of the eye. Contact dermatitis and reactions secondary to the application of drugs or cosmetics to the lids or conjunctival sac are common.

Hordeolum

Hordeolum, or sty (Fig. 7-6), is an acute suppurative inflammation of the follicle of an eyelash or the associated gland of Zeis (sebaceous) or Moll (special apocrine sweat gland). Like pustules elsewhere, the usual cause is staphylococcal infection. The initial symptom is tenderness of the lid that may become quite marked as the suppuration progresses. The initial sign is edema of the lid, which may be quite diffuse, followed by the development of a red, indurated area on the lid margin that may rupture. The main

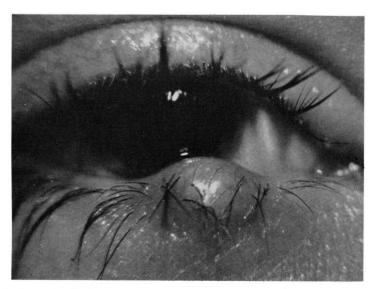

Fig. 7-6. Acute hordeolum.

differential diagnosis involves an acute chalazion that tends to point on the conjunctival side of the lid and does not involve the lid margin unless the opening duct of the meibomian gland is involved. The chalazion is preceded and followed by a shotlike tumor in the substance of the lid. Sties tend to occur in crops because the infecting organism spreads from one hair follicle to another, either directly or by the fingers. Treatment is that of acute suppurative infection elsewhere in the body. Hot compresses applied at frequent intervals hasten resolution of the lesion. When pointing occurs, incision and drainage are indicated. Frequently a sulfonamide or an antibiotic is used locally to prevent involvement of adjacent glands.

Chalazion

Chalazion (Fig. 7-7) is a chronic inflammatory lipogranuloma of one of the meibomian glands. It is characterized by a gradual painless swelling of the gland without gross inflammatory signs. Palpation indicates a small buckshotlike swelling in the substance of the lid, and this may be its only evidence. With increase in size, it may cause astigmatism by distortion of the globe or may be evident beneath the skin as a small mass. It may become secondarily infected and give rise to an acute suppurative inflammation that usually points on the inside of the lid. The lesion is a lipogranuloma resembling that seen in sarcoid or tuberculosis.

Treatment is by excision, usually through a conjunctival incision (Fig. 7-8). When small and asymptomatic, removal is not indicated, and the mass may disappear spontaneously. Some individuals tend to have a series of chalazia, apparently because of inspissation of the meibomian gland contents in the excretory ducts. If pressure upon the lid expresses a viscous secretion from the glands, massage of the lids, sometimes with a glass rod, may be helpful. Recurrence of what is believed to be a chalazion at the site where it has been excised should make one suspicious of a meibomian gland carcinoma.

Meibomianitis

In middle age a passive retention of the meibomian glands may occur with a deposition of a white, frothy secretion on the

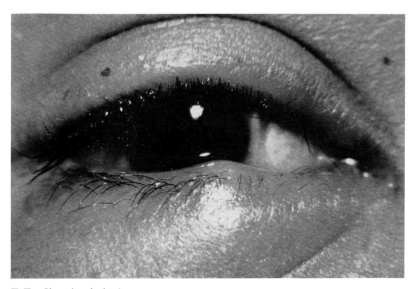

Fig. 7-7. Chronic chalazion.

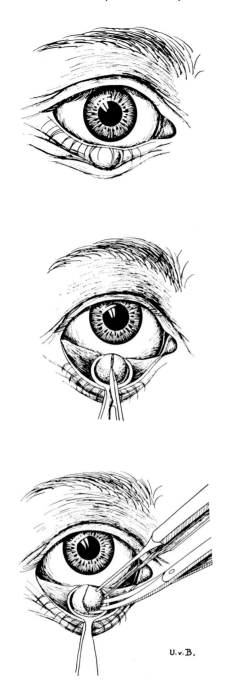

Fig. 7-8. Excision of a chalazion through a vertical conjunctival incision. Alternatively, the contents of the chalazion may be evacuated by means of a curet. (From Newell, F. W.: In Lewis-Walters practice of surgery, Hagerstown, Md., 1961, W. F. Prior Co., vol. 4, chap. 1.)

lid margins and at the canthi. The glands may be massaged to express an oily secretion, and eversion of the lids may show vertical yellowish streaks shining through the tarsal conjunctiva. Occasionally calcium is deposited in a gland, and if this material penetrates the conjunctiva, it causes a foreign body sensation and must be removed.

Meibomianitis is often associated with blepharitis and chronic conjunctivitis and may give rise to recurrent chalazia. Treatment consists of tarsal massage and removal of the secretion with a moist cotton applicator.

Blepharitis

Blepharitis is an inflammation of the lid margin that may be acute or chronic. Two forms are described: (1) simple squamous blepharitis and (2) ulcerated blepharitis.

Simple squamous blepharitis is characterized by a hyperemia usually limited to the lid margins. It is associated with scaling of the skin that may give rise to fine flakes and scales surrounding the lashes. In severe instances the lid margins may become thickened and everted. Most commonly, however, redness of the lid margins is the chief complaint. There may be burning and discomfort of the eyes and an associated chronic conjunctivitis (p. 177).

Nearly always there is an associated seborrheic dermatitis of the scalp, which may also involve the eyebrows and give rise to an erythema of the cheeks. Irritation of the lid margins by chemical fumes, smoke, and smog may aggravate the hyperemia. Frequent rubbing of the eyelids may perpetuate the inflammation. In years past, uncorrected errors of refraction have been considered an important cause.

Treatment is directed mainly toward correction of the seborrheic dermatitis of the scalp by means of one of the specific shampoos available. Scales on the lid margin should be removed twice daily by means of a moistened cotton-tipped applicator. When indicated, refractive errors and imbalances of the ocular muscles should be corrected by means of lenses. Epinephrine is commonly used to cause vasoconstriction, but its action is evanescent and becomes less effective with repeated use. Numerous antibiotics, sulfonamides, and steroids have been used locally with diminution of the inflammatory signs. For the most part, the condition tends to be arrested with treatment of the seborrheic dermatitis of the scalp and to recur when treatment is stopped.

Ulcerative blepharitis arises from acute and chronic suppurative inflammation of the follicles of the lashes and the associated glands of Zeis and Moll. *Staphylococcus aureus* is usually the causative organism. The lid margins are red and inflamed. There are multiple suppurative lesions surrounded by yellow pus that crusts and is removed with difficulty, bringing with it eyelash. Loss of lashes and the presence of necrotizing inflammation cause distortion of the lid margin, leading to ectropion, epiphora, and chronic conjunctivitis. Locally applied antibiotics such as neomycin and chloramphenicol or sulfonamides such as sulfacetamide and Gantrisin may be useful. Systemic antibiotics may be indicated in severe inflammation. In recent years ulcerative blepharitis has become uncommon.

Dermatitis

Infection of the skin of the eyelids may occur with a variety of microbial organisms and involves nearly the entire range of dermatitides. The thinness of the skin and its good blood supply allow enormous distention and injection, but more importantly, secondary infection of the conjunctiva, cornea, and intraocular contents may occur by direct extension. Conversely, inflammatory skin lesions may spread locally to the skin from the glands of the lid and from the conjunctiva, orbit, nasal accessory sinuses, or lacrimal apparatus.

Impetigo, erysipelas, anthrax malignant pustule, tuberculosis, chancre, leprosy, yaws, and tularemia may all involve the lid on occasion, often with enlargement of the parotid and submaxillary lymph glands. The term "Parinaud's oculoglandular syndrome" (p. 176) is applied to those conditions characterized by a unilateral necrotic lesion of the eyelid with preauricular adenopathy.

Accidental infection of the eyelids with the vaccinia virus (Fig. 7-9) may cause a vaccination pustule or blepharitis. Herpes zoster ophthalmicus causes a vesicular

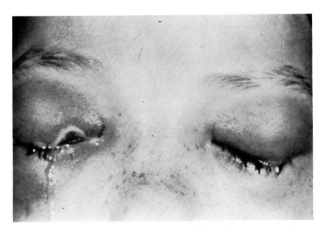

Fig. 7-9. Accidental vaccination of the upper lid with the vaccinia virus.

eruption of the eyelid which is less important than the frequent keratitis and uveitis. Verruca vulgaris and molluscum contagiosum involvement of the lid margins are important because of the resulting conjunctivitis.

Fungus infections of the eyelid may occur either as a local infection or as an involvement in the course of widespread disease.

Infection of the eyelashes by lice may cause a blepharitis or secondary infection of the skin. Primary treatment is through delousing. The parasite attached to the lashes is poisoned by anticholinesterase preparations used in the management of glaucoma and is easily removed.

Contact dermatitis

Contact dermatitis of the eyelids occurs commonly. It is characterized by a frequently recurrent, weeping, eczematous type of reaction of the skin. When chronic, the skin becomes indurated and brawny with moderate swelling and sometimes severe itching. Contact dermatitis may arise from topical compounds applied locally to relieve inflammations and infections. Particular offenders are local antibiotics, anesthetics, antihistamines, atropine, and sulfonamides. Spectacle dermatitis may arise from the nickel in frames or from plastic frames. A variety of chemicals that are used in industry, detergents, nail polishes, cosmetics, and products dispensed in aerosol cans may be implicated. Often the agent is brought to the eye by the fingers and is most marked on the side of the dominant hand, which is not usually similarly inflamed.

Treatment is unsatisfactory unless the cause is removed. This may be difficult to determine, but it is sometimes aided by the patient maintaining a diary in which he correlates his activities with the severity of the inflammation. The patient should be warned not to touch his eyelids with his fingers. In many instances it is a sound

practice to discontinue all topical medications, to proscribe cosmetics and perfumes, and to advise the use of Basis soap. Sometimes a bland ointment such as Aquaphor will relieve symptoms. A systemic antihistamine may be useful, but major reliance is placed upon removal of the cause and the application of corticosteroid preparations.

Tumors

The lids are subject to the usual tumors of the skin. If the lid margin is not involved, excision is simple. Involvement of the lid margin necessitates skilled surgery to assure excision and satisfactory closure.

Cutaneous horns

Cutaneous horns are small, cylindric epidermoid growths of unknown cause. They occur near the lid margins or the outer canthus in middle-aged or older people. They are excised easily.

Milia

Milia are small, white, round, slightly elevated cysts of the superficial dermis. They tend to occur in crops localized in a small area of the skin, sometimes on the lid. They may be derived from a hair follicle or its associated sebaceous gland. Excision may be desirable for cosmetic reasons.

Xanthelasma

Xanthelasma is a cutaneous deposition of lipid material occurring most commonly at the inner portion of the upper or the lower lid. The lesion appears as a yellowish, slightly elevated area with sharply demarcated margins tending to be approximately parallel to the lid margin. The condition occurs with primary and secondary systemic lipid anomalies, but more commonly it occurs spontaneously without evident cause. It produces only a cosmetic defect, and treatment is indicated only to remove the defect. The lesion may be excised surgically or destroyed by means of diathermy, photocoagulation, or chemicals. Recurrence is common.

Carcinoma

Basal cell carcinoma is the most common neoplasm of the lids; squamous cell carcinoma is much less common. Generally, the lower lid is involved, particularly its outer portion (Fig. 7-10). The patient may neglect the lesion for a long period inasmuch as it does not cause symptoms. There is a gradual increase in size of a typical tumor that has pearly margins and an excavated center (rodent ulcer). If the lid margin is not involved, treatment in the early stages is not particularly difficult; excision provides cure. When the lid margin is involved, surgical excision may necessitate a major plastic procedure (Fig. 7-11).

Radiation therapy may cause keratinization of the conjunctiva with chronic irritation of the cornea and keratitis. This condition is most likely to follow treatment of lesions involving the middle portion of the upper lid. When the lid margin is involved, surgical excision is preferred to radiation inasmuch as inadequate radiation may be followed by metaplasia of the tumor to the squamous cell type, and removal is more nearly assured with excision. In tumors involving the inner canthus, radiation is frequently indicated since dam-

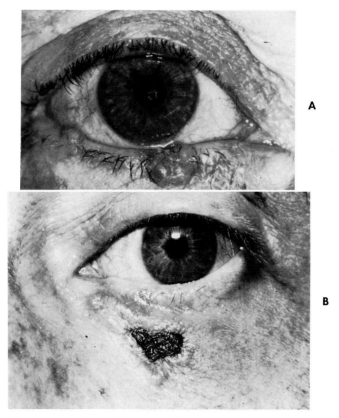

A

B

Fig. 7-10. Basal cell carcinomas of the skin of the lower eyelid, both involving the lid margin. There is great variation in the clinical appearance of these lesions, and histologic examination is required for accurate diagnosis.

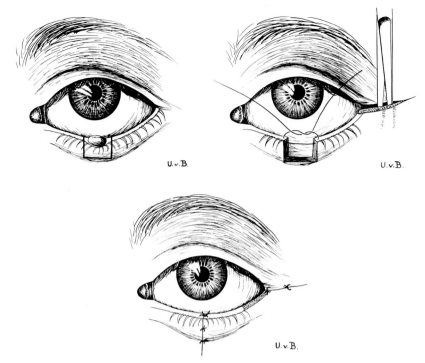

Fig. 7-11. Excision of a basal cell carcinoma of the lower lid. The incision at the lateral canthus must sever the lateral canthus ligament in order to mobilize the lid to permit closure. (From Newell, F. W.: In Lewis-Walters practice of surgery, Hagerstown, Md., 1961, W. F. Prior Co., vol. 4, chap. 1.)

age to the lacrimal drainage apparatus may be minimized. The globe is protected by means of a lead shield to prevent the formation of radiation cataract.

Neglected or mismanaged basal cell carcinoma may invade the orbit and the cranial cavity, causing a widespread destructive lesion.

The sweat glands (of Moll) of the eyelids are apocrine glands and like such glands elsewhere (axilla, surrounding the nipples, and perianal and perigenital regions) may develop a special type of carcinoma, extramammary Paget's disease. The diagnosis is usually based on the histologic appearance of the tissue, which is resected in the belief that the lesion is a basal cell carcinoma.

The meibomian glands may be involved in an adenocarcinoma, which may be preceded by a chalazion. Most commonly patients are treated for recurrent chalazion before the neoplastic nature of the lesion is evident. Such a delay may permit fatal metastasis.

Chapter 8

The conjunctiva

The conjunctiva is a thin, transparent mucous membrane that lines the posterior surfaces of the eyelids and covers the anterior surface of the globe (Fig. 1-34). It is divided into palpebral and bulbar portions and the regions connecting these two portions, the superior and inferior fornices (p. 45). Microscopically the conjunctiva consists of two or more layers of non-keratinized stratified columnar epithelium and a lamina propria composed of adenoid and connective tissue. The epithelium is continuous with the corneal epithelium and that lining the lacrimal passages and glands. The stroma is closely adherent to the tarsal plates but is thrown into many folds in the fornices and is loosely adherent to the globe. After the age of 3 or 4 months the superficial stroma in the fornices contains lymphoid tissue.

Because of its exposed position, the bulbar conjunctiva is the site of a number of degenerative changes. Inflammation may arise from exogenous microorganisms, chemical and mechanical foreign material, or electromagnetic radiation. Infection may extend from the areas adjacent to the conjunctiva or may be blood-borne, as in measles and chickenpox. Conjunctival allergic reactions may be conspicuous, as in hay fever or vernal conjunctivitis. Vascular abnormalities are readily apparent and may constitute an obvious part of systemic disease.

Symptoms and signs of conjunctival disease

Symptoms arising from disease involving only the conjunctiva are mainly ocular discomfort or burning and sometimes exudation. Severe pain suggests corneal involvement rather than origin from the conjunctiva. Itching is common in allergic conditions. Inflammatory exudates may excoriate the skin, particularly at the outer canthus, or agglutinate the eyelids together during sleep. When copious, the exudate may float across the cornea and blur vision or may even cause halos surrounding lights that disappear with rapid blinking.

The most serious symptoms of conjunctival disease arise from secondary corneal involvement by extension of inflammation, irritation by repeated contact with keratinized epithelium of the tarsal conjunctiva, exposure in cicatricial conditions that limits mobility of the lids, or failure of the goblet cells or accessory lacrimal glands to produce the secretions needed for the precorneal tear film. Visual loss from corneal involvement is common, and indeed, trachoma, an infectious disease of the conjunctiva, is probably the chief cause of blindness in the world.

The signs of conjunctival disease are mainly related to abnormalities of appearance, vascular changes, and edema (chemosis). The bulbar conjunctiva is easily inspected, but the tarsal conjunctiva can be seen only by eversion of the eyelids. Inspection of the superior fornix requires eversion of the upper eyelid by means of a retractor.

Blood vessels
Injection

The blood supply of the tarsal and palpebral conjunctiva is derived from the two arterial arcades of the lids (p. 42). The bulbar conjunctiva is nurtured by posterior conjunctival branches derived from the peripheral arterial arcades of the upper and lower eyelids. These vessels anastomose with the anterior conjunctival branches of the anterior ciliary arteries at the corneoscleral limbus (see Fig. 1-35, p. 46). Normally the posterior conjunctival arteries are nearly invisible, but in inflammations of the conjunctiva they become dilated. Conjunctival injection is characterized by superficial bright red blood vessels, most conspicuous in the fornices and fading toward the limbus. These blood vessels move with the conjunctiva and are constricted with 1:1,000 epinephrine solution instilled in the conjunctival sac (p. 131).

Both the conjunctival and ciliary vascular beds are usually injected in inflammations of the anterior segment, although one is more markedly involved than the other. In distinguishing conjunctival diseases from deeper diseases of the eye, it is wiser to direct attention to signs of corneal and iris involvement, the pupillary reaction to light, and the visual acuity.

Hyperemia of the conjunctiva

Hyperemia of the conjunctiva is a dilatation of the conjunctival blood vessels occurring without exudation or cellular infiltration. Symptoms may be absent, but frequently there is a gritty foreign body sensation that is aggravated by prolonged near work. Many patients are distressed by the conjunctival redness that becomes more marked during the day and may be further aggravated by fatigue.

The chief causes include the following: (1) irritation due to tobacco smoke, smog, and chemical fumes; (2) exposure to wind and sun; (3) inadequate ocular protection from ultraviolet radiation; (4) uncorrected refractive errors and ocular muscle imbalance; (5) prolonged topical instillation of drugs, including vasoconstrictors; (6) acne rosacea; (7) blepharitis and excessive meibomian gland secretion; and (8) ganglionic blockade in the treatment of hypertension. Chronic conjunctivitis is caused by many of the same entities (p. 177).

Treatment is directed toward removal of the cause. Temporary relief may be obtained by cold compresses or by the local instillation of weak solutions of vasoconstrictors. A large number of commercial preparations containing epinephrine or phenylephrine are available and may provide temporary relief.

Subconjunctival hemorrhage

Rupture of a conjunctival blood vessel causes a bright red, sharply delineated area surrounded by normal-appearing conjunctiva. The hemorrhage occurs beneath the bulbar conjunctiva and gradually fades in the course of 2 weeks. There are no symptoms, but many patients become alarmed by its appearance. A subconjunctival hemorrhage is caused by the same factors responsible for a black and blue spot elsewhere in the body: trauma, hypertension, blood dyscrasias, and the like. Usually no cause is found. Treatment is ineffective in hastening the absorption of blood.

Subconjunctival hemorrhage involving the entire conjunctiva follows fracture of one of the orbital bones or rupture of the posterior sclera.

Systemic disease

Typical involvement of the conjunctival blood vessels has been described in (1) sickle cell disease (p. 457), (2) diabetes mellitus (p. 385), (3) riboflavin deficiency, and (4) cryoglobulinemia (p. 461). The changes are frequently evident only with biomicroscopic examination. Inasmuch as the conjunctival blood vessels often show dilation and tortuosity with advancing age and exposure to wind, the changes with diabetes and riboflavin deficiency may be difficult to interpret.

Conjunctival vascular stasis in hemoglobin S-C disease may be characteristic of the disease. Biomicroscopic examination indicates isolated, sharply defined, twisted segments of capillaries with both the efferent and afferent connections empty of blood. The vessels are most involved in the bulbar conjunctiva adjacent to the inferior fornix. Associated with these changes may be nonspecific changes of microaneurysms, telangiectasis, and sausagelike dilation. The typical vascular stasis disappears with the local application of heat and is accentuated by cholinergic blocking.

Cryoglobulinemia is associated with stasis of blood flow in conjunctival vessels with clumping of erythrocytes. Ice water irrigation of the conjunctival sac slows the bloodstream and causes an increase in segmentation of the blood column.

Venous congestion, microaneurysms, and venous dilation have been described in the conjunctival vessels in diabetes mellitus. The changes are nonspecific and may

Clinical findings in conjunctivitis

I. Preauricular adenopathy
   A. Palpable and not tender: inclusion conjunctivitis, most APC viruses
   B. Visible and tender: APC type 8, herpes simplex, sties, acute suppurative chalazion
   C. Gross enlargement with suppuration: Parinaud's oculoglandular syndrome
II. Blepharitis and meibomianitis: *Staphylococcus*
III. Excoriation of skin of medial and lateral canthus: diplobacillus of Morax-Axenfeld
IV. Conjunctival injection
   A. Red: infectious disease
      1. Intense with petechial hemorrhages: pneumococcus or Koch-Weeks bacillus (*Haemophilus aegyptius*)
   B. Pale whitish: allergy
V. Chemosis: gonococcus, trichinosis, orbital infections
VI. Exudate
   A. Stringy, white: allergy
   B. Purulent: gonococcus, meningococcus
   C. Mucopurulent: pyogenic bacteria
   D. Scanty: virus
   E. Foamy, whitish secretion: *Corynebacterium xerose*
   F. Pseudomembrane: *Corynebacterium diphtheriae, Streptococcus,* erythema multiforme, APC type 8, vernal conjunctivitis
VII. Follicle formation
   A. Lower lid: follicular conjunctivitis, APC viruses, adult inclusion blenorrhea, molluscum contagiosum, toxic effect of pilocarpine, eserine, etc.
   B. Upper lid: trachoma
VIII. Papillary hyperplasia: vernal conjunctivitis
IX. Conjunctival scarring
   A. Upper lid: trachoma
   B. Lower lid: erythema multiforme, alkali burns, radium burns, ocular pemphigoid
   C. General: diphtheria
X. Corneal involvement
   A. Purulent: gonococcus, *Pseudomonas aeruginosa*
   B. Marginal infiltrates: *Staphylococcus,* diplobacillus of Morax-Axenfeld, punctate epithelial defects, *Staphylococcus* (lower half), trachoma (upper half)
   C. Generalized epithelial defects: Sjögren's syndrome
   D. Superior vascularization: pannus of trachoma, phlyctenular disease
XI. Unilateral inflammation: Parinaud's syndrome, adult gonococcus, contact allergy, lacrimal occlusion, viral infection

be seen with aging, arteriosclerosis, and vascular hypertension.

Conjunctivitis

Conjunctivitis is an inflammation of the conjunctiva characterized by cellular infiltration and exudation. Classification is unsatisfactory but is often based upon the cause (bacterial, viral, fungal, parasitic, toxic, chemical, mechanical, irritative, allergic, or lacrimal); the age of occurrence (ophthalmia neonatorum); the type of exudate (purulent, mucopurulent, membranous, pseudomembranous, or catarrhal); or course (acute, subacute, or chronic).

Diagnosis

The diagnosis of conjunctivitis is based upon (1) the history and clinical examination, (2) Gram's and Giemsa's stains of conjunctival scrapings, and (3) culture of the exudate.

The history of the inflammation may be helpful. Infectious disease is often bilateral and may involve other members of the family or community. Unilateral disease suggests a toxic, chemical, mechanical, or lacrimal origin. A copious exudate is more suggestive of a bacterial inflammation. A stringy, sparse exudate is more suggestive of an allergy or a viral infection.

Clinical examination requires good illumination and magnification. Attention should be directed to the presence or absence of preauricular adenopathy, involvement of the lid margins, patency of the lacrimal system, severity and nature of the conjunctival injection, occurrence of follicles or papillary hypertrophy, and the nature of the secretion. The main points of the clinical examination are summarized on p. 171.

Conjunctival scrapings are obtained with a platinum spatula, and the material is then placed on a clean glass slide. The material is fixed by drying and is not heated. It may be stained with Giemsa's stain, Wright's stain, Gram's stain, or Papa-

nicolaou's stain. Inasmuch as the conjunctiva is an exposed surface, a large number of bacteria and fungi are indigenous to the surface. Usually these are not associated with disease, but on occasion may become pathogenic. For the most part, they are present in too few numbers to be recognized readily on Gram's stain, but may be demonstrated by culture. Intraepithelial gonococci may be demonstrated some 48 hours prior to their demonstration in bacterial culture. Cytologic study of epithelial scrapings stained by Giemsa's or Wright's stain requires skilled interpretation. The main points of cytologic study are as follows:

Neutrophils: bacterial infections
  Trachoma, inclusion conjunctivitis, lymphogranuloma venereum
  Fungi
  Erythema multiforme
Eosinophils and basophils
  Vernal conjunctivitis (often fragmented)
  Hay fever conjunctivitis
  Allergies to drugs, cosmetics, etc.
Mononuclears
  Virus infections
Plasma cells
  Trachoma
Phagocytic mononuclears (macrophages)
  Trachoma (Leber's cells)
Inclusion bodies: basophilic
  Trachoma (upper tarsal), inclusion conjunctivitis (lower tarsal)
Inclusion bodies: acidophilic
  Curettings of molluscum contagiosum
Keratinized epithelium
  Sjögren's syndrome (keratoconjunctivitis sicca)
Multinucleated epithelial cells
  Virus disease

The exudate is cultured usually on blood agar and beef broth or on other media when diphtheria, gonorrhea, or fungus disease is suspected. The lids and the conjunctiva are cultured separately (different parts of the same plate may be used).

Smear and Gram's stain of the exudate are essential in the diagnosis of inflammation caused by organisms that grow relatively poorly in culture.

Clinical types

The clinical manifestations of conjunctivitis vary considerably with the cause. The onset is usually insidious. The patient notices a fullness of the lids and a diffuse, gritty, foreign body sensation. Examination indicates diffuse conjunctival injection, a clear cornea, a distinct iris pattern, and normal pupillary reaction. Within several hours of the onset, there is exudation. The type and the severity vary with the cause. There may be swelling of the lids and chemosis of the conjunctiva.

Particular emphasis in examination should be directed to the fornices to determine if there is papillary hypertrophy or follicle formation. Papillary hypertrophy is essentially a neovascularization of the conjunctival epithelium with lymphocyte infiltration occurring in chronic inflammations. It is particularly evident in vernal catarrh (p. 176). Conjunctival follicles arise in the lymphoid tissue of the substantia propria and constitute a lymphatic hypertrophy in response to chronic inflammation. The cornea should be stained with fluorescein, paying particular attention to the marginal keratitis of staphylococcal hypersensitivity. The upper and the lower lids should be everted, and the tarsal conjunctiva studied.

Bacterial inflammations. Many instances of acute conjunctivitis in the United States are caused by coagulase-producing staphylococci, hemolytic streptococci, *Diplococcus pneumoniae,* or members of the *Haemophilus* group. Almost any bacteria may be involved. Additionally, the causative organism may be one of a number of bacteria or fungi intermediate between saprophytes and pathogens. They may be recovered in culture or found in epithelial scrapings stained with Gram's iodine.

The onset is relatively acute, and both eyes are involved with a mucopurulent exudate. Drying of inspissated pus during sleep may cause the lids to be agglutinated upon awakening. Papillary hypertrophy may occur in exceptionally severe or prolonged inflammation. Conjunctivitis of bacterial origin is readily amenable to therapy: cold compresses minimize swelling and give some comfort, and a sulfonamide such as sulfacetamide instilled locally every hour is probably preferable to antibiotics. Corticosteroids should not be used. The instillation of ointment at bedtime will prevent the lids from becoming agglutinated. The eye should not be covered.

Gonococcal conjunctivitis. Gonococcal conjunctivitis is a severe, acute, purulent conjunctivitis caused by *Neisseria gonorrhoeae.* It has an incubation period of 2 to 5 days. It occurs in newborn infants, who are infected during passage through the birth canal and in adults mainly as a result of self-contamination from acute urethritis.

The inflammation may have a relatively mild onset but progresses rapidly. There are marked swelling and redness of the eyelids and severe chemosis of the conjunctiva. The exudate is first serous and then purulent. The disease is well established after 2 days, reaches its height in 4 or 5 days, and then regresses over a 4- to 6-week period. Involvement of the central cornea is common, and perforation may occur. The organism may be demonstrated in epithelial scrapings at the time of onset of the disease and in the exudate some 48 hours later. Systemic and local antibiotics and pupillary dilation by means of atropine are used in therapy.

Gonococcal urethritis is sometimes complicated by a bacteremia that causes an acute migratory polyarthritis, or a tenosynovitis. A sterile catarrhal conjunctivitis occurs in about 10% of those affected. The condition must be differentiated from Reiter's syndrome that causes a sterile urethritis, arthritis, and iridocyclitis (p. 237).

Ophthalmia neonatorum. Ophthalmia neonatorum is an acute conjunctivitis occurring within the first 10 days of life. In most states it is a reportable infectious disease. The most serious cause is *Neisseria gonorrhoeae,* which has been virtually eliminated as a cause of blindness in the United States because of Credé's prophylaxis. More common causes now are inclusion body conjunctivitis (p. 175) and bacteria, mainly pneumococcus and *Staphylococcus.* Diagnosis is based upon epithelial scrapings stained with Giemsa's and Gram's stains and upon culture. Treatment with systemic and local antibiotics is effective in bacterial disease. Inclusion conjunctivitis must be treated by means of systemic medication: sulfonamides or tetracyclines.

Credé's prophylaxis. Credé's prophylaxis consists of the instillation of 1 drop of 1% silver nitrate into the lower conjunctival sac of each eye immediately after birth. Chemical conjunctivitis occurs in about 20% of the infants thus treated, but the treatment has eliminated gonorrheal ophthalmia as a cause of blindness. Credé's prophylaxis does not prevent inclusion conjunctivitis.

Inasmuch as gonorrhea during pregnancy may be adequately treated by means of antibiotics, Credé's prophylaxis is regarded by some to be outmoded. However, gonorrhea may be undetected and unsuspected during pregnancy, with resultant contamination of the eyes in the birth canal. In some hospitals the mother and infant may be discharged during the incubation period of the infection, and the inflammation may be well established before initiation of therapy. Although many of the antibiotics have proved as adequate as silver nitrate in prophylaxis of gonococcal conjunctivitis, none has been shown to be superior.

Trachoma. Trachoma is a chronic, bilateral, infectious, cicatrizing keratoconjunctivitis caused by a member of a group of obligate intracellular organisms. Other members of this group are responsible for psittacosis and lymphogranuloma venereum. Bedsoniae has been proposed as the name of the genus and TRIC agents (*t*rachoma *i*nclusion *c*onjunctivitis) for the organisms causing eye disease. The agents are intermediate between bacteria and viruses.

Trachoma affects some 400 million persons, mainly in the Near East and Asia; in the United States it is largely confined to American Indians in the Southwest. The disease occurs among the underprivileged, in regions of poor hygiene, in countries with a warm, moist climate. Whole populations may be infected during infancy, and the trachoma is often complicated by conjunctival gonorrheal or Koch-Weeks (*Haemophilus aegyptius*) infection.

Classically the disease is divided into four stages: conjunctivitis, corneal vascularization, scarring, and scar contracture.

The diagnosis of trachoma is relatively simple in endemic areas, but isolated cases may be difficult to recognize. The severity of the disease varies markedly in different areas. However, corneal involvement associated with follicles and papillary hyperplasia occurs with no other disease. Inclusion conjunctivitis in which follicles and papillary hypertrophy occur never causes corneal changes and appears to be a distinct clinical disease. Culture studies suggest that the infectious agents causing trachoma and inclusion conjunctivitis are closely related. Inasmuch as the agent of inclusion conjunctivitis affects the uterine cervix, the possibility of a genital reservoir for trachoma has been postulated.

Clinically the organism appears as a basophilic inclusion body that is composed of elementary bodies clumped togeher in a glycogen matrix. Elementary bodies appear to develop from the conglomerations of initial bodies. Inclusion bodies are found particularly during the onset in Stage I in epithelial scrapings stained with Giemsa's stain.

The trachoma agent is sensitive to sulfonamides and broad-spectrum antibiotics. The compounds must be administered systemically. Sulfadiazine (2 to 4 Gm. daily for 14 days), oxytetracycline, and chlortetracycline (1 to 2 Gm. daily for 14 days) are the preferred agents. Entire communities may be treated prophylactically with sulfonamides, but major attention must be directed to improvement in hygiene. Active immunization by inoculation is complicated by numerous strains with poor cross-immunity and a weak immune response to the virus. Surgery is commonly required for cicatricial distortion of the eyelids.

Inclusion conjunctivitis. Inclusion conjunctivitis is an infectious disease occurring in newborn and adult forms. The agent causes a nonspecific urethritis in men and a chronic, clinically silent endocervicitis in women. Infants are infected during passage through the birth canal. Adult infection may be transmitted through nonchlorinated swimming pools (swimming pool conjunctivitis), by accidental infection in physicians' offices, by use of contaminated cosmetics for the eyelashes, and venereally.

Inclusion conjunctivitis is a cause of ophthalmia neonatorum. After a 5- to 10-day incubation period an acute conjunctivitis is characterized by marked papillary hypertrophy of the lower fornix, and a profuse exudate occurs. Inasmuch as the newborn lacks conjunctival lymphoid tissue until 4 to 6 weeks of age, follicles cannot develop. Numerous basophilic inclusion bodies together with initial and elementary bodies may be found in epithelial scrapings stained with Giemsa's stain. When untreated, the acute phase lasts 10 to 20 days and then subsides into a gradually diminishing chronic follicular conjunctivitis that persists 3 to 12 months.

Effective treatment requires systemic administration of sulfonamides for a minimum period of 7 days. Local instillation is less consistently effective, and the medication must be instilled frequently. Credé's prophylaxis does not protect against inclusion conjunctivitis.

Gonorrhea in the newborn infant may be differentiated by its shorter incubation period, by the involvement of the superior and inferior fornices, by the cytology, and by the demonstration of the causative organism.

Inclusion conjunctivitis of the adult begins as an acute follicular conjunctival inflammation that becomes chronic. The disease is identical with that of the newborn infant except that in the newborn infant an adenoid layer necessary for follicle development is lacking. Several weeks after the acute onset the inflammation subsides to a chronic conjunctival disease that persists for a period of 3 to 12 months. The cornea is never involved, and there is no residual injury. Systemic sulfadiazine, 2 to 4 Gm. for 7 days, is used for treatment.

Viral conjunctivitis. Invasion of the conjunctiva by a variety of viruses can cause conjunctivitis (p. 368). It is probable that a number of mild nonincapacitating conjunctival inflammations in which microorganisms are not demonstrated are due to viruses. Conjunctival involvement may be part of a systemic infection, or the disease may be limited to the epithelium of the cornea and conjunctiva.

Adenoviruses. The adenoviruses (adenopharyngoconjunctival, or APC) represents a group of at least 23 immunologically distinct viruses that cause inflammation of mucous membranes; they are mainly implicated in upper respiratory infections (p. 369). Some strains may cause a follicular conjunctivitis that may be associated with preauricular adenopathy and corneal infiltration with reduction of vision.

Epidemic keratoconjunctivitis. Epidemic keratoconjunctivitis (APC type 8) is an acute inflammatory disease of the cornea and the conjunctiva ushered in by a severe acute follicular conjunctivitis associated with a transient pseudomembrane, pale conjunctival chemosis, and preauricular adenopathy. After 7 to 10 days the cornea becomes involved with subepithelial infiltrates affecting the central area. The acute inflammation disappears in several weeks, and the corneal infiltrates regress over a period of months, leaving a residue of fine superficial scars that do not interfere with vision. The virus may be spread by contaminated eyedrops, eye instruments, or directly, sometimes from infected physicians. Treatment with local instillation of IDU prevents corneal involvement.

Lacrimal conjunctivitis. Lacrimal conjunctivitis is a monocular conjunctivitis secondary to infections from microorganisms in an occluded lacrimal sac. The inflammation persists until drainage is established. Usually dacryocystitis does not involve the conjunctiva. Pneumococcus infection of the lacrimal sac is a common cause of serpiginous keratitis (p. 204). Fungus occlusion of the canaliculi is often recognized because of the scraping sound when the lacrimal system is probed.

Parinaud's oculoglandular syndrome. This is a traditional ophthalmic eponym that is observed rarely. It consists of a monocular, granulomatous, necrotic conjunctival lesion associated with a suppurative preauricular adenopathy. Parinaud's syndrome must be excluded from Parinaud's sign, which is the inability to rotate the eyes upward because of midbrain neoplasms, particularly pinealoma. The chief causes of Parinaud's oculoglandular syndrome include chancre, tuberculosis, lymphogranuloma venereum, leptotrichosis, and oculoglandular tularemia.

Allergic conjunctivitis. A number of antigens may give rise to superficial conjunctival reactions. Because of the elasticity of the tissues, there may be considerable swelling. Most of the conditions are characterized by the presence of many eosinophils in the epithelial scrapings. A number of specific types are described.

Vernal conjunctivitis. Vernal conjunctivitis is a bilateral recurrent inflammation occurring during the warm months of the year, particularly in warm climates. Boys are affected more commonly than girls, usually during childhood. Two forms occur: (1) palpebral (Fig. 8-1), involving the tarsal conjunctiva of the upper lid with the formation of typical thickened gelatinous vegetations and sometimes a pseudomembrane, and (2) limbal, with inflammation of the circumference of the corneoscleral limbus with the formation of a

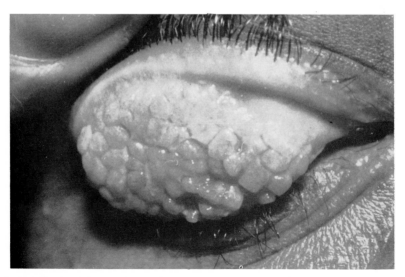

Fig. 8-1. Palpebral form of vernal conjunctivitis with marked proliferation of the conjunctiva.

gelatinous, elevated area about 4 mm. wide. The chief symptom is itching, which may be nearly intolerable. Histologically there is hyperplasia and hyalinization of connective tissue, proliferation of epithelium, and cellular infiltration with numerous eosinophils. The secretion is tenacious, stringy, and sticky. Moving to a cool climate is sometimes helpful. Treatment consists of local instillation of corticosteroids, weak solutions of epinephrine, and cold compresses. Ice compresses may give relief. Radiation therapy is now generally believed to be contraindicated. The excision of large palpebral vegetations may give symptomatic relief.

Atopic conjunctivitis. Atopic conjunctivitis is the conjunctival reaction to pollens in hypersensitive people who usually have hay fever. Atopic conjunctivitis may occur independent of pollen hypersensitivity, but there is usually a history of allergy. The onset is acute, with lacrimation, chemosis, and a watery discharge. The conjunctival secretion contains many eosinophils. The local instillation of the causative antigen causes similar symptoms. The condition responds to the local instillation of vasoconstrictors and to systemic antihistamines. Desensitization to the causative antigen may be unusually helpful. Locally applied antihistamines may cause a contact conjunctivitis.

Phlyctenular keratoconjunctivitis. Phlyctenular keratoconjunctivitis is a unilateral localized allergic conjunctival nodule about 1 to 3 mm. in size. It is considered a delayed hypersensitivity to bacterial protein, particularly tuberculoprotein. Classically it was believed to be a disease of undernourished children who had been exposed to pulmonary tuberculosis. In the United States it is mainly an inflammation affecting adults. Staphylococci are considered the most common cause. The most serious complication is corneal vascularization. The phlyctenula progresses irregularly to the central cornea and is followed by a group of blood vessels, which causes corneal scarring and reduced vision. Topical instillation of corticosteroids usually suppresses the hypersensitivity, and healing follows.

Contact conjunctivitis. Contact conjunctivitis occurs in one of two forms: (1) allergic and (2) primary irritant. Allergic contact conjunctivitis is nearly always caused by the local instillation of medication. There are itching, chemosis of the conjunctiva, and eosinophils in the scraping. The usual drugs are those used daily in the treatment of chronic ocular disease, such as pilocarpine and eserine in the treatment of glaucoma and atropine when used in the management of uveitis or retinal detachment. Local penicillin, streptomycin, sulfathiazole, local anesthetics, and antihistamines are also common offenders.

Primary irritant contact conjunctivitis is a follicular type of conjunctivitis that is particularly marked in the lower cul-de-sac. Symptoms are minimal, and the disease is often listed as a chronic conjunctivitis. Eosinophils are not present in conjunctival scrapings. Almost any compound used in the treatment of ocular disease may be a source of such irritation. The conjunctivitis disappears when the compound is discontinued, and once improved the drugs may be reinstituted without recurrence. The irritation may constitute an untoward reaction to the vehicle or a preservative rather than the active principle of the drug.

Chronic conjunctivitis. Chronic conjunctivitis is a generic term applied to persistent conjunctival inflammation that may be caused by many agents. It is characterized by bilateral conjunctival injection, scanty exudation, and a tendency to periodic exacerbation and remission. Symptoms vary from mild grittiness or foreign body sensation, with heaviness of the lids, to burning, photophobia, and irritation. The symptoms may be severe enough to handicap the patient and are often disproportionately severe for the clinical signs of disease. Examination indicates hyperemia, microscopic papillae, thickening of the conjunctiva in the fornices, and a mucous secretion.

Causes include the following:

1. *Staphylococcus aureus* infection is usually associated with a chronic blepharitis and an epithelial keratitis involving the lower one half of the cornea.

2. A variety of microorganisms often considered nonpathogenic have been implicated. These organisms often reside on body surfaces but may be found in almost pure culture, and presumably when appropriate predisposing conditions are present, they may produce inflammation.

3. The significance of viruses is not established. Virus infections tend to involve the superior conjunctiva and to be associated with filaments near the 12 o'clock meridian (see discussion on superficial punctate keratitis, p. 206).

4. Chemical and physical irritants and unsuspected foreign bodies may be a cause. The use of sun lamps without ocular protection may give rise to an actinic keratoconjunctivitis. Chemical irritation from the chlorine in swimming pools is an obvious cause. Drugs used to treat ocular disease may cause the inflammation.

5. Excessive meibomian secretion is characterized by a frothy secretion at the angles and may either cause or complicate chronic conjunctivitis.

6. Acne rosacea may have conjunctival involvement that precedes rosacea corneal vascularization.

Treatment of chronic conjunctivitis may be extremely difficult. Careful diagnosis is essential, and the cause may be eliminated when possible. Lesions of the lids and lid margins such as cysts, verruca vulgaris, and molluscum contagiosum must be eliminated. Sjögren's disease must be excluded, and the tear ducts must be tested for patency. Allergy and irritation from chemicals, smoke, and cosmetics must be minimized.

Other conjunctival disorders
Pinguecula

A pinguecula is a benign degenerative tumor of the bulbar conjunctiva that appears as a yellowish white, slightly elevated, oval-shaped tissue mass on either side of the cornea in the palpebral fissure. The lesions are usually bilateral and located nasally. They are increasingly common with advancing age. They cause a cosmetic defect and in some instances appear to precede a pterygium. Treatment is usually unnecessary, but excision is simple. Histologically a pinguecula consists of a deposition of amorphous hyaline substance in areas of degenerative elastic tissue. Rarely a pinguecula becomes inflamed, causing a foreign body sensation and a surrounding conjunctival hyperemia. The apex of the pinguecula then stains with fluorescein. The inflammation responds quickly to local antiseptics.

Pterygium

A pterygium is a triangular fold of bulbar conjunctiva that advances progressively over the cornea in the interpalpebral fissure, usually from the nasal side (Fig. 8-2). A pinguecula often precedes its development, and a pseudoelastic tissue similar to a pinguecula is present. Pterygiums occur commonly in the tropics and subtropics, particularly among those exposed to chronic conjunctival irritation from wind and sunlight.

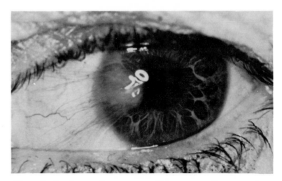

Fig. 8-2. Pterygium extending over the nasal portion of the cornea.

Symptoms are absent unless the pterygium encroaches on the visual axis. The superficial blood vessels in a pterygium may become dilated and cause a cosmetic defect.

A number of procedures for either excising or transplanting pterygiums have been proposed. Simple excision is invariably followed by recurrence. In the temperate zone of the United States they seldom progress rapidly, and they respond well to nearly any surgical procedure. In tropical areas, pterygiums progress rapidly, are commonly thick and vascular, and have a pronounced tendency to recur irrespective of the type of surgery. Repeated excision may finally result in extensive conjunctival scarring and restricted movement of the globe. Beta and grenz rays have been widely used to minimize recurrence. Beta-ray sources applied to the corneoscleral limbus may cause a sectorial radiation cataract due to interference with mitotic activity of the cells at the lens equator.

A pseudopterygium is a fold of conjunctiva that has become adherent to a marginal ulcer of the cornea. A probe may be passed beneath the head of a pseudopterygium that distinguishes it from a true pterygium. A pseudopterygium does not progress, and excision is required solely for cosmetic reasons.

Lymphangiectasis

The lymphatic channels of the conjunctiva may become dilated and give rise to clear, serous conjunctival cysts. These are approximately linear in shape and may be multiple. There is no effective treatment.

Lithiasis

Degenerations of the conjunctival epithelium in the elderly or prolonged conjunctivitis may cause yellowish to white concretions in the epithelium. The deposits may be seen in the tarsal conjunctiva or the inferior fornix. Rarely, there is dehiscence of the overlying epithelium, causing exposure of the concretion with foreign body symptoms. The area stains with fluorescein. Such concretions may be removed easily with a sharp needle-knife after the instillation of a conjunctival anesthetic.

Pigmentation

The dull, white sclera accentuates conjunctival pigmentation. A dull, grayish discoloration involving the conjunctiva in the lower fornix may follow repeated instillation of silver and mercury salts. The pigmentation arises from the deposition of the metallic ion and cannot be reversed. Epinephrine instillation may cause deep black subconjunctival deposits of melanin. Exposure to the fumes of equinone or hydroquinone may cause pigmentation of the interpalpebral bulbar conjunctiva.

A yellowish discoloration of the conjunctiva may arise from an excess of plant pigment (carotene) in food faddists who eat huge amounts of carrots. It must be distinguished from jaundice. Ochronosis and Addison's disease also cause pigmentation of the conjunctiva. The conjunctiva and not the sclera is yellow colored in jaundice.

Granulomas

Granulomas may follow faulty closure of a conjunctival incision. They occur particularly following retinal detachment and strabismus surgery. There is a formation of large, fungating, reddish masses, which bleed readily. Usually simple excision is all that is required. Retained foreign bodies may also cause a granuloma.

Tumors

Dermoid tumors. Dermoid tumors are common congenital tumors of the conjunctiva. They may be cystic or solid. A special type is a dermatolipoma, which occurs usually at the superior temporal limbus and appears as a sharply circumscribed, round, slightly yellowish, elevated mass involving the cornea and the sclera. It oc-

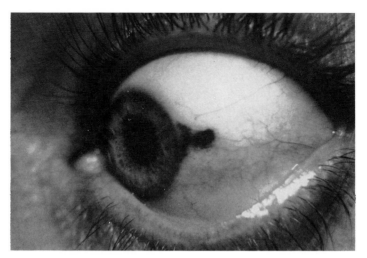

Fig. 8-3. Nevus of the conjunctiva.

curs frequently in mandibulofacial dysostosis. The lesion may be excised for cosmetic reasons.

Nevi. Nevi (Fig. 8-3) are extremely common on the conjunctiva and occur usually near the corneoscleral limbus. They appear as yellowish red areas or deeply pigmented masses usually on the bulbar conjunctiva. Malignant metaplasia occurs in about one fourth of the cases. Nevi are usually present prior to puberty but have junctional activity in adulthood. Excision is simple.

Intraepithelial epitheliomas (Bowen's disease). These slowly growing neoplasms are usually associated with chronic inflammation that occurs most commonly near the corneoscleral limbus. Men 60 years of age or older are usually affected. The tumor may give rise to an atypical squamous cell carcinoma or may metastasize without evidence of local invasion. Papanicolaou staining of scrapings may indicate carcinomatous cells.

Lymphomas. Lymphomatous disease (benign lymphoma, lymphosarcoma, and reticulum cell sarcoma) may be manifest in the adenoid layer of the conjunctiva. A smooth, elevated tumor mass, which may be widespread, develops, with protrusion of the conjunctiva. Retrobulbar extension may cause proptosis. The condition may be localized to the conjunctiva or may be a manifestation of systemic disease. The conjunctival lesion is extremely sensitive to roentgen-ray therapy.

Benign acquired melanosis (precancerous and cancerous melanosis). Benign acquired melanosis is an acquired pigmented lesion that appears at about the age of 40 to 50 years, unlike nevi that are congenital or appear before puberty. The pigmentation is diffuse, flat, unilateral, and asymptomatic. Large areas of the conjunctiva may be involved over a period as long as 20 years, but usually after 5 or 10 years the lesion imperceptibly merges into a malignant melanoma. The lesion waxes and wanes, and clinical and histologic assessment of activity is difficult. The comparable lesion of the skin is called a senile melanotic freckle of Hutchinson. Treatment is difficult. In most individuals the tumor is extremely benign, and periodic histologic study is indicated only when there is evidence of progression or activity. Exenteration of the orbit is indicated if frank malignant changes occur. Many regard the lesion as radiosensitive and believe radiation is indicated if metaplasia occurs.

Chapter 9

The lacrimal apparatus

The lacrimal apparatus consists of a secretory and a drainage portion. The secretory portion is composed of the lacrimal gland, which is divided into palpebral and orbital lobes, and the accessory lacrimal glands of Wolfring and Krause scattered through the conjunctiva (p. 43). The drainage portion consists of epithelial-lined tubes leading from the openings on the lid margins (the puncta) through the canaliculi to the lacrimal sac, which lies in the lacrimal fossa. The lacrimal sac opens into the inferior nasal meatus by its inferior continuation, the nasolacrimal duct, which lies in the bony nasolacrimal canal.

The tears (p. 74) consist of two portions, a relatively stagnant layer overlying the cornea and a fluid layer that flows in the lower fornix to the inferior punctum. The corneal layer is the precorneal film and constitutes the thin transparent layer that provides the anterior refracting surface of the eye. It is composed of a superficial oily layer derived from the meibomian glands that prevents evaporation, a middle layer of tears, and an inner mucoid layer immediately adjacent to the corneal epithelium derived from the goblet cells. The fluid layer is derived mainly from the accessory lacrimal glands and the lacrimal gland.

Symptoms and signs of lacrimal apparatus disease

Diseases of the lacrimal system are divided into those involving abnormalities of the lacrimal glands and those involving defects in the drainage system. Excessive formation of tears (see outline on p. 184) usually occurs because of reflex stimulation of the gland, whereas decreased tear formation arises either because of atrophy of glandular tissue or cicatricial occlusion of the orifices of the gland. Neoplasms and inflammatory diseases of the lacrimal gland give rise to a characteristic swelling that causes an S-shaped curve of the upper lid.

Diseases of the lacrimal drainage apparatus give rise to obstruction that causes tearing. The obstructed lacrimal sac may become acutely or chronically inflamed. The acute inflammation causes a generalized cellulitis of the sac and surrounding structures. Chronic inflammation is associated with few signs other than painless swelling with pus flowing from the puncta when pressure is applied to the sac.

The main symptoms of diseases of the lacrimal system are usually related to either an excess or a deficiency of tears or to swelling of the lacrimal gland or lacrimal sac. Excessive tear formation is a nuisance since vision is blurred by tears that overflow onto the face. Deficient tear secretion, however, may cause loss of the eye and be associated with keratinization of the conjunctiva and may give rise to almost intolerable symptoms of burning and dryness of the eyes.

Diseases of the lacrimal glands

The lacrimal glands are tubuloracemose, similar in structure to the salivary glands

—in general, they are subject to the same inflammations, diseases, and tumors. Not uncommonly the two groups of glands are involved in the same inflammatory and degenerative diseases.

The symptoms and signs of lacrimal gland disease involve oversecretion or undersecretion of tears or enlargement of the gland. In inflammation the usual signs of pain, redness, and swelling are associated with distortion of the outer one third of the lid margin, which assumes an S-shaped curve.

Inflammation

Acute dacryoadenitis. Acute dacryoadenitis (Fig. 9-1) is a rare catarrhal inflammation of the lacrimal gland that usually accompanies systemic disease. Mumps and infectious mononucleosis are the usual systemic causes of an acute process. A purulent infection may be secondary to extension of inflammation from the lids or the conjunctiva.

Pain and discomfort in the upper outer portion of the orbit are the chief symptoms. Swelling and redness of the lacrimal gland cause a mechanical ptosis of the upper eyelid and an S-shaped curve of the lid margin. Other causes of cellulitis of the skin and orbit must be considered in the differential diagnosis. Eversion of the upper lid indicates a swollen, reddened gland.

Treatment is directed to the cause. If a purulent infection is present, antibiotics and local hot compresses, possibly combined with incision and drainage, are indicated. Dacryoadenitis is usually self-limited, and therapy is directed toward preventing extension of the infection.

Chronic dacryoadenitis. Chronic dacryoadenitis is a proliferative inflammation of the lacrimal gland, usually due to specific granulomatous disease, particularly pseudotumor, Boeck's sarcoid, tuberculosis, and syphilis. Clinically, chronic dacryoadenitis is characterized by painless enlargement of the lacrimal glands, most evident when the upper lid is everted. Treatment must be directed toward the cause.

Mikulicz's syndrome is the term applied to chronic bilateral swelling of the lacrimal and salivary glands. It may occur in the course of reticuloendothelial disease, leukemias, Hodgkin's disease, sarcoid, and other granulomas. Most observers believe that it does not constitute a specific entity.

Tumors

The lacrimal gland may be involved in three types of tumor: (1) lymphomatous disease, 25%; (2) chronic granuloma arising from sarcoid or orbital pseudotumor (nonspecific granuloma), 25%; and (3) lacrimal gland neoplasm, 50%. Pseudotumor is an inflammatory granuloma usually of unknown cause (p. 194). Lymphomatous disease may vary considerably in histologic type. It may be restricted to the lacrimal gland or be but an incidental finding in the course of systemic disease. It is sensitive to radiation therapy. All are associated with a mass or fullness in the outer portion of the upper lid that may simulate the appearance of a blepharoptosis. There

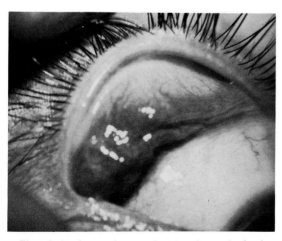

Fig. 9-1. Acute dacryoadenitis. The palpebral portion of the lacrimal gland is evident upon eversion of the upper lid.

may be proptosis with displacement of the globe down and in. Granulomas and lymphomatous disease may be associated with intermittent inflammation. Eversion of the upper lid may indicate enlargement of the lacrimal gland. Pain is a prominent symptom of all tumors. The diagnosis can be made only by means of histologic study. Inasmuch as piecemeal removal of a malignant mixed tumor may be followed by seeding and dissemination of a malignancy, the capsule must be sutured after excision and complete removal carried out within 24 hours if the mass is malignant.

Epithelial tumors of the lacrimal gland are similar in both their histologic appearance and their clinical course to neoplasms of the salivary glands. They may be classified as follows:

Benign
  Mixed tumor
  Adenoma
Malignant
  Mixed tumor
  Carcinoma unrelated to mixed tumor
    Adenocarcinoma (adenoid cystic carcinoma
      or cylindroma)
    Mucoepidermoid carcinoma
    Squamous cell carcinoma

Mixed tumor is the most common epithelial tumor of the lacrimal gland. It originates from embryonic rests, and both epithelial and mesenchymal elements are present. It is slowly progressive and involves adults of middle age. Both malignant and benign mixed tumors may erode the bone of the lacrimal fossa. Every effort must be made to excise the tumor within its capsule and to avoid seeding. If there is bony involvement, the bone should be resected. Both benign and malignant tumors recur if there is seeding, but only the malignant type metastasizes.

Adenocarcinoma occurs relatively more frequently in the lacrimal gland than in the salivary glands. It is very invasive and metastasizes by way of the lymphatics and the blood vessels. Histologically it is composed of aggregates of small undifferen-

tiated neoplastic cells separated by small and large cystoid spaces containing a mucinous material. Treatment is very unsatisfactory, although the tumor is not rapidly fatal. The preferred treatment is exenteration of the orbit with resection of the bone of the lacrimal fossa and any other involved tissues. The other types of malignant tumors listed have a similarly dismal prognosis, and radical surgery is indicated.

Tearing and dry eyes

Excessive tear formation (lacrimation) or defective drainage of tears (epiphora) is associated with blurring of vision and constant discomfort caused by tears running down the cheek. In all instances it is necessary to learn whether there is excessive production or defective drainage of tears.

Tear formation is measured clinically by the Schirmer test in which a 35 by 5 mm.

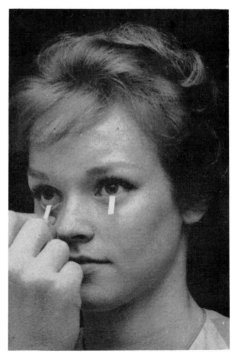

Fig. 9-2. Proper position of filter paper to measure tear formation by the Schirmer test.

strip of No. 41 Whatman filter paper is folded over the midportion of the lower lid (Fig. 9-2). Generally, if 10 mm. or more of the paper from the point of the fold becomes wet in a 4-minute period, tear formation is considered normal. More than 25 mm. of wetting indicates excessive tear formation. It may well be that the lacrimal gland secretes only under the stimulus of emotion or irritation, and that the accessory lacrimal glands and the goblet cells in the conjunctiva are largely responsible for maintaining normal moistening of the eye.

Lacrimation

Lacrimation, or the overproduction of tears, may arise because of reflex stimula-

---

Tearing and dry eyes

I. Lacrimation (excessive tear production)
  A. Psychic stimulation
  B. Parasympathetic stimulation
    1. Cholinergic drugs (Mecholyl)
    2. Anticholinesterase drugs
  C. Lacrimal gland inflammations and neoplasms
  D. Trigeminal irritation
    1. Lesions of the lids, conjunctiva, cornea, iris
    2. Glaucoma
  E. Retinal stimulation by glare and excessive light
  F. Facial nerve
    1. Sphenopalatine ganglion stimulation by inflammation and neoplasms
    2. Misdirected regeneration following seventh nerve paralysis (crocodile tears)
II. Epiphora (defective tear drainage)
  A. Abnormalities of puncta
    1. Ectropion, orbicularis oculi muscle weakness, cicatrization, occlusion
  B. Lacrimal obstruction
    1. Canaliculi—inflammation, cicatrix
    2. Lacrimal sac and duct
      a. Congenital abnormalities, inflammation, neoplasms
    3. Meatus
      a. Congenital stenosis, acquired, or local nasal disease
III. Dry eyes
  A. Conjunctival cicatrization
    1. Erythema multiforme (Stevens-Johnson disease)
    2. Trachoma
    3. Ocular pemphigoid
    4. Thermal, chemical, and radiation burns
  B. Sjögren's syndrome
  C. Lagophthalmos
  D. Riley-Day syndrome
  E. Absence of lacrimal gland
  F. Paralytic
    1. Facial nerve (between facial lacrimal nucleus and geniculate ganglion), greater superficial petrosal nerve, sphenopalatine ganglion
    2. Trigeminal nerve (decrease in reflex lacrimation)
  G. Toxic
    1. Cholinergic blockade (atropine)
    2. Deep anesthesia
    3. Debilitating disease

tion of the lacrimal gland from irritation of the conjunctival sac or the cornea or from excessive stimulation of the retina by light. Abnormal regeneration of the seventh cranial nerve following facial nerve paralysis may lead to tearing associated with salivation (crocodile tears) because of diversion of fibers from the salivary to the lacrimal gland. Cholinergic stimulation by either parasympathomimetic drugs or anticholinesterases may lead to a pharmacologic type of lacrimation. Often the cause of lacrimation can be easily identified and corrected.

Epiphora

Epiphora is that condition in which there is a faulty drainage of tears through the lacrimal passages. It arises from a variety of causes: faulty apposition of the lacrimal puncta in the lacrimal lake, scarring of the puncta, paresis or paralysis of the orbicularis oculi muscle that eliminates the suction in the canaliculi, foreign bodies in the canaliculi, and obstructions in the lacrimal sac and the nasolacrimal duct. The accumulation of tears at the inner canthus

causes irritation that reflexly stimulates additional tear formation.

The adequacy and patency of the lacrimal system may be demonstrated in several ways. Simple inspection indicates whether the puncta are in contact with the lacrimal lake. Normally, when the eye is rotated upward, the inferior punctum is not visible unless the lid is everted. Forcible closure of the eyelids indicates the adequacy of the function of the orbicularis oculi muscle.

Fluorescein solution, 2%, instilled in the conjunctival sac normally disappears within 1 minute. If the fluorescein then can be demonstrated in the nose or the pharynx, the lacrimal passages are definitely patent. Sodium saccharin, 10%, instilled in the conjunctival sac may be recognized by its sweet taste if it passes into the posterior pharynx.

Irrigation of the lacrimal system to demonstrate patency is less physiologic than instillation of drugs in the conjunctival sac. Irrigation has the advantage of rapid application and may be combined with the use of colored solutions or radiopaque sub-

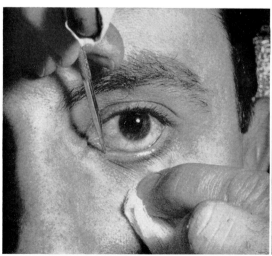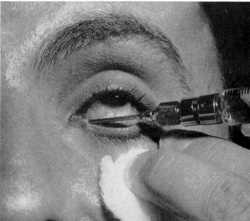

Fig. 9-3. Dilation of the inferior lacrimal punctum and irrigation of the lacrimal sac through the inferior canaliculus.

stances such as Pantopaque for subsequent roentgenographic study.

The management of epiphora depends upon its cause. Surgery of the lid is indicated if the punctum is not in contact with the lacrimal lake. Obstruction in the lacrimal sac may require anastomosis between the sac and the mucous membrane of the nose, a dacryocystorhinostomy. Atresia of the canaliculi may be difficult to correct. A large variety of surgical procedures has been described.

Decreased tear secretion

A tearing eye may be a nuisance to the patient but never causes loss of vision. A dry eye is associated with keratinization of the corneal and the conjunctival epithelium, and there may be marked corneal scarring. Removal of the lacrimal gland is not associated with particular drying of the eye, although reflex and psychic tearing are lost. The accessory lacrimal glands appear to maintain normal moistening of the globe.

Decreased tear secretion is particularly associated with conjunctival cicatrization (trachoma, chemical burns, and erythema multiforme), which occludes the orifices of the lacrimal glands, and with Sjögren's syndrome. There is less than 10 mm. of wetting of filter paper (Schirmer's test) in a 4-minute period. The eyes feel dry, burn, and have a constant foreign body sensation. Symptoms are aggravated by warmth and conditions causing rapid evaporation of tears. There may be punctate epithelial erosions of the cornea and the conjunctiva.

Conditions associated with conjunctival scarring include (1) erythema multiforme in its various ocular manifestations of Stevens-Johnson disease and Reiter's syndrome, (2) trachoma, (3) ocular pemphigoid, and (4) chemical and radiation burns of the conjunctiva. Sjögren's syndrome is a systemic disease with widespread manifestations mainly of keratoconjunctivitis sicca and arthritis with labora-

tory signs of a severe infection. It occurs mainly in women near the menopause (p. 452).

The treatment of decreased tear formation is often unsatisfactory. Artificial tears of methyl cellulose, sometimes combined with lysozyme, require frequent instillation. Obstruction of the superior and inferior puncta to conserve tears requires some moisture to be effective. Protective lenses and avoidance of dry and warm atmospheres that encourage tear evaporation are commonly the only therapy available. If parotid gland secretion is not impaired, transplantation of Stensen's duct into the conjunctival sac provides a generous salivary secretion.

Diseases of the lacrimal passages
Canaliculitis

Canaliculitis is an inflammation of the canaliculi occurring because of infection. Most attention has been directed to inflammation associated with obstruction by fungi, particularly the *Leptothrix (Actinomyces)*. Canaliculitis causes tearing and sometimes inflammation of the adjacent conjunctiva. The diagnosis is made by recovery of the fungus from the canaliculus. Probing indicates a gritty foreign body sensation in the canaliculus.

Dacryocystitis

Dacryocystitis is an acute or chronic inflammation of the lacrimal sac. The cause is obstruction of the lacrimal sac or the nasolacrimal duct followed by bacterial infection.

Acute dacryocystitis. Acute dacryocystitis is a suppurative inflammation of the lacrimal sac with an associated cellulitis of the overlying tissues (Fig. 9-4, *A*). The onset is acute, with major symptoms of a suppurative infection at the inner canthus. There is painful swelling of the tissues overlying the lacrimal sac. There is exquisite tenderness in the region that is often combined with widespread cellulitis associated with constitutional symptoms. The main differential diagnosis involves other causes of acute suppurative inflammation in the area. Local hot compresses and systemic antibiotics are used in treatment. Incision and drainage are indicated if there is abscess formation.

Chronic dacryocystitis. Chronic dacryocystitis occurs because of obstruction of the nasolacrimal duct, and it is seen most frequently in newborn infants and in middle life (Fig. 9-4, *B*). The chief symptoms are epiphora and regurgitation of pus through the puncta when the lacrimal sac is massaged.

Infantile stenosis. Dacryocystitis in infants arises because of failure of the nasolacrimal duct to open into the inferior meatus as normally occurs about the third week of life. The initial symptom is constant tearing of one eye. This is followed by regurgitation of pus through the puncta. Acute dacryocystitis may occur, but this is exceptional.

The treatment of the stenosis has been debated extensively. There is a strong tendency toward spontaneous patency with drainage and disappearance of the condition. The majority of instances are rectified spontaneously by the age of 6 months without treatment. Generally, a medication such as sulfacetamide is used locally to prevent lacrimal conjunctivitis. While awaiting spontaneous correction, the parents are instructed to massage the lacrimal sac daily to keep it empty of pus.

If the obstruction persists after the age of 6 months, lacrimal probing is indicated inasmuch as spontaneous patency is unlikely. Usually the patient is mummified in a blanket, and a local anesthetic is instilled into the conjunctival sac. The superior

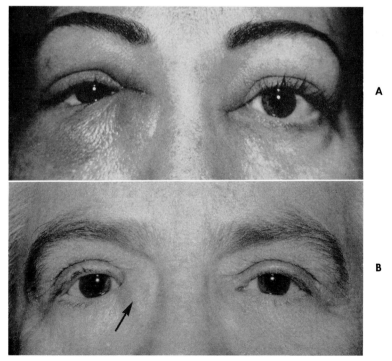

Fig. 9-4. A, Acute dacryocystitis with cellulitis of the eyelids. **B,** Chronic dacryocystitis with a mucocele of the lacrimal sac.

punctum is manipulated inasmuch as it is probably without function, and if subsequent atresia or stricture occurs, it is not symptomatic. A lacrimal probe is inserted into the upper punctum, directed medially and into the lacrimal sac, and then turned at right angles into the nasolacrimal canal and the inferior meatus. The nose is inspected to be certain that the tip of the probe is not covered by mucous membrane. In exceptional instances more than one probing must be done. In rare instances there is failure of the nasolacrimal duct to form, and it is necessary to perform dacryocystorhinostomy. Such surgery is wisely deferred until the child is 3 or 4 years old. It is an uncomplicated procedure in the very young because of the softness of the bone.

Adult chronic dacryocystitis. Adult chronic dacryocystitis follows occlusion of the lacrimal sac that may occur spontaneously or follow injury or nasal disease in this region. Spontaneous atresia is more common in women in middle life. An annoying epiphora occurs initially, and as the occlusion continues, there is regurgitation of pus from the lacrimal sac. If neglected, an extraordinary dilation and thinning of the lacrimal sac occurs that is known as mucocele or hydrops of the lacrimal sac. Acute suppuration is unusual. Differential diagnosis involves mainly the various causes of tearing and granulomatous infections of the lacrimal sac.

Surgery is the only satisfactory treatment. When not severe, instillation of zinc and epinephrine collyria may be helpful in the elderly. Probing of the lacrimal passages with probes of successively greater size may be useful, but for the most part relief is transient, and the procedure is painful. The threading of fine polyethylene tubes through the lacrimal passages has had a transient popularity.

The surgical procedure of choice is a dacryocystorhinostomy in which a communication is established between the lacrimal sac and the nose. Many procedures have been recommended. If the bony opening into the nose is large enough, the majority of patients improve. Extirpation of the sac (dacryocystectomy) should not be carried out. In exceptional elderly patients in whom intraocular surgery is required, the lacrimal sac is removed to eliminate the regurgitation of pus into the conjunctival sac.

Neoplasms

Tumors of the lacrimal sac are rare. The majority of neoplasms are squamous cell carcinomas, with lymphosarcomas and granulomas occurring as in lacrimal gland tumors. The initial symptom is tearing that may be followed by the signs of chronic dacryocystitis with regurgitation of pus and mucus through the punctum. Regurgitation of blood is nearly always due to a malignant tumor of the lacrimal sac. A painless, nonreducible swelling then occurs in the region of the sac, with eventual extension of the tumor outside the lacrimal fossa. Tumors can be demonstrated roentgenographically by injection of contrast media into the lacrimal passageways. Squamous cell tumors must be completely excised. Excision followed by radiation therapy is recommended for lymphomatous disease.

Chapter 10

The orbit

Each orbit is approximately pear shaped. The stem contains the attachment of the rectus muscles together with the blood vessels and the nerves. The middle portion is expanded to make room for the eye. The base forms the thick orbital margins for protection. Adjacent to the inferior wall of the orbit is the maxillary sinus. Adjacent to the medial wall is the ethmoid sinus. Laterally the temporalis muscle fossa is located anteriorly, whereas the temporal lobe of the brain is adjacent to the posterior part. Superiorly the frontal sinus is located anteriorly, and the frontal lobe of the brain is located posteriorly. At the apex of each orbit is the junction of the anterior and middle cranial fossa.

As indicated in the outline on p. 191, affections of the orbit constitute a heterogeneous group of abnormalities occurring within a bony cavity that permits expansion only anteriorly. The orbit contains tissue of both ectodermal and mesodermal origin that may be primarily or secondarily affected. Tissues from the intracranial cavity or sinuses may herniate through bony defects into the orbit and present orbital symptoms. Tumors from surrounding tissues may extend to the orbit, the initial symptom often arising because of displacement of the globe or involvement of the motor nerves to the eye. Additionally, the venous drainage of the orbit is into the cavernous sinus, and orbital infections may cause a cavernous sinus thrombosis. An increase in the intravascular pressure of the cavernous sinus from a carotid-cavernous fistula may cause a pulsating protrusion of the globe.

Symptoms and signs of orbital disease

Diseases of the orbit often manifest themselves by pain, redness, and swelling with displacement of the globe. Proptosis usually refers to unilateral displacement and exophthalmos to bilateral protrusion of the eyes. Abnormalities at the apex of the orbit may involve the motor and sensory nerves of the eyes and the optic nerve.

In proptosis or exophthalmos there is usually increased width of the palpebral fissure, with the scleral rim (p. 39) visible above or below. In thyroid disease (p. 395), retraction of the upper lid accentuates the appearance. In enophthalmos the palpebral aperture is more narrow and a blepharoptosis may appear to be present.

Proptosis of an eye is appreciated best by viewing the eyes from above and behind by looking over the brow of a patient (p. 134). A number of devices are available to measure the distance between the anterior surface of the cornea and the bony margin of the orbit. The measurements with the usual exophthalmometers are accurate to within 1 to 2 mm. An exophthalmometer may be improvised by viewing the front surface of the cornea over a ruler held against the zygoma or the maxilla.

Orbitometry is used to measure the ease with which the orbital contents are compressed. This may be estimated by means of palpation or may be measured by determining how much displacement of the globe occurs when a definite force is applied.

Proptosis may cause double vision, which may be the initial symptom and occur prior to the development of gross protrusion of the eye. The direction of displacement of the eye may be of value in suggesting the most likely cause of proptosis. Proptosis of thyroid disease is usually symmetric unless muscle involvement occurs. Tumors within the muscle cone cause a symmetric proptosis, whereas those outside of the muscle cone may cause the eye to be deviated up or down, in or out, in addition to forward.

The chief signs in ocular proptosis are discussed in the following paragraphs.

Displacement of the eyeball. A relatively small mass in the muscle cone causes early symmetric displacement of the globe. Masses outside the muscle cone must be larger to displace the globe—the proptosis is asymmetric. Tumors of the lacrimal gland may cause no proptosis or may displace the globe down and in. The lacrimal gland itself may be proptosed when there is a marked increase in the volume of the orbital contents.

Palpable tumors. Tumors located in the anterior one half of the orbit may be palpated through the lids. Often a lateral canthotomy or a conjunctival incision in the lower, outer canthus will permit the surgeon to palpate deep in the orbit. Such an incision should never be used in the upper lid because of the damage to the levator palpebrae superioris muscle and possible subsequent ptosis. It may be easy to palpate retrobulbar tumors through an inferior incision when the globe is proptosed. The tactile sensation of a tumor may be simulated by the tendon of the superior oblique muscle, by localized fat in the lids, and by indurated inflammatory tissue.

Congestion and edema of the lids and conjunctiva. Marked congestion of the vessels of the globe is most suggestive of an inflammation, a thyroid abnormality with rapid progression of the exophthalmos, a carotid-cavernous sinus fistula, or an orbital inflammation.

Bruit in the head. This classical sign of carotid-cavernous sinus fistula is usually associated with noises in the head such as the sound of running water or the swishing of water. It may be most marked on the side of a cavernous sinus fistula, but it has a scant localizing value. The bruit is synchronous with the heart and may disappear with pressure applied to the internal carotid artery. Bruits occur normally in many infants, in some orbital tumors that have no vascular component, and rarely are a sign of intracranial tumor.

Visual abnormalities. Diplopia is often an early sign of proptosis and may occur prior to development of gross displacement of the globe. Indentation of the posterior sclera by a tumor causes increased hyperopia. This is often associated with decreasing visual acuity. There may also be striae of the fundus that appear ophthalmoscopically as faint parallel lines extending temporally from the optic disk.

Miscellaneous signs. Interference with the venous drainage of the optic nerve may cause a papilledema or papillitis that may be followed by optic atrophy. Marked congestion of the orbit may severely restrict ocular movements. The prominence of the globe causes increased exposure of the cornea with lacrimation and photophobia. An exposure keratitis may develop.

Diagnosis

An initial decision must be made as to whether ocular proptosis is actually present or whether the appearance is simulated by some other condition. Retraction of the upper lid causes the eye to appear more prominent, although it is not displaced. Lid retraction is a common sign of thyroid disease (p. 395). A slight blepharoptosis, as occurs in Horner's syndrome (p. 221), may simulate an ocular proptosis

Diseases of the orbit (excluding eyeball)

I. Development abnormalities of size, shape, and position
  A. Craniosynostosis
  B. Craniofacial dysostosis
  C. Mandibulofacial dysostosis
  D. Hypertelorism
  E. Failure of eye to develop or enucleation in infancy

II. Developmental anomalies of contents
  A. Hemangiomas
  B. Lymphangiomas
  C. Dermoid cysts
  D. Lipomas
  E. Choristomas

III. Herniation of adjacent structures through wall
  A. Mucocele
  B. Meningocele
  C. Encephalocele

IV. Inflammation of walls or contents
  A. Cellulitis
  B. Abscess
  C. Periostitis
  D. Chronic granuloma (pseudotumor)
  E. Gumma
  F. Tuberculoma
  G. Sarcoid granuloma

V. Vascular abnormalities
  A. Carotid-cavernous sinus fistula
  B. Cavernous sinus thrombosis
  C. Orbital aneurysm
  D. Hemorrhage
  E. Angioneurotic edema

VI. Tumors
  A. Primary
    1. Bone
      a. Chondrosarcoma
      b. Osteosarcoma
    2. Muscle
      a. Rhabdomyosarcoma
    3. Optic nerve
      a. Meningioma
      b. Glioma
    4. Lacrimal gland
      a. Benign: mixed, adenomas, cysts
      b. Malignant: mixed, adenocarcinoma, mucoepidermoid, squamous cell

VI. Tumors—cont'd
    5. Connective tissue
      a. Fibroma
      b. Neurofibromatosis
    6. Vascular
      a. Hemangioma
  B. Direct extension
    1. Eyelids
      a. Squamous cell
    2. Eyeball
      a. Malignant melanoma
      b. Retinoblastoma
    3. Intracranial cavity
      a. Meningioma
    4. Nasal accessory sinuses
      a. Osteoma
      b. Chondrosarcoma
      c. Malignancies
  C. Metastatic
    1. Sympathicoblastoma (neuroblastoma)
    2. Chloroma (in myeloblastic leukemia)
    3. Lymphoma (in lymphatic leukemia)
    4. Hypernephroma
    5. Carcinoma: breast, uterus, thyroid, prostate, lung

VII. Systemic disorders
  A. Thyroid disease
  B. Osteitis deformans (Paget's disease), osteosarcoma following osteitis deformans
  C. Histiocytosis
    1. Nevoxanthoendothelioma
    2. Eosinophilic granuloma
    3. Hand-Schüller-Christian disease
    4. Letterer-Siwe disease
  D. Hematopoietic system
    1. Lymphoma (diffuse or follicular)
      a. Lymphatic cell
      b. Reticular cell
      c. Mixed
      d. Hodgkin's type
    2. Plasma cell
      a. Primary
      b. Metastatic

VIII. Injuries

of the opposite side. Abnormalities of orbital structure causing a shallow orbit, as in Crouzon's disease, simulate proptosis. Marked enlargement of the eye such as occurs in congenital glaucoma (p. 317) makes the eye more prominent without displacement.

Physical examination should be directed to possible neoplasms in areas adjacent to the orbit, notably the nasopharynx and the intracranial cavity. Thyroid disease, lymphomatous disease, and pseudotumor must always be excluded. A chest roentgenogram is desirable to exclude metastatic malignancy, although a normal chest film does not exclude this possibility. Roentgen-ray studies of the orbit are essential. Blood tests should exclude hematopoietic disease and syphilis, and attention should be directed to the causes of other chronic granulomas. Removal of a portion or all of a tumor may provide both cure and a diagnosis. It is essential that every precaution be taken to avoid seeding of a neoplasm. Following excisional biopsy, it is desirable to base the decision concerning further therapy upon the best possible histologic sections and not upon frozen sections.

Roentgenography is essential in the diagnosis of orbital disease. The standard frontal projection permits a composite view of the bones forming the orbit. When both orbits are photographed on the same film, their dimensions and density can be compared. Water's technique is necessary for detail of the roof of the orbit. Separate oblique views are required for examination of the inner and the outer walls. The Caldwell position is required for demonstration of the superior orbital (sphenoidal) fissure. Visualization of the inferior orbital (sphenomaxillary) fissure requires a special posteroanterior projection. This view is necessary to demonstrate fractures of the floor of the orbit.

A number of special methods are used in combination with positioning of the head and often the subtraction technique to demonstrate particular defects: (1) cerebral arteriography to demonstrate the ophthalmic artery and its branches in the orbit; (2) orbital phlebography by means of catheterization of the angular vein at the medial canthus or the frontal vein on the forehead to demonstrate displacement of the ophthalmic vein; (3) laminography to study the details too small to be visible on a conventional roentgen-ray study and to visualize orbital structures without superimposition of surrounding structures; and (4) injection of radiopaque material into the orbit to demonstrate its escape into adjacent nasal sinuses in fractures or to outline structures within the orbit.

Developmental anomalies

The orbit and its contents may be affected by a number of congenital abnormalities involving the bones of the skull or the face. Frequently there is a characteristic shape of the head or facial appearance associated with exophthalmos, optic atrophy, papilledema, and strabismus. The common abnormalities may be classified as follows:

Craniosynostosis
    Brachycephaly (short head): fusion of the coronal suture
    Oxycephaly (tower head): fusion of the coronal and other sutures
    Plagiocephaly (slanting, asymmetric head): fusion of a portion of a suture
    Scaphocephaly (boat head): fusion of the sagittal suture
Craniofacial dysostosis (Crouzon's disease)
Mandibulofacial dysostosis (Franceschetti)
Hypertelorism (Greig)

Craniosynostosis

Craniosynostosis (Fig. 10-1) follows premature closure of a cranial suture. The closure causes a complete arrest of bone growth perpendicular to the closed suture, and compensatory growth of the cranium in other diameters causes anomalies in the shape of the skull. The deformity pro-

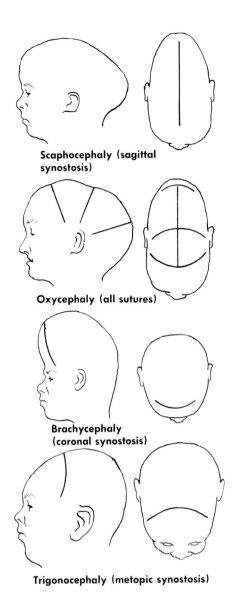

Scaphocephaly (sagittal synostosis)

Oxycephaly (all sutures)

Brachycephaly (coronal synostosis)

Trigonocephaly (metopic synostosis)

Fig. 10-1. Shape of the head in some common types of premature fusion of a cranial suture.

gresses until the brain ceases growth at about the age of 8 years.

Increased cerebrospinal pressure is common and may be followed by secondary optic atrophy. Primary optic atrophy may occur because of traction on the nerve by downward displacement of the base of the brain or compression of the nerve in the optic foramen. The orbit may be unusually shallow because of an abnormality of the lesser wing of the sphenoid bone. Esotropia or exotropia may occur. The strabismus may be secondary to optic atrophy or may be due to anatomic changes in the orbit.

Increased cerebrospinal pressure, papilledema, or optic atrophy are indications for cranial surgery. Craniectomy in the early months of life is advocated by some in all instances of craniosynostosis to prevent mental retardation and the cosmetic defect. Others believe that the procedure should be individualized, that a cosmetic defect is not constantly produced, and that mental retardation is not due to the abnormality of the bone.

Craniofacial dysostosis (Crouzon's disease)

Craniofacial dysostosis is an abnormality in which brachycephaly (short head) is combined with hypoplasia of the maxilla. The nose is broad and hooked. The palate is high, and the maxillary dentition is irregular. The earlobes are often large, and atresia of the external auditory canal is frequent.

The eyes are widely separated. A shallow orbit simulates an exophthalmos. Exotropia is common. The optic nerve may be involved as in other forms of craniosynostoses. Exposure keratitis may necessitate a lateral blepharoplasty.

Mandibulofacial dysostosis (Franceschetti)

Mandibulofacial dysostosis is a hereditary abnormality of the facial bones with hypoplasia of the zygoma and the mandible that causes a birdlike face. The inferior orbital margin is indistinct, and malformations of the lower lid are common. The palpebral fissure slants downward to the temporal side (antimongoloid), and there may be an ectropion. The external ear may be abnormally small (microtia), and there may be atresia of the external auditory canal. Atrophy of the mandible causes a prognathism of the upper jaw and an open bite. Associated skeletal anomalies are common, and dermolipomas of the conjunctiva occur.

Hypertelorism (Greig)

Hypertelorism is an abnormality of the bones of the skull often associated with facial clefts and other malformations. The orbits are widely separated, and an extreme exotropia is often present. Optic atrophy occurs rarely. There is much question as to whether the abnormality constitutes an independent entity. Hypertelorism may be associated with a congenital type of glaucoma in Axenfeld's syndrome (Fig. 10-2).

Orbital inflammation
Acute inflammation

Acute inflammations of the orbit are mainly curiosities now. Most originate from the adjacent sinuses, usually in individuals with a long history of neglected sinusitis. A cellulitis may arise from rupture of the sinus into the orbit or as an extension of thrombophlebitis. The symptoms are due to an acute increase in the volume of the orbital contents combined with inflamma-tion. Proptosis is accentuated by severe swelling of the lids and chemosis. Movements of the eye may be limited. Pressure upon the globe causes severe pain. The constitutional signs of infection occur: fever, malaise, and prostration. Exposure of the cornea may occur, and the orbit may provide a source of metastatic infec-tion or may cause a cavernous sinus thrombosis. Treatment is directed toward eradi-cation of the source of infection. A puru-lent nasal sinus must be drained, as must an abscess in the orbit.

Chronic (pseudotumor) inflammation

Chronic granulomas of the orbit are called pseudotumors and include a wide variety of chronic inflammations. A minority arise because of specific granulo-matous infection of the orbital tissues: tuberculosis, syphilitic gumma, sarcoid, and mycotic infections. The majority are non-specific reactions and histologically are composed of fibroblasts combined with perivascular lymphocytic infiltration. Often there is a large eosinophilic component. The inflammation has no pathologic coun-terpart elsewhere in the body.

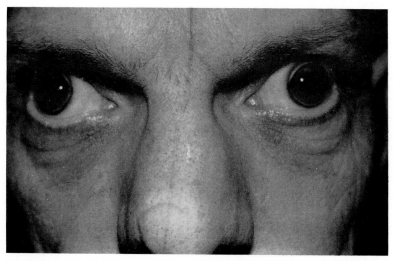

Fig. 10-2. Hypertelorism (Greig) with exotropia and Axenfeld's syndrome of congenital glaucoma and posterior embryotoxon simulating an arcus senilis.

Middle-aged men are involved predominantly. The signs and symptoms are those of an orbital tumor. The onset is acute, with a rapid development of proptosis and an associated diplopia. Often there is congestion of superficial orbital vessels. A tumor may be palpated. Extreme proptosis may develop rapidly with optic atrophy. Pain in the orbit is common.

The treatment is unsatisfactory, but often there is spontaneous remission. Excision is always incomplete and is followed by recurrence. A variety of surgical procedures may be used to protect the cornea from exposure, thus preventing keratitis e lagophthalmos. The chief treatment is systemic administration of corticosteroids in large doses. The fellow orbit becomes involved in about 25% of the cases.

Cavernous sinus thrombosis

Cavernous sinus thrombosis is an acute thrombophlebitis originating from an infection in an area having venous drainage to the cavernous sinus. There are severe constitutional symptoms of fever, malaise, and sometimes meningitis. There is involvement of the structures traversing the cavernous sinus and the orbit, pain in the ophthalmic division of the trigeminal nerve, ocular muscle palsies, and sometimes papilledema and visual failure. Proptosis with chemosis occurs. The disease originally is unilateral, but it soon becomes bilateral. Treatment is by means of antibiotics combined with anticoagulants.

Injuries

Blunt trauma to the orbit may cause severe intraorbital hemorrhage that suffuses readily beneath the conjunctiva and under the lids and may limit ocular movement markedly. Severe hemorrhage may also be a sign of fracture of the wall of the orbit and may be associated with serious brain damage. Penetrating injuries of the orbit may perforate its thin posterior walls to enter the brain or the sinuses.

The most common fracture of the orbit involves its medial margin and the nose and is particularly likely to occur in automobile accidents. Fractures of the superior margin of the orbit may damage the trochlea and may cause the symptoms of a superior oblique muscle paralysis. Fractures of the lateral margin are fairly common and give rise to an asymmetry of the face with loss of the cheekbone. Early care with elevation of the zygomatic arch can prevent the need for much corrective surgery. Fractures of the inferior margin are frequently comminuted and associated with fractures of other facial bones. The medial wall of the orbit may be ruptured, with emphysema of the tissues occurring. This may be recognized by the peculiar crepitation of the skin of the lids or the orbit to palpation. Marked increase in intraorbital pressure may cause a blowout fracture of the floor of the orbit with prolapse of orbital contents into the maxillary sinuses (p. 343). Early treatment is indicated to prevent permanent extraocular muscle damage.

Tumors and related conditions

A large variety of new growths, inflammations, congenital abnormalities, and systemic diseases may reflect themselves by orbital involvement. Diagnosis is always complicated by the frequency with which the ocular manifestations of thyroid gland abnormalities and pseudotumors cause similar symptoms and signs. The medical history is helpful. A sudden onset and a rapid progression suggest a pseudotumor or other inflammatory process rather than a tumor. Orbital pain most commonly arises from inflammation rather than from a neoplasm, although tumors of the lacrimal gland are almost invariably painful. A history of thyroid diseases suggests a thyroid abnormality even though the patient may be euthyroid or hypothyroid. A complaint of noise in the head is suggestive of a carotid-cavernous sinus fistula. Intermittent proptosis

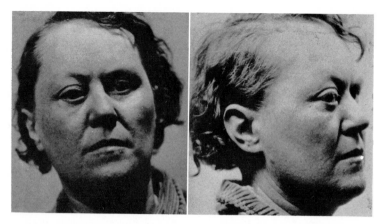

Fig. 10-3. Meningioma of the sphenoidal ridge causing a proptosis and a fullness of the temporal fossa. (From Newell, F. W., and Beaman, T. C.: Amer. J. Ophthal. **45**:30, 1958.)

may be due to varices of the orbit, and congestion is aggravated by increased venous pressure brought about by coughing or bending over.

The most common causes of proptosis in the adult orbit are thyroid disease, lymphomatous disease, pseudotumor, hemangioma, and mucocele of the frontal sinus. There is considerable variation in the orbital diseases encountered in different institutions, and this most likely reflects the interests of the staff and the type of patient referred for care.

Meningioma of the sphenoidal region (Fig. 10-3) causes a slight proptosis, often combined with fullness of the temporal fossa. This is a brain tumor readily amenable to palliative surgery. Meningioma of the lateral one third of the sphenoidal region is particularly common in middle-aged women. It is diagnosed by roentgen-ray studies of the orbit.

The most common cause of proptosis in children is a dermoid cyst. Neuroblastomas metastasize readily to the orbit. Gliomas of the optic nerve may be associated with other signs of neurofibromatosis either in a patient or in the parents. Rhabdomyosarcoma occurs more frequently in the orbit than elsewhere in the body and is the most common primary orbital malignancy in children.

The superior orbital fissure syndrome is characterized by local pain, proptosis, paralysis of cranial nerves III, IV, VI, and the ophthalmic division of nerve V. Blepharoptosis is present, with the eye usually turned down and out. There is anesthesia in the area of distribution of the trigeminal nerve. The most common cause is a neoplasm that involves the apex of the orbit, but in many instances a pseudotumor is responsible.

Surgery of the orbit

Removal of all of the orbital contents is a mutilating procedure indicated mainly for malignancies of the lacrimal gland, for extension of lid malignancies into the orbit, for malignant melanoma of the conjunctiva, occasionally when a malignant melanoma or a retinoblastoma has burst through the globe and has caused marked orbital involvement, and for primary intraorbital malignancies such as rhabdomyosarcoma. The procedure may be lifesaving in lacrimal gland tumors in which areas of bony involvement must be removed, which usually necessitates exposing the dura mater. In other malignancies there has often been extension into adjacent nasal sinuses and the intracranial cavity, and the procedure is mainly palliative.

Tumors of the orbit may be approached from its anterior margin or the lateral or superior wall. The anterior approach is made with an incision through the eyebrow, taking care not to injure the levator palpebrae superioris muscle. This approach has relatively limited application and is used solely for palpable tumors.

The lateral approach to the orbit is usually combined with a lateral canthotomy and horizontal incision extending from the lateral canthus toward the tragus of the ear. The lateral bony margin of the orbit is incised with a Stryker saw that does not cut soft tissues, and the lateral wall is reflected backward, using the temporalis muscle as a hinge. Exposure of the lateral orbital contents is good, and this is the procedure of choice (among ophthalmologists) for the treatment of benign tumors confined to the orbit. The anterior and the lateral approaches are combined for removal of benign lacrimal gland tumors, particularly the benign mixed cell tumor, which may recur or seed the operative area.

The superior orbital approach requires a craniotomy and retraction of the frontal lobe to expose the posterior portion of the orbit. Immediately beneath the periorbita of the superior wall is the levator palpebrae superioris muscle and the superior rectus muscle. This approach is mainly indicated in diseases involving both the cranial and the orbital cavities, such as a meningioma. It is extremely difficult to remove orbital tumors through a superior approach without damaging the ocular muscles.

Decompression of the orbit is carried out when increased pressure or volume of the orbital contents threatens the integrity of the globe. All four walls of the orbit have been used for the procedure. The lateral approach is the most satisfactory to ophthalmologists, and neurosurgeons favor the superior approach.

Protection to the globe in proptosis may be provided by adhesions created between the upper and lower lids or by a lateral blepharoplasty. In a desperate situation in which the cornea is exposed and the lids cannot be drawn into position to protect it, the entire cornea may be covered with a conjunctival flap.

Chapter 11

The cornea

The cornea forms the anterior one sixth of the globe. The stroma constitutes 90% of its structure and is covered anteriorly by epithelium 5 to 6 cell layers thick and posteriorly by a single cell layer of endothelium. The stroma is composed of 100 to 200 regularly arranged corneal lamellas and contains a scattering of compressed keratocytes. The central cornea is avascular, and the periphery is nourished by episcleral branches of the anterior ciliary arteries. The cornea is innervated by sensory fibers from the long and short ciliary nerves derived from the ophthalmic division of the trigeminal nerve.

The cornea is the main refracting surface of the eye because it separates air with an index of refraction of 1.0 and aqueous humor with an index of refraction of 1.34. It is transparent because of the regular arrangement of the corneal lamellas, the paucity of cells, the absence of blood vessels, and its mechanism for dehydration. The method by which the cornea maintains this deturgescence is not known, but intact epithelium and endothelium are required. The corneal epithelium must remain moist, a function maintained chiefly by secretion of tears from the accessory lacrimal glands, the conjunctival goblet cells, and the meibomian glands (p. 41). The precorneal tear film is relatively stagnant and is absent in areas where the epithelium is not intact.

Inasmuch as the corneal epithelium is continuous with that of the conjunctiva (but does not contain goblet cells), infectious diseases of the conjunctiva often extend to the cornea. As is also true of the conjunctiva, inflammations of the eyelids or abnormalities in their position cause inflammation or irritation of the cornea. A deficiency of tears (p. 210) may cause corneal disease that dominates the clinical picture.

Symptoms and signs of corneal disease

The two main symptoms of corneal disease are visual abnormalities and pain. Interference with the cellular regularity of the cornea by edema, scar tissue, or new blood vessels causes diminished central visual acuity. Corneal edema causes the tissue to act as a diffraction grating so that light is broken into its component colors, as occurs with a prism. The affected individual observes a halo surrounding lights (iridescent vision). Pain in corneal diseases arises from exposure of delicate nerve endings in the epithelium. It is described as a foreign body sensation or burning and is often severe enough to incapacitate the patient. There may be an associated reflex lacrimation.

The cornea is in an excellent position for biomicroscopic study, and magnification is required to see many abnormalities. Illumination with a penlight combined with inspection through a condensing lens frequently provides adequate magnification. Attention is directed particularly to its size and shape and the presence or absence of opacities in the grossly transparent corneal tissue. Normally the convex surface of the cornea provides a sharp image of the examining light; in areas of disease, the light is distorted or dull.

A solution of 2% sterile fluorescein (p. 108) may be instilled to observe loss of corneal epithelium. Corneal sensitivity is measured by touching the cornea with a wisp of cotton and observing the lid closure reflex. Inflammation of the cornea may be associated with ciliary injection (p. 131).

Scars

It is customary to describe three degrees of scars in the cornea: (1) leukoma, in which the involved portion of the cornea is entirely opaque, (2) macula, in which the involved cornea is translucent, and (3) nebula, which is a mild loss of corneal transparency that is nearly impossible to see without magnification. If the iris has become adherent to a corneal scar, the condition is referred to as an adherent leukoma. Corneal opacities arise because of irregularity in the arrangement of corneal lamellas combined with fibroblastic proliferation. As we have seen (p. 71), epithelial defects heal quickly without scarring, whereas Bowman's membrane and the underlying stroma heal with permanent opacification. Endothelial defects also heal quickly, but the cut edges of Descemet's membrane may curl and subsequent regenerative activity of the adjacent endothelial cells sometimes lays down several new layers of "glass membranes."

Corneal vascularization

The normal central cornea is without blood vessels and depends upon atmospheric oxygen for its aerobic metabolism (p. 68). Neovascularization of the cornea may follow any condition that reduces the compactness of the corneal lamellas, for example, corneal infection, inflammation, and those conditions causing stromal edema. The neovascularization may be sub-

epithelial (superficial), arising from the superficial corneal plexus; interstitial, arising from the deep corneal plexus; or deep, arising from apposition of the major arterial circle of the iris or radial vessels of the iris to the cornea. The blood vessels may extend from the entire corneal circumference or extend radially from a portion of the corneal margin (fascicular). Superficial neovascularization associated with fibroblastic proliferation is termed "pannus."

The blood vessels extend a varying distance into the cornea and are associated with a varying degree of corneal clouding. In the acute stage the vessels are prominent, easily recognized, and associated with ciliary injection. After subsidence of the condition causing neovascularization they may appear as fine lines unfilled with blood (ghost vessels).

Neovascularization is unquestionably a reparative process in response to a noxious stimulus, and the primary corneal abnormality often resolves quickly after vascularization. The most serious consequence is loss of corneal transparency combined with a biochemical modification of the corneal tissue, changing it from an avascular tissue not participating fully in the body's tissue immunity to one requiring a direct blood supply and one allowing an antigen-antibody reaction.

Corneal edema

As we have seen (p. 69), the corneal stroma may swell to three times its normal thickness when its cut edges are immersed in fluid, a property that permits a rapid watertight wound in corneal transplantation. Such swelling is normally prevented by the metabolism of the epithelium and endothelium. During waking hours, anterior aqueous humor flows through the stroma to the tears. If the endothelium is damaged or diseased, the overlying stroma becomes edematous and presents a grayish white opacification. In epithelial defects the edema is prevented from extending deeper than Bowman's membrane and the cornea appears dull, uneven, and hazy. The most prominent symptoms are decreased visual acuity and the appearance of halos around lights (iridescent vision). The source of the subepithelial fluid is debated; presumably when the epithelial layer is intact, it is derived from the aqueous humor and when it is damaged, from the tears.

Pigmentation

A Hudson-Stähli line is a subepithelial deposit of iron-containing pigment, probably hemosiderin, that forms a minute horizontal line. A Fleischer ring is the deposition, probably of a similar iron compound, at the base of the cone in keratoconus (p. 202). Stocker described a similar deposit at the head of a pterygium (p. 178). In Wilson's hepatolenticular degeneration (p. 448) there is a deposition of a copper-containing material in the inner layers of the cornea that extends into the trabecular meshwork of the anterior chamber recess (Kayser-Fleischer ring). The ring is often incomplete—it may be concealed in its early stages by the corneoscleral limbus and require gonioscopy for demonstration.

Krukenberg's spindle is a vertical pigment deposit on the endothelial surface of the cornea, probably derived from uveal pigment. It is deposited by convection currents in the anterior chamber and is usually arranged in an approximately triangular pattern, with the apex near the center of the cornea and the base in the 6 o'clock meridian.

Keratic precipitates, which are epithelioid inflammatory cells adherent to the endothelium in inflammations of the anterior segment, may occasionally become pigmented.

Blood staining of the cornea usually follows injuries in which there has been bleeding into the anterior chamber followed by an increase in intraocular pressure. The anterior layers of the cornea are transparent, but the endothelium becomes glazed with a brownish tan pigment, which may obscure the iris entirely. If the cornea is incised for a third or more of its circumference, as is done in cataract extraction, blood staining may occur without increased intraocular pressure, although blood must be present in the anterior chamber.

Heavy metals such as silver (argyria), iron (siderosis), gold (chrysiasis), copper (chalcosis), and mercury may be deposited in the stroma adjacent to Descemet's membrane. They are caused by local medication (silver), intraocular foreign bodies (iron or copper), intraocular blood (iron), systemic therapy (gold), toxic vapors (mercury), or a disordered metabolism (copper in hepaticolenticular degeneration).

Abnormal deposits in systemic disease

The cornea is frequently the site of deposition of abnormal metabolic products circulating in the blood. Often the disorder is not particularly conspicuous and may be overlooked if special magnification is not used.

In corneal arcus (arcus senilis, gerontoxon) (see Fig. 27-2) there is a lipid infiltration (neutral fats, phospholipids, and steroids) at the corneal periphery. It consists of two concentric areas separated by a clear interval of about 1 mm. and occurs almost universally after 60 years of age, although often involving only a sector of the cornea.

Corneal arcus tends to develop more commonly and earlier in life in Negroes than in Caucasians. Both races show a tendency to develop the lesion with increasing age. The condition is not a useful predictor of vascular hypertension, myocardial infarction, or strokes; heredity appears most important in its development. It does not occur invariably in familial hypercholesterolemia, and there is no relationship between corneal arcus and secondary types of hypercholesterolemia such as occur in diabetes mellitus, lipoid nephrosis, and myxedema. Previous vascularization of the cornea leads to the deposition of lipid adjacent to the blood vessels in some patients with hypercholesterolemia. Juvenile gerontoxon is seen in Axenfeld's syndrome (p. 194) and may occur in association with megalocornea. The optical zone of the cornea is not involved, there are no symptoms, and treatment is not indicated.

The cornea has been described as becoming black in color as a result of melanin synthesis associated with frequent local instillation of epinephrine in the treatment of glaucomas. In Negroes there is often deposition of melanin in the superficial layers of the peripheral cornea. These appear as extensions of conjunctival pigmentation and are irregularly arranged peninsulas of pigment.

Calcium may be deposited in the cornea in a variety of conditions. Hypercalcemia (p. 399) due to any cause may result in the deposit of calcium crystals in the cornea and conjunctiva. The calcium is subepithelial and usually appears in a horizontal band that begins at the corneal margin (band keratopathy). There are also subconjunctival opacities, consisting of glasslike, glistening crystals, associated with a diffuse conjunctival hyperemia.

Band keratopathy of the cornea and calcification of the conjunctiva may be observed in (1) hyperparathyroidism, (2) vitamin D poisoning, (3) sarcoidosis and multiple myeloma, (4) renal disease, and (5) milk-alkali syndrome (ingestion of milk and calcium carbonate). Band keratopathy occurs without an increase in blood calcium in old and degenerated eyes. It rarely follows severe interstitial keratitis.

Still's disease (p. 236) in children may be associated with a gradually progressive iridocyclitis with band keratopathy. The calcium may be removed chemically by chelation, but generally no improvement in vision occurs.

In some types of mucopolysaccharidosis (gargoylism) (p. 445) the cornea, among other tissues, accumulates an abnormal amount of the compound. The cornea is cloudy, not unlike the appearance in corneal edema, and the iris is seen with difficulty.

In cystine storage disease (p. 434), cystine crystals in the conjunctiva and cornea appear as tinsel-like, fine refractile crystals uniformly scattered through the tissue.

In paraproteinemia (p. 460), particularly multiple myeloma, iridescent crystals may be scattered through the cornea and conjunctiva. Deep deposits giving rise to an appearance similar to that occurring in corneal dystrophy may be present in cryoglobulinemia (p. 461).

Abnormalities of size and shape
Microcornea

In microcornea the cornea has a diameter of less than 10 mm. with a decreased radius of curvature. The majority of these eyes are hyperopic, and the development of glaucoma in later years is common. The term is reserved for eyes in which the small corneal diameter is the sole abnormality. When the entire eye is small, the condition is described as microphthalmia. Vision is reduced, and ocular nystagmus and strabismus may occur. Usually there are numerous associated developmental abnormalities, and sometimes only cystic remnants of the eye are present.

Megalocornea

Megalocornea (keratoglobus) is a bilateral abnormality in which each cornea has a diameter of more than 14 mm. (Fig. 11-1). Glaucoma is not present, but many authorities believe that the corneal enlargement is secondary to an arrested congenital glaucoma. The anterior chamber is deep, the iris stroma atrophic, and the iris

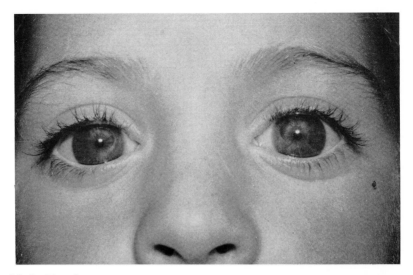

Fig. 11-1. Megalocornea.

tremulous. Posterior subcapsular cataract occurs with aging. Megalocornea must be differentiated from congenital glaucoma. Measurement of the intraocular pressure and study of the anterior chamber angle by means of a prism (gonioscopy) are essential in the differential diagnosis.

Keratoconus

Keratoconus (conical cornea) is an abnormality in which the symmetric curvature of the cornea is distorted by an abnormal thinning and forward bulging of the central portion of the cornea (ectasia) (Fig. 11-2).

The condition is usually bilateral, but one eye may be involved long before its fellow. Its onset is usually at the time of puberty. Women are involved more frequently than men. It progresses slowly over many years but may become stationary at any time. The chief symptom is decreased visual acuity for far and near combined with marked astigmatism, which as it progresses becomes irregular and cannot be improved with spectacles. Contact lenses, by providing a regular anterior curvature, frequently provide visual improvement.

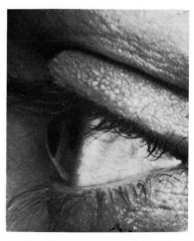

Fig. 11-2. Abnormal corneal profile in keratoconus.

Diagnosis may be difficult in the early stages. Viewing the cornea from above, looking down from behind the patient and over the brow, as is done in the diagnosis of proptosis (p. 134), may indicate the corneal cone. The corneal cone distorts the pattern of Placido's disk, a flat disk having concentric black and white circles with a central opening to observe their corneal reflection. Bowman's membrane at the base

Table 11-1. Corneal inflammation

Type	Etiology
Infectious	
Bacterial	
Acute serpiginous ulcer	Trauma and *Diplococcus pneumoniae; Streptococcus hemolyticus*
Indolent ulcer	*Moraxella liquefaciens*
Pseudomonas aeruginosa ulcer	Trauma and contaminated eyedrops
Virus	
Dendritic keratitis	Herpes simplex *(Herpesvirus hominis)*
Epidemic keratoconjunctivitis	APC type 8
Pharyngoconjunctival fever	Exogenous APC types 3, 7, and 18
Trachoma	Psittacosis–lymphogranuloma venereum–trachoma group (Bedsoniae or TRIC group)
Superficial punctate keratitis	Considered virus
Herpes zoster ophthalmicus	Varicella virus involving ophthalmic branch of N V
Keratitis vaccinia and variola	Vaccination or smallpox
Fungi	
Keratomycosis	Injury by plant material; prolonged local antibiotic and corticosteroid therapy
Treponema pallidum	
Interstitial keratitis	Congenital syphilis (rare in acquired type)
Hypersensitivity	
Marginal catarrhal ulcer	Staphylococcic conjunctivitis and blepharitis
Phlyctenular keratoconjunctivitis	Delayed hypersensitivity to tuberculoproteins and other bacterial proteins
Vascular disease	
Ring-type ulcer	Failure of corneal nutrition secondary to disease involving the corneal capillaries: (1) lupus erythematosus and (2) periarteritis nodosa, etc.
Interstitial keratitis with vertigo, tinnitus, and deafness (Cogan)	Vascular inflammatory disease?
Nutritional deficiency	
Keratomalacia (xerophthalmia)	Vitamin A deficiency
Acne rosacea	Nutritional?
Chronic serpiginous ulcer (Mooren's)	Nutritional? Elderly
Interruption of fifth cranial nerve	
Neurotrophic keratitis	Usually surgical section of trigeminal nerve
Exposure of cornea	
Keratitis e lagophthalmos	Failure of lids to cover eye: (1) proptosis, (2) facial nerve paralysis, (3) severe ectropion, and (4) absence of blinking
Decreased lacrimation	
Keratoconjunctivitis sicca	Conjunctival scarring in erythema multiforme, ocular pemphigoid, and Sjögren's disease

of the cone may be infiltrated with an iron pigment, Fleischer's ring. Breaks in Descemet's membrane cause aqueous humor to enter the stroma and to produce a severe corneal edema, hydrops of the cornea.

Contact lenses frequently maintain visual acuity at a useful level. If useful vision is not obtained, a penetrating corneal trans-plant is indicated. Usually the entire thinned cornea must be removed, necessitating a graft of 7 to 8 mm. in diameter.

Staphyloma

An ectasia or bulging of the cornea that is lined with uveal tissue is an anterior staphyloma. It occurs, with iris prolapse, most commonly in degenerated eyes following perforation of a corneal ulcer. The anterior chamber is obliterated, and a secondary glaucoma is present. Often enucleation is required.

Inflammation (keratitis)

An etiologic classification of various types of corneal inflammation is presented in Table 11-1. The microbial causes are similar to those of conjunctivitis, and often the cornea and conjunctiva are similarly affected, although the corneal involvement is far more serious because of interference with its optical function. In addition to infectious causes, inflammation occurs with hypersensitivity, vascular disease with ischemia affecting the peripheral corneal arcade of blood vessels, nutritional deficiencies, exposure, anesthesia following interruption of the trigeminal nerve, and decreased lacrimation.

Most inflammations cause a cellular infiltration of varying severity combined with a loss of corneal luster and transparency. Loss of the corneal epithelium causes a defect that stains with fluorescein. Ciliary injection occurs, and severe pain is often a prominent symptom. Blood vessels may invade the normally avascular stroma and cause marked decrease in vision.

Bacterial infections

The corneal epithelium constitutes a barrier to invasion by microorganisms. Bacterial inflammations are thus preceded by removal of the epithelium or damage by adjacent infection in the conjunctiva. The infecting organism may be introduced by a foreign body; may be present in the lacrimal system, conjunctiva, or eyelids; or may be introduced into a damaged cornea by contaminated medication. The causative organism may be difficult to demonstrate, but cultures and smears stained with Gram's iodine and Giemsa's stain should be made before treatment is instituted. Usually a broad-spectrum antibiotic such as chloramphenicol or a mixture of antibiotics such as Neosporin should be instilled every 1 or 2 hours during the waking hours until specific antimicrobial therapy may be instituted. Local instillation of atropine solution is commonly used to combat the secondary inflammatory response of the anterior uvea. Bandaging the eye is always contraindicated as it increases the temperature within the closed eyelids and provides an efficient incubation for the multiplication of organisms.

Acute serpiginous ulcer. Acute serpiginous ulcer is usually caused by *Diplococcus pneumoniae* (pneumococcus), and the organism often has a focus in the lacrimal sac. (Chronic serpiginous ulcer, p. 208, is a nonmicrobial disease.) The ulcer is of a dirty gray color with overhanging margins, and it causes marked thinning of the cornea. Penetration of bacterial toxin into the anterior chamber stimulates a copious exudate of leukocytes that collect in the anterior chamber to form a sterile hypopyon. Leukocytes may coalesce on the endothelium posterior to the ulcer (Fig. 11-3). If untreated, the cornea may perforate, and the eye may be lost because of a purulent inflammation.

The bacteria are sensitive to many antibiotics or sulfonamides, and the ulcer responds quickly to treatment. A concurrent pneumococcal dacryocystitis may necessitate dacryocystorhinostomy or temporary occlusion of the canaliculi.

Pseudomonas aeruginosa ulcer. *Pseudomonas aeruginosa* ulcer is caused by a gram-negative aerobic bacillus found on the normal skin and intestinal tract of man. It is a common cause of corneal ulceration. The bacteria may be introduced by contaminated fluorescein solution used to examine an injured eye. The lesion usually begins centrally, spreads quickly, and may cause perforation and loss of the eye within 48 hours. Treatment is by means of frequent instillation of polymixin B or E

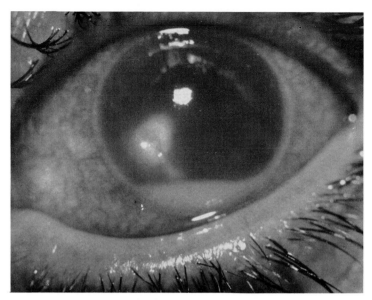

Fig. 11-3. Acute serpiginous ulcer with leukocytes in the anterior chamber (hypopyon).

(colistin), sometimes combined with sub-conjunctival injection.

Viral infections

The cornea may be involved in a wide variety of exogenous or endogenous viral infections. Because of the difficulty in demonstrating the causative organisms, viral infections are diagnosed mainly by their morphologic appearance and sometimes by the systemic immune responses.

Dendritic keratitis. Dendritic keratitis (from *dendri-* [Greek], tree) is an acute and chronic corneal disease secondary to infection of the corneal epithelium with herpes simplex virus, of which there are a number of strains. The initial infection arises because of corneal invasion by the virus from the outside. It is usually transmitted by an individual with an acute herpes infection of the lips or mouth. Following infection, the virus often resides in the lacrimal gland and is continuously secreted. Thereafter, minor trauma, menstruation, and physical or mental stress may trigger sudden replication of the virus in the epi-

thelium, with recurrence of the disease. Usually one eye is involved in repeated corneal inflammation.

The epithelial disease is ushered in with minute vesicles that rupture, leading to superficial dots in the early stages. These coalesce to form a branchlike (dendritic) ulcer that stains with fluorescein. Late in the disease the epithelium between the branches may be lost, resulting in the sharply demarcated, irregularly shaped area of a geographic ulcer.

The symptoms of dendritic keratitis are foreign body sensation, lacrimation, and reduction of vision if the optical area of the cornea is involved. After repeated attacks, the patient is quite aware of recurrence early in the course of the disease. Giant multinucleated cells are demonstrated with Giemsa's stain. Corneal material will cause inflammation of the abraded rabbit cornea, and the virus may produce cytopathogenic effects on HeLa cell cultures.

The treatment of epithelial dendritic keratitis is by instillation of drops of IDU (idoxyuridine) every hour during the day and every 2 hours during the night. The lesion heals within 7 to 14 days in 80% of the cases, commonly leaving a subepithelial opacity in the region of involvement that disappears in the course of several weeks. Treatment with IDU must be continued for about 14 days, but as the lesion heals, the frequency of instillation may be reduced. If there is an associated uveitis, atropine instilled locally may relieve symptoms.

Stromal involvement occurs in several forms. Disciform keratitis is a central corneal, disk-shaped, gray area that forms beneath the epithelial ulcer after 5 to 10 days. It is presumably due to a toxic or hypersensitivity response to the virus. After healing, the stromal opacity gradually fades, but if healing is delayed, there may be corneal vascularization. IDU has no effect on the disciform keratitis, but it may be used to combat the epithelial disease, combined with cautious local instillation of corticosteroids to combat the hypersensitivity reaction.

Active multiplication of the virus in the stroma occurs when epithelial disease has been treated with corticosteroids that reduce tissue immunity. There may be gradual increase in depth and diameter of the corneal ulcer. The eye is often less red and less uncomfortable than prior to the use of corticosteroids, and the patient may instill the medication frequently. Eventually a descemetocele develops in which Descemet's membrane bulges into the ulcer, creating a shining, dark area. Aqueous humor leaking through this opening creates the impression of tearing. With rupture of the descemetocele, the eye may be lost.

Corticosteroids should never be used in epithelial dendritic keratitis. Persistent stromal keratitis is best treated by lamellar keratoplasty with removal of all diseased tissue. A descemetocele requires either a penetrating or a lamellar transplant.

Recurrent inflammation of the stroma and epithelium with corneal vascularization, redness, discomfort, and a prolonged course is usually classified as keratitis metaherpetica. It is presumably due to previous damage to the cornea with virus infection and not to active virus multiplication. The inflammation commonly recurs until the abnormal tissue is excised and replaced with normal cornea in a lamellar transplant.

Involvement of the iris in stromal keratitis may be due to direct invasion of the virus or to a toxic effect. Superinfection, particularly that resulting from fungus invasion, may also occur.

Superficial punctate keratitis. Superficial punctate keratitis is probably a specific viral infection of both eyes characterized by a punctate epithelial keratitis that persists from 6 months to 4 years. There are numerous remissions and exacerbations and eventual healing without corneal scars. Patients complain of intermittent burning, irritation, tearing, and blurred vision. Magnification is required to see from 1 to 50 (usually about 20) minute, oval, corneal opacities composed of a conglomeration of minute dots. New lesions appear as old ones heal, so that their distribution varies from examination to examination. There is hyperemia of the conjunctiva in the 12 o'clock meridian. Topical steroids have a dramatic suppressive effect, and other medications are of no particular value.

A recurrent punctate erosion of the corneal epithelium may follow inadvertent injury to the eyes with aerosal products. The patient is usually unaware of the injury, but the cornea is studded with minute epithelial defects that stain with fluorescein solution. Once the cause is learned, more cautious use of aerosols prevents recurrence.

Systemic virus diseases. Corneal inflammation occurs in a large number of virus diseases (p. 368) and may or may not be associated with systemic abnormalities that dominate the clinical picture. Many of the adenoviruses (p. 369) cause ocular signs with corneal inflammation. Herpes zoster ophthalmicus (p. 371) caused by *Herpesvirus varicellae* may cause severe anterior uveitis and keratitis. Smallpox (p. 373) is a common cause of blindness in countries where it is epidemic, and accidental inoculation of the cornea may follow vaccination. The photophobia observed in measles (p. 372) is due to a frequently undiagnosed keratoconjunctivitis, whereas mumps (p. 372) may cause a transient corneal edema.

Other infections

Keratomycosis. Infection of the cornea with fungi has increased some fifteenfold since the introduction of local therapy with corticosteroids and antibiotics. The infection occurs when a fungus is introduced into the cornea by injury, frequently by a corneal abrasion with a tree branch, shrub, or other vegetable matter. Keratomycosis may also complicate prolonged therapy with corticosteroids and antibiotics and should be considered in every persistent corneal ulceration.

The keratitis appears as a fluffy, white, elevated protuberance surrounded by a shallow crater, which in turn is surrounded by a grayish, sharply demarcated halo persisting for months (Fig. 11-4). There is no corneal vascularization. There may be

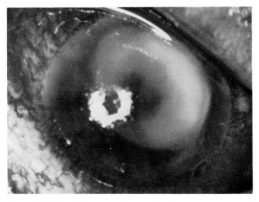

Fig. 11-4. Fungus ulcer of the cornea with a deep infiltrate and ciliary injection.

bilateral anterior uveitis followed by intermarked conjunctival injection, which is disproportionately severe for the amount of keratitis present. It may be difficult to demonstrate the fungi on culture and smear. Many different fungi have been described as causing inflammation.

Treatment consists of local instillation of antifungal agents such as nystatin, 100,-000 units/ml., or a sulfonamide such as Gantrisin or sulfacetamide solution. Many eyes do not heal until a conjunctival flap is drawn over the cornea surgically.

Interstitial keratitis. Congenital syphilis was formerly the most common cause of interstitial keratitis. It resulted in a severe bilateral anterior uveitis followed by interstitial corneal vascularization between the ages of 5 and 20 years. At the present time the disease may be entirely prevented by adequate treatment of congenital syphilis, but once the inflammation has developed, antisyphilitic therapy is of no value.

Today interstitial keratitis is a relatively uncommon disease. It is described as a complication of tuberculosis or leprosy or as a trophic disturbance following vaccination and as a portion of Cogan's syndrome. There is usually a relatively small amount of inflammation of the anterior segment. The disease is ushered in by a foreign body sensation and opacities in the peripheral cornea followed by vascularization arising from blood vessels in the pericorneal arcade that push the opacities ahead of them as they grow into the cornea. In many instances only a sector of the cornea may be involved. The treatment is directed to the cause.

Interstitial keratitis and deafness (Cogan) is a rare disease affecting young adults. The major symptoms arise from interstitial keratitis and involvement of the vestibuloauditory system. Either the eye or the ear may be affected initially, but involvement of the other organ follows within 2 months.

The ocular involvement consists of

patchy, deep, peripheral corneal infiltrates that fluctuate in intensity and distribution and are accompanied by interstitial corneal vascularization. Vestibuloauditory symptoms consist of the simultaneous onset of vertigo, tinnitus, and deafness. Complete nerve deafness and nonresponsive labyrinths usually result.

The disease presumably does not arise from drug sensitivity but is a vascular hypersensitivity of unknown cause. Several cases have been reported that resembled periarteritis nodosa. One patient had an unclassified aortitis without involvement of small vessels.

Treatment is symptomatic. Systemic corticosteroids have been reported to be of value.

Hypersensitivity

Marginal catarrhal ulcers. Marginal catarrhal ulcers are attributed to a hypersensitivity to the exotoxin of *Staphylococcus aureus*. They are always associated with conjunctivitis or blepharitis (Fig. 11-5) in which the staphylococci can be isolated and demonstrated with ease

(p. 173). The inflammation responds rapidly to the topical instillation of corticosteroids, which must be administered with appropriate medication to combat the bacterial source of the toxin.

Phlyctenular keratoconjunctivitis. Phlyctenular keratoconjunctivitis was described earlier (p. 177). The condition is a common cause of decreased vision among Eskimos, presumably because of their sensitivity to tuberculosis.

Vascular disease

Ring-type ulcer. A ring-type ulcer is a sterile necrosis of the peripheral cornea that appears to melt away gradually. It is due to systemic disease, particularly connective tissue disorders that obliterate the blood vessels in the peripheral corneal arcade. Blindness occurs commonly. Local therapy is generally ineffective.

Chronic serpiginous ulcer (Mooren's ulcer). Chronic serpiginous ulcer (Mooren's ulcer) is a slowly progressive necrotic lesion of the cornea near the periphery. Its cause is not known, but it presumably arises because of sclerosis of pericorneal

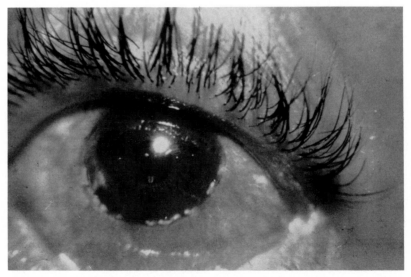

Fig. 11-5. Acute *Staphylococcus aureus* conjunctivitis with marginal corneal ulcers due to hypersensitivity to the exotoxin of *Staphylococcus aureus*.

blood vessels with ischemia of the peripheral cornea. The disease begins with the appearance of an ulcer about 1 mm. within the corneoscleral limbus, which gradually spreads along the corneal margin and toward the central cornea. Perforation of the cornea is rare unless there is secondary infection. Pain and photophobia are disproportionately severe in comparison to the mild tissue reaction. Treatment is often unsatisfactory and is directed toward reducing intraocular pressure and preventing infection. The intraocular pressure may be reduced by an incision on the central side of the ulcer (a delimiting keratotomy), by repeated emptying of the anterior chamber, or by making a fistulous tract in the ulcer with cautery.

Other disorders

Neurotrophic keratitis. Neurotrophic keratitis arises because of anesthesia of the cornea, which allows trauma and desiccation of the corneal epithelium without reflex protection. In addition, the trigeminal nerve may play a role in the metabolism of the cornea. Inasmuch as the cornea is anesthetic, there is no pain, but the eye is injected, and there may be marked loss of vision. The lesion begins inferiorly with exfoliation and ulceration, and it may progress until there is loss of the globe. Tarsorrhaphy is the usual method of treatment. If it is probable that both the trigeminal and the facial nerves will be sacrificed in a neurosurgical procedure, as in a cerebellar angle tumor, the keratitis should be anticipated, and tarsorrhaphy should be performed before the cornea ulcerates. Neurotrophic keratitis does not constantly follow section of the gasserian ganglion.

Exposure keratitis. Exposure keratitis, sometimes called keratitis e lagophthalmos, is an inflammation due to failure of the lids to cover the globe (p. 159). There is exfoliation of the corneal epithelium followed by secondary infection. The condition is most commonly associated with paralysis of the facial nerve in which the function of the orbicularis oculi muscle is absent. The cornea may be similarly exposed following blepharoptosis surgery or in severe proptosis.

Keratitis e lagophthalmos causes pain and ciliary injection. It is evident upon examination that the cornea is not protected by closure of the lids. Treatment is directed toward prevention of corneal drying. In mild cases the instillation of an ointment at bedtime and protection of the globe is all that is required. In facial nerve paralysis a lateral blepharoplasty may be carried out. If the paralysis is permanent and there is no likelihood of restoration of the facial nerve function, a permanent type of blepharoplasty is carried out. In instances of proptosis with exposure keratitis, a central tarsorrhaphy is required.

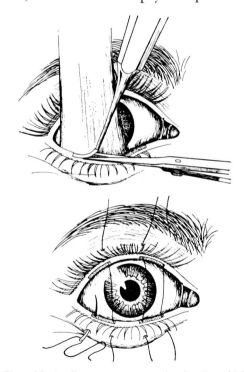

Fig. 11-6. Temporary tarsorrhaphy in which posterior portions of the upper and lower lid margin are denuded and brought together with sutures to prevent exposure of the cornea.

Keratomalacia. Keratomalacia arises from vitamin A deficiency, which causes desiccation and necrosis of the cornea and the conjunctiva. Vitamin A is a fat-soluble vitamin derived either from conversion of carotene or from preformed vitamin in the diet. Carotene occurs in many plants, particularly leafy greens and yellow vegetables. Preformed vitamin A is derived from butterfat, cheese, and liver. Failure to ingest adequate vitamin A or its precursor is commonly associated with other dietary deficiencies, notably inadequate protein. Secondary deficiency occurs because of inadequate saponification of vitamin A in the gut and is observed in sprue, celiac disease, and cystic fibrosis of the pancreas. In cirrhosis of the liver, there is a failure to store vitamin A.

Vitamin A deficiency in the retina has been studied carefully, particularly in animals in whom nutrition can be supported by administration of vitamin A acid, which is not converted to the prosthetic group of retinene. In man, vitamin A deficiency causes blindness by the following: (1) destruction of the cornea in xerophthalmia (dry eye) and keratomalacia (corneal softening), (2) loss of retinene in the visual pigments of the retina, (3) faulty growth of bone with optic nerve compression in the optic canal, and (4) faulty fetal development in a vitamin-deficient mother.

In children with acute but not chronic deficiency, dryness of the conjunctiva (xerosis conjunctivae) is the initial external sign of the deficiency. It is paralleled by a decrease in dark adaptation, which may give rise to no complaint. Bitot's spot is seen, particularly in male children, and occurs on the exposed bulbar conjunctiva, usually in the palpebral fissure on the temporal side. It appears as a highly refractile mass with a silvery gray hue and a foamy surface. It is extremely superficial, and the foam may be rubbed off, leaving a roughened conjunctival surface that fills with foam in several days.

The keratomalacia or softening of the cornea may be generalized or localized. It may lead to destruction of the eye if infection occurs. It is particularly common with an associated protein deficiency. Generally, it occurs in infants and not in adults.

Acne rosacea. Acne rosacea is a chronic disorder of the skin of the face characterized by erythema, erythematous papules, telangiectasia, and occasionally tissue hypertrophy, particularly of the nose. The conjunctiva may be injected, and ultimately there may be peripheral corneal vascularization. A variety of disorders may be associated: vitamin deficiency, alcoholism, and vascular, endocrine, and gastrointestinal instability. Treatment is directed toward a stable dietary and personal regime. This is often unsatisfactory.

Keratoconjunctivitis sicca. Keratoconjunctivitis sicca is a symptom complex due to a deficiency in tear secretion arising from atrophy of the lacrimal glands or from scarring of their ducts so that the eye becomes dry (p. 186). The corneal epithelium lacks luster, and the cornea stains with fluorescein. There are burning, fullness, and a gritty foreign body sensation. Filaments of corneal epithelium may form, but often they are wiped off by blinking and are not observed.

The chief causes of keratoconjunctivitis sicca are trachoma (p. 174), erythema multiforme (p. 120), cicatrizing conjunctivitis, Sjögren's syndrome (p. 452), and vitamin A deficiency. Keratoconjunctivitis sicca is a common cause of ocular symptoms, and severe forms may result in blindness through corneal keratinization.

Dystrophies

Corneal dystrophy is an abnormality characterized by a loss of clarity of a portion of the cornea without preceding inflammation. A true dystrophy is always bilateral, involves the central portion of the cornea and not the peripheral portion, is not associated with inflammation or vascularization, and is frequently familial.

Cornea guttata

Cornea guttata is a dystrophy in which there are hyaline deposits on the endothelium. These normally occur as a degenerative change with aging, are located at the periphery of the cornea, and are called Hassall-Henle bodies. They are of no clinical significance except as an indication of aging. In central cornea guttata (Fuchs' dystrophy) there are hyaline endothelial deposits in the central area of the cornea, and there may be gradual deterioration of vision. The deposits may act as a diffraction grating and may cause iridescent vision. In a small proportion of patients there is a disturbance in corneal hydration and the development of a subepithelial edema followed by epithelial erosions and bullae (bullous keratopathy). There is a marked loss of vision. On occasion a cornea guttata involving only the endothelial surface may be aggravated into epithelial involvement by surgical trauma to the eye, prolonged tonography, corneal contact lenses, or other inadvertent minor corneal injury. In recent years early endothelial and epithelial dystrophy have responded well to partial penetrating transplant, provided all of the diseased tissue has been removed.

Hereditary dystrophy

A variety of hereditary dystrophies involving the stroma are described, largely on the basis of their morphologic characteristics. Many do not interfere with vision but create an interesting display of patterns in the usually structureless cornea. If visual acuity is reduced, a corneal transplant may be carried out with good results.

Keratoplasty

Corneal transplant, or keratoplasty, is the excision of opaque corneal tissue and its replacement by a clear cornea from a human donor. One of two techniques is used: (1) the penetrating graft, in which the entire thickness of cornea is removed and replaced by transparent corneal tissue, and (2) the partially penetrating, or lamellar, keratoplasty, in which a superficial layer is removed and replaced without entering the anterior chamber. The graft may vary in size from replacement of the entire cornea to one with a diameter of 5 mm., the minimal size that will remain transparent.

With improved surgical techniques and correspondingly better visual results, the indications for transplant have been defined in terms of the condition of the recipient cornea rather than central visual acuity. The likelihood of visual improvement with transplant is related more to the disease causing the corneal abnormality than to the preoperative visual acuity. In diseases such as keratoconus in which there is no corneal vascularization the likelihood for marked improvement in vision is excellent. In corneal leukomas, particularly those following alkali burns in which there is superficial and deep vascularization, there is little likelihood of the graft remaining transparent. In every case, light preception and projection must be normal. The prognosis is much less favorable in degenerative conditions such as corneal dystrophy (p. 210) but varies with the type and extent of the corneal abnormality.

Donor material is obtained preferably from an adult between 25 and 35 years of age who has died of an acute disease or injury. Eyes from stillborn infants are least desirable. Eyes from individuals more than 60 years of age must be used with considerable caution in penetrating keratoplasty but are useful in the lamellar type. Eyes of patients who have been ill for a long period prior to death frequently respond poorly in a transplant. Suitable transplant material should be obtained from nonsyphilitic donors.

The donor eye should be enucleated, using sterile instruments and a sterile technique, within an hour after death, although if the eyelids are closed carefully and the body refrigerated, delays up to 5 hours are permissible. The donor eye should be used within 2 or 3 days unless specially prepared for long-term storage. Most eyes in this country are stored in a tightly closed sterile container with the cornea resting uppermost on sterile gauze moistened with normal saline solution and refrigerated at 4° C. Persons wishing to donate their eyes for use in keratoplasty should contact an eye bank that is a member of the Eye Bank Association of America.

Penetrating keratoplasty

The excision of all layers of the cornea and replacement with a clear donor cornea is the traditional type of keratoplasty. Frequently it is preceded by a lamellar keratoplasty to minimize vascularized and opaque areas. A penetrating transplant is complete when the entire cornea is excised and incomplete when it is not.

The operation is usually performed using topical and retrobulbar anesthesia and akinesia. The graft is removed from the donor eye using a trephine. The same trephine is used to remove the diseased area from the recipient eye. The donor cornea is then sutured into position using fine sutures. These are usually removed 35 to 42 days postoperatively when healing is far advanced.

Lamellar keratoplasty

Since all layers of the cornea are not removed in nonpenetrating, or lamellar, keratoplasty (Fig. 11-7), it has a more limited application than the penetrating type. Conversely, the procedure is associated with fewer postoperative complications than penetrating keratoplasty, may be repeated with a good chance of success even after earlier failures, and does not complicate a subsequent penetrating graft. The indications for lamellar keratoplasty are the following: (1) optical, in super-

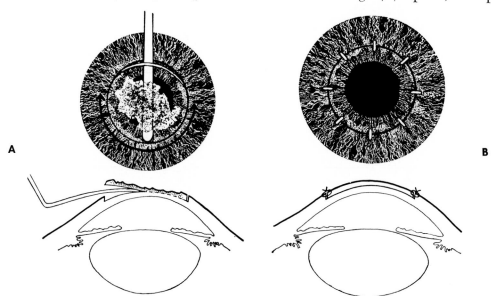

Fig. 11-7. Lamellar keratoplasty. **A,** The diseased area is demarcated with a trephine and then removed by dissection. **B,** The diseased cornea is replaced with cadaver cornea maintained in position with interrupted sutures. (From Hogan, M. J.: Amer. J. Ophthal. **45:**106, 1958.)

ficial corneal opacities that do not involve the innermost layers of the cornea; (2) therapeutic, in inflammatory disease of the cornea, particularly herpes simplex involvement of the corneal stroma; and (3) to prepare the cornea for subsequent penetrating keratoplasty in instances in which the entire cornea is involved in opacity. In addition to these usual indications, early lamellar keratoplasty has been used successfully in severe corneal injuries due to chemicals and multiple foreign bodies.

Keratoprosthesis

The recent development of new plastics has led to new corneal implants (keratoprostheses) that hold much promise for individuals in whom corneal transplantation was previously contraindicated or foredoomed to failure because of excessive scarring or neovascularization. A thin transparent sheet of Silastic rubber placed in the corneal stroma adjacent to Descemet's membrane often leads to disappearance of stromal edema. In densely scarred corneas a central optical cylinder of plastic surrounded by a cuff of Dacron or dentin from a tooth extracted from the patient may provide a marked improvement in vision.

Injuries

Foreign bodies of the cornea (p. 335) constitute about 25% of all significant eye injuries.

Abrasions

Removal of the corneal epithelium by an abrasion or ultraviolet light causes considerable pain and lacrimation, but the lesion heals quickly and is of little clinical importance unless infection occurs. The abraded area stains with fluorescein. The eye is usually more comfortable if tightly patched, and the majority of corneal abrasions heal with no treatment other than patching. Ointments should not be used in this condition. Local anesthetics are contraindicated because they delay epi-

thelization. If infection is feared, it is probably better to use sulfacetamide solution locally than to use a wide-spectrum antibiotic.

Recurrent corneal erosion

Occasionally following uncomplicated corneal abrasion, the regenerated epithelium does not appear to adhere to the underlying basement membrane. In such an instance the patient, on awakening in the morning and opening his eyes or rubbing his eyes, will remove the epithelium, and there is sudden onset of a foreign body sensation and lacrimation. Examination with high magnification between attacks shows a minute opacification in the subepithelial area. This area stains with fluorescein when the epithelium is removed. The disorder is disabling because of recurrent pain, but it causes no visual disability. Treatment is difficult. Some cases are caused by the subepithelial inclusion of ointment in the treatment of corneal abrasion. Once recurrent corneal erosion has occurred, it is treated by removal of the abnormal epithelium and pressure dressing in the hope that the epithelium will attach itself normally to the underlying tissue. In some cases corticosteroids are used locally following removal of the epithelium. Often several treatments are required. The instillation of an ointment at bedtime may prevent the lid from adhering to the loose epithelium and may prevent flicking it off when the eyes are opened.

Lacerations

Corneal lacerations (p. 339) are of unusual seriousness because the interior of the eye is opened to infection and there is likelihood of additional injury to intraocular structures. Treatment is directed toward prevention of infection by administration of an antibiotic, avoidance of prolapse of intraocular contents that may occur with repeated examinations, and closure of the laceration with sutures after excision of prolapsed intraocular tissue.

Chapter 12

The sclera

The sclera is a dense, fibrous structure composed of elastic and collagen tissue and constituting the posterior five sixths of the globe. Its anterior portion is visible beneath the transparent conjunctiva as the white of the eye. It has a paucity of cells and only a few blood vessels. The sclera may be regarded as essentially a collagen tissue, and it may be involved in rheumatoid arthritis, polyarteritis nodosa, erythema multiforme, and congenital abnormalities involving the skin, vessels, joints, and bones.

Symptoms and signs of scleral disease

The symptoms of scleral disease may be minimal. With inflammation there may be severe or dull pain, which may be aggravated by contraction of an ocular muscle if the sclera is inflamed near its insertion. Anterior inflammations may be evident by generalized or localized areas of deep, reddish injection. These areas may be painful to palpation. Posterior inflammations cannot be seen. In thinning or necrosis of the sclera the bluish black choroid may be exposed.

Intrascleral nerve loop

An intrascleral nerve loop is an anatomic variation sometimes confused with a pigmented neoplasm of the eye. Usually a long posterior ciliary nerve loops into the sclera about 4 mm. from the corneoscleral limbus, giving rise to a minute pigmented dot on the sclera. Its unchanging appearance and location should suggest the diagnosis.

Staphylomas

Staphylomas or ectasias of the sclera are bulgings or enlargements occurring because of increased intraocular pressure or local defects in the resistance of the sclera to stress.

Total staphylomas occur in congenital glaucoma when the entire globe is enlarged. It is postulated that a similar mechanism may be involved in pathologic myopia.

Partial staphylomas involve localized segments of the globe, mainly in areas in which the sclera is penetrated by blood vessels or nerves. Anterior staphylomas are divided into ciliary, which occur in the region of the ciliary body, and intercalary, which involve the area between the ciliary body and the corneoscleral limbus. These staphylomas occur in far-advanced glaucoma or following injury to the eye.

Equatorial staphylomas involve the areas near the points of exit of the four vortex veins from the eye. Equatorial staphylomas may be a factor in retinal separation, but the localized bulging of sclera is often not seen until the area is exposed surgically to correct the separation.

Posterior staphylomas occur at the lamina cribrosa, secondary to the optic atrophy occurring as the result of prolonged increase in intraocular pressure.

Inflammations

The sclera has a poor blood supply and a relatively inactive metabolism. Inflammations are not common and tend to be torpid. Many, apparently, are examples of a delayed type of hypersensitivity reaction. Scleritis tends to be associated with rheumatoid arthritis and may be similarly difficult to manage. Those involving the anterior segment respond to steroids applied locally.

Scleritis

Scleritis is an inflammation of the sclera that involves adjacent tissue; therefore uveitis is often associated. In anterior scleritis the anterior portion of the globe is mainly involved, with small, deep, painful, red infiltrations developing that coalesce to form nodules. Prior to the introduction of corticosteroids the inflammation could persist for months or years. When adjacent to the cornea, a sclerosing keratitis may occur in which the cornea is transformed into a tissue indistinguishable from the sclera.

Annular scleritis may involve the entire corneoscleral limbus and cause corneal vascularization. It appears as a gelatinous, reddish infiltration of the conjunctiva, episclera, and sclera, adjacent to the corneoscleral limbus. There is severe ocular pain, and the condition may spread relentlessly to involve the cornea and the uveal tract.

Posterior scleritis causes inflammation of the choroid and the retina with disturbances of vision. There may be severe pain and signs suggestive of cellulitis of the orbit. The disease may progress to perforation of the sclera that may require enucleation. Treatment is mainly corticosteroids, antibiotics, and drugs to relieve pain.

Previously scleritis was attributed to tuberculosis, syphilis, gout, sarcoid, and similar granulomatous infections. There is a tendency now to regard most cases as a manifestation of collagen diseases, particularly arthritis, and systemic corticosteroids constitute the main therapy.

Episcleritis

Episcleritis (Fig. 12-1) is an inflammation that tends to involve the episclera between the insertion of the rectus muscles and the corneoscleral limbus. It usually occurs in a nodular form with a purplish, round to oval elevation a few millimeters in diameter. The cause of the inflammation is not known. Most frequently middle-aged men are affected. There may be a deep, boring pain, most severe at night, but the inflammation tends to disappear spontaneously, leaving a residue of a faintly pigmented patch to which the conjunctiva is adherent. The nodules may involve both eyes and tend to be recurrent, involving adjacent areas. Treatment is by instillation of local corticosteroids.

Episcleritis periodica fugax is characterized by diffuse congestion and edema of a localized area of the episclera, with a tendency to spontaneous remission within a period of a few hours or days. Clinically it typifies a localized sensitivity of the tissue.

Scleromalacia perforans

Scleromalacia perforans (p. 452) is a rare necrotizing disease of the sclera asso-

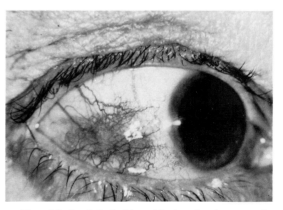

Fig. 12-1. Episcleritis with localized area of injection.

ciated with rheumatoid arthritis. The anterior sclera is usually involved in the development of several areas of staphyloma in which the sclera appears almost entirely absent and the dull black-blue choroid bulges forth. The disease often proceeds relentlessly to blindness, but a variety of ingenious implants of sclera and fascia lata have been described.

Degenerations
Senile hyaline plaque

Senile hyaline plaque is a misnomer applied to a darkish deposition in the sclera (Fig. 12-2) located immediately anterior to the insertion of the medial or lateral rectus muscle. It appears as an area of translucency in the sclera and was formerly thought to be due to thinning of

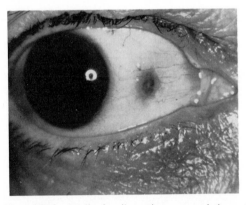

Fig. 12-2. Senile hyaline plaque consisting of a deposition of calcium sulfate crystals immediately anterior to the insertion of the medial rectus muscle.

the sclera because of traction of the rectus muscles. However, histochemical examination shows it to be an area of deposition of calcium sulfate crystals. Treatment is not indicated.

Osteogenesis imperfecta

Osteogenesis imperfecta (p. 444) is a relatively common disorder of connective tissue in which the scleras are a uniform and impressive blue color. This arises from thinning of the sclera, which permits the underlying choroid to shine through. Similar blue scleras are also seen in other connective tissue disorders, notably Marfan's syndrome.

In *ochronosis* (p. 432) there is a deposition of melanin in the sclera that must not be mistaken for a neoplasm.

Injuries

Injuries of the sclera are always associated with injury to adjacent tissues, and the involvement of the sclera is seldom considered separately. Laceration of the anterior sclera causes a prolapse of ciliary body and choroid. Frequently enucleation of the eye is required.

Injuries of the posterior sclera are usually the result of contrecoup by blunt trauma and often are not diagnosed. The history of blunt trauma associated with a severe subconjunctival hemorrhage and a persistently soft globe suggests the diagnosis. There is usually an associated severe injury of the retina and the choroid.

Chapter 13

The pupil

The iris contains a central aperture, the pupil, which controls the amount of light entering the eye, constricting in bright illumination and dilating in the dark. Pupillary size is controlled by the opposed actions of two nonstriated muscles, both derived from the cells of the secondary optic vesicle, the sphincter pupillae (N III parasympathetics), and the dilatator pupillae (sympathetic). The two layers of secondary optic vesicle fuse to form the pigment layer of the iris, and its most anterior portion at the pupillary margin forms the pigment frill that is conspicuous in ectropion uveae.

Normal pupils are round, nearly equal in size, and regular in shape. Each is located with its center a little below and slightly to the nasal side of the cornea. The pupils are constricted in infancy and in old age and are at their maximal size during childhood and adolescence. Myopic eyes have slightly larger pupils than hyperopic eyes, blue eyes have larger pupils than brown eyes, and women have slightly larger pupils than men. In bright illumination the pupils are constricted (miotic), and in dim illumination the pupils are dilated (mydriatic). Pupils are considered miotic if less than 2 mm. in diameter and mydriatic when more than 6 mm. in diameter. Unequal size of the pupils is called anisocoria.

The sphincter pupillae (p. 17) is a typical annular sphincter muscle located next to the pupillary margin deep in the iris stroma. It is innervated by efferent visceral fibers that originate in the Edinger-Westphal nucleus. These fibers enter the orbit with the inferior branch of the oculomotor nerve. A short motor branch is sent to the ciliary ganglion where synapse is made with postganglionic fibers. Six postganglionic short ciliary nerves run from the ganglion, divide, penetrate the sclera around the optic nerve, and pass forward in the suprachoroidal space to the ciliary and the sphincter pupillae muscles.

The dilatator pupillae muscle (p. 17) is arranged radially in the iris stroma. It extends from the outer edge of the sphincter muscle to the root of the iris, and it contains pigment. It is innervated by sympathetic fibers that probably originate in the hypothalamus. From here they descend in the lateral columns of the cervical cord and emerge with the eighth cervical and first thoracic ventral nerve roots. The fibers then ascend the sympathetic chain to the superior cervical ganglion where they synapse. Postganglionic fibers extend cranially along the internal carotid artery and reach the dilatator pupillae muscle mainly with the two long ciliary nerve branches of the nasociliary branch of the fifth (trigeminal) cranial nerve. Sympathetic fibers pass through but do not synapse in the ciliary ganglion.

Inasmuch as the sphincter pupillae and the dilatator pupillae are an integral part of the iris (p. 15), their function may be markedly altered in iris inflammations, de-

217

generations, and congenital abnormalities. Additionally, the pupil provides the passageway for aqueous humor to reach the anterior chamber from the ciliary body. If aqueous humor is prevented from passing through the pupil, iris bombé ensues with a secondary glaucoma (p. 316).

Symptoms and signs of pupillary abnormalities

The chief symptoms arising from abnormalities of the pupil relate to its function as a diaphragm in controlling the amount of light entering the eye. When the pupil is dilated, approximately 50 times as much energy enters as when it is constricted. Dilation and constriction occur constantly in the normal eye (p. 90) in response to the amount of light stimulating the retina.

Conditions associated with mydriasis cause photophobia because of excess light entering the eye. There is also more chromatic and spherical aberration and less depth of focus, as is true of a camera with the diaphragm opened widely. (The normal eye is about f 5.6.)

Miosis interferes with vision in dim illumination because of failure of the pupil to dilate in response to the reduced lighting. Visual loss arising from minor opacities of the lens may be severely aggravated by pupillary constriction, which is often a serious problem in the treatment of open-angle glaucoma (p. 314).

Openings in the iris in addition to the pupil may cause monocular double vision (diplopia). Surgical iridectomies are usually located near the 12 o'clock meridian and are covered by the upper lid and cause no symptoms. In conditions such as polycoria (multiple pupils) or iridodialysis (Fig. 13-2), diplopia may be an annoying symptom.

The signs of pupillary abnormalities arise from its shape, position, and response to stimulation. The pupils of the two eyes are usually of about equal size and respond similarly to stimulation. Distortion and ir-

regularity of the pupil may arise from disease or injury involving the iris itself. In abnormalities reflected in differences in size of the two pupils (anisocoria, p. 221) or in disturbances of pupillary reflexes (p. 90), one must determine if the condition arises from a localized iris abnormality, a lesion in the retina or optic nerve and its central connections, or an interruption of the sympathetic or parasympathetic efferent innervation.

Pupillary reflexes

The pupillary reflexes have been described in detail previously (p. 90). When light is directed into one eye, the pupil constricts (direct light reflex) and the opposite pupil simultaneously constricts (consensual light reflex). The receptors for the light reflex are the retinal rods and cones. The afferent axons responsible for conduction of the impulse are separate from the visual fibers but follow the same course in the optic nerve and chiasm; they separate from visual fibers at the level of the lateral geniculate body to pass through the brachium of the superior colliculus and synapse in the pretectal region. Here fibers pass with partial decussation to the Edinger-Westphal portion of the oculomotor nucleus (N III). Visceral motor efferent fibers pass from the nucleus in the oculomotor nerve to synapse in the ciliary ganglion (p. 50). Postganglionic fibers reach the sphincter pupillae muscle by the long and short posterior ciliary nerves.

In an eye blind from disease of the retina or the optic nerve, the direct light reflex is abolished, and there is no consensual reflex in the opposite eye. However, the blind eye has an intact consensual reflex when the normal fellow eye is stimulated with light. In an eye with hemianopsia arising from an optic tract lesion, light stimulation of the portion of the retina corresponding to the field defect is characterized by a diminished or absent direct light reflex. This is called the hemianopic pupillary reflex. Detection requires a small bundle of light rays so that the uninvolved side is not stimulated by scattered light within the eye. In hemianopsia due to involvement of the visual fibers posterior to the lateral geniculate body, the pupillary reaction to light is intact since the afferent pupillary fibers have already separated from the visual fibers.

When an individual focuses upon a nearby object, the pupil constricts via a reflex that follows visual fibers to the calcarine cortex, then areas 19 and 22, the cortico-tectal tract, and finally the oculomotor nerve. This accommodative reflex may be separated from convergence by covering one eye or by prisms to eliminate convergence.

Synkinetic or associated constriction of the pupil occurs with convergence and is not a true reflex but reflects an associated reaction involving the common innervation of the medial rectus muscle involved in convergence and the sphincter pupillae muscle. A less commonly observed synkinetic reaction is the pupillary constriction that may follow contraction of the orbicularis oculi muscle innervated by nerve VII. Stimulation of the trigeminal nerve from painful stimuli of the cornea, conjunctiva, or skin of the face may also cause reflex pupillary constriction.

Hippus, a rhythmic dilation and contraction of the pupils, may be a normal reaction associated with respiration. It also may be associated with multiple sclerosis or with meningitis, or it may follow oculomotor paralysis.

Congenital abnormalities

Inasmuch as the pupil is but the aperture of the iris, it is evident that developmental pupillary abnormalities arise in the iris. In many, however, the most striking change is the alteration in the appearance of the pupil. In aniridia (p. 225) the iris is rudimentary and the cornea area appears to be jet black with no iris present. A coloboma of the iris (Figs. 13-2 and 14-2) may be associated with faulty closure of the embryonic fissure with typical defects in the optic nerve and choroid. More common is simple coloboma of the iris in which a single or all layers of the iris are absent in a localized area, either extending as far as the ciliary body (total) or involving only a portion of a sector (partial). The pupil is pear shaped (Fig. 13-2) because of the absence of iris, but the usual layers are retained in the normal sector, which shows normal reflexes. Colobomas may be surrounded by iris tissue (Fig. 13-2) and appear as additional pupils (pseudopolycoria). Conspicuous displacement of the pupil from its normal position is corectopia, or ectopic pupil (Fig. 13-2). Except for the cosmetic variation, it causes no symptoms.

Miosis and mydriasis

Constriction of both pupils to less than 2.0 mm. with failure to dilate in the dark most commonly follows the instillation of drugs used in the treatment of glaucoma. Accidental or therapeutic systemic administration of these compounds may cause miosis, depending upon the dose. Morphine causes extreme constriction of the pupil. During sleep the pupils constrict, and this may distinguish true sleep from simulated sleep (as does involuntary fluttering of the eyelids in simulated sleep). With aging, the pupils normally become smaller (senile miosis), but normal reflexes are retained. Bilateral adhesion of the iris to the lens (posterior synechiae, p. 232) may cause small pupils that are usually irregular. Congenital absence of the dilatator pupillae muscle results in marked miosis due to unopposed action of the sphincter pupillae.

Miosis is characteristic of acute lesions of the pons and is associated with disturbance of the conjugate ocular movements. Removal of the cerebrum results in miosis, with both eyes turned to the right or left (conjugate deviation).

Blinking or closure of the eyes is associated with constriction of the pupil. Irritation of the conjunctiva or the cornea may cause miosis.

Dilation of both pupils to more than 6.0 mm. combined with failure to constrict when stimulated with light follows local instillation of drugs that paralyze the sphincter pupillae. Usually systemic administration of these compounds has a minimal pupillary effect, and their chief action involves the ciliary muscle, resulting in decreased accommodation. In bilateral blindness due to lesions anterior to the lateral geniculate body the pupils are dilated and, of course, fail to constrict with light stimulation.

In coma due to alcohol, diabetes, uremia, postepilepsy, apoplexy, or meningitis, the pupils are usually equally dilated and do not constrict with light stimulation.

During general anesthesia the pupils are usually dilated in Stages I and II, constricted in Stage III, and Stage IV is usu-ally heralded by sudden, wide pupillary dilation. Surprise, fear, and pain cause dilation of the pupil, as does any strong emotion, pleasant or unpleasant, or vestibular stimulation.

Argyll Robertson pupil

The Argyll Robertson pupil is a bilateral abnormality characterized by failure of the pupils to constrict with light but by retention of pupillary constriction with convergence and accommodation. The entire syndrome includes miotic, irregular, and unequal pupils, the presence of some vision in each eye, failure of the pupils to dilate with local scopolamine instillation, and further miosis with eserine instillation. When all signs are present, they characterize tabes dorsalis of central nervous system syphilis. The lesion is thought to be in the pretectal region where the afferent pupillary fibers synapse. Hemorrhage and tumors involving the pretectal region may be associated with failure of the pupils to react to light and retention of the reaction to accommodation. How-

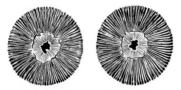

Argyll Robertson pupil
Miotic, irregular, unreactive to light,
reacts to accommodation

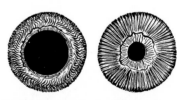

Oculomotor paralysis with fixed
dilated pupil likely with lost accommodation

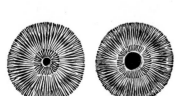

Horner's syndrome
Miosis, ptosis, anhidrosis on side of
sympathetic innervation interruption

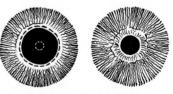

Adie's syndrome
Pupil larger or smaller than fellow,
reacts slowly to light and accommodation

Fig. 13-1. Neurologic causes of anisocoria.

ever, the pupils are not miotic, unequal, or irregular and are not typical of those described by Argyll Robertson pupil.

Anisocoria

Anisocoria, or unequal size of the pupils, is a relatively common normal variation. The normal difference in diameter, however, is slight, and often it is not noted. About 2% of apparently normal individuals have a 0.5 to 2.0 mm. difference in the size of the pupils with normal pupillary reflexes. The cause is unknown but may have an hereditary transmission.

Inequality in size of the pupils or a difference in their reflex reactions or responses to locally instilled drugs may indicate serious ocular or neurologic disease demanding careful study (Fig. 13-1). If the afferent pupillary fibers in one eye and optic nerve are intact, the pupils remain equal in size because of the decussation of the second-order neurons and the efferent outflow so that the iris muscles of the involved eye are normally innervated. Anisocoria thus mainly reflects an abnormality either involving the iris musculature of one eye with the eye itself or in the efferent parasympathetic or sympathetic motor innervation. The involved pupil may be either smaller or larger than the fellow. Irritative lesions of the parasympathetic pathway cause constriction, whereas paralytic lesions cause dilation. Irritative lesions of the sympathetic pathway cause dilation, whereas paralytic lesions cause constriction.

Tonic pupil (Adie's syndrome)

Tonic pupil is an abnormality in which disturbances of pupillary reaction are associated with abnormalities of tendon reflexes in patients who do not have syphilis. The shape of the pupil is slightly irregular, and one pupil is larger than the other. Although the condition is limited mainly to one side, it may be bilateral. In the complete form of Adie's syndrome the pupil reacts barely, if at all, to light. When the patient makes an attempt to fix a near point, a slow and delayed pupillary constriction appears. This response may be very marked and may exceed that of the normal pupil. After the pupil constricts with near vision, it redilates very slowly and may remain smaller than the normal pupil for some time. There is an associated diminution, or absence, of tendon reflexes; however, the pupillary signs may occur without involvement of the deep tendons.

There is a supersensitivity to cholinergic stimulation, and the pupil may constrict with 0.25% physostigmine and 2.5% Mecholyl, which do not affect the normal eye. This suggests that the lesion is either at the level of the ciliary ganglion or its postganglionic outflow. The disease is entirely benign, and no treatment is indicated.

Horner's syndrome

Interruption of the sympathetic nerve supply to the dilatator pupillae muscle results in a constricted pupil. The miosis is not marked and is often not noticed. Interruption of the sympathetic nerves anywhere in their course from the hypothalamus to the orbit results in Horner's syndrome. In addition to the miosis, there are ptosis, anhidrosis, and in experimental animals but not man, an enophthalmos.

The blepharoptosis is the result of loss of sympathetic nerve supply to Müller's smooth muscle of the upper lip, which provides its "tone." The lid droops only 1 or 2 mm. The anhidrosis follows loss of the sympathetic nerve fibers to the face and neck. The sweating fibers follow the external carotid artery, and in lesions occurring between the bifurcation of the common carotid artery and the orbit, they are not affected. The enophthalmos is not present in man but is simulated by the slight ptosis. It is marked in animals that have much smooth muscle in the orbit.

Horner's syndrome is usually due to interruption of the cervical sympathetic

Some causes of inequality of pupil size (anisocoria)

I. Local ocular causes
  A. Drugs topically instilled: mydriasis or miosis
  B. Injury
    1. Rupture of iris sphincter with contusion (traumatic iridoplegia)
    2. Adhesions between iris and cornea following laceration (adherent leukoma or anterior synechiae)
  C. Inflammation
    1. Keratitis (miosis)
    2. Acute iridocyclitis (middilation)
    3. Adhesions between iris and lens (posterior synechiae)
  D. Angle-closure glaucoma (middilation)
  E. Ischemic anterior ocular segment
    1. Retinal separation surgery
    2. Internal carotid artery insufficiency
  F. Diseases of iris
    1. Essential atrophy
    2. Aniridia
    3. Congenital variation

II. Paralysis of sphincter pupillae muscle (pupil dilated)
  A. Cerebral disease
    1. Neoplasm
    2. Aneurysm
    3. Degenerations
    4. Infectious disease: syphilis, herpes zoster ophthalmicus, encephalitis, botulism, diphtheria
    5. Cavernous sinus thrombosis
    6. Subdural and extradural hemorrhage
  B. Toxic polyneuritis (alcohol, lead, arsenic, carbon dioxide)
  C. Diabetes mellitus (pupil spared in 75% of cases of diabetic ophthalmoplegia)

III. Paralysis of dilatator pupillae muscle (pupil contricted)
  A. Horner's syndrome

IV. Lesion of intercalated neuron
  A. Argyll Robertson pupil (tabes dorsalis, pupil constricted)
  B. Midbrain lesions (pupil dilated)

trunk or the lower cervical and upper thoracic anterior spinal roots. The most common causes are mediastinal tumors, particularly bronchogenic carcinoma, Hodgkin's disease, and metastatic tumors. Large adenomas of the thyroid gland and neurofibromatosis may be causes. Surgical and accidental trauma to the neck are the next most common causes. Diseases within the central nervous system that may cause this syndrome include occlusion of the posterior inferior cerebellar artery, multiple sclerosis or syringomyelia involving the reticular substance of the pons, and tumors of the cervical cord. Congenital Horner's syndrome may be associated with less pigment in the iris on the affected side than in the fellow eye (heterochromia iridis) (p. 226).

The affected pupil does not dilate following the local instillation of 4% cocaine solution, but the normal pupil does. If the

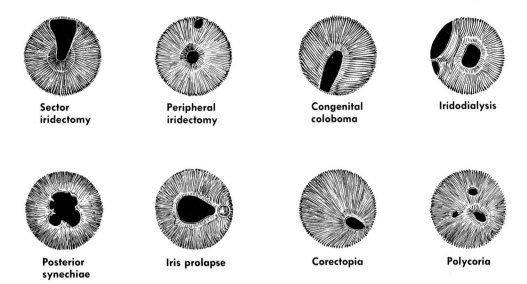

| Sector iridectomy | Peripheral iridectomy | Congenital coloboma | Iridodialysis |
| Posterior synechiae | Iris prolapse | Corectopia | Polycoria |

Fig. 13-2. Irregularity of the pupil in various disorders.

lesion causing Horner's syndrome involves the sympathetic nerves between the synapse in the superior cervical ganglion and the eye, the pupil will be supersensitive to epinephrine and will dilate with the instillation of 1:1,000 epinephrine hydrochloride, a concentration that does not affect the normal pupil. This reaction distinguishes between pre- and postganglionic lesions causing Horner's syndrome.

Irregularity

The pupils may be of irregular shape in a variety of disorders (Fig. 13-2). Following a corneal laceration, the iris prolapses into the wound, causing a tear-shaped pupil. The appearance is quite characteristic of corneal lacerations. Following blunt trauma to the eye, the iris may be torn from its insertion at the scleral spur, causing an iridodialysis. The sector of the pupil corresponding to the iridodialysis is flattened and becomes a chord of the circular pupil.

In uveitis the iris may be bound to the lens by posterior synechiae. These may be evident only when the pupil is dilated, but if they formed when the pupil was miotic, the irregularity of the pupillary margin will be marked.

Surgical colobomas of the iris may be recognized by their usual location near the 12 o'clock meridian and by the deficiency of the iris pigment frill at the edges of the incision. A congenital coloboma usually involves the inferior nasal iris, and the frill of pupillary pigment lines the margins.

Chapter 14

The uvea

The middle coat of the eye, the uvea (from *uva* [Latin], a grape), is composed of the iris, the ciliary body, and the choroid. The iris, a diaphragm located about 3 mm. behind the cornea, separates the anterior and posterior chambers. It contains a central aperture, the pupil, which regulates the amount of light entering the eye and contains two muscles: (1) the sphincter pupillae (N III, parasympathetics) and (2) the dilatator pupillae (sympathetics). The ciliary body secretes aqueous humor and contains the ciliary muscle (N III) that governs accommodation. The choroid extends from the margin of the optic nerve forward to become continuous with the ciliary body. The blood supply of the outer one half of the retina is provided by the adjacent choroid.

The iris contains a variable amount of pigment in its anterior stroma. The anterior stroma is absent in some areas, forming iris crypts. The stroma rests upon a layer of pigment epithelium that is continuous with the retina and that contains the dilatator muscle. The sphincter muscle is located near the pupil in the stroma. The iris is divided into an inner pupillary zone concentric with the pupil and an outer ciliary zone by the collarette, the remnant of the minor vascular circle of the iris. The blood vessels of the iris are arranged in a radial pattern and have a thick adventitia.

The ciliary body is composed of (1) a corona ciliaris that contains ciliary processes and (2) an orbicularis ciliaris, or pars plana, that is the area transitional with the choroid. The ciliary processes secrete the aqueous humor into the posterior chamber.

Located within the ciliary body is the ciliary muscle, divided into well-defined longitudinal and circular fibers and poorly defined radial fibers. Zonular fibers connect the equator of the lens with the ciliary muscle, and with contraction of the muscle there is increased refractive power of the lens known as accommodation.

The choroid consists first of a layer of capillaries separated from the retinal pigment epithelium by a glass membrane, the lamina vitrea, and then of veins of increasingly larger size as they approach the sclera. The blood supply is derived from the short and long posterior ciliary arteries. There are many anastomoses between the posterior and the anterior groups of vessels. The choroidal blood vessels are subject to the same intraocular pressure as the retinal blood vessels and have much the same intravascular pressure.

Symptoms and signs of uveal disease

The symptoms and signs vary considerably with the disease. Abnormalities of the iris may distort the shape of the pupil or may interfere with dilation and constriction (p. 90). Inflammations of the iris and the ciliary body cause a ciliary type of injection (p. 131). Diseases of the ciliary body and the iris may be associated with severe, deep, boring, dull, aching pain within the eye. Inflammation of the posterior choroid occurs without ciliary injection or pain.

Most local diseases of the ciliary body cause contraction of the ciliary muscle with disturbed accommodation. Diseases affecting the oculomotor nerve supply result in pupillary dilation and a loss of accommodation. Diseases of the choroid often affect overlying retina and cause interference with visual function. The disturbance in visual function reflects the layer of the retina impaired. Widespread disturbances of the retinal pigment epithelium and photoreceptor layer of the neural retina cause impaired dark adaptation (night blindness) described as a tapetoretinal degeneration (p. 265). If the portion of the choroid providing nutrition to the fovea centralis is involved, there are abnormalities of central vision. Peripheral visual field changes follow interference with the extracentral retina. Inflammations of the uvea cause exudation of inflammatory cells and a protein-rich fluid into the eye, which decreases visual acuity.

The iris may be examined directly, with the cornea providing magnification for study. The ciliary body can be seen only with a gonioscope after maximal pupillary dilation.

Ophthalmoscopic visualization of the choroid is usually prevented by the pigment epithelium of the retina that causes the fundus to appear reddish brown in color. Sometimes a portion of the choroid is visible at the temporal side of the optic disk as a choroidal crescent. In lightly pigmented subjects, details of the choroid may be observed. A whitish sclera may be observed between blood vessels. These vessels usually belong to the outer vessel layer of Haller and consist of veins that have a considerably greater diameter than the corresponding retinal vessels. The choriocapillaris is never seen ophthalmoscopically in health. In choroidal sclerosis the choriocapillaris layer atrophies and the

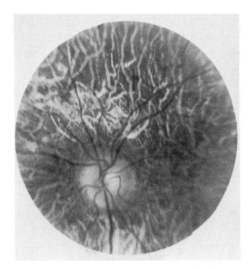

Fig. 14-1. Choroidal sclerosis with the veins of the choroid visible through the attenuated pigment epithelium of the retina.

veins are seen as a dense network of whitish vessels (Fig. 14-1).

The pigment of the choroid is more brownish than the jet black retinal pigment. The choroidal pigment does not proliferate in inflammatory irritation as does the retinal pigment. Deficiencies in the elastic layer of the lamina vitrea (Bruch's membrane) have been described as the cause of a variety of ocular abnormalities, for example, disciform macular degeneration, angioid streaks, and rare hereditary diseases.

Congenital and developmental anomalies
Aniridia

Aniridia is a hereditary, usually dominant, abnormality in which the anterior growth and differentiation of the optic cup fail. This results in a rudimentary iris, which is concealed behind the corneoscleral limbus. Bilateral involvement is usual. The eye appears black with no iris visible. Photophobia may be present. The rudimentary iris tissue can be seen only with a gonioscope. Visual acuity is reduced to about 20/100, and an ocular nystagmus is present. Glaucoma often develops in adolescence. The glaucoma is difficult to correct surgically, and medical treatment is preferred. Provision of an artificial pupil by means of an iris painted on a contact lens reduces photophobia but does not improve vision.

Congenital aniridia occurring in families without other affected members may be associated with a variety of systemic disorders: mental retardation, microcephaly, hemihypertrophy, horseshoe kidney, and genital abnormalities (cryptorchidism, hypospadias, and pseudohermaphrodism). A Wilms' tumor may develop by the age of 3 years. Rhabdomyosarcoma, nephroblastoma, adrenal tumors, hepatoblastoma, and gonadoblastoma have also been described, although less commonly than Wilms' tumor.

Coloboma

Failure of the optic cup (p. 61) to close in the region of the fetal fissure gives rise to a coloboma. Typically these are located in the inferior nasal sector and extend from the optic nerve to the iris. Uveal tissue is entirely absent in the area of coloboma. The pigment epithelium of the retina is missing—the sensory retina is present but is transparent and cannot be seen with the ophthalmoscope.

The white sclera is seen ophthalmoscopically at the base of choroidal colobomas. A scleral ectasia may be present. The appearance of a coloboma may be simulated by maldevelopment arising because of prenatal inflammation, particularly toxoplasmosis. A coloboma of the ciliary body may be associated with a notching defect of the lens corresponding to the deficient area.

Typical congenital colobomas of the iris involve the inferior nasal portion and give rise to a defect in the shape of the pupil (Fig. 14-2). The edges of the coloboma show the pupillary frill with pigment epi-

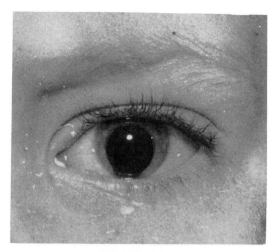

Fig. 14-2. Congenital coloboma of the iris in the characteristic down and in position in the region of the site of closure of the fetal fissure.

thelium, unlike surgical colobomas. Many different shapes, sizes, and locations of colobomas are described.

Heterochromia iridis

The color of the two irides is often slightly different. In simple heterochromia iridis there is a relative hypoplasia of the lighter colored iris combined with a relative hyperplasia of the iris architecture on the side of the darker colored iris. The abnormality may be transmitted as an autosomal dominant trait or may be associated with displacement of the medial canthi, hypertrophy of the nasal bridge, albinism, and inner ear alterations (Waardenburg-Klein syndrome).

In hypochromic heterochromia the eye with the lighter colored iris is abnormal. The difference between the two eyes may be extremely slight if blue irides are involved. The condition may be associated with Horner's syndrome of paralysis of the sympathetic nerves to the dilatator pupillae (p. 221); with Fuchs' heterochromic cyclitis; with mild iridocyclitis with ciliary injection, often with cataract and sometimes with glaucoma (p. 316); with glaucomatocyclitic crises; with diffuse iris atrophy secondary to inflammation, trauma, or ischemia of the iris; and with infiltration of a nonpigmented tumor into the iris.

In hyperchromic heterochromia the iris on the side of the anomaly or disease is darker than its fellow. The condition occurs with retention of an iron foreign body in the eye (siderosis), with malignant melanoma of the iris, in monocular melanosis in which there are excess chromatophores in the iris stroma, following anterior chamber hemorrhage from any cause, following perforating injuries or contusion of the globe occurring before the age of 10 years, and in association with microcornea.

Iris atrophy

As we have seen (p. 15), the pupillary zone of the iris is relatively flat because of atrophy of the anterior leaf of the stroma. The delicate gossamer appearance of the ciliary zone may be lost in a variety of conditions in which the fine collagen fibers atrophy and disappear with the blood vessels and are replaced by a network of minute sclerosed lines. Hypochromia iridis causes such an atrophy together with a loss of chromatophores, but if there is no pigment loss, the iris appears dull and patternless but has the same color as its fellow. Such atrophy may be diffuse or localized. It occurs to a minor degree with aging and may be severe following ocular inflammation, trauma, ischemia, and glaucoma. It may follow interruption of the ciliary ganglion and may occur in tabes dorsalis not associated with the pupillary signs.

Essential iris atrophy. Essential iris atrophy is a rare progressive unilateral vascular disease affecting young women predominantly. It is characterized by patchy loss of all layers of the iris, a distorted and migrating pupil, and secondary glaucoma (Fig. 14-3). The onset is gradual, with the patient aware only of a change in

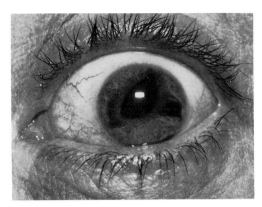

Fig. 14-3. Essential atrophy of the iris with the formation of additional pupils—polycoria.

shape or position of the pupil. During the next several years holes develop in the iris. Secondary glaucoma then ensues from peripheral anterior synechiae and damage to the trabecular meshwork from a cuticular membrane. The disease may be diagnosed by direct inspection of the iris. Treatment is directed toward the secondary glaucoma and is often not effective.

Secondary iris atrophy. Secondary iris atrophy does not cause the frank holes seen in the essential type. The atrophy is caused by ischemia of the iris secondary to infarction of the iris arteries. The vascular insufficiency may follow carotid artery insufficiency, lupus erythematosus, and similar widespread arterial disease.

Iridoschisis

Iridoschisis is a rare progressive bilateral degeneration of the anterior stromal leaf of the iris. It involves both sexes, usually after the age of 65 years. It is characterized by preferential involvement of the lower half of the iris; the remainder of the iris is normal and the pupil is not displaced. The anterior stromal layer in the involved sector becomes detached from the posterior layer and disintegrates into fibrils that remain attached at one end while the other floats free in the anterior chamber. Treatment is not indicated.

Rubeosis of the iris

New blood vessel formation on the surface of the iris may occur spontaneously in diabetes mellitus (p. 385) or follow central retinal vein closure (p. 260). New blood vessels may be seen on the surface of the iris, particularly in the region adjacent to the pupil. They must be distinguished from dilation of preexisting blood vessels, which often accompanies the same diseases. Gonioscopy indicates the anterior chamber recess to contain minute blood vessels arising from the root of the iris. Vision is usually reduced because of retinal changes secondary to the initiating cause. Hemorrhage into the anterior chamber (hyphema) is frequent. Severe glaucoma, usually resistant to either medical or surgical therapy, may necessitate enucleation for relief of pain.

Rubeosis iridis occurs in a large variety of abnormalities, presumably secondary to anoxia of the iris: aortic arch syndrome, carotid occlusive disease, carotid fistula, temporal arteritis, anterior ocular segment ischemia, retinal arterial and venous occlusion, retinal disease associated with neovascularization, intraocular tumors, and following radiation and intraocular inflammation.

Inflammatory disorders

Inflammation of the uveal tract includes a variety of conditions that vary in severity from abscess formation, which may follow exogenous or endogenous introduction of pyogenic bacteria, to the widespread but minimal inflammation of the choroid in miliary tuberculosis. Because of their common blood supply, inflammations of the iris, the ciliary body, and the anterior choroid tend to be involved to a greater or lesser extent in the same inflammatory process. Inflammation of the posterior choroid, however, unless exceptionally severe, does not involve the structures of the anterior uveal tract. Inflammatory reactions are frequently designated as acute, recurrent, or chronic, or they may be designated according to the site of the most severe reaction: iritis, cyclitis, iridocyclitis, choroiditis, anterior uveitis, or posterior uveitis.

Exogenous and endogenous uveitis

Inflammation of the uveal tract may be divided into exogenous and endogenous types. In exogenous disease the causative agent is introduced directly into the eye by penetration of the cornea or the sclera. Endogenous inflammations may arise from an abnormality within the eye itself such as cataract, necrosis of an intraocular tumor, or by participation of the uveal tract in a systemic inflammatory reaction. Many workers in the past have regarded most instances of endogenous uveitis *without systemic disease* to be the result of an interaction of antigen with antibody in a previously sensitized uvea. Currently, most authorities agree that the causative mechanism is unknown but involves complex cellular and humoral reactions combined with factors of ocular reactivity.

The inflammation may be purulent or nonpurulent. Nonpurulent inflammations are often divided clinically into granulomatous and nongranulomatous types, but the pathologic lesion, when available for histologic study, does not parallel the clinical type. Additionally, nongranulomatous lesions with persistence or recurrence may merge into the granulomatous type. Purulent and nonpurulent types may be exogenous or endogenous.

Purulent uveitis

Purulent uveitis is caused by pyogenic bacteria and rarely by fungi. The organisms are introduced into the eye through a laceration, a surgical incision, or by perforation of a corneal ulcer. In years past a septicemia, particularly during the bacteremic stage of meningococcus meningitis (p. 365), was a cause. Common organisms include *Staphylococcus aureus, Bacillus subtilis* (a contaminant of operating room air-conditioning systems), *Pseudomonas aeruginosa, Proteus,* coliform bacilli, and fungi. The purulent inflammation is classed as either a panophthalmitis or an endophthalmitis.

Panophthalmitis. Panophthalmitis is an acute inflammation of the intraocular contents, with necrosis of the sclera or the cornea and extension of the inflammation to the orbital contents. The disease is fulminating, with an incubation period of only a few hours. The lids are red and swollen, and there is marked chemosis of the conjunctiva. Involvement of orbital tissues may cause proptosis. The cornea is usually a whitish mass of inflammatory tissue, and if there has been a laceration or surgical incision, pus is dripping from the wound. There may be severe ocular pain until the globe ruptures. When treatment is ineffective, the signs gradually subside, and the eye becomes a shrunken mass of fibrous tissue, a phthisis bulbi.

Endophthalmitis. Purulent endophthalmitis is a suppurative inflammation of the intraocular contents in which all layers are not affected and in which the globe does not rupture. The onset is less violent than that of panophthalmitis, but there is a gradual increase in severity of the inflammation. Fungi, necrosis of intraocular tumors, and retained intraocular foreign bodies often cause a purulent endophthalmitis. Leukocytes may accumulate in the anterior chamber (hypopyon), and the vitreous body may be filled with inflammatory cells. The inflammation frequently causes destruction of the eye.

Treatment. Treatment of purulent endophthalmitis is often heroic and frequently unsuccessful. The main effort is directed toward obtaining a high intraocular concentration of an antibiotic specific for the causative organism. Inasmuch as the causative organism and its antibiotic sensitivity are not known until cultured, a broad-spectrum antibiotic to which penicillinase staphylococci and gram-negative bacteria

are sensitive is used systemically, topically, and subconjunctivally. Systemic corticosteroids may minimize the fibroblastic response to inflammation. Once it is evident that a useful eye will not result, the entire intraocular contents are removed (evisceration), leaving only the scleral shell covered by conjunctiva.

Nonpurulent uveitis

Nonpurulent inflammations of the uveal tract are often classed as granulomatous or nongranulomatous. The use of these terms, associated with definite histologic lesions, to describe clinical disease is protested by those who believe they are cumbrous expressions for acute (nongranulomatous) and chronic (granulomatous) uveal inflammation. The present tendency is toward a more precise description of the inflammatory involvement, emphasizing the morphology of the lesion without attempting to classify or to imply the underlying mechanism of the inflammation. Nonpurulent uveitis may involve either the anterior or posterior uvea, and many times both are involved (Table 14-1).

Chronic (granulomatous) uveitis. A granulomatous uveitis is a chronic, usually progressive inflammation in which there is cellular infiltration, chiefly by mononuclear cells, macrophages, and epithelioid cells, with tissue necrosis and repair by fibrosis. Involvement of the anterior uvea in granulomatous inflammation is characterized by a torpid, chronic course with minimal signs of infection. Mutton-fat keratic precipitates form, and there is only a mild aqueous flare with few cells in the aqueous humor. There is a marked tendency to the formation of posterior synechiae and interference with ocular function.

In the posterior ocular segment, granulomatous disease is associated with marked vitreous clouding with heavy, veil-like opacities, with one or more choroidal exudative areas that involve the overlying pigment epithelium of the retina.

Table 14-1. Characteristics of acute and chronic uveitis

	Chronic (granulomatous)	Acute (nongranulomatous)
Anterior uvea		
Pain, photophobia	Minimal or absent	Severe
Vision	Gradual reduction	Abrupt reduction
Course	Protracted, remissions and exacerbations	Self-limited (1-6 weeks), often recurrent
Keratic deposits	Heavy, coalesce, often "mutton fat," crenated margins, macrophages, phagocytized pigment	Pinpoint, lymphocytes and plasma cells
Aqueous humor	Few cells, often large, little aqueous flare	Many cells, monocytes, intense aqueous flare, sometimes coagulation
Iris nodules and precipitates	Frequent	None
Posterior uvea		
Retinal and subretinal edema	Usually slight or moderate and localized around exudates	Marked and generalized, with blurring of neuroretinal margins and retinal vascular bed
Choroidal exudates	Heavy massive exudates, edges possibly blurred by surrounding retinal and subretinal edema	No heavy massive exudates, occasionally localized areas of deeper infiltration
Secondary retinal involvement	Almost invariable, with retinal destruction	None or limited to pigment epithelium and rods and cones
Residual organic damage	Heavy glial scars with massive pigment surrounding the lesion	None or fine granular changes in pigment epithelium with damage to neuroepithelium and superficial gliosis
Anterior segment changes	Sometimes epithelioid or mutton-fat keratic deposits	Usually none
Vitreous changes	Usually heavy vitreous blurring, heavy, veil-like opacities frequent	Slight to intense general blurring, fine muscae or stringlike, fibrinous opacities

Granulomatous uveitis characterizes diseases in which granuloma formation is prominent elsewhere: syphilis, tuberculosis, sarcoid, and toxoplasmosis. A granulomatous type of inflammation is also seen in sympathetic ophthalmia, phacoanaphylactic uveitis, following recurrent attacks of nongranulomatous uveitis, and ocular infection with most nonpyogenic microorganisms. The inflammation has been considered a manifestation of a delayed type of hypersensitivity or a bacterial type of hypersensitivity.

Acute (nongranulomatous) uveitis. Nongranulomatous uveitis is an acute, self-limited, often recurrent inflammation of the uveal tract characterized by edema, capillary dilation, and an exudation of polymorphonuclear leukocytes that are quickly replaced by lymphocytes and plasma cells. Nongranulomatous inflammation of the anterior segment is characterized by punctate keratic precipitates, acute and severe inflammatory signs with a sudden onset, severe symptoms with a minimal tendency toward formation of posterior synechiae, and a tendency to spontaneous remission.

Nongranulomatous lesions are rare in the choroid. They are associated with fine cells in the vitreous body and retinal edema without exudation.

Nongranulomatous uveitis has been regarded as an example of the immediate type of hypersensitivity reaction. Sensitivity to the alpha strain of beta hemolytic streptococci was formerly regarded as the chief cause, but this has not been confirmed.

Symptoms and signs

The symptoms of nonpurulent uveitis vary with the portion of the uveal tract involved. Visual loss is the main symptom of posterior inflammations, while anterior uveitis may initially cause pain, photophobia, and lacrimation. Pain is more common in acute iridocyclitis than in chronic iridocyclitis and is particularly severe when associated with keratitis. It is referred to the periorbital and ocular region and is aggravated by exposure to light and by pressure. Photophobia varies in severity and may be so marked that the lids cannot be opened to examine the eye. Lacrimation is usually proportionate to the degree of photophobia. Decreased vision arises because of exudation of cells and protein-rich fluid and fibrin into either the anterior chamber or vitreous body or because of involvement of the overlying retina in posterior uveitis. Inflammation of the choroid beneath the fovea centralis causes an early loss of visual acuity that is often disproportionately severe in comparison to the amount of choroidal involvement. Uveitis adjacent to the disk (juxtapapillary) may cause a nerve fiber bundle defect (p. 308). Choroidal inflammation distant from the posterior pole, although affecting the overlying retina, may cause only minimal changes in the peripheral visual field. Toxic edema of the posterior pole of the eye with swelling of the optic disk (papillitis) and macular edema may occur with severe inflammations of both the anterior and posterior uvea and cause decreased visual acuity.

Anterior uveitis. The signs of anterior uveitis include ciliary injection, exudation into the anterior chamber, iris changes, and posterior synechiae (adhesions between the iris and lens).

Ciliary injection. Ciliary injection (p. 131) is the result of extension of the inflammation to the anterior conjunctival branches of the anterior ciliary vessels that form the superficial and deep pericorneal plexus (p. 46). The severity varies with the degree of inflammation. Very little or none occurs in chronic iridocyclitis, while in severe acute inflammation there may be associated episcleral and conjunctival injection and conjunctival edema. In less acute inflammation there is a deep, circumcorneal injection with a violet hue. The injection fades in the conjunctival fornix and does not bleach with the instillation of 1:1,000 epinephrine.

Exudation into the anterior chamber. The inflammation of the iris and ciliary body causes a breakdown of the blood-aqueous barrier, so that there are increased protein and fibrin in the aqueous humor as well as inflammatory cells. The protein gives rise to a translucence of the aqueous humor, which can be seen with the biomicroscope and is described as aqueous flare. Fibrin may be present in such an excessive amount that the inflammatory cells present do not move. The cells are suspended in the aqueous humor and, because of thermal convection currents, rise when close to the iris and descend at the cooler cornea. Inflammatory cells adhere to the endothelial surface of the cornea, giving rise to keratic precipitates (K.P.). Two main types of keratic precipitates occur:

(1) large, heavy, greasy, fat keratic precipitates (mutton-fat K.P.) composed of macrophages and phagocytized pigment and (2) small, white punctate accumulations composed of lymphocytes and plasma cells. Similar cellular accumulations may occur at the pupillary margin (Koeppe nodules), on the surface of the iris (floccules of Busacca), on the lens surface, and in the anterior chamber angle. Occasionally in severe acute iridocyclitis so many cells are present that a hypopyon forms, or rarely diapedesis of erythrocytes causes a hyphema.

Inflammations of the anterior choroid and the ciliary body cause minimal external signs of inflammation. Epithelioid cells escape into the anterior chamber to form mutton-fat keratic precipitates that gradually increase in number, although the aqueous flare and the number of cells in the anterior chamber are minimal.

Iris changes. In acute iridocyclitis the pupil may be constricted or in middilation. The iris may be edematous with its pattern blurred ("muddy") and the capillaries engorged. In chronic iridocyclitis, nodules may arise from proliferation of the iris pigment epithelium or infiltration of the iris with round cells and macrophages. Rarely typical granulomatous nodules such as tubercles or sarcoid nodules may be found. These may be followed by a patchy area of iris atrophy. Diffuse iris atrophy (p. 227) with loss of iris pattern follows prolonged iridocyclitis and may involve both the stroma (mesodermal) and pigment (ectodermal) layers.

Posterior synechiae. Severe inflammations cause the iris to become adherent to the lens, resulting in the formation of posterior synechiae. This may give rise to a small, irregular pupil that does not react to light in the area of adhesion. The adhesion arises initially because of apposition of the iris to the lens, which is brought about by inflammatory cells and fibroblasts from the iris. Sometimes a large clump of iris pigment remains on the anterior lens capsule, a sign pathognomonic of past or present inflammation. If posterior synechiae involve the entire pupillary margin, aqueous humor cannot flow from the posterior chamber into the anterior chamber, and the resultant iris bombé causes a severe glaucoma.

Posterior uveitis. The two most important signs of posterior uveitis are vitreous opacities and chorioretinal lesions.

Vitreous opacities. A variable degree of cloudiness of the vitreous arises in posterior uveitis because of exudation of inflammatory cells and a protein-rich fluid combined with erythrocytes and tissue cells. Vitreous opacities consist of aggregates of cells, coagulated exudate and fibrin, and strands of degenerated vitreous body that are visible with the ophthalmoscope. They appear as black dots against the red background of the fundus or may be so numerous as to make all fundus details indistinct. They are best studied by means of the biomicroscope combined with a concave contact lens to neutralize the refractive power of the cornea.

Choroiditis. In the acute stage, choroiditis appears ophthalmoscopically as an ill-defined grayish yellow or grayish white area surrounded by the normal colored fundus. The lesions may be single or multiple. The adjacent neural retina becomes edematous and opaque and is so commonly inflamed that the lesion is described as chorioretinitis (Fig. 14-4). Inflammatory cells and exudate may burst through Bruch's membrane and cause vitreous clouding, which further obscures the ophthalmoscopic details of the lesion.

With healing, the margins of the lesion become more sharply defined and the vitreous clouding clears. If the choroid has been the main site of the lesion, it appears as a whitish yellow area delicately stippled with pigment. When the retina has been destroyed, a whitish patch of scar appears that consists of either a fibrous replacement of retina and choroid or stark, white sclera over which both the retina and choroid have been destroyed. The retinal pigment epithelium proliferates particularly at the margins of the lesions, and the final ophthalmoscopic appearance is often one of white sclera surrounded by black pigment. Pigment proliferation does not always occur following severe inflammation, presumably because of destruction of the retinal pigment epithelium.

Following healing, particularly in toxoplasmosis, an acute area of chorioretinal inflammation, a satellite lesion, may occur adjacent to a healed area, often with a zone of normal fundus separating the two (Fig. 14-4).

A minute hemorrhage between Bruch's

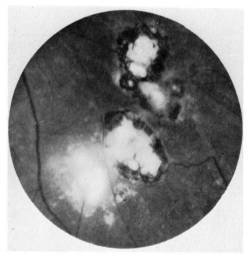

Fig. 14-4. Healed and active chorioretinitis. In the lesions above, destruction of the retina and choroid has made the sclera visible. The retinal pigment epithelium proliferated with healing to give the black margins. The lesion below is active, has poorly defined margins, and the blood vessel crossing it is obscured by the retinal edema. The multiple lesions, their appearance, and the occurrence of an active satellite inflammation adjacent to an apparently healed area are characteristics of the retinochoroiditis of toxoplasmosis.

membrane and the pigment epithelium at the posterior pole may signal the onset of a fairly typical ophthalmoscopic lesion that has been attributed to histoplasmosis. In the foveal region one sees ophthalmoscopically a dark grayish, well-defined lesion without any vitreous body reaction. Occasionally the hemorrhage breaks into the neural retina to form an arc of bright red blood adjacent to the primary lesion.

Diagnosis and etiology

The diagnosis of nonpurulent uveitis presents no marked difficulties. Acute iridocyclitis presents the signs and symptoms of the red eye (p. 131), and angle-closure glaucoma, keratitis, or conjunctivitis is usually easily excluded. The diagnosis is confirmed by biomicroscopic examination and observation of keratic precipitates, aqueous flare, and cells. Neither does posterior uveitis with clouding of the vitreous and ophthalmoscopic observation of a chorioretinal inflammatory lesion present diagnostic problems.

The etiologic factor causing nonpurulent uveitis may be immediately evident when associated with systemic disease but in other instances may be impossible to demonstrate. The problem of diagnosis is enormously complicated by the inability to secure uveal tissue for study, so that even after effective specific therapy the cause remains presumptive. Additionally, the response of the uveal tract to inflammation is often histologically nonspecific even in well-defined systemic disorders. In many patients the etiologic factor is diagnosed only by exclusion of other possible causes; in others, such as patients with arthritis or genitourinary tract disease, one learns only that the uveal tissue is participating in an abnormality that possibly is also affecting other portions of the body. In some patients, too, the uveitis is not causally related to any systemic disorder present, even in conditions in which the disease is often associated with uveal inflammation.

In many cases the cause of uveitis is often immediately apparent, and appropriate specific treatment is initiated. Many patients in whom a cause is not found have only a single attack, and others are seen with chorioretinal scars or anterior segment lesions from asymptomatic inflammations that have occurred previously. In conditions such as heterochromic cyclitis (p. 226) and glaucomatocyclitic crises, no systemic abnormality has ever been found and etiologic studies are usually not emphasized. Virtually every systemic infection may cause a uveitis, but often attention is not directed to the eyes unless there is a disturbance in vision.

Local ocular disease with uveitis. A variety of inflammations and diseases primarily involving the eye or its adnexa may be associated with uveitis:

1. Severe infection of the conjunctiva or cornea involving the uvea by direct contiguity or by entry of an exotoxin into the eye (The infection may be bacterial, viral [often herpes simplex], or fungal. An orbital abscess may involve the vortex veins, or a meningitis may extend along the sheaths of the optic nerve. Involvement of the nasociliary branch of the ophthalmic nerve in herpes zoster ophthalmicus, p. 371, is associated with both uveitis and keratitis.)

2. Disease of the lens
   a. Hypermature cataract with release of toxic products within the eye
   b. Endophthalmitis phacoanaphylactica, an autoimmune process in which the eye has become sensitive to its own lens protein (Usually the sensitization occurs when one lens is removed extracapsularly so that lens protein is retained in the eye and gives rise to antibody production. With extracapsular extraction of the lens in the fellow eye, an antigen-antibody reaction occurs.)

3. Trauma
   a. Sympathetic ophthalmia, a rare bilateral granulomatous panophthalmitis or endophthalmitis that follows lacerations of the globe and possibly constitutes an autosensitization to uveal pigment
   b. Retained intraocular foreign body
   c. Contusion damage from blunt trauma
   d. Chemical injury
   e. Perforation of the lens

4. Heterochromic cyclitis, a nongranulomatous iridocyclitis occurring in an eye lighter in color than its fellow eye, often complicated by posterior subcapsular cataract and secondary glaucoma (Some question exists as to whether this is a distinct disease or a depigmentation occurring secondary to recurrent uveitis.)

5. Blind eyes with degenerative changes (Often these eyes have a chronic uveitis, and a decision must be made as to whether it is worthwhile to retain or enucleate the eye.)

6. Necrosis of intraocular tumor (In most instances the diagnosis of the cause of uveitis may be readily made in such eyes.)

7. Free blood within the eye following trauma or hemorrhagic intraocular disease

Systemic disease with uveitis. As suggested in the chapter concerning ocular infections and granulomas (p. 363), nearly any bacteria, virus, fungus, rickettsia, protozoa, spirochete, or worm causing a systemic infection may cause a uveitis. Sarcoid, collagen diseases, immediate and delayed hypersensitivity, autoimmune diseases, and chronic infection in a number of distant organs have been implicated.

The etiologic diagnosis of uveitis is often based upon the following:

1. A uveitis of a type associated with a particular systemic disease
2. A positive focal reaction occurring

following the diagnostic or therapeutic administration of an antigen when there is a marked aggravation of the inflammation—a dangerous test usually observed inadvertently and not always accurate

3. Exclusion of all other likely causes of the uveitis

4. Therapeutic improvement with specific medication (Nongranulomatous uveitis, particularly, is self-limited, and a diagnosis based upon improvement with specific medication may be erroneous.)

The major systemic conditions considered in the diagnosis of uveitis without obvious cause vary from place to place and from time to time. Currently major attention is directed to the diagnosis of toxoplasmosis, tuberculosis, syphilis, histoplasmosis, sarcoidosis, arthritis, and genitourinary tract disease.

Toxoplasmosis (p. 376). The primary lesion is a retinitis with secondary choroidal involvement. The disease may be congenital or acquired. In both types the retinochoroidal inflammation is multiple, with prominent pigment proliferation particularly involving the posterior pole. The congenital type may cause cerebral calcification, hydrocephalus, and mental retardation. The methylene blue antibody titer in both mother and child is almost always positive.

Tuberculosis (p. 365). Patients with pulmonary tuberculosis have a remarkably low incidence of uveitis except in terminal miliary disease when ocular involvement is only incidental. Tuberculosis usually causes a granulomatous inflammation of the posterior or anterior segment. The tuberculin test is positive, and a healed primary lesion may be seen on chest roentgenograms. Often there is a history of tuberculosis in other family members. There may be a beneficial response to the administration of isoniazid. This is obviously tenuous evidence upon which to base a diagnosis of tuberculosis and to undertake prolonged therapy, for if there is improvement with isoniazid therapy it must be continued for a year to avoid producing a resistant strain of tubercle bacilli.

Syphilis (p. 380). The development of the *Treponema pallidum* antibody tests has renewed interest in syphilis as a cause of uveitis in patients in whom the history suggests the possibility of latent syphilis. Uveal syphilis causes a large variety of lesions that vary in severity from the transient hyperemia (roseola) of the iris in the early secondary stage to gummata in the late tertiary stage. Acute iridocyclitis occurs in the early secondary stage and may be combined with a generalized severe uveitis in the tertiary stage with widely disseminated multiple lesions extending from the optic disk to the equator. A ring scotoma is typical. A marked pigmentary proliferation may occur, causing a condition resembling retinal pigmentary degeneration (p. 265).

In congenital syphilis, acute iridocyclitis may occur when the infant is about 6 months old. Choroiditis often occurs before birth and gives rise to a variety of atrophic scars and pigment clumps that are moderately typical (salt and pepper fundus). Interstitial keratitis that occurs 10 to 15 years after birth is always associated with an acute, severe anterior uveitis.

Recently a spirochete morphologically indistinguishable from *Treponema pallidum* has been found in the aqueous humor of patients who received presumably adequate penicillin therapy for congenital or acquired syphilis. Routine serologic tests for syphilis were negative, but the serum fluorescent treponemal antibody absorption test was usually positive. Final proof that these spirochetes are virulent and cause syphilis or ocular signs is not yet available.

Histoplasmosis. Histoplasmosis is a fungus infection caused by *Histoplasma capsulatum* endemic in the Mississippi Valley and occurring mainly as a subclinical disease demonstrable only by skin hypersensitivity and positive complement fixation. The organism has not been found in the eye except in endophthalmitis, and its role in causing chorioretinal disease is entirely speculative.

The ocular disease attributed to histoplasmosis is initially diagnosed because of loss of vision due to an elevated macular lesion. Recurrent hemorrhage beneath the retinal pigment epithelium is common. Blood sometimes seeps into the neural retina, giving rise to a dark lesion due to the deeper blood and a bright red lesion due to blood in the neural retina. There are multiple, small, discrete areas of healed chorioretinitis at the equator and a healed pigmented area at the disk resembling a choroidal crescent). There is a minimal cellular reaction.

Although the ophthalmoscopic appearance of the lesion is similar in different patients, the role of histoplasmosis is entirely speculative. Moreover, histoplasmosis infections are so ubiquitous in the Midwest that positive diagnostic tests are not significant in this region.

Differential diagnosis involves malignant melanoma (which is uncommonly associated with hemorrhage or occurrence in the fovea), choroidal vascular anomalies (central serous detachment of the retina, central hemorrhagic detachment, and angiospastic retinopathy), and chorioretinitis from other causes.

Sarcoidosis (p. 383). Probably in every case of sarcoid there is involvement of the uveal tract at some time. The disease often excites a minimal inflammatory reaction, and attention is not directed to the eyes. Anterior inflammation is associated with a granulomatous type of inflammation with numerous mutton-fat keratic precipitates and a few cells evident by means of microscopic examination of the anterior chamber. There is a tendency toward the formation of broad, flat posterior synechiae that cause distortion of the pupil. Involvement of the posterior ocular segment may simulate a variety of inflammations. Periphlebitis with neovascularization may occur. This may be difficult to distinguish from sickle cell abnormalities in Negroes, in whom both diseases are common. The choroidal lesion causes destruction of the overlying retina, and there may be a fairly severe inflammatory reaction with exudation of cells into the vitreous body and the formation of veils and membranes. The lesion shows little tendency to heal, and pigment proliferation is minimal.

Diagnosis of sarcoidosis is based upon evidence of its many clinical manifestations, an anergy to tuberculin, and histologic demonstration of the disease. The conjunctiva may be a source of a typical nodule, although it is so small that serial sections are required. Biopsy of involved skin is much more likely to indicate the disease than an enlarged lymph node.

Treatment is based mainly upon use of corticosteroids locally and systemically.

Arthritis. Patients with ankylosing spondylitis (Marie-Strümpell disease) develop an intermittent nongranulomatous anterior uveitis in 15% of the cases. The ocular disease is never particularly severe and responds readily to local medication. Ocular inflammation may precede joint disease. Young men are mainly affected; often there is a family history of ankylosing spondylitis or rheumatoid arthritis. The involvement of cervical vertebrae often makes it difficult for such a patient to place his head in position for biomicroscopy. However, the lumbosacral spine is initially involved and the disease may easily escape diagnosis.

Juvenile rheumatoid arthritis (Still's disease) may also be associated with uveitis, although band keratopathy is more common. The initial sign of the disease may, however, be uveitis with minimal inflammatory signs but leading to many complications.

Patients with uveitis as a group have a higher percentage of positive blood tests for various rheumatoid factors than the normal population. Many of these patients do not have signs or symptoms of arthritis. Because of such tests, the occasional instances of uveitis with rheumatoid arthritis (p. 451), and the beneficial effects of corticosteroids, attention has been directed to uveitis as a collagen disease. There seems to be no question that many patients with uveitis, particularly the nongranulomatous type, have an abnormality of their immune mechanisms. However, it has not been possible to learn its nature, and the positive tests are significant mainly in population studies and not in individual patients.

Genitourinary tract disease. In the period when focal infection was considered a source of many ocular infections, the genitourinary tract was second in importance to the nasal accessory sinuses and nasopharynx. An occasional patient is seen in whom a chronic prostatitis appears to play a role in uveitis, but such instances are so uncommon that a causal relationship is unlikely. Uveitis may complicate a metastatic gonorrhea (p. 363) in which there is an acute or chronic urethritis followed by arthralgia and ocular inflammation. Even prior to specific treatment for gonorrhea, such instances were uncommon.

Two uncommon syndromes are related to genitourinary tract disease: (1) Behçet's disease and (2) Reiter's syndrome.

Behçet's disease classically consists of aphthous mouth and genital lesions and hypopyon iritis. Numerous other signs are described: repeated sore throats followed by malaise and fever, migratory arthralgia and myalgia, inflammation of the choroid or retina, erythema nodosum and a hypersensitive reaction of the skin to a needle prick, and acute involvement of the brain stem with death.

The aphthous lesions consist of super-ficial discrete ulceration surrounded by a red areola and normal mucous membrane. They may involve the mouth or the pharynx. The genital lesions are usually confined to the labia or the scrotum. The iritis is acute with severe inflammatory signs but is usually self-limited.

Reiter's syndrome consists of a sterile urethritis, polyarthritis, and ocular involvement of conjunctivitis or iritis. Cutaneous lesions may occur in about 25% of the patients. The cause of the disease is not known. The iritis or iridocyclitis may not be diagnosed, and undoubtedly many instances of conjunctivitis reported are examples of ciliary injection secondary to iridocyclitis. The urethritis may be erroneously diagnosed as gonorrheal in origin. The arthritis varies in severity and is migratory. The uveitis is often not severe and cannot be diagnosed without biomicroscopic examination. The disease is characterized by remissions and recurrences and is refractory to therapy.

Hypersensitivity. The specific diagnosis of the cause of uveitis is complicated by the inability to fulfill Koch's postulates without destroying the eye. In many instances it seems likely that initial invasion of microorganisms into the uveal tract causes a sensitization of the tissues. Subsequent entry of the microorganisms into the eye causes a hypersensitivity reaction with the signs and symptoms of uveitis. In other instances the eye appears to demonstrate an autoimmune reaction. An ocular antigen-antibody reaction is easily produced in the laboratory and is described as immunogenic uveitis.

Immunogenic uveitis. Immunogenic uveitis may be produced by inducing either a systemic or ocular hypersensitivity to an antigen. The antigen selected is usually an animal serum albumin, whole blood, egg albumin, antitoxin, or a similarly well-defined protein. If the animal is sensitized by means of a systemically administered antigen, subsequent injection of the same antigen into the vitreous body causes a severe self-limited uveitis.

If the antigen is injected initially into the vitreous body, there is an immediate inflammatory response, presumably to the trauma of injection, which persists several days and then subsides. A uveitis of several days' duration occurs 7 to 14 days later. This delayed inflammation can be prevented by whole-body x-radiation, but it is not prevented by x-radiation of the eye only. The uveitis is likely due to the reaction of antibody to antigen that is still retained within the eye. If the animal is not treated with x-radiation, systemic administration of the antigen many months after initial sensitization will cause an immediate violent uveitis.

It is postulated that following injection of the antigen into the vitreous body, it slowly diffuses out and gives rise to immunologically competent cells elsewhere in the body. These cells in turn return to the uveal tract, enhance the migration of other immunologically competent cells, and imprint the response to the antigen upon them. The whole-body x-radiation prevents the development of immunologically competent cells. Inasmuch as these are initially produced outside the eye, radiation of the eye does not affect their production. It is suggested that any microorganism or antigen that enters the eye may sensitize the eye, and subsequent systemic exposure to the antigen may produce uveitis. Inasmuch as the ocular cells have had an abnormal response to the antigen impressed upon them, there is no necessity to postulate the continued presence of antigen within the eye.

Diagnostic measures

Until recently there was a tendency to apply an elaborate battery of diagnostic tests to each patient with uveitis not obviously of ocular origin or complicating a readily evident systemic disease. Many of these surveys were either negative or suggested so many possible causes for uveitis that the findings were not helpful. The topic is in a changing state currently, and only general principles can be presented.

Frequently the etiologic factor is not actively sought in acute inflammations in that they are often self-limited and respond readily to corticosteroids. When such inflammations are recurrent, as they often are, attention is usually directed to a possible anaphylactic type of hypersensitivity, mainly caused by streptococci, and to systemic diseases such as rheumatoid arthritis or infections of the genitourinary tract.

In chronic inflammations the etiologic diagnosis is based on the characteristics of the eye involvement in toxoplasmosis and histoplasmosis. Sarcoid is sought in Negro patients. If the inflammation is unusually severe and requires systemic corticosteroids for suppression, the drugs are not discontinued to determine bacterial hypersensitivity by means of skin testing.

In many patients the following diagnostic steps are carried out: (1) a serologic test for syphilis is made (a history of treated syphilis necessitates the serum fluorescent treponemal antibody absorption test even though routine serologic tests are negative); (2) chest x-rays are studied, with particular attention directed to healed primary tuberculosis, to sarcoid, and to histoplasmosis; (3) the white blood count and sedimentation rate are determined; (4) often tests for various immunologic abnormalities of connective tissue diseases are done; (5) skin testing with tuberculin and histoplasmin are frequently done routinely; (6) the methylene blue test for toxoplasmosis is not widely available but may be correlated with ocular changes suggestive of toxoplasmosis; and (7) the complement fixation test for histoplasmosis is usually not done unless the skin test is positive. In patients sensitive to histoplasmin, skin testing may markedly increase the complement fixation titer.

The history and systemic physical examination are often noncontributory. Exposure to puppies and kittens is important in *Toxocara* infections (p. 379), and there may be a marked eosinophilia. Recurrent infections associated with upper respiratory or renal infections may suggest a streptococcal sensitivity, but often the history is misleading. Physical examination should be directed particularly to evidence of infection in the teeth, pharynx, nasal accessory sinuses, and genitourinary tract. In patients with uveitis, elimination of any infection is desirable on a general hygienic basis. Cutaneous and mucous membrane lesions should be sought. Involvement of joints in arthritic lesions should be excluded.

Treatment

If possible, specific treatment is carried out. Local and not systemic treatment is indicated for inflammation of unknown etiology confined to the iris and the ciliary body. Cycloplegic drugs are used to dilate the pupil and paralyze accommodation. Maximal pupillary dilation is desired to prevent posterior synechiae, and atropine or scopolamine solution are customarily used. Corticosteroid preparations are instilled at frequent intervals. On occasion they are injected subconjunctivally. Care must be taken not to produce glaucoma in genetically sensitive persons (p. 306).

Posterior uveitis is treated mainly by the administration of systemic corticosteroids and rarely by the use of other anti-inflammatory agents such as chloroquine or compounds that interfere with the synthesis of immune globulins. Desensitization to specific microorganisms to which the patient is hypersensitive is now seldom recommended. The administration of "foreign proteins" containing pyrogens or endotoxin stimulates the corticotropin system and results in an increased endogenous secretion of corticosteroids. Possibly the stimulation of the reticuloendothelial system by pyro-

gens contained in these products also results in a desensitization to endotoxins. Pyrogens and similar products should not be injected in patients in whom adrenal cortical function has been suppressed by systemic administration of corticosteroids.

Specific therapy is usually not possible. Early syphilitic inflammations respond readily to penicillin. Toxoplasmosis responds to systemic administration of pyrimethamine (Daraprim) combined with a sulfonamide. However, systemic corticosteroids are preferred by many. Tuberculosis responds to isoniazid and similar agents, but there are few cases in which they are indicated. Antibiotics are never administered on an empiric basis.

Complications

The tendency for inflammation of the uveal tract to involve adjacent tissues leads to many complications. Often the complications dominate the disease picture and may lead to marked loss of vision.

Keratitis and keratopathy. Corneal involvement may occur in several ways. The cornea and anterior uvea may be nearly simultaneously inflamed in herpes zoster ophthalmicus and syphilitic interstitial keratitis. In severe herpes simplex keratitis, iridocyclitis, sometimes with hemorrhage, is a late complication.

Prolonged iridocyclitis causes damage to the corneal endothelium with folds, haziness, and edema in Descemet's membrane and subepithelial edema. Continued edema is followed by vascularization of the cornea.

Band keratopathy (p. 201), in which there is a progressive, superficial deposition of calcium in a horizontal band across the cornea, often complicates any uveitis in young persons. It has been described principally in juvenile rheumatoid arthritis (Still's disease, p. 236), but it also occurs in older individuals when the inflammation has caused severe ocular damage.

Intraocular pressure. Uveitis causes a

hyposecretion of aqueous humor, and the intraocular pressure is usually low. Glaucoma may occur by one or more mechanisms. The corticosteroids (p. 306) in genetically susceptible individuals may lead to a glaucoma with decreased outflow identical to that in the open-angle type except that it disappears when the drug is stopped. The trabecular meshwork may be occluded with inflammatory cells and exudate in acute, severe iridocyclitis or may partake of the inflammation itself. Repeated or prolonged inflammation may permanently damage the trabecular meshwork and lead to a permanent glaucoma not unlike open-angle glaucoma.

Occlusion of the pupil by posterior synechiae causes a glaucoma by preventing the aqueous humor from passing from the posterior to the anterior chamber (iris bombé). Peripheral anterior synechiae may form between the iris and the cornea because of a shallow anterior chamber, exudate between the two tissues, or intense edema of the root of the iris and cause a glaucoma due to an angle-closure mechanism (p. 309).

The treatment of glaucoma complicating uveitis necessitates a delicate balance between measures directed against the increased intraocular pressure and those used to treat the inflammation. The use of corticosteroids is minimized and the pupil is not constricted. Carbonic anhydrase inhibitors (p. 106) are used systemically and often combined with the local instillation of epinephrine salts. Removal of the anterior aqueous humor by means of paracentesis not only provides material for microscopy and microbial culture but temporarily reduces ocular pressure and sometimes is followed by decrease in inflammation. Iris bombé may necessitate a procedure in which the iris ballooning forward is opened with a knife passed from the corneoscleral limbus (iris transfixation). Surgical procedures necessitated because of peripheral anterior synechiae or damage to the trabecular meshwork should be postponed as long as possible after cessation of the inflammation.

Cataract. The systemic administration of steroids for a long period, particularly in patients with rheumatoid arthritis, may cause posterior subcapsular cataracts identical to those caused by uveitis. The typical cataract in uveitis occurs in long-standing cyclitis and involves the posterior subcapsular region in a lens opacity that has many colors (polychromatic). In particularly severe cyclitis the cataract may involve both the anterior and the posterior subcapsular regions. Cataract commonly develops when there is an inflammation with a depigmentation of the iris, leading many to believe that this constitutes a specific entity of cyclitis, heterochromia iridis, cataract, and glaucoma.

Edema of the macula and optic nerve. Swelling of the retina at the posterior pole may occur in severe inflammation involving either the anterior or posterior uvea. Often it is difficult to evaluate with the ophthalmoscope because of clouding of the vitreous, but it leads to a marked diminution in central visual acuity. The optic nerve may be similarly involved, with engorgement of its blood vessels, edema, and blurring of its margins. Edema of the macula commonly complicates uveitis occurring in the region of the ora serrata. The inflammation is so peripheral that it can be seen only by means of indirect ophthalmoscopy or biomicroscopy combined with a contact lens and prism; therefore it is not readily diagnosed, and attention is directed to the loss of vision arising from the macular edema. The combination is designated as peripheral uveitis, pars planitis, or cyclitis.

Severe choroiditis may cause a papillitis as a toxic phenomena. In Jensen's choroiditis juxtapapillaris (adjacent to the disk) the optic nerve involvement is so marked that the choroiditis may be unrecognized.

Retinal separation. Secondary retinal separation may involve one of several mechanisms. Severe exudative changes of the vitreous body may be followed by traction bands and a retinitis proliferans. Severe diffuse uveitis may cause an elevation of the retina that may simulate a tumor. Bilateral exudation with uveitis and retinal separation associated with vitiligo, alopecia, localized whiteness of hair (poliosis), and often deafness constitutes Vogt-Koyanagi disease. Retinal separation occurs similarly in Harada's disease, but anterior uveal involvement is rare and the visual prognosis is much better than in Vogt-Koyanagi disease. Additionally, skin, hair, and hearing signs are exceptional, but a sterile meningitis with increased intracranial pressure and pleocytosis of the cerebrospinal fluid occurs commonly.

Periphlebitis may occur following any retinal inflammation. It is considered particularly common in tuberculous uveitis but may complicate a variety of diseases, notably sickle cell trait.

Injuries
Contusions

Blunt trauma to the eye is best tolerated by individuals younger than 30 years of age. In persons older than this, blunt trauma is often followed by a severe intraocular hemorrhage that does not absorb.

Contusion to the eye may cause a number of changes in the iris: (1) rupture of the sphincter pupillae muscle with a dilated, unresponsive pupil; (2) iridodialysis, in which the root of the iris is torn from its insertion, causing an extra pupil at the periphery and the pupil in the sector of the defect to become a chord rather than an arc (Fig. 341); and (3) hemorrhage into the anterior chamber (hyphema, p. 342).

The ciliary body is seldom grossly involved. Many hyphemas probably originate from a separation of the ciliary body from the scleral spur, but this is not diagnosed. Ciliary body injury may well be the chief cause of a unilateral glaucoma,

similar to open-angle glaucoma, which occurs many years after injury. The possibility of a unilateral glaucoma being traumatic in origin must always be considered.

The choroid is bound tightly to the sclera at the posterior pole because of the entrance of the short posterior ciliary arteries. Thus the choroid cannot "slip" easily, and when the eye is contused, the posterior pole is often involved.

Hemorrhage into the choroid may vary from a small intrachoroidal hemorrhage to a massive expulsive hemorrhage of the type that may occur with intraocular surgery. Bleeding occurring secondary to trauma gives rise to no particular problems of differential diagnosis. When located in the choroid, the hemorrhagic area is dark brown with pinkish to red edges evident in retroillumination. Hemorrhagic areas frequently absorb very slowly over a long period of time and disappear, leaving a residue of marked pigment disturbance.

Choroidal tears (Fig. 14-5) are a common result of severe contusions to the anterior segment of the eyeball. They occur most frequently on the temporal side of

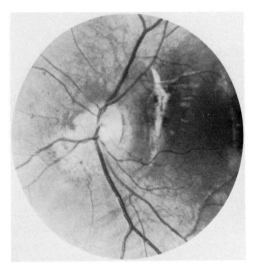

Fig. 14-5. Choroidal tears following blunt trauma to the anterior portion of the eye.

the eye and are concentric with the disk, usually located between the disk and the macula or temporal to the macula. They may be single or multiple. They probably result from stretching of the posterior choroid as a result of compression of the eye, the temporal side being more vulnerable because of its greater extent and the blow being more commonly directed from the less-protected temporal side.

The tears are crescentic, vertical, and of variable length. Hemorrhage into the choroid, the subretinal area, or into the retina frequently accompanies a disruption of the tissue. As hemorrhage and edema absorb, the yellowish gray lesions become well defined. When the tear is between the disk and the macula, vision is usually reduced, but it may be little affected if the tear affects the area temporal to the macula. Disruption of the overlying retina may give rise to a typical nerve fiber type of defect in the visual field.

Treatment is complete bed rest, instillation of a cycloplegic, and binocular patching of the eyes for 1 to 2 weeks.

Serous choroidal detachment

Serous choroidal detachment occurs frequently as a complication of intraocular surgery. Clinically the disease is usually found after an uncomplicated cataract extraction in which there has been prompt re-formation of the anterior chamber and apparent uncomplicated convalescence. In 5 to 10 or 15 days after the procedure the anterior chamber is observed to be extremely shallow or flat. There are many folds in Descemet's membrane. The tension is low, and occasionally there is demonstrable leakage of aqueous humor in the corneoscleral wound. Through a widely dilated pupil, the detachment of the choroid may be visible by oblique illumination and appears as a dark gray-brown mass. On ophthalmoscopy the detachment is seen to be a smooth, rounded swelling, extending hemispherically into the vitreous

humor. The lesion may be single or multiple and usually rises anterior to the equator on either side of the midline. The borders are dark and well defined. The retinal vessels appear normal as they course over the elevated lesion.

Trauma combined with decreased intraocular pressure (hypotony) is required to produce choroidal detachment. There is a disturbance of the normal pressure relationships within the choroid, producing a transudation of fluid in the suprachoroidal space and resulting in choroidal detachment. The serous choroidal detachment recedes once the wound heals, and the injury from the surgical manipulation subsides. This may occur within several days or, occasionally, weeks. One of the most common reasons for a serous choroidal detachment not receding rapidly is persistence of a small fistula permitting loss of aqueous humor. If this cause can be excluded, it is possible that the persistence may be due to hemorrhage. The latter complication may take months to resorb or may persist, owing to organization of blood in the suprachoroidal space.

Lacerations

A laceration of the cornea is followed immediately by prolapse of the iris into the wound. If the wound is small, the pupil is distorted and has a teardrop shape. If extensive, the entire iris may be prolapsed (p. 339).

Prolapse of the ciliary body through a scleral or corneal laceration is particularly serious inasmuch as vitreous humor is lost, and the zonule is additionally involved. Neglected prolapse of the ciliary body is considered much more likely to cause a sympathetic ophthalmia (p. 341) than prolapse of other portions of the uveal tract.

Tumors of the choroid
Malignant melanoma

Malignant melanomas of the choroid (Fig. 14-6) are the most common intra-

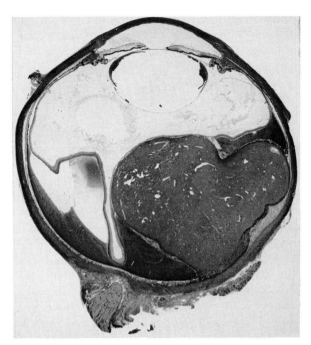

Fig. 14-6. Malignant melanoma of the choroid that has ruptured through Bruch's membrane into the eye. (Hematoxylin and eosin stain; ×5.)

ocular tumors. They occur after puberty and show an increase in incidence with advancing age. They are rare in Negroes and are slightly more common in men than in women. They arise from the Schwann cell, a cell originating from the neural crest and having the potentiality of forming a variety of neuroectodermal and peripheral end organs. They are found in approximately 10% of eyes blind from injury or inflammation, a finding suggesting that irritation may play a role in their formation.

Malignant melanomas originate most frequently in the outer layers of the choroid and may spread carpetlike between the sclera and the lamina vitrea. Tumors may remain quiescent for long periods and then apparently without reason suddenly begin rapid growth. With increase in size, there may be globular growth inward. Eventually the lamina vitrea is perforated, and there is sudden growth of a mushroom or collar button shape.

Symptoms and signs

The chief symptoms of malignant melanomas arise from the retinal detachment caused by the increase in volume of the choroid. Early there may be metamorphopsia associated with macropsia or micropsia. This is followed eventually by a loss of visual field in the sector corresponding to the tumor. The visual field loss is larger than anticipated from the size of the tumor. Glaucoma occurs late in the course of the disease and in the early stages a decreased tension may occur. Intraocular inflammation occurs frequently, and a malignant melanoma must be considered in the diagnosis of the cause of any obscure intraocular inflammation, particularly when opaque media make it impossible to inspect the fundus.

Sudden loss of vision suggests that a lesion is not a malignant melanoma, as does a sudden increase in the size of a mass over several days' time. A drawing of the tumor, with emphasis upon the blood vessel distribution, and photography of the lesion may be helpful in making an exact diagnosis and in observing slight increases in size of the tumor. Physical examination should be done to exclude metastatic disease, although the presence of a malignancy elsewhere does not exclude malignant melanoma as the ocular tumor. Neovascularization or vasodilation of episcleral vessels in the quadrant of involvement suggests a neoplasm, as does melanosis oculi. A vascularized mass on the sclera suggests an extraocular extension. Anesthesia of the cornea, partial paralysis of the iris, or dilated iris vessels occurring in the sector of tumor involvement have been noted uncommonly.

Ophthalmoscopy indicates a retinal detachment of grayish brown color. The pigmentation is distinctly lighter than the jet black color seen in inflammatory retinal pigment proliferation. Discrete areas of light-colored pigmentation may occur some distance from the detachment. The retina is smoothly elevated, with little tendency to form traction folds, and is usually without a break. There may be two areas of detachment, seemingly not connected. With increase in size, a malignant melanoma becomes more distinct, whereas with other diseases the lesion becomes less distinct with increase in size. Rest in bed with binocular patches fails to reduce the extent of a detachment in malignant melanoma.

Vessels on the retinal surface not associated with the retinal vasculature are suggestive of tumor. Hemorrhage is uncommon in malignant melanoma. The only exception is in large necrotic tumors that have burst through the lamina vitrea.

Slit lamp examination of the fundus should be carried out with a Goldmann or Hruby lens with the pupil well dilated. An increase in thickness of the retina suggests a hemangioma. Cystoid degeneration of the overlying retina suggests a malignant melanoma. Conversely, a fine sprinkling of lipoid deposits in the retina (edema residues) is never present immediately overlying the melanoma. Cells in the vitreous body with the retina indistinctly seen suggest an inflammatory lesion, unless a tumor has broken through the lamina vitrea and necrotized. Study of the border of the elevated lesion may indicate a reddish or pink halo, suggesting a hemorrhage rather than a tumor.

Transillumination is of questionable diagnostic value. The transscleral method is employed as follows: A point source of light is placed on the scleral surface behind the lesion, and the general illumination of the widely dilated pupil is observed. Alternatively, the fundus may be observed with the unilluminated ophthalmoscope. If the lesion is far posterior, it is necessary to incise the conjunctiva in order to place the light source behind the lesion. Patients may be able to note an inability to observe the light when it is at the site of a malignant melanoma due to failure of the rods and cones in the area. Marked pigmentation of a normal eye, hemorrhage, and dense inflammatory areas may give rise to faulty interpretation of decreased transillumination. Similarly, small tumors and lightly pigmented neoplasms will not interfere with light transmission.

Visual field studies are chiefly of value in differentiating a benign nevus and a malignant melanoma. Usually the choriocapillaris is intact when a nevus is present; there is no field defect, or the defect is proportionately smaller than the lesion. In a malignant melanoma the field defect is proportionately larger and is progressive. A hemangioma causes a sector-shaped field defect associated with thickening of the retina.

Biopsy of an intraocular tumor is never indicated and may cause seeding of tumor cells along the needle tract.

There is considerable evidence to indicate that malignant melanomas smaller than 5 disk diameters in size have a significantly better prognosis than larger tumors. Thus in the event of difficulty in exact diagnosis it is permissible to procrastinate and observe until the clinical course of the disease makes the diagnosis evident.

Treatment

The treatment of malignant melanoma is enucleation once the clinical diagnosis has been clearly established. If the eye is blind and painful, particularly if the media are opaque, early enucleation is indicated. In eyes with good vision and small tumors, enucleation is not an emergency procedure.

The treatment of a malignant melanoma in the only useful eye is a particular problem. There is obviously no effective therapy for a large, rapidly growing tumor except enucleation. In the case of small, flat, slowly progressive growths, however, focal irradiation by means of a radiation source sutured to the sclera, diathermy, or light coagulation have all been reported to arrest the growth effectively. It is evident that for successful results the tumor must be small, and inasmuch as histologic diagnosis is impossible there is no certainty about the nature of the tumor. Additionally, like malignant melanomas elsewhere in the body, the tumor cells may remain quiescent for long periods and then show renewed activity without known cause.

Benign melanoma

Benign melanomas of the choroid (Fig. 14-7) occur most commonly in the posterior half of the fundus, are oval or circular in outline, and vary from 0.5 to 4 disk diameters in size. The lesion is sharply demarcated from the surrounding fundus, but the contrast between the melanoma and the adjacent choroid may be so slight that detection requires careful ophthalmoscopic examination. The lesion usually becomes pigmented between the sixth and the tenth years of life.

The tumor varies in color from "slate gray" to "blue ointment." There is no overlying retinal abnormality, and the choroidal pattern can easily be seen surrounding,

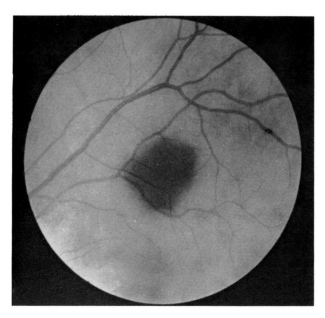

Fig. 14-7. Benign melanoma of the choroid.

but not over, the tumor. There may be single or multiple lesions. Since a benign melanoma does not involve the choriocapillaris layer, there is usually no field defect, which is an important distinction from malignant melanoma.

Benign melanomas may become malignant, a change that may be recognized by stippling or irregular pigmentation over the tumor. This stippling should be distinguished from drusen, which occur with great frequency (p. 269). Increase in size, of course, is an ominous sign, and for this reason the lesion should be followed by means of serial photographs.

Hemangiomas

Hemangiomas (angiomas) of the choroid are a rare condition associated in about one half of the cases with skin nevi elsewhere in the body, frequently in the area innervated by the first or second branch of the trigeminal nerve. Secondary glaucoma is often associated with them. A monocular buphthalmos is commonly associated with either choroidal or retinal hemangiomas, or with von Recklinghausen's neurofibromatosis. Neurologic signs may occur occasionally, with the hemangiomas then being a manifestation of the Sturge-Weber syndrome.

Choroidal hemangiomas may vary in size from 2 to 17 mm. in diameter and from 1 to 9 mm. in thickness. They may increase slowly in thickness, giving rise to a progressive hyperopia when the hemangioma involves the posterior pole. Rarely, both eyes may be involved in a similar process.

Metastatic carcinoma

The breast is the most common primary site of malignant disease that metastasizes to the choroid. Other structures that may be involved include the lung, kidney, and stomach, and there are reports citing nearly every area and type of malignancy. The complication is fairly common in the terminal stages of a malignant disease; frequently, however, patients are so ill at this period that the diagnosis is not made. The left eye is affected more frequently than the right eye, probably because the left carotid artery is a direct branch of the aorta, whereas the right carotid artery is a branch of the innominate artery. In a large proportion of cases the disease is bilateral, although further advanced in one eye. Involvement of the choroid in preference to the retina probably reflects the greater number of blood vessels going to the choroid from the ophthalmic artery.

Metastasis to the choroid leads to retinal detachment with loss of vision in the area of involvement. Probably because of the large number of blood vessels to the area, the posterior segment is involved preferentially, and early loss of central vision occurs. The ophthalmoscopic appearance is characteristic. There is a sharply circumscribed detachment with abrupt delineation and no retinal breaks. There may be rapid growth of the tumor anteriorly, but usually there is a rim of undetached retina between the tumor and the periphery. The color of the detachment is much lighter than that seen in malignant melanoma.

The diagnosis depends to a large extent upon accurate history and physical examination. The primary malignancy may have been removed from 1 or 2 months previously to many years prior to the onset of symptoms. There may be no evidence of metastasis elsewhere in the body, but commonly osteolytic or pulmonary lesions can be demonstrated.

Treatment of a metastatic malignancy to the choroid must be directed to the primary disease. Certain tumors arising from the male and female breast and the prostate are functionally dependent upon the same hormones as their parent cells, and their growth may be inhibited or accelerated by withdrawal or administration of these hormonal substances. At present the treatment of choice for metastatic car-

cinomas of the prostate is orchiectomy
and the administration of estrogens. Some
metastatic carcinomas of the breast are
benefited by surgical oophorectomy, adrenalectomy, or hypophysectomy.

In patients with metastatic disease of the
eye, which is responsive to these procedures, there may be dramatic remission of
the secondary retinal detachment. The central vision improves, and there is no ophthalmoscopic evidence of the disease. The
remission may be incomplete, however, so
that the detachment does not progress but
does not disappear entirely.

In tumors that are not hormonal dependent, the ocular treatment is related to the
life expectancy and whether or not both
eyes are involved. Enucleation is generally
not indicated. Radiotherapy with a tumor
dose of 2,500 to 3,500 r may be used, with
appropriate precautions to protect the lens.
However, the adult lens is resistant enough
to radiation that cataract formation will
probably not be a problem in view of the
limited life expectancy of the patient. If
the metastasis is binocular and the patient
is not within the final weeks of life, radiotherapy may be carried out on both eyes.

Ciliary body tumors
Malignant melanoma

These tumors occur less frequently in
the ciliary body than in the choroid. They
tend to extend to involve either the choroid, the iris, or both. They may spread
ringlike around the ciliary body, following
the course of the major arterial circle of
the iris. Because of their location, symptoms are minimal, and diagnosis may be
delayed until the tumor has caused a retinal detachment or has become visible in
the anterior chamber, especially by gonioscopy (Fig. 14-8). The mass may be demonstrated by transillumination, and with
maximal pupillary dilation, it may be observed directly. The treatment is enucleation. Inasmuch as benign melanomas of the
ciliary body are more common than benign

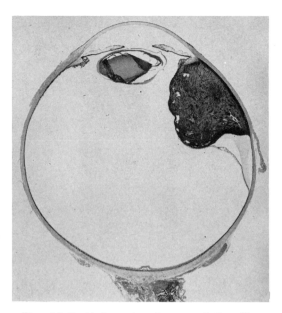

Fig. 14-8. Malignant melanoma of the ciliary
body that has detached the peripheral retina.
(Hematoxylin and eosin stain; ×4.)

tumors of the choroid, and because the
tumor is often relatively small, there have
been renewed attempts to resect the tumor
rather than to remove the eye. The initial
reports indicate this to be a promising
method of treatment.

Medulloepitheliomas

Inasmuch as pigmented and nonpigmented epithelium of the ciliary processes
is derived from the primitive optic vesicle, tumors arise in the pars ciliaris retina
that are comparable to retinoblastomas.
The neoplasm corresponds to the primitive
embryonic retina. It does not metastasize.
It may cause uveitis because of necrosis,
secondary glaucoma, and staphyloma.
Symptoms usually occur between the third
and the sixth years. Enucleation is required.

Tumors of the iris

There is considerable variation in the
amount of pigment in the anterior stroma

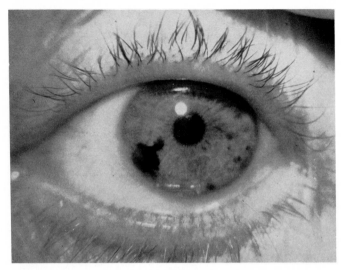

Fig. 14-9. Benign melanoma of the iris. There are freckles in the temporal portion of the iris. Gonioscopy indicates that the benign melanoma does not extend to the insertion of the iris.

of the iris. About one half of all Caucasians have pigment flecks on the surface of the iris that are of no pathologic significance. Histologically they belong to the group of benign melanomas. The term "benign melanoma" is preferably not applied to these freckles of the iris, but it is limited to slightly elevated, localized pigmented areas extending deep into the stroma. These benign melanomas are not progressive and do not cause pupillary distortion (Fig. 14-9).

Malignant melanoma of the iris often originates from benign melanoma. There are usually no symptoms, and the tumor is diagnosed by the patient or a friend who notices the brownish mass on the iris sur-

face. A malignant melanoma is progressive and extends into the filtration angle. It has blood vessels growing in it, and there may be associated seeding of the remaining iris. The pupil is distorted, and this defect is accentuated when the pupil is dilated. In some patients the malignant melanoma is diffuse and causes an increasing pigmentation of the iris with an associated glaucoma. If the tumor is localized and confined to the iris, it may be treated by iridectomy. Diffuse tumors require enucleation. The tumors are but minimally malignant, and with careful observation, enucleation may be deferred until there is obvious progression.

Chapter 15

The retina

The eye is so arranged that light falling upon the retina induces a chemical reaction that initiates a nervous impulse that is transmitted to the brain, where it is perceived (p. 85). Embryologically the invagination of the optic cup gives rise to the two main layers of the retina: the outer pigment epithelium and the inner nervous layer. The two layers must be in apposition for normal retinal function. The lamina vitrea (Bruch's membrane, p. 11), which is derived from both the retina and the choroid, separates the retinal pigment epithelium from the choriocapillaris.

The innermost nervous layers of the retina are transparent, and light passes through to cause a photochemical reaction in the outer segments of the rods and cones. This reaction causes a nervous reaction that is amplified within the retina. The photoreceptors synapse with bipolar cells, which in turn synapse with the ganglion cells, whose axons pass to the optic nerve and synapse in the lateral geniculate body (vision) or pass to the pretectal region (pupil).

Only cones are present in the foveal region. The innermost layers of the retina in this region are displaced temporally; therefore light falls directly upon the cones without transversing the full thickness of the retina. This region functions in bright illumination (photopic vision), central visual acuity, and color vision; the number of cones decreases rapidly away from the fovea. The rods are most numerous in the peripheral retina and are functional in dim illumination (scotopic vision).

The blood supply to the retina (p. 26) in man is derived primarily from the ophthalmic artery from two sources: (1) the choriocapillaris, which nurtures the retinal pigment epithelium and the outer half of the neural retina adjacent to the choroid, and (2) the branches of the central retinal artery, which supply the innermost half of the retina. Both systems are necessary for retinal function.

The central retinal artery is a medium-sized artery that branches from the ophthalmic artery immediately after its entry into the orbit; consequently, its intravascular pressure is high. The central retinal artery has the usual three layers of intima, media, and adventitia, with well-developed elastic and muscular components. As the artery passes through the lamina cribrosa the internal elastic lamina is reduced to a single layer and is entirely lost after the first or second bifurcation. Within the eye the smooth muscle of the medial coat is markedly decreased, although contractile elements persist to the precapillary arterioles. The diameter of the retinal arteries beyond the optic disk is 65 to 135μ. Thus, both in diameter and in structure, these retinal vessels may be classified as arterioles.

The retinal arteriovenous crossings share a common adventitial sheath. A similar anatomic arrangement is seen elsewhere only in the afferent and efferent arteries of the glomerulus. The common adventitial sheath is the anatomic basis for some retinal vein occlusions and the signs of arteriolar sclerosis at arteriovenous crossings.

Symptoms of retinal abnormalities

The symptoms of retinal abnormalities involve mainly disturbances in vision. Interference with cone function causes diminished central visual acuity and decreased color vision. Similar symptoms may arise from optic nerve disease, particularly that which involves the papillomacular nerve fiber bundle. Opacities of the ocular media that interfere with image formation at the fovea cause a generalized depression of vision. Localized disturbance in the fovea centralis area such as hemorrhage, edema, deposits, or tumors may cause micropsia (small images) or macropsia (large images). Interference with rod function causes defective dark adaptation. Retinal disease is characterized by a defect in the visual field that corresponds to the affected area.

Traction upon the retina gives rise to photopsia, sparks, rings, lightning flashes, or luminous bodies observed when the eyes are closed. Their occurrence in one eye only serves to distinguish them from visual hallucinations arising from lesions in the temporal or the occipital lobes. Frequently the patient is unaware of retinal disease, and the abnormality is detected by means of functional testing or ophthalmoscopic examination.

The function of the retina is determined by measurement of (1) form sense (central visual acuity), (2) light sense (dark adaptation), (3) color vision, (4) central and peripheral visual fields, (5) electroretinography, and (6) electro-oculography. The measurement of central visual acuity is meaningful only when determined with the patient wearing the best

possible corrective lenses to exclude refractive errors as a cause of decreased vision. The light sense is seldom tested clinically (p. 77). Color vision, when abnormal due to retinal disease, usually parallels the decrease in visual acuity and involves all colors. Hereditary color blindness, as a rule, is associated with good central visual acuity, and there is specific involvement of the perception of certain colors, particularly red and green (p. 83). Measurement of the central visual field tests the integrity of the retina within an area of 30° from the fixation point. Measurement of the peripheral visual field is usually a more gross test than that of the central area and determines the function of the entire retina. Inasmuch as the optic nerve consists of axons of ganglion cells that form the nerve fiber layer of the retina, optic nerve abnormalities may give rise to many of the same symptoms as retinal disease.

Electroretinography (p. 81) is the measurement of an action potential evoked by the stimulation of the retina with light. It is a mass response and not diagnostic in small retinal lesions. It may be subnormal or completely absent when the entire retina is disturbed. In disturbances of the retinal pigment epithelium it is often extinguished even though some vision remains.

Electro-oculography in the measurement of a standing potential present between the cornea and the retina which varies as the patient moves his eyes. It is measured by means of electrodes placed on the eyelids, and it reflects most accurately abnormalities in the retinal pigment epithelium. For the most part, these tests are used in research studies.

Ophthalmoscopic findings

The retina may be examined with a direct or an indirect ophthalmoscope, or with the slit lamp combined with a –40 diopter contact lens placed on the patient's eye to neutralize the refractive power of the cornea. The technique of ophthalmoscopy and the features of the normal fundus are described on p. 142. The main ophthalmoscopic abnormalities of the retina include the following: (1) disturbances of blood vessels, (2) opacities of the neural retina, (3) disturbances in the position of the neural retina, (4) derangements of the retinal pigment epithelium, and (5) abnormalities of the lamina vitrea (Bruch's membrane).

Disturbances of blood vessels

The ocular fundus is the sole place in the body that small arteries, arterioles, and their accompanying veins may be directly observed. They are subject to the same diseases as elsewhere in the body but constitute a highly specialized vascular bed that has no other counterpart. Thus changes observed ophthalmoscopically must be extrapolated to similar changes in blood vessels of comparable size elsewhere in the vascular tree only with considerable caution.

The main changes observed in the retinal blood vessels include arteriolar constriction, variations in caliber, tortuosity, abnormal arteriovenous crossings, vascular pulsation, venous dilation, neovascularization, hemorrhage, microaneurysms, perivasculitis, and retinal artery (p. 258) or vein (p. 260) occlusion.

Arteriolar constriction. A marked increase in the systolic blood pressure causes a generalized constriction of the retinal arterioles. When the blood pressure returns to normal, the constriction disappears. Focal constriction is not caused by experimental elevation of the blood pressure, and in hypertensive cardiovascular disease, localized constrictions persist clinically after the blood pressure is normal. Extreme arteriolar constriction is seen in tapetoretinal degenerations and following occlusion of the central retinal artery. In these conditions it indicates retinal atrophy.

Variations in caliber. Variations in arterial caliber are essentially a sign of arteriosclerosis and arise because of irregular thickening of the medial wall of the arteriole. Inasmuch as arteriosclerosis is not distributed uniformly throughout the body, one cannot draw parallels concerning the state of other vascular beds.

Tortuosity. Tortuosity of arterioles may be caused by both arteriosclerosis and arteriolar sclerosis. There are so many normal variations in the course of blood vessels that it is often difficult to recognize tortuosity. Congenital heart disease causes a cyanosis retinae in which there is marked tortuosity of blood vessels that persists after correction of the cardiac defect.

Abnormal arteriovenous crossing. Abnormal arteriovenous crossings arise because the retinal arterioles and venules have a common sheath at points where they cross. They are discussed on p. 404.

Vascular pulsation. Vascular pulsation occurs when the intraocular pressure equals the pressure within the vessel. There is normally a pulsation of the central retinal vein synchronous with the heart. It arises from pulsation in the central retinal artery that is transmitted to the vein. If the pulsation cannot be detected, gentle pressure upon the globe will elicit venous pulsation. Venous pulsation cannot be elicited in impending central vein closure, and it usually cannot be elicited in papilledema.

Arterial pulsation is always pathologic. It occurs when the intraocular pressure is equal to the diastolic blood pressure and in an aortic regurgitation in which there is a high pulse pressure.

Venous dilation. The veins may become dilated in any condition in which there is increased venous pressure (Fig. 15-1). Thus dilated veins are a constant feature of papilledema. Dilated veins are also seen

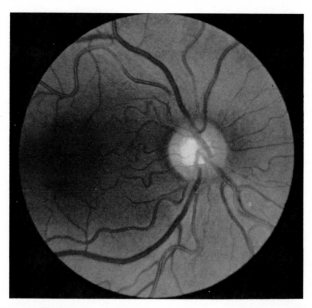

Fig. 15-1. Venous dilation due to superior vena cava syndrome, which causes increased venous pressure in the head.

in diabetes, impending obstruction of the central retinal vein, angiomatous tumors of the retina, and polycythemic states.

Neovascularization. The growth of blood vessels into the vitreous body, over the surface of the optic disk, or into the retina reflects a change in the nutrition of these tissues in which the direct blood supply has been restricted (Fig. 15-4). Blood vessels may grow into the vitreous body, with accompanying glial tissue (proliferative retinopathy), or as delicate, web-like, naked vessels (rete).

Neovascularization occurs in a variety of diseases: in retinal vein occlusion, in diabetes mellitus, in sickle cell trait, in Eales' disease, following vitreous hemorrhage, in the aortic arch syndrome, in retrolental fibroplasia, and in Coats' disease.

Hemorrhage. Hemorrhages within the retina assume different shapes, depending upon the layer in which they occur. Preretinal hemorrhages (Fig. 15-2) occur between the retina and the vitreous body. They are characteristically large with a tendency to meniscus formation inasmuch

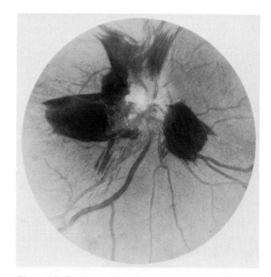

Fig. 15-2. Preretinal hemorrhage in diabetes mellitus. Venous dilation is also present.

as the blood is not clotted and is only loosely restricted. Flame-shaped hemorrhages occur at the level of the nerve fiber layer and tend to parallel the course of the nerve fibers in the region of the retina where they occur. Round hemor-

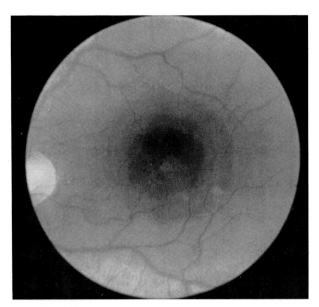

Fig. 15-3. Retinal hemorrhage in the macular area.

rhages originate from the deep capillaries of the retina, and they are confined by Müller's cells and the axons of the inner and outer plexiform layers. Hemorrhages in the neural layer of the retina have a bright red color and tend to absorb slowly without glial tissue formation. Hemorrhage between the pigment epithelium and Bruch's membrane is dark colored, well circumscribed, elevated, and may simulate a neoplasm.

A retinal hemorrhage (Fig. 15-3) is a signal to learn if the cause is within the eye itself or reflects systemic disease. Numerous hemorrhages occur in retinal vein closure, and there may be a few evident in macular degeneration. Systemic causes of hemorrhage include diabetes, blood dyscrasias, atherosclerosis, and hypertension. A preretinal hemorrhage adjacent to the disk may be a sign of subarachnoid hemorrhage.

Microaneurysms. Microaneurysms constitute one of the most common retinal abnormalities. Large numbers form in diabetes mellitus, and these are characteristically on the venous side of the capillary network. Microaneurysms may be seen in most of the conditions associated with retinal venous stasis—central or branch vein closure, Coats' disease, periphlebitis, and hyperviscosity of the blood. Microaneurysms can be identified with certainty by fluorescein angiography and histologic examination. Ophthalmoscopically they appear as minute red dots of unchanging appearance, which are unrelated to visible blood vessels. They appear to remain for months but are eventually converted to minute, white dots. Small, deep, round hemorrhages with similar appearance absorb more rapidly and disappear without leaving a residue. Although microaneurysms occur in a large variety of conditions, it is only in diabetes mellitus that large numbers occur predominantly at the posterior pole.

The resolving power of the direct ophthalmoscope is about 75μ. The majority of microaneurysms that occur in the retina are smaller than this and are invisible ophthalmoscopically. They may be demonstrated in large numbers in histologic flat preparations of the retina.

Perivasculitis. Inflammation of the retinal vessels leads to localized thrombus formation followed by neovascularization, often with a tendency for hemorrhage into the vitreous. The affected vessels appear initially to be sheathed with a white band and eventually are converted to fibrotic cords. The most frequent cause is posterior uveitis, usually by direct involvement in the inflammation, but sometimes there is apparently a toxic reaction to the uveitis. Other causes include giant cell arteritis (p. 454), nonspecific retinal periphlebitis (Eales' disease, p. 273), sarcoidosis (p. 383), and carotid artery insufficiency.

Opacities of the neural retina

The neural retina is normally transparent ophthalmoscopically, and the sheet of blood in the choriocapillaris is viewed through the retinal pigment epithelium. Inflammation, anoxia, or metabolic products in the retina cause a loss of transparency, the normal reddish appearance of the retina being replaced by a whitish or yellowish opacity.

The term "deposit" is usually applied to the condition arising from localized patches of retinal anoxia occurring mainly in retinal vascular disease (Fig. 15-5). If the anoxia is chronic, the deposits are sharply defined, whereas acute anoxia is characterized by localized retinal edema with ill-defined margins. Persistent anoxia is followed by replacement of ischemic retinal cells by lipid-laden macrophages that give a bright and refractile ophthalmoscopic appearance.

The term "exudate" is usually applied to the retinal response to acute inflammation. The involved area is frequently obscured by inflammatory cells in the vitreous body. It is usually a dirty white color, has ill-defined margins, and is often associated with destruction of the underlying choroid.

In some abnormalities characterized by the accumulation of abnormal metabolic products in nervous tissue, for example, Tay-Sachs disease (p. 441), the cell bodies in the retina, often ganglion cells, become filled with opaque material. Inasmuch as this layer is pushed aside in the foveal

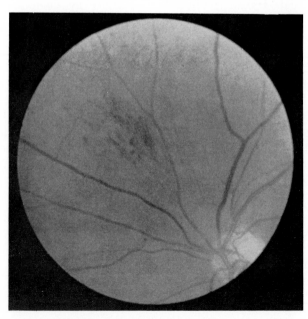

Fig. 15-4. Rete neovascularization in diabetes mellitus.

area the choroidal circulation can be seen here, causing a cherry red spot.

Cotton-wool patches (cytoid bodies). Cotton-wool patches ophthalmoscopically appear as indistinct, white retinal opacities with a hazy, irregular outline (Fig. 15-6).

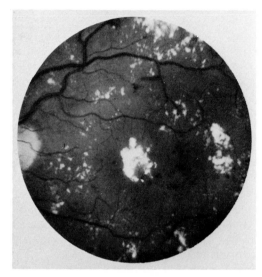

Fig. 15-5. Deposits and hemorrhages of the retina in diabetes mellitus.

They vary in size and shape, are usually ovoid, rarely exceed the diameter of the optic disk, and generally are limited to the posterior segment. Their main component is commonly referred to in ophthalmic pathology as a cytoid body.

Cotton-wool patches occur in the retina during the course of severe arterial hypertension and bacterial endocarditis (Roth's spots), following retinal trauma, and in severe anemia, papilledema, diabetic retinopathy, generalized carcinomatosis, acute systemic lupus erythematosus, and dermatomyositis.

Microscopically, cotton-wool patches are limited to the nerve fiber layer. They are most likely an infarct followed by nonspecific deposit of acellular origin and probably follow damage to the terminal arterioles in the nerve fiber layer.

Generalized edema. Retinal edema mainly affects the inner retinal layers closest to the ophthalmoscope. The deeper, outer layers are too compactly arranged to respond with edema. The most common cause of generalized edema is arterial occlusion, in which the retina

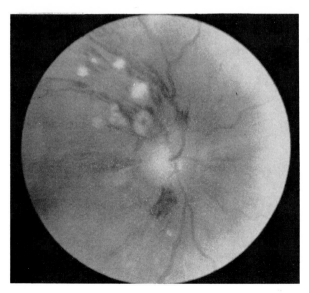

Fig. 15-6. Cotton-wool deposits at the posterior pole in hypertensive retinopathy. There are flame-shaped hemorrhages in the nerve fiber layer. The arterioles are attenuated.

appears pale white and watery, with retinal blood vessels barely visible. The foveal region, which lacks the inner retinal layers, is never involved in retinal edema and may appear normal; the pallor of the surrounding retina makes the normal fovea appear as a cherry red spot.

Gliosis. Retinal scarring results from the the proliferation of glial cells, especially astrocytes, and retinal pigment epithelium. Glial proliferation causes a diffuse, white, usually well-defined retinal opacity. It may accompany new blood vessels into the vitreous body.

Disturbances in the position of the neural retina

The normal neural retina lines the globe smoothly without elevation or distortion. In a variety of serious abnormalities the neural retina is separated from the retinal pigment epithelium by a serous fluid or blood, and inasmuch as the outer layers no longer derive adequate nutrition, vision is lost in the region of the abnormality. The entire neural retina or a localized portion may be involved. The major ophthalmoscopic alterations are a diminished red reflex and inability of the observer to focus upon adjacent portions of the retina simultaneously. The major causes of abnormal position are proliferative retinopathy (p. 391), retinal separation (p. 262), retinoschisis (p. 265), retrolental fibroplasia (p. 258), retinal dysplasia (p. 257), persistent primary vitreous (p. 257), and tumors (p. 274).

Derangements of the retinal pigment epithelium and abnormalities of the lamina vitrea

The retinal pigment epithelium obscures the view of the choriocapillaris, and the amount of melanin in its cells largely determines the degree of redness of the normal ocular fundus (p. 142). A decrease in pigmentation occurs in sclerosis of the choriocapillaris (p. 225), albinism

(p. 430), and progressive myopia. In destructive inflammatory lesions involving both the choroid and the retina, all retinal and choroidal layers may be destroyed so that the dead-white sclera is visible. Proliferation of the retinal pigment epithelium is stimulated in inflammatory processes, with resultant deep black pigmentation that commonly surrounds an area of chorioretinitis. In tapetoretinal degenerations the pigment often has a central nucleus with dendrites and is most marked at the equator. Degenerative disease at the fovea may also be associated with pigment proliferation.

The cuticular layer of Bruch's membrane may form hyaline masses or excrescences (drusen, p. 269) that appear as small, bright dots deep in the retina. The elastic layer may degenerate, causing radial streaks that form bizarre patterns (angioid streaks, p. 272).

Congenital and developmental abnormalities

Myelinated nerve fibers. Myelination of of the optic nerve proceeds from the optic chiasm to the lamina cribrosa. Normally myelination is not complete until 2 or 3 months after birth. Sometimes it continues to the retinal surface (Fig. 15-7). Ophthalmoscopy indicates an area of white, opaque, glistening appearance and feathered edges continuous with the optic disk.

Usually the area of myelination involves only a small sector of the retina and does not extend beyond the second arteriolar bifurcation. The absence of pigment proliferation and the normal visual field differentiate myelinated nerve fibers from a chorioretinitis. There are no symptoms or treatment.

Grouped pigmentation. Grouped pigmentation of the retina is a rare, nonfamilial retinal abnormality characterized by grayish to black, small, pigmented spots scattered throughout the fundus. They are sometimes grouped to resemble animal

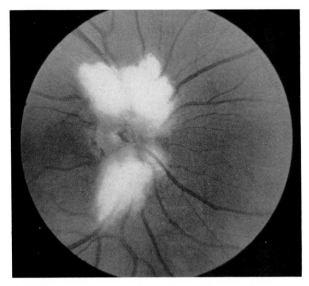

Fig. 15-7. Myelinated nerve fibers on the surface of the retina.

footprints (bear tracks) in the retina. There are no symptoms.

Persistent hyperplastic primary vitreous. Persistent hyperplastic primary vitreous is a unilateral ocular abnormality resulting from failure of the tunica vasculosa lentis, which provides nutrition for the lens in utero, to regress. The lesion occurs in full-term infants and is usually diagnosed shortly after birth. The involved eye is usually slightly smaller than the fellow eye and has an abnormally shallow anterior chamber. Immediately behind the lens is a whitish, fibrous tissue mass with long ciliary processes extending to its periphery. The easily visible ciliary processes distinguish persistent hyperplastic primary vitreous from microphthalmia and from retinal dysplasia. Cataract, followed by swelling of the lens due to rupture of the posterior capsule, and secondary glaucoma with buphthalmos may occur. At about the fourth month, spontaneous deep vitreous and posterior chamber hemorrhages occur.

The differential diagnosis involves retinoblastoma that is not associated with cataract and retrolental fibroplasia that is bilateral and is associated with premature birth. Treatment is ineffective.

Retinal dysplasia. Retinal dysplasia is a a developmental aberration present at birth and characterized by bilateral ocular anomalies, systemic malformations, and a familial tendency. Most infants with the abnormality are born at term—the entity is not related to prematurity.

Microphthalmia is common, the anterior chamber is shallow, and broad posterior synechiae may be present. A white, vascularized mass is situated behind the lens, and remnants of primitive hyaloid blood vessels may be evident. Secondary glaucoma may develop. There may be associated mental retardation, hydrocephalus, congenital heart disease, polydactylism, cleft palate, umbilical hernia, and malrotation of the intestines.

The ocular differential diagnosis includes other causes of a white mass behind the lens such as retrolental fibroplasia, retinoblastoma, and persistent primary vitreous. Usually the occurrence of a whitish mass behind the lens in both eyes, evident at birth in full-term infants, serves to distinguish the condition.

Pseudoglioma. Pseudoglioma is an old, mainly obsolete, term used to describe any eye, but particularly that of an infant in which there is a white mass behind the lens that is not a retinoblastoma. The term may be applied to persistent hyperplastic vitreous, retrolental fibroplasia, retinal dysplasia, and a host of other diseases.

Retrolental fibroplasia. Retrolental fibroplasia, or retinopathy of prematurity, is a primary retinal abnormality involving both eyes. It results from disordered retinal vascularization and occurs almost exclusively in premature infants having a birth weight of less than 1,500 grams who have been subjected to a high oxygen environment during the first 10 days of life.

Between 1943 and 1953, nearly 7,000 premature infants in the United States were blinded because of development of total retinal detachment and formation of a dense fibrous membrane behind the lens. In man the retinal blood vessels normally reach the ocular periphery at the ninth gestational month. With premature birth, retinal vascularization is incomplete, and with excess oxygen there is patchy overgrowth of capillary endothelium combined with areas of avascularity. The retina becomes elevated, with neovascularization into the vitreous body combined with retinal and vitreous hemorrhages, and in the most severe cases the retrolental space is filled with a mass of fibrous tissue containing disorganized retina. The mechanism of injury by excess oxygen is still not clearly understood, but presumably it removes the stimulus for orderly growth of blood vessels.

In the fully developed condition the diagnosis is evident. The eyes are small and sunken, with faded, fetal, grayish blue irides. A white mass presses against the lens, and frequently glaucoma will develop accompanied by tearing and corneal edema but no enlargement of the globe. The infant will often sit, rocking back and forth and grinding his eyes with his fists.

Incomplete retrolental fibroplasia may be associated with gradual ocular deterioration in adolescence. Central visual acuity may be reduced and macular pigmentation and esotropia occur. Myopia is common. The minimal scarring in the peripheral retina may give rise to retinal separation requiring surgical correction.

In recent years the idiopathic respiratory distress syndrome was recognized as affecting some 10% of all infants weighing less than 2,500 grams at birth. High concentrations of oxygen are required for several days after birth. The cardiac and pulmonary deficiencies may disappear at any time, but the high oxygen concentration of the arterial blood causes retinal damage. Ophthalmoscopic examination for retinal vasoconstriction may aid in judging a safe amount of oxygen. If the blood level of oxygen has been excessive, the retinal vessels will show a proportionate degree of vasospasm. If the constricted vessels dilate 10 to 15 minutes after removal of the infant from the incubator, permanent damage may be avoided by reducing the incubator oxygen level. If vasoconstriction persists, some retrolental fibroplasia will develop, and the incubator oxygen level must be lowered to minimize further damage. If the retinal vessels are normal, safe arterial oxygen levels have not been exceeded.

Other retinal disorders
Retinal artery occlusion

Occlusion of the central retinal artery (Fig. 15-8) causes sudden, painless loss of vision. Occlusion of a branch causes a sector defect in the field of vision. The main causes of the condition are arterial disease with vasospasm or thrombus formation or an embolus, particularly associated with endocarditis or following cardiac surgery.

A number of other conditions may cause arterial occlusion. Atheroma formation complicated by subintimal hemorrhage

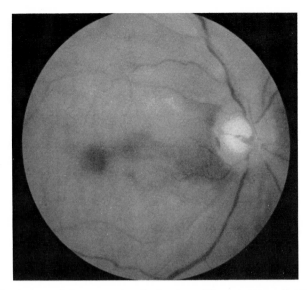

Fig. 15-8. Occlusion of the central retinal artery. The veins are slightly attenuated, but the arteries are maximally constricted and visible only as indistinct white lines. The retina is edematous, and the choroidal circulation visible at the fovea centralis causes a cherry red spot.

and vascular spasm is a demonstrated cause, as is a dissecting aneurysm of the central retinal artery. Arterial emboli may develop in patients with chronic rheumatic valvulitis (particularly mitral stenosis) and in coronary occlusion with mural thrombi. More commonly occlusion results from vasospasm secondary to arteritis in the elderly or from vasomotor instability such as that associated with migraine in younger individuals.

The ischemia of arterial occlusion initially causes cloudy swelling of the inner portion of the retina that receives its nutrition from the central retinal artery or its tributaries. This is followed by autolysis and macrophages loaded with fat granules. In the final stages the inner retinal layers are replaced with glial tissue that rests upon the outer nuclear layer.

Embolic disease causes a sudden, complete loss of vision without premonitory symptoms. Vasospastic disease is usually preceded by repeated transient episodes of decreased vision or blindness in the affected eye (amaurosis fugax), and finally there is an attack in which vision does not return. The symptom of unilateral periodic blindness must be differentiated from internal carotid-basilar occlusive disease (p. 419). Ophthalmodynamometry is normal in central artery occlusion but is frequently decreased on the side of carotid occlusion. Visual loss in carotid occlusive disease is seldom permanent or complete, even though the vessel becomes completely occluded.

On ophthalmoscopic examination in central retinal artery occlusion the retina is opaque and white due to ischemia. The fovea stands out conspicuously as a cherry red spot. The retinal arteries appear as thin, red threads. The blood column may be fragmented so that there are segments with blood interspersed with apparently empty spaces. After a week the retina resumes its normal ophthalmoscopic appearance, but the arteries remain thin lines that, in time, may develop parallel sheathing to appear as white threads. The optic nerve becomes atrophic and appears dead-white against the normally red fundus background.

The cherry red spot may occur in Tay-Sachs disease and other degenerations of ganglion cells, but these are bilateral conditions occurring early in life.

The prognosis is related to the length of time the occlusion has persisted. Relief within 1 hour may restore all vision, whereas relief within 3 or 4 hours may restore peripheral vision, with a defect of central vision persisting. After this period has elapsed, the visual defect is likely to be permanent.

Treatment is directed toward relief of vasospasm or an attempt to dislodge an embolus to a more peripheral and smaller vessel. Immediate intermittent massage of the globe is indicated. Moderate pressure is applied to the globe for a period of 5 seconds, then suddenly released for 5 seconds, and then repeated. If available, 5 or 10% carbon dioxide and 90% oxygen are administered. The carbon dioxide causes vasodilatation and, in this concentration, will cause severe respiratory acidosis, a condition that is usually prevented because of inefficient administration. Breathing into a small paper bag may well be as efficient as the carbon dioxide and oxygen combination. Hyperbaric oxygen may be helpful. Stellate ganglion block with procaine or Xylocaine may be helpful, as may retrobulbar injection with the same drugs or with acetylcholine, tolazoline, or papaverine. Anticoagulants may be helpful in the early stage of occlusion; intravenous heparin is the drug of choice.

Retinal vein occlusion

Retinal vein occlusion (Fig. 15-9) is a local circulatory disturbance characterized by retinal edema, hemorrhage, and engorgement of the venous tree. It involves the central retinal vein or a major branch. There is gradual (2 to 3 hours) loss of

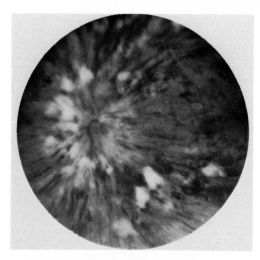

Fig. 15-9. Occlusion of the central vein of the retina. The old term "retinal apoplexy" is highly descriptive.

central and peripheral vision, producing markedly depressed central visual acuity and a peripheral vision defect corresponding to the retinal sector affected. The superior and the inferior temporal branches are the most common sites of branch closure.

The pathogenesis is complex, but one of three occlusive mechanisms usually dominates the clinical and histologic picture:

1. External compression of the vein arises (a) from an atherosclerotic process affecting the central retinal artery where it is adjacent to the central retinal vein. (b) from a connective tissue strand within the floor of the physiologic excavation, or (c) from the cribriform plate. On the retinal surface, occlusion is favored by multiple crossings of the same artery and vein or congenital venous loops or twists. In some patients the initial event may be an arterial occlusion, the vein being also involved because of edema of the surrounding retina.

2. Degenerative venous disease affects the venous endothelium and causes detachment, proliferation, and hydrops. It is associated with severe systemic disease:

arterial hypertension, cardiac decompensation, and diabetes mellitus. Inflammatory venous disease may be due to optic nerve inflammation or to systemic granulomatous disease, particularly tuberculosis.

3. Thrombosis from venous stagnation is caused by reduced intravenous pressure, which results in collapse of the vein. The stagnation is due to spasm of corresponding retinal arterioles, blood dyscrasias, increased viscosity of the blood, or sudden reduction of systemic blood pressure from cardiac decompensation, surgical or traumatic shock, or therapy for arterial hypertension. Glaucoma with increased intraocular pressure obviously predisposes.

The pathologic changes are dominated by hemorrhage, neovascularization, and glaucoma. There is secondary destruction of the retina, which is replaced with fibrous tissue. Some affected eyes ultimately require removal because of neovascularization of the iris (rubeosis iridis, p. 228), which causes a painful, hemorrhagic glaucoma.

The main symptom is painless loss of vision, which involves all function or corresponds to the affected retinal sector. Transient decrease of vision occurs frequently prior to complete occlusion. This decrease is never as complete as that in occlusive carotid-basilar disease. Visual loss with frank venous occlusion develops over a period of several hours and not suddenly as it does in retinal artery closure. Vision tends to remain poor or to deteriorate following occlusion.

Ophthalmoscopic examination indicates engorgement of the venous tree, or portions of it, associated with edema of the corresponding sector of the optic disk and the retina along involved tributaries. Physiologic pulsation of the involved vein is absent and cannot be elicited by pressure upon the eye. If venous circulation has been impaired for an extended period, the optic disk shows fine, veil-like neovascularization or dilatation and tortuosity of the vessels on its surface.

When complete occlusion takes place, the involved retina is splashed with numerous superficial and deep hemorrhages. The disk may be covered with hemorrhages that may break into the vitreous body. The veins are enlarged, engorged, tortuous, and dark blue in color, with streaks of yellowish retinal edema paralleling them.

With or without therapy, the hemorrhages tend to clear very slowly and to leave a residue of grayish white retina, frequently having a fine network of gliosis on its surface. Often there is a marked degree of neovascularization with fine blood vessels about the optic disk or adjacent to the involved vein. The veins become narrowed and in many cases are obscured by white streaks.

The main differential diagnosis includes those conditions causing dilatation and tortuosity of retinal veins in the prodromal stage and the same vascular signs associated with hemorrhage after frank occlusion has occurred. The best diagnostic sign is the absence of spontaneous or induced venous pulsation in occlusion. Those conditions that may cause venous dilatation include diabetes mellitus, blood dyscrasias (particularly those with associated increased blood viscosity), congenital tortuosity of retinal vessels, arteriovenous aneurysms of the retina, angiomas of the retina, papilledema, and congenital heart disease. Retinal hemorrhages are rarely as marked in any other condition as in vein closure.

Treatment is directed toward (1) removal of the underlying cause if possible, (2) use of anticoagulant drugs to permit collateral venous channels to develop, and (3) recognition and treatment of preexisting glaucoma.

The main causes of retinal vein occlusion that can be specifically treated include granulomatous infections, particularly tuberculosis and syphilis. Sudden reduction of blood pressure in individuals with advanced arterial disease should be avoided as much as possible.

Anticoagulation is usually carried out with bishydroxycoumarin (Dicumarol) or a related drug combined with careful observation of the prothrombin level, which is usually maintained at about the 10 to 20% level. Anticoagulation is generally contraindicated in occlusion secondary to venous inflammation in which secondary venous thrombosis tends to diminish hemorrhage. Best results are obtained when therapy is carried out in patients who are in good health, have only a mild degree of retinal atherosclerosis, and have had a sudden onset of occlusion suggestive of a stagnation factor. Impending occlusion is the chief indication for anticoagulation. Patients and physicians must be on the alert for transient diminution of vision and signs of venous engorgement, particularly if one eye has been lost from a venous occlusion. Anticoagulation may have to be continued indefinitely. Venous occlusion during therapy suggests failure to maintain the prothrombin level in a therapeutic range. Primary glaucoma must always be excluded as the cause.

Retinal separation (detachment)

The invagination of the optic vesicle gives rise to two primitive retinal layers: the outer pigment epithelium and an inner sensory layer. The potential space between these layers persists except at the site of exit of the optic nerve and at the ora serrata. A break or a hole in the inner sensory layer permits the accumulation of fluid between the two primitive layers of the retina that separate with loss of retinal function. This is a serous separation or detachment (Fig. 15-10). The subretinal fluid that accumulates between the layers contains much more protein than does the vitreous, and it is derived in large part from blood plasma.

Tumors of the choroid may elevate both primitive layers of the retina, causing a

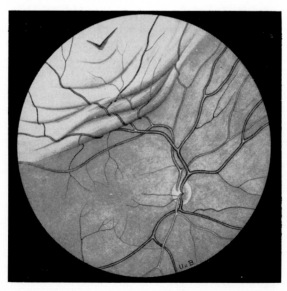

Fig. 15-10. Retinal detachment with horseshoe-shaped hole in the superotemporal quadrant. (From Newell, F. W.: In Lewis-Walters practice of surgery, Hagerstown, Md., 1961, W. F. Prior Co., Inc., vol. 4. chap. 1.)

"solid" detachment, or may produce a toxic fluid that also elevates the retina in an area distant from the actual tumor (malignant melanoma, p. 242). The exudate occurring in severe inflammations of the choroid or retina may cause a similar elevation. Bilateral elevation may occur as the result of a transudate produced in eclampsia or sudden, severe vascular hypertension from other causes. Traction bands sometimes form within the eye, as in retinitis proliferans, with the sensory retina pulled inward following intraocular hemorrhage, trauma, or inflammation.

Serous retinal separation occurs secondary to the formation of breaks or holes in the sensory layer of the retina or because of separation of this layer at the ora serrata, a retinal dialysis, or disinsertion. Retinal breaks occur because of degenerative changes in either the retina or the adjacent vitreous body, or because of ocular trauma. Retinal disinsertion occurs mainly in youthful individuals and may constitute either a congenital or a traumatic defect.

Retinal separations occur more commonly in men than in women, in eyes with degenerative myopia, and in the aged. The separation tends to be bilateral in about one third of the patients with retinal degenerative changes. The time interval between separation in the first and then in the second eye may be as long as 10 years. The role of trauma is obvious when there is a direct ocular contusion or a penetrating injury with a retinal break in an otherwise healthy retina. Often, however, the history of trauma is obscure, and enough degenerative changes are present in each eye to account for the retinal separation. In such eyes the role of trauma in precipitating the detachment is difficult to assess, particularly if the trauma has not involved the eye directly. Retinal separation may occur after an uncomplicated cataract extraction, but it is seen more often if vitreous humor has been lost during surgery. Congenital cataract extraction is prone to be complicated by retinal separation that may occur many years after surgery.

Retinal breaks may follow penetrating ocular injuries, but in other instances the cause of the break is not clear. They may result from retraction of the vitreous body if retinovitreal adhesions are present, may arise from degenerative changes following minute retinal or choroidal vascular obstructions, or may follow retinal inflammations. In youthful eyes the rupture of a congenital retinal cyst is an etiologic factor, whereas in senile eyes there may be rupture of peripheral degenerative cysts.

The two main premonitory symptoms of retinal separation are (1) photopsia, or flashes of light without retinal stimulation by light due to vitreous traction on the retina, and (2) a sudden shower of black dots in the peripheral visual field arising from a minute vitreous hemorrhage at the point of a retinal break. In many patients, premonitory symptoms are either absent or ignored, and the first symptom is a progressive defect in the visual field corresponding to the area of detachment.

The diagnosis of retinal separation is based upon the ophthalmoscopic appearance of the retina. Indirect ophthalmoscopy has its greatest application in this condition—when combined with gentle scleral depression the examiner can study the retina from the optic disk to the ora serrata. Maximal pupillary dilation is required—10% phenylephrine and 1% Mydriacyl are frequently used. The peripheral retina may also be studied with a biomicroscope and a concave corneal contact lens containing prisms that allow visualization of the periphery.

On ophthalmoscopic examination the detached retina appears dark red to gray, with the normal choroidal pattern absent. The retina may be thrown into folds that change in location or shape with changes in position of the eye or the head. Fixed folds, the result of alterations in the vitreous body, do not change with position. The retinal vessels are dark red in the area of detachment and have an undulating course over its surface. The arteries and veins appear to have blood of the same color.

Retinal breaks are recognized by the bright red reflex of the choroid shining through the grayish, opaque veil of surrounding retinal tissue. Noncontributory holes may be found in areas of attached retina. Horseshoe-shaped tears with their base anterior are most common in the superior temporal quadrant near the equator. Small round holes may be found anywhere but are frequently seen in the extreme peripheral retina. Retinal dialysis usually occurs in the inferior quadrants, and it is most often single, semilunar, and at the extreme retinal periphery. Retinal detachments with hole formation are readily diagnosed. However, in serous detachments, holes are not found in 5 to 15% of the patients, depending upon the skill of the observer.

Visual field examination is useful in delineating the extent of retinal involvement and in indicating whether or not the separation regresses with bed rest.

The most important differential point is the solid detachment caused by tumor, particularly malignant melanoma of the choroid. Failure of the detachment to regress with bed rest, the darker color, the failure to transilluminate, and absence of hole formation serve to characterize tumor formation.

The treatment of serous retinal detachment is essentially surgical and is directed toward closure of breaks in the retina and toward drainage of subretinal fluid. Once the diagnosis has been established, treatment must be started immediately.

Retinal breaks are closed by producing an area of chorioretinitis in the region of the defect so that adhesions forming between the edges of the break and the underlying choroid will obliterate the opening. The inflammation is produced by the application of diathermy or intense cold (-70° C.) to the sclera in the region of the hole. Subretinal fluid is often removed by perforating the choroid, but it will absorb spontaneously if the pigment epithelium is brought into contact with the retinal hole.

A number of operations are employed to decrease the size of the sclera so that a smaller or shrunken retina will fit the smaller scleral shell (Fig. 15-11). In shortening procedures, one or more quadrants of the sclera are resected and shortened. This may be combined with the implantation of a foreign material such as various-shaped pieces of silicone to cause further indentation of the choroid. There may be buckling of a segment of the sclera, or an engirdling rod may be placed around the entire circumference of the eye.

Failure to obtain anatomic reattachment of the retina usually is due to failure in obliterating the causative retinal break. Because of the frequency with which the

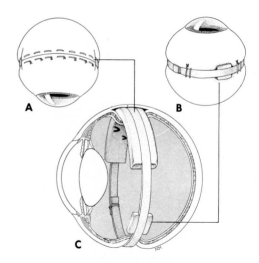

Fig. 15-11. Encircling silicone band with two grooved silicone plates. The sclera has been resected in the region of the retinal breaks. (From Boyd, B. F.: Highlights Ophthal. **10:**89, 1966.)

fellow eye is involved, every attempt must be made to secure correction, even if several reoperations are required.

Retinoschisis

Retinoschisis develops because of splitting of the neural layers of the retina. This split usually occurs in the outer plexiform layer. Central vision is rarely affected by the condition, and attention is usually directed to the area of involvement because of a defect in the peripheral visual field.

At its onset, retinoschisis affects the extreme retinal periphery, most commonly in the inferior temporal quadrant. It gradually extends nasally to encompass the entire periphery and progresses from the temporal region toward the fovea. Finally, it forms a huge, cystlike elevation.

Prognosis in retinoschisis is good. It seems likely that in many instances it remains undiagnosed indefinitely. In advanced cases, however, central visual acuity may be lost. The development of a break in the retina may lead to retinal detachment.

Retinoschisis, in its early stages, appears to be an exaggeration of cystoid degeneration of the retina. If the sclera of the area is indented, the affected retina appears to have lost some of its transparency (white with pressure). In later stages the inner layer forms a fixed, smooth, convex, sharply limited, transparent elevation.

No treatment is indicated if the condition does not extend to the equator, although annual ophthalmoscopic and perimetric examinations are advised. Extension beyond the equator calls for limitation of extension of the process by means of photocoagulation, surface diathermy, or cryotherapy at the advancing edge of the elevation in normal retinal tissue. Good results have been reported by photocoagulation of the base of retinoschisis itself.

Pigmentary degenerations of the retina*

A large variety of hereditary, noninflammatory deteriorations of the photoreceptors and pigment epithelium are characterized by the premature death of normally formed cells as a result of inherited, innate fragility that limits their life-span. Night blindness is the most common initial symptom. The rod and cone layer of the retina is characteristically involved, and there is early extinction of the electroretinographic response to weak stimuli. Ophthalmoscopically there are often changes in the pigment epithelium. The age of onset is usually between 10 and 20 years, and all light perception may be lost between 50 and 60 years of age. The inheritance pattern differs. Generally, sex-linked forms are most severe.

There is frequent association with systemic defects: obesity, polydactyly, hypogenitalism and mental retardation (Laurence-Moon-Biedl syndrome), renal abnormalities, deafness, convulsions, ophthalmoplegia, cerebellar ataxia, and progeria.

There is no effective treatment.

---

*The terminology of these conditions is difficult. They are not inflammations and the use of the word "retinitis" is unsatisfactory. The retinal pigment epithelium is the tapetum and the term "tapetoretinal degeneration" has been proposed. Despite the similar ophthalmoscopic appearance in their end stages, it seems likely that further study will indicate that in some individuals the primary defect is in the photoreceptor layer, while in others it is in the retinal pigment epithelium. However, "degeneration" in the sense of a change of tissue to a less active form and "pigmentary" to emphasize the involvement of the retinal pigment epithelium can provide a temporary nomenclature until the nature of the conditions is determined. In addition, occlusive vascular disease of the choriocapillaris may be mainly reflected in the pigment epithelium and photoreceptors, and because of the similarity of symptoms to primary diseases of these structures, some choriocapillary abnormalities are discussed in this section, in addition to Chapter 14.

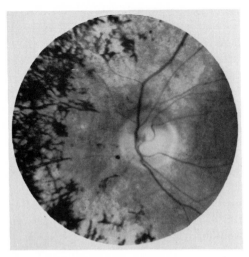

Fig. 15-12. Pigmentary degeneration of the retina.

Retinitis pigmentosa. Retinitis pigmentosa (Fig. 15-12) is a primary pigmentary degeneration of the retina. It is a hereditary abnormality, nearly always bilateral, affecting retinal rods predominantly. The disease begins in youth with the development of night blindness and a ring scotoma that expands peripherally and centrally until only a small contracted visual field remains (tubular vision). The remaining vision may be obliterated at the age of 50 or 60 years.

Ophthalmoscopic examination reveals the following: (1) marked narrowing of the retinal arteries and veins; (2) waxy, yellowish appearance of the optic disk; and (3) pigment deposits that have a dense center and irregular processes similar in appearance to bone corpuscles. The narrowing of the retinal arteries is most characteristic and aids in the diagnosis, even when pigment is sparse or absent. The pigment usually begins in the equatorial region with fine speckling, which becomes more dense and advances centrally but never involves the macular region. It may lie on top of blood vessels and completely obscure the blood column.

Central visual acuity remains in the 20/30 to 20/50 range until middle life, although the markedly restricted visual field limits the patient's mobility. Posterior subcapsular cataract may reduce central vision and require extraction. Pathologically the condition is characterized by disintegration of the rod and cone layer of the retina, patchy areas of increased and decreased pigment epithelium, and migration of pigment into the retina.

Secondary pigmentary degeneration occurs in choroiditis, particularly that due to syphilis. At times it is difficult to distinguish the syphilitic chorioretinitis from retinitis pigmentosa. However, in secondary pigmentary degeneration the pigment is less regular, is distributed beneath blood vessels, is associated with areas of chorioretinitis, and produces a less definite ring scotoma.

Choroideremia. Choroideremia is a sex-linked tapetoretinal degeneration in which there is atrophy of the choroid with secondary atrophy of the retina, causing night blindness.

In the female carrier the condition is asymptomatic and is associated with a nonprogressive pigmentation and depigmentation of the fundus that is most marked in the equatorial region. The pigment granules have an irregular, square appearance like a large chunk of coal, and their size is about the diameter of the central retinal artery. Under or adjacent to the groups of pigment are depigmented areas up to ½ disk diameter in size, and they appear paler than the rest of the fundus or have a bright yellow color.

Choroideremia in male individuals is progressive and usually has its onset between the ages of 10 and 13 years. The initial symptom is night blindness, which becomes complete in about 10 years. The peripheral field then begins to contract and finally, after about 35 years, all vision is lost. The earliest fundus changes are pigmentary and resemble the changes found in the fundi of female carriers.

However, atrophic changes then dominate the fundus picture, and the white sclera becomes exposed in the equatorial region. At this time, night blindness occurs. Eventually the sclera is entirely exposed, and an annular scotoma is present. The atrophy then extends toward the ora serrata and the macula until all vision is lost. The retinal vessels are normal.

The differential diagnosis involves the following: (1) retinitis pigmentosa, which is excluded by the absence of retinal vessel changes, the late onset of optic atrophy, and the clear-cut choroidal vessels at the edge of normal fundus; (2) gyrate atrophy may be confused in the early stages of choroideremia when there is patchy atrophy, but the pigment changes in choroideremia should aid in distinguishing the condition; (3) widespread choroidal sclerosis appears as a thick, whitish veil and not as bare sclera as occurs in choroideremia; (4) the atrophy of pathologic myopia involves the posterior pole rather than the equator, but the occurrence of such myopia in choroideremia may make the distinction difficult; and (5) Oguchi's disease.

There is no effective treatment.

Gyrate atrophy. Gyrate atrophy of the choroid is a tapetoretinal abnormality with onset in childhood. It is characterized by the presence of irregularly shaped areas of retinal and choroidal atrophy in which white sclera is seen with strands and islands of apparently uninvolved retinal and choroidal tissue between. The involved area usually surrounds the disk and the macula, and the extreme peripheral fundus is not involved. Night blindness occurs constantly, and vision may be markedly reduced with foveal involvement. The disease is slowly progressive. There is no treatment.

Macular disease

We have seen (p. 24) that the macular region is located temporal to the optic disk and surrounds the fovea centralis, which contains the cones mainly responsible for central visual acuity and color vision. The area is involved in the same vascular, inflammatory, and degenerative diseases that affect the retina and underlying choroidal vasculature elsewhere. Several factors so modify disease in the macular region that its abnormalities are often considered apart from diseases of the remainder of the retina. A minute lesion that would not affect visual function if located elsewhere may cause a profound loss of central visual acuity. Additionally, the spreading of the inner layers of the retina to expose the cones in the fovea centralis favors swelling of Henle's layer of the retina, which is seen particularly in neuroretinitis with the formation of a circular area of deposits surrounding the fovea centralis. The optical system of the eye focuses light energy in this region so that degeneration of the area may follow unwise exposure to the light of the sun as occurs in eclipse retinopathy. Moreover, the macular area, for reasons still unexplained, appears to be preferentially involved in a variety of degenerative conditions.

Macular degenerations

Abnormalities affecting the fovea centralis and causing a defect in central visual acuity with depressed color vision have been classified broadly as macular degenerations. For the most part, the lesions are easily seen with the ophthalmoscope. Degeneration of the macula can be divided into primary and secondary types. The primary type results from a genetically transmitted defect. It is familial and not exogenous and is bilateral and progressive. The secondary type follows vascular or inflammatory disease, is commonly unilateral, and frequently does not progress after the cause has been removed. The secondary type is at times amenable to therapy, although in many diseases, particularly vascular degenerations, therapy is not successful.

Primary macular degenerations may be subdivided into those with central nervous system involvement and those confined to the eye. Central nervous system involvement arises because of abnormalities affecting the ganglion cells of both the retina and the brain. Cerebromacular degenerations include amaurotic familial idiocy (Tay-Sachs disease) and the late infantile and juvenile types. Involvement of the central nervous system frequently leads to early death of these children, and many cases are not diagnosed because the fundi have not been examined.

The most important entity of the group without central nervous system involvement is the hereditary macular degenerations classified as dystrophies of the macula. The genetic behavior, age of onset, course, and effect upon vision are poorly understood. However, members of the same family tend to have a similar age of onset and ophthalmoscopic lesion, although the appearance is not necessarily identical. The lesion covers an area of ½ to 5 disk diameters. When large, the area of involvement is not sharply defined, although the central area may be well demarcated. The damage varies in severity from a loss of macular luster to a considerable pigmentary reaction with an atrophic scar. Optic atrophy is not associated with the macular lesion—thus the ganglion cells of the retina are not involved. Three types of the condition occur: (1) the pigmented, which may represent an inverse retinitis pigmentosa, (2) the exudative, and (3) the atrophic. The heredodegenerations of the retina have been classified by age of onset as infantile, juvenile, adolescent, adult, presenile, and senile. The outstanding symptom is loss of central vision that may precede ophthalmoscopic changes. The visual defect may be relatively mild or extremely severe. A central scotoma with normal peripheral isopters is present. There may be progressive deterioration of vision throughout life.

The secondary group of macular degenerations occurs because of severe ocular trauma, inflammation involving the macular area, distant inflammation causing edema of nerve fibers in direct contact with the vitreous body, and vascular disease affecting the area.

The most common cause of secondary macular degenerations is alteration of the blood supply from the choriocapillaris. The layers of the retina adjacent to the choriocapillaris receive from it their entire nutrition. Since the choriocapillaris cannot be seen with the ophthalmoscope, it is not immediately evident that the lesions are secondary. This problem is not generally so difficult with other types of secondary macular degeneration in which the cause becomes evident, either by a

---

Primary macular degeneration

I. With central nervous system involvement
  A. Cerebromacular degeneration
    1. Amaurotic familial idiocy
      a. Infantile (Tay-Sachs)
      b. Late infantile
      c. Juvenile
  B. Niemann-Pick disease
II. Without central nervous system involvement
  A. Heredodegeneration of the macula
    1. Dystrophies
      a. Pigmented
      b. Exudative
      c. Atrophic
    2. Infantile
      a. Congenital macular
    3. Juvenile
    4. Adult
    5. Presenile
    6. Senile
    7. Honeycomb choroiditis
  B. Central choroidal sclerosis
  C. Angioid streaks

Secondary macular degeneration

I. Inflammatory
   A. Choroid
   B. Retina
   C. Distant intraocular
II. Vascular
   A. Choriocapillaris
      1. Senile degeneration
      2. Hyaline degeneration
         (drusen)
      3. Senile disciform
         (Kuhnt-Junius)
III. Retinal
   A. Venous occlusion
   B. Arterial occlusion
   C. Angiospastic
IV. External
   A. Blunt trauma
   B. Radiant energy (eclipse blindness)
V. Refractive
   A. Myopia (malignant myopia)
   B. Hyperopia

careful history or from observation of the ophthalmoscopic signs.

The macular changes due to sclerosis of the choriocapillaris are diagnosed as senile macular degeneration. Central visual acuity diminishes gradually, with involvement of one eye preceding the other by months or years. Ophthalmoscopic examination may indicate minimal change considering the severity of visual loss. There may be fine pigmentary deposits in the macula, with discrete, minute yellowish exudative areas. There may be hyaline deposits (drusen) on the cuticular layer of Bruch's membrane.

Medical therapy is of no value. The visual loss occurs because of a diminution of blood supply to the fovea centralis, and function cannot be restored to the delicate cones once it is lost. Some patients obtain useful vision with telescopic lenses, special magnifying lenses, and similar optical aids. Although the proportion of patients who obtain satisfaction is disappointingly small,

each patient should have a trial opportunity with these lenses before it is concluded that they are of no use. Physicians must reassure these patients that the condition will not progress to complete blindness. Although central vision is lost, the disease never involves the peripheral retina sufficiently to eliminate so much of the peripheral vision that the patient becomes helpless.

Senile disciform degeneration. This secondary type of macular degeneration begins with a choroidal hemorrhage that may extravasate between the retinal pigment epithelium and Bruch's membrane. Gradually a localized mass of connective tissue proliferates from the choroid, giving rise to an elevated macula. The typical case develops in a patient past middle life who has arterial disease. It is most common in the sixth decade, men are more commonly affected than women, and in more than half the cases the condition is bilateral. It commences with a hemorrhage at the macula and terminates with the presence of tumorlike masses of organized tissue at the macular region that abolish central vision.

Frequently the other macula betrays choroidal sclerosis: pigmentary changes, drusen, white exudative spots, etc. In all unilateral cases observed that have become bilateral, the second eye has shown similar changes. Thus it seems quite possible that choroidal sclerosis may be a constant precursor. Treatment is ineffective.

Hyaline deposits of the lamina vitrea (drusen) may, when large or centrally located, cause a form of central retinopathy due to pressure on visual cells. Additionally, the drusen are seen in angioid streaks of the retina, disciform degeneration, and many diseased eyes.

In the common senile macular degenerations arising from alterations in the blood supply to the choroid, there is, unfortunately, very little that can be done.

Systemic vasodilators, iodides, vitamins, and many other compounds have been used, but there seems to be nothing that will stem the inexorable course of the affliction. Iodides are not without risk and, although widely used, they have never been proved valuable. Leopold showed that most compounds that cause systemic vasodilatation either have no effect on the choroidal circulation or cause vasoconstriction. Thus, until an effective treatment is devised for combating the vascular degenerative changes, therapy must be limited to symptomatic measures.

Serous chorioretinopathy

This is an abnormality in which there is an accumulation of serous fluid or blood between the pigment epithelium and the rods and cones in the macular area. There is elevation of the macula, reduction in the central visual acuity, and a central scotoma. A positive scotoma may follow exposure of the eye to bright light.

A large number of terms are used to describe the condition: central serous retinopathy, central serous choroidosis, serous or hemorrhagic disciform detachment of the macula, and central angiospastic retinopathy. Headache is often associated with the onset. The headache is unilateral, on the side of the ocular lesion, and may be associated with retrobulbar pain. Many patients have a variety of allergies, and there is a prominent psychosomatic element in their complaints.

Ophthalmoscopically the fundus lesion is characterized by a circumscribed elevation of the retina or pigment epithelium in the macular region. There may be a serous or hemorrhagic extravasation. The lesions tend to remain unchanged for long periods. Histologically there is dilation and stasis in the orbital and vortex veins and their tributaries, and the lesion is suggestive of a widespread hemodynamic disturbance. The lesion may involve the retina only or the choroid only; more commonly, both are involved. There may be active proliferation of the pigment epithelium, producing elevated, pigmented lesions suggesting a chorioretinitis. The lesions tend to disappear, leaving a residue of mounds of pigment proliferation. A tumor may be suspected, although hemorrhage and involvement of the posterior pole are both unusual with tumor.

An area of leakage in the choriocapillaris may be demonstrated with fluorescein angiography. Photocoagulation of this area may be followed by complete resolution of the lesion. Usually vision tends to return to normal levels without treatment, but careful testing indicates a persistent central scotoma when the fovea has been stimulated with a bright light. There tend to be recurrent attacks.

Coats' disease

Coats' disease is a chronic, progressive retinal abnormality characterized by retinal exudates and usually associated with malformation of retinal blood vessels. It begins early in youth (average, 16 years), involves male patients predominantly, and is usually unilateral, but when both eyes are involved one is affected more severely than the other.

The main symptom is decrease in central or peripheral vision. In the very young, attention may be directed to the abnormality because of a white mass behind the lens suggesting a retinoblastoma. Enucleation is frequent in youthful patients. Pathologic examination indicates initial rod and cone degeneration followed by exudates, extensive detachment, and neofibrovascularization.

Ophthalmoscopic examination reveals yellowish white exudative patches beneath retinal blood vessels. These wax and wane and may disappear in one area while occurring in another. Subretinal hemorrhages are frequent and are usually associated with numerous glistening deposits,

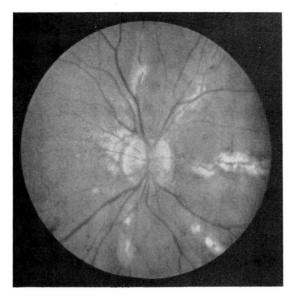

Fig. 15-13. Marked angioid streaks.

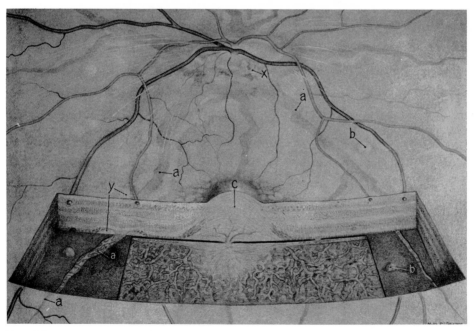

Fig. 15-14. Mechanism of angioid streaks. Diagram illustrating the histopathologic change that produces the fundus appearance of angioid streaks: **a,** angioid streak; **b,** drusen of Bruch's membrane; **c,** mound of vascularized scar tissue at the macula; **x,** hyaline body of the optic disk; **y,** fibrous tissue cuffing of an angioid streak. In the lower part of the diagram between two angioid streaks, Bruch's membrane and the choriocapillaris have been cut away, showing the pattern of underlying choroidal vessels. (From Goodman, R. M., Smith, E. W., Paton, D., Bergman, R. A., Siegel, C. L., Otteson, O. E., Shelley, W. M., Pusch, A. L., and McKusick, V. A.: Medicine **42:**297, 1963.)

presumably cholesterol. The retinal vessels may have a tortuous course, aneurysms, fusiform dilatations, loops, and glomerulus-like formations. Hemorrhage into the vitreous body may occur with subsequent development of retinitis proliferans. Eventually there may be detachment of the entire retina, iritis, cataract, and glaucoma.

Treatment is frequently ineffective, but diathermy may be helpful in some instances, either by means of the photocoagulator through the pupil or by high-frequency current through the sclera.

Derangements of the elastic membrane: angioid streaks

Angioid streaks (Figs. 15-13 and 15-14) consist of a bizarre network of pigmented striations that, on ophthalmoscopic examination, appear to lie between the retinal and choroidal vascular beds. They may occur with pseudoxanthoma elasticum, Paget's disease (osteitis deformans), sickle cell disease, and generalized vascular disease involving the elastic coat of blood vessels. In a typical case the fundus presents a more or less complete peripapillary pigmented ring, with offshoots extending toward the equator in a radial distribution. In the early stages the streaks usually appear red but later may assume a gray, brown, or black color. At times, a white sheathing, probably connective tissue, is seen in conjunction with the streaks. The striations are flat, serrated, and may be several times wider than a retinal vein. They gradually taper off toward the periphery of the fundus, where they then may appear as thin lines. They do not branch dichotomously, as do retinal vessels, and they give the appearance of cracks in dry mud. The macular region is usually involved to a varying degree, with the appearance of fresh hemorrhages, exudates, or scars with clusters of pigment. The periphery of the fundus may show an occasional chorioretinal lesion. There is

frequently a dustlike pigment stippling that appears to be peculiar to the condition. Both sexes are affected equally. The disease is most commonly found between the second and fifth decades of life. Both eyes are invariably involved. The visual fields remain normal, but central vision is reduced because of the eventual severe macular degeneration, resembling disciform senile degeneration.

Angioid streaks originate because of tears in Bruch's membrane of the choroid. Histologic studies show a diffuse degeneration of the elastica layer of Bruch's membrane, characterized by numerous ruptures and calcium deposits. There is no effective treatment.

Inflammations

The retina may be involved in exogenous and endogenous inflammations of the vitreous body or the choroid. Probably the main cause is an inflammatory lesion in the adjacent choroid. Retinal inflammation leads to an exudation of cells into the vitreous body, and if marked, this may cause diffraction of light and interference with vision. Inflammations affecting the posterior pole disturb the fovea centralis and disturb central visual acuity. Ophthalmoscopically the inflamed area appears yellowish white with ill-defined borders in the acute stage. When healed, the choroid or the sclera may be exposed, but the lesion may be surrounded by proliferated pigment epithelium.

Toxoplasmosis. Toxoplasmosis (p. 376) is likely the main infectious cause of retinitis and occurs in both a congenital and an acquired form. There tends to be secondary involvement of the choroid with destruction of both the retina and the choroid, producing the ophthalmoscopic appearance of a sharply defined area of dull white sclera surrounded by irregular areas of pigment proliferation. The congenital form of the disease is associated with cerebral calcification and internal hydrocephalus. The topic is discussed on p. 376.

Eales' disease. Eales' disease is a non-specific inflammation of peripheral retinal veins that mainly affects male individuals between the ages of 15 and 30 years. It is characterized by recurrent retinal hemorrhage adjacent to the involved veins and by vitreous hemorrhage. Both eyes are involved in about one half of the cases. The cause is not known, but the condition may result from sensitivity to tuberculoprotein, to which nearly all of these patients react. Thromboangiitis obliterans has been observed in several patients. Sickle cell disease may cause nearly identical involvement. The chief symptom is loss of vision due to vitreous hemorrhage. Although this hemorrhage tends to absorb rapidly, repeated hemorrhages result in vascularization of the vitreous body, chronic uveitis, and glaucoma.

Ophthalmoscopic examination indicates segmental, dilated, beaded, occluded veins, with sheathing or exudation, and blood in the vitreous body and the retina.

Occlusion of the affected vessels by means of photocoagulation is remarkably effective in preventing progression. Photocoagulation may have to be repeated.

Injuries

Contusions and retinal breaks. Contusion of the eye may cause retinal breaks leading to retinal separation. A traumatic retinal break occurs in an otherwise healthy retina—it is usually single, is often horseshoe shaped, and is located in the superior temporal quadrant. Eyes that have been subject to severe contusions should be studied carefully 3 and 6 months after the injury to be certain a retinal break has not developed. It is necessary to study the fundus with wide pupillary dilation, directing particular attention to the periphery.

Commotio retinae. Commotio retinae is a contrecoup phenomenon in which the posterior pole develops edema and hemorrhages because of a blunt contusion of the anterior segment. Vision is markedly reduced and often does not improve. Ophthalmoscopically there are hemorrhages and generalized edema that obscure fundus details.

Macular hole. Macular hole is a term applied to round, red defects of the fovea centralis that measure about ¼ disk diameter in size and are associated with marked reduction in vision. Ophthalmoscopically, they appear to be holes in the retina, yet retinal separation follows only exceptionally. Examination with a biomicroscope indicates that the majority of them are cysts with a translucent anterior wall. There is no treatment.

Lacerations of the retina. Lacerations of the retina are usually associated with loss of vitreous and considerable disorganziation of the globe. Retinal separation is uncommon following such injury inasmuch as the trauma stimulates proliferation of glial tissue, which closes the defect.

Purtscher's injury. Purtscher's injury is a rare abnormality in which the sudden increase in intravascular pressure associated with crushing injury of the chest causes hemorrhages and edema of the retina.

Fat emboli. Fat emboli of the retinal blood vessels may be seen in fractures of long bones.

Radiant energy. The cornea and the lens transmit infrared rays with nearly 100% efficiency. These rays are absorbed by the pigment epithelium of the retina, and ordinarily the increased heat is dissipated by the choroidal circulation. If intense heat is applied, the temperature of the retina is increased, and at 62° C. there is coagulation of retinal proteins. At 100° C. the blood in the choroidal vessels boils. During a solar eclipse with the visibility screened by the moon, an infrared burn of the fovea centralis may occur. There is immediate reduction in vision that does not improve. During subsequent days, the fovea centralis becomes discretely pigmented, and there may be areas of depigmentation. The condition in many respects resembles that seen in senile macular degeneration. A similar lesion was observed in servicemen using a telescope for long periods in tropical areas with the sun's rays focused on the fovea centralis. The lesion may also occur from the infrared rays of an atomic explosion. Controlled photocoagulation is the basis of the therapy in which light energy from a xenon tube or a laser is directed into the eye.

Tumors
Retinoblastomas

Retinoblastomas are malignant tumors arising in the nuclear layers of the retina. They are always congenital and are usually observed shortly after birth, although their appearance may be delayed until late childhood. They are characterized by multiple origins within the eye, and in about one third of the patients they involve both eyes. There is a strong hereditary tendency, and the tumors are transmitted as an autosomal dominant trait in individuals who survive the disease following enucleation, spontaneous regression, or enucleation combined with radiation. Individuals who have

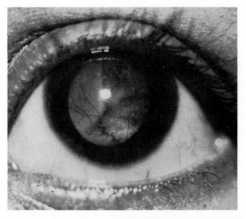

Fig. 15-15. Advanced retinoblastoma with the tumor adjacent to the lens.

survived the tumors should be warned of the dangers of transmission to their offspring. In normal parents who have already had one child with a tumor and who presumably do not carry a dominant gene for retinoblastoma, there is a likelihood of less than 4% that a subsequent child will have a tumor.

The tumor generally is first diagnosed when it has protruded far forward into the vitreous body and is visible in the eye as a grayish yellow reflex behind the lens (Fig. 15-15). Usually by this time the pupil is fixed, the eye is blind, and the term "cat's eye" has been applied to the clinical appearance. If the growth continues, buphthalmos, secondary glaucoma, cataract, and perforation may ensue. The most important diagnostic step to be taken when retinoblastoma is suspected in one eye is careful ophthalmoscopic examination of the opposite eye with the pupil widely dilated and the patient anesthetized. All portions of the retina must be inspected, with particular emphasis on the periphery. Careful study of the fellow eye, when there is no involvement, must be carried out at 6-week to 8-week intervals until late childhood.

Unilateral tumors. Because unilateral retinoblastomas are always far advanced when diagnosed, enucleation with as long a section of the optic nerve as possible is the treatment of choice. Generally, a much longer portion of the optic nerve than usual may be obtained at the time of surgery by putting traction sutures on the insertions of each of the rectus muscles, drawing the eye far forward and nasally, and placing the enucleation scissors as far posterior as possible. At the time of surgery, histologic study should be made ·of the resected portion of the optic nerve to be certain that there is no tumor extending beyond the point of excision (Fig. 15-16). If there is no evidence of tumor in the orbit, an implant may be used after the enucleation. If residual tumor is found in the optic nerve remaining in the orbit, the orbit should be treated with massive doses of radiation similar to those given when the tumor is diagnosed in the fellow eye. In recent years the amount of radiation given has been reduced to approximately 3,500 r in air.

Bilateral tumors. Bilateral retinoblastomas are best treated by enucleation of the most-advanced eye and medical and radiation therapy to the opposite eye. When both eyes are involved with far-advanced tumors, it is probably kindest to the patient and to all concerned to proceed with bilateral enucleation because radiation is almost certain to destroy an eye with an advanced tumor. The eye that is most advanced is enucleated and is managed exactly as if the tumor were unilateral. The opposite eye is then treated by means of intracarotid tetraethylmelamine (TEM) given continuously or immediately prior to, and at the conclusion of, radiation therapy; 3,500 r of radiation measured in air are given through divided portals to the involved eye.

In recent years the technique of light coagulation developed by Meyer-Schwickerath has been used in the treatment of retinoblastomas involving less than one third of the retina. The therapy is not superior to radiation, particularly because it does not sterilize tumor nests as yet invisible ophthalmoscopically as is possible with radiation therapy. Nevertheless, it is a valuable adjunct to treatment. Since the tumor itself is too pale to absorb much light energy, treatment must be directed to the surrounding choroid, using high-intensity radiation.

Phakomatoses

This group of interrelated diseases is characterized by skin lesions and wide-

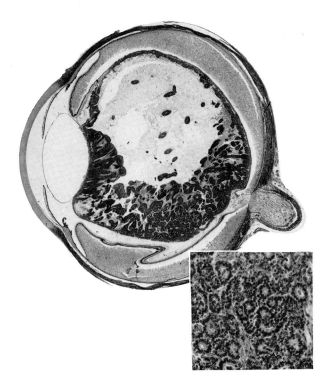

Fig. 15-16. Eye of patient shown in Fig. 15-15. Inset shows typical rosette formation in the tumor.

spread tumors. Neurofibromatosis (Recklinghausen's disease) is associated with widespread cutaneous and central nervous system abnormalities. Multiple astrocytomas may occur in the retina, although a more common ocular manifestation of the disease is an orbital tumor or glioma of the optic nerve. Astrocytomas also may occur in the fundus. They appear as hemispheres placed against a refractile white and slightly uneven base. Tuberous sclerosis (Bourneville's syndrome) is a clinical syndrome of mental deficiency, epilepsy, and adenoma sebaceum. Lindau–von Hippel disease is a familial, often bilateral, angioblastic retinal tumor with associated lesions in the viscera and the brain. On ophthalmoscopic examination there is a reddish, slightly elevated tumor, about the size of the optic disk or smaller, that is nourished by a large artery and vein. Coagulation of the tumor by means of photocoagulation or transscleral diathermy prevents the formation of hemorrhages and deposits and a secondary glaucoma. Sturge-Weber syndrome (encephalofacial angiomatosis) is characterized by a nevus flammeus in the area of distribution of the trigeminal nerve, angioma of the choroid causing a buphthalmos, and venous angioma of the meninges of the cerebral cortex. Focal epilepsy and mental retardation are common. This is the most common cause of monocular glaucoma in infants.

Chapter 16

The vitreous body

The vitreous body is a transparent gel having a volume of about 4.5 ml. that entirely fills the vitreous cavity. In health it is in contact with the retina throughout. It is attached firmly at the optic disk and in the region of the ora serrata. The vitreous body may be divided into a peripheral cortical portion that entirely surrounds it and a central portion that is a true gel. The gel is composed of a collagen-like fibrous meshwork that contains hyaluronic acid and in which a large amount of water is suspended. The cortical layer contains a few large, flat cells and a fibrous network that extends fanlike into the central gel. There is a diffusional exchange between blood vessels on the disk and the retina and the vitreous body. Additionally, aqueous humor secreted by the ciliary processes in the posterior chamber diffuses through the vitreous body toward the optic nerve.

The vitreous body is a true physical and biologic gel. With disease, aging, and injury, the delicate balance maintaining water in suspension is disturbed, and the vitreous liquefies. With loss of the gel structure, fine fibers, membranes, and cellular aggregates become visible, although they are seen only with difficulty inasmuch as they are nearly transparent.

Symptoms and signs of diseases of the vitreous body

Abnormalities in the vitreous body manifest themselves by two main symptoms: (1) floaters and (2) photopsia, or light flashes observed with the eyes closed when the eyes move. The vitreous body may be studied with the ophthalmoscope, and when there are large or numerous opacities, they appear black against the red fundus background. More details are seen when the vitreous body is studied with a biomicroscope using a −40 diopter lens to study the posterior structure.

Degenerations

Liquefaction (syneresis). With aging, the vitreous body tends to become partially or completely fluid. This liquefaction begins in the center of the vitreous body and tends to strip it from the superior and posterior portions of the retina. Liquefaction creates the appearance of delicate membranes or strands floating freely in the fluid. On ophthalmoscopy, fine opacities may be seen that move freely with ocular rotation. Opacities are more easily demonstrated with a biomicroscope. Liquefaction also follows injury and inflammation. It constitutes a degenerative condition and leads commonly to vitreous detachment.

Vitreous detachment. With syneresis, a membrane may appear that seems to separate the vitreous gel from an optically empty space in front of the retina. The membrane often contains a small opacity. Middle-aged patients frequently notice the sudden appearance of a relatively large, fixed floater near their point of fixation.

277

There may be associated subjective lightning flashes, so that with the eyes closed, or in a dark room, a sudden movement of the eye causes a flash of light due to the intact vitreous body bumping the retina. Examination with a biomicroscope and a concave lens indicates a membrane in the posterior viteous body with a floater in front of an optically empty space adjacent to the retina. The fellow eye tends to be involved within months. There is no treatment. The symptoms gradually subside, although the membrane remains unchanged.

Vitreous shrinkage. Vitreous shrinkage is a destructive phenomenon in which contraction of the vitreous body causes traction upon retinal areas to which it is fixed. Shrinkage in the macular area causes central flashes of light and may produce a macular cyst. Traction in the region of the ora serrata may be a factor in the production of holes and retinal dialysis.

Vitreous opacities

A larger variety of foreign substances may be suspended in the vitreous body, including (1) exogenous material such as parasites or foreign bodies or (2) endogenous substances such as cellular elements derived from the blood or from the intraocular contents. Pigment, exudates, tumor cells, cholesterol, or calcium salts may be present. Symptoms vary with the location of the opacities, with their number, and with their density. If very numerous, there may be diffraction of light with marked reduction in vision.

Muscae volitantes. These opacities consist of fine aggregates of vitreous protein that occur in all persons. One may observe muscae volitantes when looking at a brightly illuminated field such as a blue sky or a pastel wall. They are seen drifting in and out of the visual field and tend to dart out of the field of vision when one attempts to fix upon them directly. Rarely, a patient becomes disturbed by these floaters and requires reassurance. Correction of any refractive error present makes the floaters more difficult to observe.

Hemorrhage. A minute hemorrhage into into the vitreous body adjacent to the peripheral retina is often the initial sign of retinal hole formation and may be followed by retinal separation. Bleeding into the vitreous body may occur from newly formed blood vessels, in inflammations, from the rupture of subhyaloid hemorrhages through the limiting face, and in subarachnoid hemorrhages. The blood may be evenly dispersed through the vitreous body or may be distributed in sheets. Absorption is often good, but repeated hemorrhage is followed by fibroplastic organization in the vitreous body. In diabetes mellitus, vitreous hemorrhage may be followed quickly by retinitis proliferans. Diminished vision is the chief symptom of vitreous hemorrhage. Treatment is difficult. A retinal hole must be closed to correct retinal detachment. Photocoagulation of newly formed blood vessels often prevents further bleeding in inflammatory diseases. For the most part, blood absorbs fairly well in young people, but the rate of absorption becomes increasingly slower with aging. Vitreous withdrawal and replacement with transparent cadaver vitreous is usually not successful. Systemic medications are of no value.

Asteroid hyalitis. In this condition, stellate or discoid opacities are suspended in a normal vitreous body. They may be present in part or all of the vitreous body. They appear creamy white when viewed with the ophthalmoscope but sparkle in the illumination of a biomicroscope. They are usually unilateral and usually occur in men at an average age of 60 years. There are no symptoms, and the patient is not aware of the disorder. The opacities consist of a calcium-containing lipid and appear to arise from degeneration of vitreous fibrils. There is no treatment. Unlike the opacities of synchysis scintillans, the material is distributed uniformly through the vitreous body and does gravitate.

Synchysis scintillans. Synchysis scintillans is a condition in which a vitreous body that has liquefied contains numerous crystals composed of cholesterol. They occur in eyes that have had recent recurrent uveitis or vitreous hemorrhage, and they constitute a degenerative change in the fluid vitreous body. The crystals gravitate to a dependent position in the eye and with movement fill the globe with a snowstorm of brilliant crystals that gradually settle. If the ocular disease is bilateral, the crystals are bilateral; they occur at any age. There is no treatment.

Amyloidosis. Amyloid is a homogeneous, eosinophilic material composed of glycoproteins that may be deposited in almost any body tissue (p. 449). It may occur secondary to chronic systemic disease or as a familial disease with distinctive variations. Amyloid may be deposited in every ocular tissue and give rise to proptosis, ophthalmoplegia, anterior uveitis, unequal pupillary size, and perivasculitis with retinal hemorrhages.

Opacification of the vitreous with fibrillar "glass-wool" deposits is the most characteristic ocular involvement. The opacities are gray or yellowish white in color, and vitreous fibrils are thickened and opaque, with many smaller round opacities attached to the fibrils. Vision is reduced to hand movements or light perception. The opacities prevent visualization of the retina with the ophthalmoscope. Excision of the opaque vitreous and replacement with saline solution at present appears to be the treatment of choice.

Chapter 17

The optic nerve

The optic nerve is morphologically and embryologically a tract of the central nervous system. It is organized like the white matter of the brain and contains true neuroglial cells but no sheaths or cells of Schwann; within the orbit the optic nerve is surrounded by the meninges. It is composed mainly of the axons of the ganglion cells of the retina, and these make synapse in the lateral geniculate body (vision) and pretectal region (pupil). Behind the lamina cribrosa of the eye the fibers are myelinated as far as the optic disk, but in the retina they are bare axons constituting the nerve fiber layer of the retina. In addition to these fibers there are photostatic fibers that extend to the superior colliculus, autonomic fibers, and efferent fibers extending to the retina that have no known function.

The intraocular portion of the optic nerve is the optic disk or papilla. The distribution of the retinal nerve fibers forming the papilla is shown in Fig. 19-3, and its ophthalmoscopic appearance is described on p. 142. All fibers arising nasally to the fovea centralis decussate in the optic chiasm, including those in the fovea (see Fig. 1-41). Temporal fibers do not decussate.

Symptoms and signs of optic nerve disease

The symptoms of optic nerve disease are related mainly to loss of vision. If the papillomacular bundle that is composed of fibers from the fovea centralis is involved, there is decrease of central vision. This is associated with a central scotoma (p. 126), an island of blindness involving the fixation point and surrounded by a seeing area. Involvement of peripheral fibers gives rise to defects in the peripheral visual fields. The nerve fibers in the optic tract have not yet synapsed and therefore diseases affecting them can cause a retrograde optic atrophy, but the visual field abnormality involves both eyes. Inflammation or atrophy of the optic nerve due to toxic chemicals may be associated with abnormal color vision and combined with a scotoma that involves the central fixation area and the physiologic blind spot (cecocentral scotoma, see Fig. 4-2). Inflammations of the optic nerve within the orbit may be associated with deep orbital pain aggravated by movement of the eyes.

Ophthalmoscopy plays a major role in the diagnosis of optic atrophy, papilledema, and papillitis. Attention is directed particularly to the margin of the disk, the presence or absence of a physiologic cup, pulsation of the central retinal vein, and the color of the disk (p. 142). Measurement of the central visual acuity and determination of the central visual fields, usually by means of a tangent screen, are essential to accurate diagnosis. As indicated in the outline on p. 286, the variety of diseases affecting the optic nerve is extremely large, and accurate diagnosis requires considerable attention to the history, neurologic examination, evidence of systemic disease, and awareness of the large variety of diseases that may cause similar findings.

Developmental anomalies

Hyaloid artery. The nutrition of the lens lens during the first 10 weeks of fetal development is provided mainly by the hyaloid artery, which subsequently atrophies. Occasionally a short stub of this vessel projects into the vitreous body from the center of the optic disk. It is of no clinical significance but has been a source of recurrent vitreous hemorrhage. The hyaloid artery at the 100 mm. stage of fetal development forms a fusiform enlargement, the bulb, from which arise retinal vessels. The bulb is surrounded by a small mass of neuroglial cells, Bergmeister's papilla, which may persist and give a slight elevation to the central portion of the disk.

Pits in the optic disk. Pits in the optic disk are probably atypical colobomas of the optic nerve. They are usually single and located in the inferior temporal margin of the optic disk. The pit is darker than the surrounding tissue and is usually round or oval. The pit may be shallow or as deep as 8 mm. It is from one eighth to one third the size of the disk. A small central scotoma is often present. In some 30% of the patients a typical serous chorioretinopathy (p. 270) (disciform detachment of the macula) develops.

Hyaline bodies. Hyaline bodies or drusen are bilateral, waxy, pearl-like whitish irregularities on the surface of the optic disk, usually on the nasal side (Fig. 17-1) They are formed by a deposition of hyalin that increases in size by accretion, giving a laminated structure. They have been described in association with tuberous sclerosis, angioid streaks, pseudoxanthoma elasticum, pigmentary degeneration of the retina, optic atrophy, and nervous and renal dysfunction. They may simulate

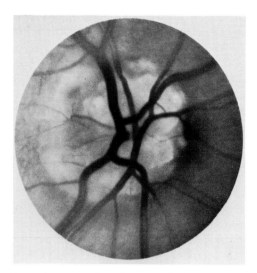

Fig. 17-1. Hyaline bodies of the optic disk. They have been described as resembling tapioca pudding.

the appearance of papilledema and may give rise to field defects.

Colobomas. Colobomas of the disk are usually associated with defective vision. The disk appears enlarged, and the nerve tissue is often displaced to the upper portion. The blood vessels may be distributed normally or may be displaced to either the periphery of the disk or to its lower portion.

Conus. Normally the choroid and the retina stop abruptly at the margin of the optic disk. Commonly the retinal pigment epithelium is heaped up at the disk margin, usually on the temporal side, and appears as a dark pigment ring. Less frequently the retinal pigment epithelium stops short of the disk, and ophthalmoscopically the choroid or the bare sclera is seen through the transparent nerve fiber layer of the retina. This usually occurs at the temporal edge of the disk and gives rise to a temporal crescent, or conus, which is often seen in myopia. When such a crescent is present at the inferior portion of the disk, it often constitutes an incomplete coloboma of the disk.

A conus surrounding the entire disk may develop in glaucoma, sclerosis of choroidal vessels, and pathologic myopia. The changes may be associated with visual field defects. In general, the disk varies little in size from patient to patient, and when it appears large, a circumpapillary conus is present.

Myelinated nerve fibers. Myelination of the optic nerve begins at the chiasm about the twenty-fourth week of fetal life and by birth has reached a point immediately behind the lamina cribrosa. In rare cases the myelination continues beyond this, and the nerve fiber layers of the retina are white in the region immediately surrounding the disk (see Fig. 15-7). When thick, a scotoma may be present, but it is always smaller than the appearance of the lesion would suggest. The condition is of no pathologic significance but should be distinguished from edema of the retina or swelling of the disk.

Optic neuritis

The optic nerve may be involved in inflammatory, degenerative, or demyelinating disease any place in its course, from the ganglion cells in the retina to the synapse of these fibers in the lateral geniculate body. The causes of optic neuritis are approximately the same irrespective of the portion of the nerve involved. The main symptom is loss of central visual acuity and a central scotoma. In retrobulbar neuritis the inflammation affects the optic nerve behind the optic disk. The ophthalmoscopic appearance of the disk is normal, although optic atrophy (p. 285) may follow. If the inflammation involves the intraocular portion of the nerve, the abnormality is called papillitis, and inflammatory changes of the disk are evident ophthalmoscopically. When the disk and the retina are both involved, the condition is termed neuroretinitis.

Optic neuritis may be an acute or a chronic process characterized by loss of central vision and development of a central scotoma demonstrated by visual field examination. The loss of vision varies from a very slight depression to complete loss of light perception. The loss of vision may occur abruptly over a period of a few hours, and recovery may be equally precipitous. In other patients the visual decrease develops slowly. The disease may be unilateral or bilateral.

Retrobulbar inflammation of the optic nerve in the posterior portion of the orbit where it is in close relationship with the superior rectus and medial rectus muscles gives rise to pain on movement of the eye. There may be tenderness on palpation. This pain combined with loss of central vision, a central scotoma, and the absence of any ophthalmoscopic changes often suggests the diagnosis of retrobulbar neuritis. If the causative agent is removed or if the condition occurs in the course of a demyelinating disease, the inflammation may run its course in 2 to 6 weeks, and a complete recovery ensues. A residue of optic atrophy affecting the papillomacular bundle, however, may remain and be combined with decreased central visual acuity.

Some causes of optic neuritis

I. Demyelinating disease
II. Vascular disease
   A. Atherosclerosis
   B. Arteriolar sclerosis (hypertension)
   C. Giant cell vasculitis
III. Nutritional disease: pellagra, beriberi
IV. Toxic substances
V. Infectious disease: syphilis, tuberculosis, malaria, pneumonia, measles
VI. Pernicious anemia
VII. Blood loss
VIII. Orbital disease: thyroid tumors
IX. Lactation
X. Malignant disease
XI. Diabetic neuropathy
XII. Intracranial disease: tumors, meningitis, etc.

An optic neuritis involving the intra-ocular portion of the optic nerve causes hyperemia and edema of the disk known as papillitis. Central vision is reduced, and a central scotoma is present. The disk appears much smaller than normal because the contrast with the surrounding fundus is diminished. The disk margins are obscured, and there is venous dilation. The physiologic cup is obliterated. Flame-shaped hemorrhages may occur on the surface of the disk and the adjacent retina. In severe inflammations, retinal deposits occur, and these may be grouped about the fovea centralis in a circinate pattern. The swelling of the disk seldom exceeds 2 diopters. With persistence of the swelling, there may be glial tissue proliferation from the disk along the retinal vessels and the development of a secondary optic atrophy (p. 285). Papillitis is distinguished from papilledema by the early decrease in central visual acuity, its unilaterality, the limited elevation of the disk, and the occurrence of inflammatory cells in the vitreous body.

In individuals aged 20 to 44 years, demyelinating disease is considered the chief cause of optic neuritis, although it may not be demonstrated until some time has passed after the initial attack. An individual in this age group having an initial bout of optic neuritis has a 40 to 50% chance of multiple sclerosis developing within 10 to 15 years. In those instances in which there is a single attack that never recurs, an infection with a neurotrophic virus is assumed to be the cause.

After the age of 45 years, the most common cause of optic neuritis is vascular disease affecting the blood supply of the optic nerve. This may involve atherosclerosis, arteriolar sclerosis in hypertension, or giant cell vasculitis.

It is often impossible to find the cause of optic neuritis. In eyes enucleated because of inflammation of the retina or the choroid, there is often an extension of the inflammatory process to the optic nerve. The primary disease dominates the clinical picture, and the optic neuritis is incidental.

Vitamin B deficiency may give rise to a bilateral optic neuritis, particularly in individuals in whom alcohol is the main source of calories. Vision improves if vitamin B is provided, even though the alcohol consumption is unrestricted. Patients with pellagra and beriberi may have a similar bilateral optic neuritis.

Pernicious anemia, diabetic neuropathy, exophthalmic thyroid disease, severe hemorrhage, lactation, infectious diseases, and toxic substances may be associated with optic neuritis. Sinus disease and foci of infection are considered unlikely causes, although in previous years the spontaneous improvement often seen in optic neuritis was attributed to treatment of these infections.

Treatment must be directed to the cause. In those numerous instances in which a cause cannot be demonstrated, the main reliance is upon administration of systemic corticosteroids and vitamin B.

Pseudoptic neuritis. Pseudoptic neuritis or pseudopapillitis is the name given to congenital abnormalities of the optic disk in which the disk margins are blurred by the heaping up of nerve fibers, accentuated by an excess of glial tissue. The disk has a dirty, grayish appearance with ill-defined margins, frequently most marked on the nasal side. It occurs most commonly in eyes that are hyperopic. There is no interference with vision, and the blood vessels are normal. The condition is not progressive and requires no treatment.

Papilledema

The optic nerve is surrounded by the meningeal sheaths of the brain. Increased intracranial pressure thus may be transmitted to the subarachnoid space surrounding the optic nerve. The central retinal vein, which courses from the retina through the optic nerve, turns abruptly about 12 mm. behind the globe and exits from the nerve, passing through the meningeal sheaths. It is postulated that the vein is compressed by the high pressure as it passes through the subarachnoid space and that there is interference with normal venous drainage. This in turn causes a passive edema of the optic nerve and disk without interference of vision.

Papilledema (Fig. 17-2) begins at the superior and inferior disk margins, then involves the nasal side, and finally involves the temporal side. The physiologic cup becomes obliterated, and there is anterior displacement of the central vessels on the surface of the optic disk. The retinal veins become markedly dilated, and there is nearly always a loss of spontaneous or induced venous pulsation. The disk becomes elevated and occupies a larger area than usual. This displaces the retina from the disk margins and causes the physiologic blind spot to be enlarged on perimetric measurement. Hemorrhages may occur on the surface of the disk and in the nerve fiber layer of the retina. These may break through into the vitreous body. A retinal edema may develop, combined with exudates in the macular region. In the early stages, central visual acuity is not affected, in contrast to inflammations of the optic nerve. If papilledema persists, there is ultimate interference with central visual acuity and the development of a secondary type of optic atrophy.

The degree of papilledema is often pro-

A
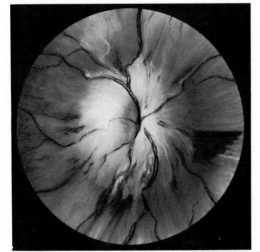

B
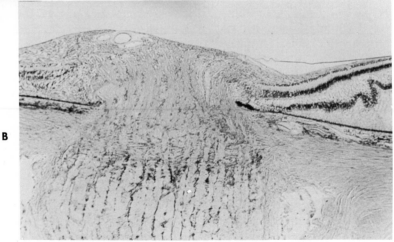

Fig. 17-2. Papilledema. **A,** Note preretinal hemorrhage adjacent to the disk. **B,** Note how the swollen optic disk has pushed the retina from the disk margins. This accounts for the enlargement of the blind spot demonstrated with tangent screen perimetry. (Hematoxylin and eosin stain; ×47.)

portionate to the increase in the intracranial pressure. However, papilledema does not always accompany increased intracranial pressure. When papilledema does not occur in increased intracranial pressure, it is postulated that the subarachnoid space surrounding the optic nerve is not in free communication with the intracranial subarachnoid space. When lumbar puncture does not demonstrate increased intracranial pressure, a block in the brain stem may be the cause of the low intraspinal pressure.

Brain tumors located below the tentorium are considered to be more likely to produce papilledema than those located above. Papilledema may occur in blood dyscrasias and in hypertensive cardiovascular disease. In hypertensive cardiovascular disease the occurrence of cottonwool spots in the retina and the arteriolar constriction serve to distinguish hypertensive papilledema from that due to intracranial neoplasms. Papilledema is seen in pseudotumor cerebri, congenital hydrocephalus, craniosynostosis, and following head injury. Pulmonary insufficiency, particularly that associated with cystic fibrosis of the pancreas, may cause the condition.

Papilledema is usually bilateral. Marked unilateral swelling of the optic disk is more likely due to an optic neuritis that involves the nerve between the globe and the exit of the central retinal vein. Vision is reduced, and a central scotoma is present. When unilateral optic atrophy occurs prior to a condition causing papilledema to develop, the atrophic nerve does not swell.

Treatment must be directed to the cause. Persistent papilledema is associated with ultimate loss of vision and secondary optic atrophy. Decompression procedures are indicated to preserve vision.

Optic atrophy

Optic atrophy is the end result of diseases or injuries of the optic nerve causing loss of axis cylinders and myelin sheaths. There is always an associated change in the visual field or in the central visual acuity or in both. If the lesion causing the optic atrophy is in the retina, an ascending optic atrophy occurs, terminating in the lateral geniculate body. Descending optic atrophy follows diseases of the optic nerve in the cranium or in the orbit.

The disease is called primary if the optic nerve is atrophic and is without evidence of preceding edema or inflammation. It is called secondary if there is gliosis with tissue overgrowth, causing blurred, irregular disk margins. The same disease, however, may cause either a primary or a secondary optic atrophy, the only difference being an inflammatory or edematous disturbance of the disk prior to the onset of the optic atrophy.

The chief symptom of optic atrophy is loss of vision. Depending upon the disease, this may involve central or peripheral vision. Commonly it may require examination of the visual fields to demonstrate. The failure to demonstrate a defect by means of confrontation fields does not exclude a field defect that may require extremely small stimuli to detect.

Primary optic atrophy. In primary optic atrophy the number of nerve fibers in the optic nerve is reduced, and there is a loss of the capillaries nourishing the optic disk. The disk appears distinct with sharp margins, and it has a pale pink to white color. The amount of pallor does not parallel the severity of the atrophy. The atrophy may be limited to only a portion of the nerve.

Primary optic atrophy is seen most commonly in glaucoma in which there is also cupping of the nerve. It occurs in the late stages of retinitis pigmentosa and diffuse chorioretinitis. In macular lesions the optic atrophy may be limited to the papillomacular bundle. In central artery closure and following quinine poisoning the optic nerve may be waxy white, and the retinal vessels are small, white cords in which blood cannot be seen. In tabes dorsalis, following methyl alcohol poisoning, in brain tumors affecting the axons anterior to the synapse of the lateral geniculate body, and following trauma to the optic nerve posterior to the globe, the disk is sharply defined and dirty white in color, with no ophthalmoscopic evidence of the cause.

Secondary optic atrophy. In secondary optic atrophy there is preceding swelling of the optic disk, arising either from papilledema or papillitis. Ophthalmoscopically the disk margins appear blurred, the lamina cribrosa is obscured, and there is gliosis over the surface of the disk and extending to the retina. The blood vessels may be distorted by this scar tissue. Secondary optic atrophy may be observed following papillitis, prolonged papilledema, and occlusion of the central vein.

Optic nerve tumors

Optic nerve tumors are exceedingly uncommon. Retinoblastomas, retinal gliomas, and malignant melanomas of the choroid may extend to involve the optic nerve. A melanocytoma of the optic disk has an ophthalmoscopic appearance of a black minute mass lying upon the optic disk. It is entirely benign.

Gliomas. Gliomas of the optic nerve and and chiasm are associated with neurofibromatosis in 16% of the cases. The remainder are mainly astrocytomas, but all types may occur. The tumor usually originates in the orbital portion of the optic nerve during the first decade of life. Loss of vision occurs early, and there may be an associated optic atrophy or edema of the disk. Proptosis is usually straight forward or down and forward. The optic foramen may be markedly enlarged.

Meningiomas. Meningiomas of the optic optic nerve arise either in the meninges

Etiologic classification of optic atrophy

I. Compression
   A. Tumors: neoplastic, aneurysm
   B. Bony overgrowth: Paget's disease, craniosynostosis
   C. Adhesions: opticochiasmic arachnoiditis
II. Following retinal ganglion cell disease
   A. Chorioretinal inflammations, degenerations, atrophy
   B. Primary pigmentary degeneration of the retina
   C. Cerebromacular degenerations
III. Hereditary
   A. Leber's disease
IV. Inflammatory
   A. Demyelinating disease
   B. Meningitis, encephalitis, abscess
   C. Syphilis
   D. Optic neuritis
   E. Metastatic septicemia
V. Ischemic
   A. Arterial occlusive disease: retina, disk, nerve or tract
      1. Arteriosclerosis
      2. Giant cell vasculitis
      3. Lupus erythematosus
   B. Blood loss
   C. Glaucoma
VI. Following papilledema
VII. Toxic
   A. Chemical: arsenic, lead, methyl alcohol, quinine, tobacco and alcohol (?)
   B. Vitamin B deficiency
      1. Beriberi
      2. Thiamine deficiency
VIII. Miscellaneous
   A. Diabetes mellitus
   B. Pernicious anemia
   C. Lipoidoses
   D. Mucopolysaccharidosis

surrounding the nerve or extend from the cranial cavity. They produce proptosis, optic atrophy, and visual loss. Occasionally the optic nerve may be involved in its intraocular portion.

Chapter 18

The lens

The lens is a transparent, avascular, biconvex structure held in position behind the pupil by the zonular fibers. It is entirely surrounded by a capsule and has a single layer of epithelial cells beneath the anterior capsule. A "nucleus" located centrally is surrounded by a cortex consisting of more recently formed lens fibers. Throughout life new lens fibers are formed at the equator, migrate inward, and ultimately become compressed at the nucleus. The old lens fibers are never lost but form the inelastic nucleus. Inasmuch as the lens has no blood supply, its metabolism is mainly anaerobic, and most of its energy is derived from glycolysis. The lactic acid formed is not metabolized further but is excreted into the aqueous humor.

The lens and the cornea are the main refracting surfaces of the eye. The inherent elasticity of the lens causes it to become more spherical when zonular fibers relax after the ciliary muscle contracts, a process known as accommodation (p. 86). Because of compression of mature fibers in the nucleus, the lens gradually loses its inherent elasticity, and usually by the age of 45 years the change in shape in response to ciliary muscle contraction is too slight to provide additional refractive power for near work, a condition of presbyopia (p. 352).

The lens is transparent because it contains only a few cells and because all of its components have approximately the same index of refraction. Any loss of transparen-cy is called cataract or, less alarmingly to a patient, a lens opacity. Cataracts essentially arise from protein denaturation and the accumulation of water.

Symptoms and signs of diseases of the lens

The symptoms of diseases of the lens are entirely related to vision. With presbyopia, there is failure of near vision. With cataract formation, there may be a decrease of vision for far and near. Lens opacities in the nucleus cause an increase in the index of refraction and increased refractive power of the anterior segment. This may cause a myopia so that the patient unexpectedly is able to read again without glasses, although, of course, the myopia reduces uncorrected distant visual acuity. Rarely, lens opacities in the visual axis cause an optical defect in which two blurred retinal images are formed, a monocular diplopia. An opacity due to increased water content is often reversible, causing a variation in visual acuity. The coincidence of visual improvement while using a proprietary medication to treat cataract has led to a number of cataract remedies, all inefficacious.

Dislocation of the lens so that it is not in the visual axis eliminates its refractive power, and the eye is comparable to one from which the lens has been removed. A convex lens is required for clear distant vision, and an additional convex lens is needed for near work. In subluxation of the lens the visual axis passes through the edge of the lens so that the refractive power is reduced and an irregular astigmatism occurs; these may vary as the lens changes in position. A dislocated lens may cause a secondary glaucoma if it lodges in the anterior chamber. A markedly swollen lens may also interfere with aqueous humor drainage and may cause a secondary glaucoma. Rupture of the lens capsule causes a cataract but also an inflammatory reaction in the anterior segment that may be complicated by glaucoma.

Inspection of the details of the lens structure usually requires examination with a biomicroscope. Inspection using a penlight and a condensing lens will indicate only gross abnormalities. When the lens is examined with an ophthalmoscope and the pupil is widely dilated, cataracts are seen as dark opacities against the red background of the fundus reflex. If the lens is displaced, the iris loses support and becomes tremulous, the condition of iridodonesis; the anterior chamber is deeper. The image normally reflected from the anterior lens surface is absent. If a lens is dislocated into the vitreous body, it may be seen with the ophthalmoscope in the region to which it has gravitated as a circular, dark area, if it is cataractous, or as a black-rimmed globule magnifying the retina beneath it, if it is transparent.

The number of abnormalities possible for the lens is limited. It may have variations in size, shape, or position, or it may have a loss of transparency. It may reflect metabolic, cutaneous, and connective tissue disturbances as well as being a sensitive index of aging.

Developmental anomalies
Coloboma

In this condition there is a minute notch in the equator of the lens. The defect is not primarily in the lens—it is in a failure of zonular fibers to develop in a sector, permitting relaxation of a portion of the lens periphery. A retinal detachment may occur. A similar coloboma may follow blunt contusion to the eye. The condition is observed only with the pupil maximally dilated. Treatment is not indicated.

Spherophakia (microphakia)

In this condition the lens is small and has increased anterior and posterior curvature. The zonular fibers are easily visible with pupillary dilation, and since the iris lacks support, it is tremulous. Subluxation is common, apparently because of the weakened zonule. Glaucoma occurs because the small lens blocks the pupil. The increased refractive power of the lens causes a myopia.

Spherophakia may be part of a hereditary syndrome (Weil-Marchesani) in which there is short stature, short, stubby fingers, and mental retardation. The syndrome constitutes a hyperplastic form of congenital mesodermal dystrophy in contrast to Marfan's syndrome, which is hypoplastic. Treatment is directed mainly toward the prevention of a pupillary-block glaucoma by means of an iridectomy.

Lenticonus

Lenticonus is a familial abnormality in which there is a variation in curvature of the lens, with the formation of a cone at the posterior or anterior pole. Ophthalmoscopy shows a dark disk present in the center of the pupil. The condition involves male individuals predominantly and is often bilateral. Nephritis occurs commonly.

Ectopia lentis

When the lens loses the support provided by the zonular fibers, it dislocates either into the vitreous cavity or into the anterior chamber (Fig. 18-1). If some, but not all, of the zonular fibers remain attached, they act as a hinge so that the lens is subluxated from its usual position. Examination indicates the anterior chamber to be deeper than normal and the iris

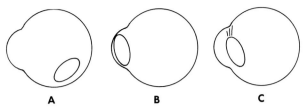

Fig. 18-1. A, Dislocation of the lens into the vitreous cavity. **B,** Dislocation of the lens into the anterior chamber, an abnormality that leads to pupillary-block glaucoma. **C,** Subluxation of the lens with the remaining zonular fibers acting as a hinge.

to be tremulous (iridodonesis) because it has lost its posterior support. The symptoms are mainly optical since absence of a major refracting element causes the eye to become markedly hyperopic and to lose the accommodation provided by the lens. Migration of a dislocated lens into the anterior chamber causes an acute secondary glaucoma. Often glaucoma occurs with a lens in the vitreous cavity, although the mechanism is unclear. A subluxated lens may with time become dislocated, but this course is not inevitable.

The same conditions are responsible for either subluxation or dislocation: ocular trauma, particularly in an individual with latent syphilis; deliberate dislocation as a surgical procedure (couching); and a variety of hereditary diseases, aniridia, Marfan's syndrome, homocystinuria, spherophakia, and sometimes an autosomal recessive abnormality without other defects.

Treatment is directed toward correction of the optical defect by means of spectacles or contact lenses. The optical results of lens extraction are often poor.

Marfan's syndrome. Marfan's syndrome (p. 444) is a widespread systemic abnormality of connective tissue transmitted as an autosomal dominant defect. Ectopia lentis occurs in many but not all cases. The lens is often subluxated upward and nasally so that its equator can be seen in the pupil. Severe myopia is common. The systemic manifestations include aortic dilation, dissecting aneurysms of the aorta,

muscular underdevelopment, femoral and diaphragmatic hernias, and multiple skeletal defects, particularly arachnodactyly (spider-fingers).

Homocystinuria. Homocystinuria (p. 433) is a widespread abnormality characterized by dislocation of the lens, mental retardation, and the excretion of an excessive amount of homocystine in the urine. The latter defect is qualitatively detected by a cyanide-nitroprusside test of the urine, and cystinuria and homocystinuria are differentiated by paper electrophoresis. Excessive amounts of homocystine in the urine result from a deficiency in the enzyme cystathionine synthetase, which is involved in the conversion of homocystine to cystathionine.

Ectopia lentis is progressive, and the dislocated lens commonly causes a pupillary-block glaucoma. Myocardial infarction, stroke, and other manifestations of arterial or venous thrombosis are extremely common. Many clinical features suggest Marfan's syndrome, but demonstration of the inborn error of metabolism distinguishes the two conditions. Unlike other inborn errors of metabolism, homocystinuria is transmitted as an autosomal recessive. A variety of therapeutic attempts to prevent the development of the defects through supplementation of the diet are currently under study.

Dislocation of the lens. Dislocation of the lens into the vitreous body is usually a result of trauma. Curiously, syphilis is common in individuals with traumatic dislocation of the lens. Deliberate dislocation (couching) is as ancient a surgical procedure as circumcision and trepanation, and it is still performed illegally in the treatment of cataract in remote parts of India. The lens in the vitreous body may be tolerated for long periods or may cause an inflammation or a secondary glaucoma. An immediate and severe glaucoma occurs if it is trapped in the anterior chamber. When necessary to remove a dislocated lens, the surgery is difficult. Often the patient is placed face downward, causing the lens to gravitate into the anterior chamber. It is trapped in the anterior chamber by placing needles through the sclera so as to pass either through the lens or behind it. Some surgeons make a corneoscleral incision as for cataract extraction, remove the vitreous body with a large needle, pluck out the lens, and return the vitreous body to the eye. Liquid nitrogen or carbon dioxide snow devices used to freeze the lens may be of unusual value in the removal of dislocated and subluxated lenses. The lens freezes before the surrounding vitreous body and adheres to the probe, allowing it to be lifted from the eye through a cataract incision.

Cataract

A cataract is any opacity occurring in the normally transparent lens. It arises either because of hydration or denaturation of the lens protein; often both processes occur. Many classifications are used:

1. According to the age of onset
   a. Congenital d. Adult
   b. Infantile   e. Senile
   c. Juvenile
2. According to the location of the opacity
   a. Nuclear   c. Capsular
   b. Cortical   d. Subcapsular
3. According to the degree of opacity present
   a. Immature when transparent lens fibers are present
   b. Mature when the entire lens has become opaque
   c. Hypermature when liquefaction of the opaque lens fibers occurs
4. According to the rate of development
   a. Stationary
   b. Progressive
5. On the basis of appearance with the biomicroscope
   a. Lamellar
   b. Coralliform
   c. Punctate and many others
6. On the basis of the etiology
   a. Hereditary
   b. Traumatic
   c. Metabolic
   d. Rare types often occurring with specific syndromes

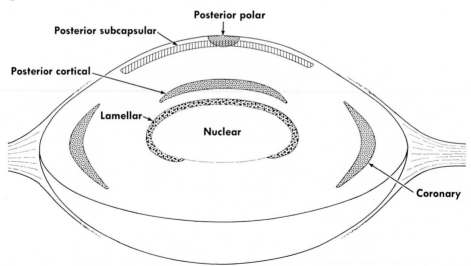

Fig. 18-2. Location of lens opacities.

No classification of cataract is entirely satisfactory. Most cataracts can probably be described loosely as congenital, senile, traumatic, or secondary to a systemic or an ocular disorder. The most significant clinical points are the following: (1) whether visual improvement will follow surgery if required and (2) whether or not a systemic disease is present and, if present, whether it has a causal relationship with the cataract.

Congenital cataract

At least 90% of the general population have minute opacities in their lenses that can be seen only with the biomicroscope (Fig. 18-2). These never progress and do not interfere with vision. Such minimal opacities are of some medicolegal importance in the differentiation of traumatic cataract, which they do not resemble. They consist of multiple, fine, irregularly shaped opacities in the central or peripheral areas of the lens. The diagnosis is based upon their morphologic characteristics as seen with a slit lamp.

Congenital cataracts severe enough to reduce vision to an extent that surgery is considered are relatively uncommon. Many hereditary types of cataract are not present at birth but develop months and years later, often paralleling the rate of development observed in other members of the family. Severe cataract present at birth suggests severe maternal infection during the first trimester of pregnancy.

History and examination. In any patient in whom a congenital cataract is diagnosed, a family history should be obtained. There is no quicker way of initiating a study of the family than observing the eyes of the parents accompanying a young patient. In some families there is a similarity of the type and progress of the cataract and associated ocular defects.

The maternal history of infection during gestation may be helpful in the diagnosis of congenital cataract. Maternal rubella during the first trimester of pregnancy is the most significant disease, although cataract may be associated with other virus infections and with toxoplasmosis.

Congenital cataracts often occur with other ocular defects and systemic abnormalities. Hearing should be tested. The occurrence of supernumerary fingers and toes, gross abnormality in the development of the bones of the face or skull, or disproportion of the bones of the extremities should be sought. Flaccidity of the muscles should be investigated. Evidence of mental retardation and delayed physical development should be sought, particularly with reference to delayed psychomotor development such as failure to sit or stand or talk at anticipated age levels.

Urinalysis is the single most important laboratory study. A reducing substance in the urine may occur with galactosemia, and further progression of the cataract and mental retardation may be prevented by removing galactose from the diet. Test tapes usually are directed to glucose solely and do not measure other reducing substances. Reducing substance and albumin may occur in the urine in the oculocerebrorenal syndrome, a moderately common cause of congenital cataract. Aminoaciduria occurs in a variety of congenital disorders associated with cataract.

Examination and evaluation of the extent and density of the lens opacity is the most important part of the ocular examination. This determines the method and the time of surgery of congenital cataract. In very young infants, examination is based upon the ophthalmoscopic pattern and whether or not any portion of the fundus is visible when the pupils are dilated. The response to opticokinetic nystagmus is a gross test, but if a nystagmus can be elicited, surgery probably will not be required. In older children, disproportionate reduction of vision for the severity

Classification of cataract

I. Eye otherwise healthy and no systemic disease
  A. Nearly all senile cataracts
  B. Most adult cataracts
  C. Some congenital cataracts
  D. Premature infants (develop about the age of 3 years)

II. Additional ocular defects present but no systemic disease
  A. Microphthalmia
  B. Aniridia
  C. Many congenital cataracts
  D. Retinitis pigmentosa
  E. Glaucoma, absolute
  F. Intraocular inflammation
  G. Retrolental fibroplasia
  H. Retinal detachment

III. Cataract and systemic disorders (associated ocular defects common)
  A. Generalized
    1. Maternal rubella, other viral infections, and toxoplasmosis in first trimester of pregnancy (associated deafness, heart defects)
    2. Marfan's syndrome (arachnodactyly, ectopia lentis, mesodermal hypoplasia)
    3. Laurence-Moon-Biedl syndrome (retinitis pigmentosa, obesity, polydactyly, hypogenitalism, mental retardation)
    4. Infections, granulomas, etc. causing uveitis with complicated cataract
  B. Cutaneous
    1. Atopic dermatitis (15 to 25 years of age)
    2. Rothmund's syndrome (onset 3 to 6 months)
    3. Congenital ichthyosis
    4. Incontinentia pigmenti
    5. Werner's syndrome (onset after puberty)
  C. Neurologic
    1. Mental deficiency
    2. Mongolism
  D. Metabolic
    1. Diabetes mellitus (solely in growth-onset diabetes)
    2. Galactosemia (never at birth; shortly after)
    3. Lowe's syndrome (oculocerebrorenal syndrome)
    4. Hypocalcemia (with tetany)
    5. Pituitary disease (rare)
    6. Cretinism
  E. Muscular
    1. Myotonic dystrophy (20 to 30 years of age)
  F. Bone
    1. Mandibulofacial dysostosis
    2. Osteitis fibrosa and skin pigmentation
    3. Stippled epiphysis

IV. Miscellaneous
  A. Senile
  B. Toxic
    1. Corticosteroids systemically for long periods
    2. Corticosteroids locally
    3. Ergot
    4. Naphthalene
    5. Dinitrophenol
    6. Triparanol (Mer/29)

C. Traumatic
    1. Ruptured capsule (with retained foreign body)
    2. Intact capsule
        a. Vossius ring (anterior)
        b. Posterior subcapsular
D. Electromagnetic radiation
    1. Infrared (iris absorption with heat coagulation of underlying lens; also true exfoliation of lens capsule)
    2. Microwaves (focused, high energy, a heating effect)
    3. Ionizing radiation (cataractogenic dose varies with energy and type; younger lens more vulnerable)

of the lens opacity suggests amblyopia ex anopsia or associated defects.

Nonsurgical treatment. If visual acuity with lenses is better than 20/70, surgery is not indicated in eyes that are normal except for the congenital cataract. This amount of vision permits schooling with individuals who have normal eyesight. Near, rather than distant, vision is the critical measurement. Not uncommonly a disproportion exists between near and far vision, and these children can often see much smaller print than anticipated from their distance central acuity.

If there are associated ocular defects such as retinal or choroidal abnormalities, strabismus, nystagmus, or microphthalmia, it is unwise to recommend surgery if corrected vision is better than 20/200. It is unlikely that such eyes will show a significant improvement even with a perfectly black pupil and unhindered light transmission.

Surgery is not indicated to improve vision in monocular congenital cataract inasmuch as vision is rarely improved to more than 20/200 with correction. On occasion, lens extraction may be necessary in monocular opacities because of glaucoma, intraocular inflammation induced by maturity of the lens, or for cosmetic purposes, but significant improvement in vision is uncommon.

Surgical treatment. Most attention is devoted to patients in whom the opacity is marked enough to interfere with central vision. Such cataracts may be classified as follows: (1) bilateral complete cataract, either present at birth or developing during the first few months of life; (2) severe involvement of both eyes without complete opacification of the lenses; (3) mild involvement of the lens of one eye and severe involvement of the other; (4) bilateral, dense central opacities allowing adequate vision with dilated pupils but inadequate vision when pupils are small; and (5) moderate involvement of both eyes.

In the first and second groups, operation is indicated when the density is severe enough to preclude useful vision. In the third group, if vision is better than 20/70 in one eye under all conditions, the patient will lead a fairly normal life if no surgery is done. In the fourth group, satisfactory vision may be obtained by keeping the pupils dilated and by prescribing suitable lenses. This is not feasible over a long period of years, and surgery will ultimately have to be done. In the fifth group there are many borderline cases, and if vision is 20/70 or better in both eyes under all conditions, surgery should not be done.

There are several methods of removing congenital cataracts. Usually surgery is deferred until at least the child's second year, when more adequate evaluation of vision can be made. The selection of the procedure is governed to some degree by whether or not the eye is of normal size and whether the pupil can be widely dilated. If the pupil does not dilate well or if the eye appears small, it is necessary to do a complete iridectomy. Inasmuch as this necessitates corneoscleral incision, the anterior lens capsule may be opened at this time and the lens cortex removed either by irrigation or by suction.

If the pupil dilates widely and the eye is of normal size, an opening may be made in the anterior capsule with a needle-knife and the lens permitted to absorb. The cortex and the nucleus, which is insoluble in the adult, are dissolved by the proteolytic enzymes present in the aqueous humor, which produce rapid absorption. Repeated needlings are frequently necessary. Later the anterior capsule may proliferate, causing continued opacification of the pupillary area. If too large an opening is initially made in the lens capsule, the rapid hydration of lens cortex may cause a severe secondary glaucoma that necessitates immediate removal of the lens material. In recent years techniques designed to remove the lens by aspiration have become popular.

A congenital cataract is never removed intracapsularly because the posterior capsule is frequently bound to the anterior vitreous face, and it is impossible to remove the lens without disturbing or removing much of the vitreous body from the eye.

Complications. The complications following surgery for congenital cataract involve a number of conditions:

1. Glaucoma may be due to iris bombé arising from postoperative iridocyclitis.

2. Peripheral anterior synechiae may arise from delayed formation of the anterior chamber and cause glaucoma.

3. Detachment of the retina is a common cause of blindness following congenital cataract surgery. It often occurs 20 or more years later.

4. Loss of vitreous humor at the time of surgery leads very frequently to retinal detachment and to an occluded pupil. Vitreous humor in the anterior chamber interferes with the absorption of lens cortex and frequently results in persistent cortex in the anterior chamber, with an unsatisfactory visual result.

Results. The visual results of surgery for congenital cataract are poor. Poor vision often is the result of ocular defects present in addition to the congenital cataracts. In one series of 233 eyes, 35.5% had vision of 20/40 or better, whereas 25% had vision of 20/200 or less, and 6% were blind. In another series, only 11% obtained a vision of 20/70 or better, whereas 42% had vision of less than 20/200. Some 37% of patients with congenital cataracts were found to have serious associated ocular defects.

Special types. Special types of congenital cataract include lamellar cataract (zonular) and those associated with maternal rubella, Lowe's syndrome, mental retardation (Sjögren), mongolism, and galactosemia.

Lamellar cataract (zonular). Lamellar cataract is a common type of cataract and

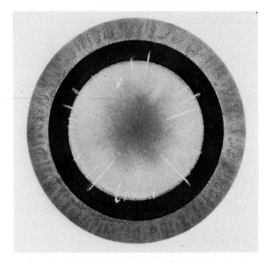

Fig. 18-3. Lamellar (zonular) cataract with riders.

may develop up to a year after birth (Fig. 18-3). It is usually bilateral and is often transmitted as a dominant trait without other abnormality. It consists of a series of concentric, thin sheets (lamellas) of opacities surrounded by clear lens. At the edge of the opacity there may be U-shaped riders extending from the anterior nucleus face to the posterior surface. Vision may be quite good or markedly reduced, depending upon the density of the opacity. Vision may become worse at puberty, necessitating surgery. A similar opacity occurs in hypocalcemia in infancy. A unilateral lamellar cataract may follow contusion of the eye.

Maternal rubella. Maternal rubella during the first trimester of pregnancy may cause widespread ocular and systemic defects. The incidence of complications varies with different strains of the virus and are more severe the earlier in pregnancy the rubella occurs. The lens may be entirely opaque or there may be a central pearly white opacity. Nystagmus, strabismus, corneal opacities, microphthalmia, retinal pigmentation, and glaucoma have been described in addition to cataract. The pupil dilates poorly, and surgical results have not been satisfactory.

A similar embryopathy has been reported as occurring with maternal herpes zoster and toxoplasmosis acquired during the first trimester. It seems likely that in many instances of maternal infection causing severe deformities, spontaneous abortion occurs.

Oculocerebrorenal syndrome (Lowe). Lowe's syndrome is a familial disease associated with a renal tubular lesion, a vitamin-resistant renal rickets, retarded physical and mental development, hypotonia, and cataracts or glaucoma. The cataract is present at birth, and several different types have been described: complete, nuclear, and posterior polar. Glaucoma may occur independently or may be associated with cataract. There are aminoaciduria, albuminuria, and intermittent glycosuria. Bony and constitutional changes occur, and there may be many constitutional signs. Only occurrences in males have been described thus far.

Congenital cataract with mental retardation (Sjögren). Congenital cataract with mental retardation is an autosomal recessive abnormality in which the cataract develops during the first year of life, and deficient mentation develops after the fourth year. The cataracts are usually lamellar and often progress to involve the entire lens. Skeletal deformities, epilepsy, and deafness have been reported. Congenital cataract, spinocerebellar ataxia, and mental retardation (Marinesco and Sjögren) are transmitted as an autosomal recessive, and consanguinity of the parents is frequent. There may be widespread bony and central nervous system changes.

Mongolism. Mongolism is a frequent type of mental retardation that is associated with widespread systemic and ocular defects. There is both physical and mental retardation. The stature is small, the face is round and mongoloid in appearance, the skull is small, there is obesity, hypogenitalism is common, and there is generalized laxity of ligaments and hypotonia. The intelligence quotient is between 20 and 50.

The eyes are widely separated, and the palpebral fissures are narrow and run obliquely down and inward. Epicanthus is common. The free edge of the upper lid is markedly arched. The iris is light blue in color with speckled white or light-colored dots in the ciliary portion (Brushfield's spots). These occur in normal individuals and are said to be present at birth in all mongoloids. They tend to disappear with increasing pigmentation of the iris.

Various types of cataract may occur: lamellar, posterior polar, sutural, and peripheral. For the most part, the opacities are not marked. Nystagmus may occur, and high myopia is common.

Two types of chromosomal abnormality occur. The most common is trisomy of the 21 chromosome pair, resulting in a total of 47 chromosomes. The involvement of children of older mothers is related to the tendency for nondisjunction of older ova. The other type of chromosomal anomaly is translocation, which is the exchange of chromosomal segments between nonhomologous chromosomes. This abnormality appears to be genetic and occurs in children of younger mothers.

Galactosemia. Galactosemia is a congenital and hereditary abnormality of lactose metabolism in which there is impairment of enzymatic conversion of galactose to glucose (p. 437). The children are normal at birth but soon develop feeding problems, with vomiting, diarrhea, and failure to thrive. Bilateral cataracts develop in lenses that were entirely normal at the time of birth. In the early stages there appears to be an oily drop in the center of the lens. A zonular cataract may develop. Treatment involves exclusion of milk and other sources of galactose from the diet. Cataract, mental retardation, and liver impairment may be avoided by early recognition of the disorder. The cataracts respond well to surgery when it is required.

Acquired cataract

Acquired cataracts include those that occur sporadically as a result of toxins, systemic disease, injury, damage from intraocular inflammation, and aging. Many abnormalities cause characteristic morphologic changes that may be distinguished by biomicroscopic examination.

Symptoms. The chief symptom of acquired cataract is a gradual decrease of vision that is not associated with pain or inflammation of the eye. There may be early unilateral diplopia due to the lens opacity splitting light bundles, but this disappears with further decrease in vision.

Vision is often better in dim illumination in which there is dilation of the pupil. Patients may complain of spots in the visual field that, unlike those arising from vitreous floaters, remain fixed and do not dart about with movements of the eye. In nuclear cataracts there is often a marked increase in the refractive power of the lens, and patients may discover that they are able to read once again without glasses. The improvement is transient and is associated with a decrease of uncorrected vision for distance.

Examination. Examination of the lens with the ophthalmoscope may indicate a gross opacity filling the pupillary aperture or an opacity silhouetted against the red background of the fundus. A nuclear opacity is located centrally and usually appears larger than a posterior subcapsular opacity. A peripheral cortical opacity gives rise to the appearance of spokes, with only their periphery evident. Usually pupillary dilation is necessary to examine the lens adequately.

Ocular examination is particularly directed to evidence of injury or inflammation to account for the lens opacity. Usually these factors are brought out in the history. Roentgen-ray examination to dem-

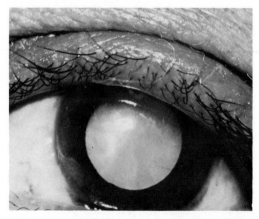

Fig. 18-4. Cataract visible with direct illumination.

onstrate a foreign body is indicated if there is a history of injury followed by lens opacity. General physical examination and laboratory studies do not indicate the etiology except in the relatively youthful. Diabetic cataracts occur usually about the age of 20 years. Hypocalcemic opacities are associated with tetany. The main differential diagnosis involves determining whether the cataract is due to toxins, trauma, or senile changes.

Medical treatment. There is no treatment that will restore the denatured protein of the cataractous lens to its original transparent state. However, lens vacuoles may at times disappear spontaneously and give rise to a transient improvement in vision. Because of this spontaneous improvement, a number of remedies have been used but with no evidence that they are of any value. The word "cataract" connotes eventual surgery or blindness to so many people that a euphemism such as lens opacity is substituted.

During the period of decreasing vision, frequent and accurate refraction will maintain vision at the best possible level. When minute opacities involve the axial area, dilation of the pupil by means of a weak solution of phenylephrine (Neo-Synephrine, 2.5%) or 2% homatropine may provide visual improvement. Pupillary dilation must not be used in patients with a shallow anterior chamber in whom there is danger of precipitating angle-closure glaucoma.

Surgical treatment. Cataract extraction is indicated in the following instances: (1) when the opacity has advanced to the stage that it causes a visual defect that interferes with an individual's vocation or avocation and (2) if the lens threatens to cause a secondary glaucoma or a uveitis.

Vision is evaluated in terms of both eyes with the best possible correcting lenses worn. As long as there is adequate vision in one eye, surgery is seldom indicated in the poorer eye. Cataract extraction is often not recommended if either eye has corrected vision of better than 20/70. There are many exceptions, however, and the vision required by an active middle-aged individual may be quite different from that required by a sedentary elderly housewife.

In recent years an increasing number of ophthalmic surgeons advocate surgery for advanced monocular cataract in active individuals irrespective of the vision in the opposite eye. Binocular vision may be restored postoperatively by means of a contact lens on the operated eye. The decision whether to operate is based on the predicted ability of the patient to wear a contact lens. In those patients who are unable to wear a contact lens, the monocular aphakia may cause an annoying diplopia.

A cataract may cause glaucoma by one of the following two mechanisms:

1. An immature cataract may imbibe a large quantity of fluid and become intumescent, with marked increase in volume of the lens. This may produce a secondary angle-closure glaucoma.

2. Hypermaturity of the lens in which the opaque cortex becomes fluid, with the nucleus floating in the shrunken capsule, may cause a glaucoma through an inflammatory reaction by the release of a toxic fluid. Such lenses should be removed prior to the onset of glaucoma. Thus opacification of the entire lens protein is considered an indication for cataract extraction.

The contraindications to cataract surgery are optic nerve atrophy, detachment of the retina, extensive chorioretinitis, and any disease of the anterior or posterior ocular segment that has destroyed vision and makes lens extraction unlikely to provide improvement in vision. If the light projection is faulty, it is likely that cataract extraction will not materially improve vision.

An acquired cataract may be removed in one of two ways: (1) intracapsular, in which the entire lens (including its capsule) is removed, and (2) extracapsular, in which a large portion of the anterior capsule is excised, the nucleus removed, and the cortex irrigated from the eye, leaving the posterior capsule in position. The extracapsular extraction has been largely supplanted by the intracapsular extraction, and many surgeons believe that there is no indication for extracapsular extraction in the adult.

Adequate anesthesia and akinesia have probably been the most important factors in improving the visual results of cataract extraction. Akinesia of the orbicularis oculi muscle is produced by means of a block of the facial nerve just anterior to the tragus or by infiltration of the muscle fibers with a local anesthetic. An anesthetic is also injected into the muscle cone and causes anesthesia of the uveal tract and akinesia of the ocular muscles. Following the retrobulbar injection, massage of the globe for 5 minutes reduces the intraocular pressure and decreases the danger of vitreous loss.

An incision is made at the superior corneoscleral limbus, extending from the 9 to the 3 o'clock meridian. Delicate sutures of catgut or silk are usually prepared and looped out of the way, ready to be tied after the lens is delivered. A complete iridectomy or a peripheral iridectomy in the 12 o'clock meridian may be performed. A complete iridectomy gives rise to a cosmetic defect, but it is associated with fewer complications than a peripheral iridectomy. The peripheral iridectomy provides a cosmetically pleasing eye with a round pupil, but it may be associated with more complications than a complete iridectomy.

Intracapsular lens extraction depends upon a nicety of balance between the resistance of the capsule and the zonule to rupture and the tendency for the vitreous body to extrude from the eye. A number of techniques have been devised to provide a safe intracapsular extraction.

The lens capsule may be grasped with a delicate forceps, either at the equator or on the anterior surface, and may be de-

livered from the eye by sliding or by tumbling. In the sliding technique the lens is lifted from the eye with the 12 o'clock meridian presenting in the wound first. In the tumbling procedure the lens is rotated with the 12 o'clock meridian as the fulcrum, so that the 6 o'clock meridian presents in the wound first. Instead of forceps, a suction cup may be used to grasp the lens. Many types are available, some utilizing a vacuum pump, and in others the vacuum is provided by a rubber suction tip. The lens may be frozen to a probe cooled to –35° C. and lifted from its position. The zonular fibers supporting the lens are usually quite fragile after the age of 55 years, and they may be ruptured by pressure applied through the corneoscleral limbus or by traction transmitted through the lens capsule. The zonule may be dissolved by alpha chymotrypsin, a proteolytic enzyme that is injected into the posterior chamber and causes dissolution of the zonule within 2 minutes. The enzyme is not indicated in patients less than 20 years of age because the vitreous body is adherent to the lens and may be removed in toto. After this age the adhesion disappears. Its main indication is in lens extraction in patients between the ages of 20 and 50 years.

Complications. Cataract extraction may be associated with many complications that interfere with a successful result. At the time of surgery, the lens capsule may rupture before the lens is removed, and the operation is converted to an inadvertent extracapsular extraction. Unlike the planned extracapsular extraction, the anterior capsule is removed inadequately or not at all. The cortex freed with capsule rupture may cause uveitis and may lead to the complications of intraocular inflammation. Proliferation of the anterior lens capsule remaining within the eye may obscure vision.

Pyogenic bacteria introduced into the eye at the time of surgery cause a panophthalmitis; fungi cause an endophthalmitis.

Loss of vitreous body at the time of surgery leads to both immediate and delayed complications. The vitreous body prevents apposition of the wound edges of the corneoscleral incision and causes faulty healing. The wound heals by secondary intention, with much fibrous tissue proliferation. This in turn causes the pupil to become drawn up and gives rise to a characteristic boat-shaped appearance of the pupil. Eyes in which there has been a loss of vitreous body are particularly prone to develop retinal detachment in later years. Apposition of the vitreous face to the endothelium of the cornea may give rise to localized areas of edema that interfere with vision.

Very rarely in the course of a cataract extraction a major vessel within the eye may rupture, causing a massive hemorrhage, with extrusion of the intraocular contents. More frequently there may be bleeding into the anterior chamber between the third and the fifth day after surgery. This hyphema is seldom severe and absorbs spontaneously.

Faulty apposition of the wound edges may cause the anterior chamber not to reform, subsequently producing an angle-closure type of secondary glaucoma with adhesions between the peripheral iris and the cornea (peripheral anterior synechiae). More frequently the anterior chamber forms normally and then is lost 7 to 14 days after the surgery. This may be due to a fistula or an internal cyclodialysis. If the condition persists, the trabecular meshwork may be damaged, with the consequent production of glaucoma. Faulty wound healing may cause the inclusion of epithelium in the anterior chamber, leading to epithelium growing over the surface of the iris and the posterior surface of the cornea. This complication may be noted many weeks after the cataract operation when there is an onset of tearing of the eye. Treatment is usually unsatisfactory.

Despite the long list of complications associated with cataract extraction, the operative results are excellent. In average surgical practices, some 95% of all patients having cataract extraction have improvement of vision, and the large majority have normal vision restored.

Removal of the lens causes a marked reduction of the refractive power of the eye and a severe impairment of the efficiency of the eye as an optical instrument. The most evident change is a marked hyperopia that cannot be neutralized by accommodation because the lens is absent. Additionally, there is an increased spherical and chromatic aberration and magnification of images upon the retina when the condition is corrected with lenses. The usual incision at the limbus causes astigmatism. The larger pupillary aperture caused by a sector iridectomy results in increased size of diffusion circles on the retina and in diminution in the depth of focus. Additionally, the correcting lenses worn in aphakia are maximally effective only when the patient looks through the optical center of the lens. There is also an annular area of blindness from 30° to 60° in the field of peripheral vision, and objects dart in and out of this area of vision. Because of the magnification, patients have a moderately difficult time in becoming adjusted to the glasses, particularly in walking. Conversely, because of the magnification, they are frequently able to read unusually small print. Since accommodation is absent, it is necessary to wear bifocal or trifocal lenses, and because of the decreased depth of focus, the range of clear vision for near is limited. Usually the refraction following a cataract extraction does not stabilize for several months, and a final type of lens is not prescribed until that time.

Many of the optical disturbances created by aphakia may be minimized, although not eliminated, by wearing contact lenses. Probably because of the interruption of the nerve supply by the corneal section, contact lenses appear to be somewhat better tolerated by cataract patients than by other patients. Frequently balancing this tendency, however, is the advanced age of the patient, which makes him unwilling to attempt the care that contact lenses require.

Special types. A large variety of acquired types of cataract have been described: senile, toxic, traumatic, diabetic, and hypocalcemic. Some have a characteristic appearance in the early stages, but with progression it is not possible to distinguish the various types.

Senile cataract. With aging, the lens gradually tends to become opaque. Virtually everyone past the age of 65 years has evidence of lens opacity. Such opacities may be divided into those involving the nucleus, the cortex, and the capsule. Not infrequently these changes occur concurrently.

Nuclear, or hard, cataract is an accentuation of the normal sclerosing process of the lens nucleus. It becomes evident about the age of 50 years and progresses slowly until the entire nucleus is opaque. Not uncommonly the earliest change is an increase in the index of refraction, so that there is a decrease in hyperopia and an increase in myopia. The gradual progress of this lens opacity may be associated with improved vision for near. This may lead to a mistaken subjective impression that vision has permanently improved—"second sight" of the aged. However, as the opacity progresses, there is a gradual deterioration of vision for both near and far. Inasmuch as the opacity is located centrally, there may be marked variations of vision, depending upon the diameter of the pupil.

A cortical, or soft, cataract involves the lens cortex. There is either opacification of proteins or imbibition of fluid into the cortex, giving rise to clefts that run radially between the lamella of the lens, creating a spokelike pattern. These opacities tend to involve the periphery initially and may become very marked without interference with vision. Gradually, however, the opacities involve the central area, causing interference with central vision.

Cataracts involving the capsule only are usually congenital. A posterior subcapsular opacity is the most common type of senile change. This usually develops gradually and causes a beaten-gold appearance of the involved area. It involves the central visual axis early and, though minute in extent, may cause a maximal disturbance of vision.

Toxic cataract. A large variety of compounds may cause lens opacity that is often not attributed initially to the drug. Some of this difficulty arises because cataractogenic substances may not cause lens opacities in experimental animals, whereas in other instances there seems to be a toxicity of the drug combined with a metabolic abnormality of the patient.

Toxic cataracts resemble mainly senile peripheral cortical or posterior subcapsular opacities. In some instances the opacity goes on to maturity even though the drug is withdrawn, but it may not progress when the drug is stopped.

Currently the corticosteroids, when administered in high doses for long periods, especially in arthritis patients, are particularly prone to cause cataracts. Usually the drug has to be administered for more than a year. Patients with asthma and ulcerative colitis receiving similar quantities of the drug develop opacities much less commonly. The opacity begins at the posterior pole as a highly refractile, multicolored dot that interferes early with vision. Peripheral cortical opacities then develop, and cataract extraction may be required.

Traumatic cataract. Contusion of the eye may cause a posterior subcapsular cataract many months after the original injury, even though the lens capsule has not been grossly injured.

Rupture of the lens capsule invariably

causes a cataract. If the opening is microscopic in size, there may be a minute linear opacity corresponding to the opening. More commonly, however, there is an initial posterior subcapsular opacity that extends forward to involve the entire lens, with grayish lens material extruding into the anterior chamber. An inflammation of varying severity results, and in individuals less than 25 years of age the entire lens may be autolyzed. In patients older than this the nucleus remains and causes a continuing inflammation.

The effects of a foreign body within the lens depend upon its size and rate of oxidation. Glass and plastics are well tolerated. Iron and copper cause characteristic opacities.

Diabetic cataract. Diabetic cataract is a rare lens opacity occurring in growth-onset diabetes, usually in poorly controlled diabetics about 20 years of age. The opacity closely resembles "sugar" cataracts in experimental animals. The opacities are bilateral, cortical, involve the anterior and posterior subcapsular region predominantly, and consist of minute dots of varying size, usually called "snowflakes." A diabetic cataract may go to complete opacity (maturity) in less than 72 hours. Surgery is often disappointing inasmuch as the cortex absorbs from the anterior chamber slowly. Adult diabetics appear to have a slightly earlier onset of senile cataract than do nondiabetics, but this has not been proved. Surgery is usually uncomplicated, but retinopathy may prevent visual improvement.

Hypocalcemic cataract. A hypocalcemic cataract occurs only if the blood calcium is in a range where tetany occurs. If the underlying disorder is corrected, the cataract is often arrested. The opacity may be lamellar or may resemble a diabetic cataract.

Chapter 19

Glaucoma

Glaucoma is an ocular abnormality in which the intraocular pressure is so elevated as to cause organic changes in the optic nerve and typical defects in the visual field. The degree of increased pressure causing organic change is not the same in every eye, and some individuals may tolerate for long periods a pressure that would rapidly blind another. There are two major factors involved in this individual variation: (1) the rate of production of the aqueous humor and the ease of excretion of the aqueous humor through the trabecular area, which provide the homeostatic control of the level of the intraocular pressure, and (2) the adequacy of the blood supply to the intraocular portion of the optic nerve (papilla), which governs whether or not the optic nerve atrophies with accompanying visual changes. The healthy eye tolerates indefinitely a pressure of 20 mm. Hg, as measured with the Schiøtz tonometer, without damage to the optic nerve.

Glaucoma is customarily divided into primary and secondary types, depending upon the obviousness of the ocular disease present. Primary glaucoma is a bilateral disease that is divided into two types: (1) angle-closure glaucoma, which in past years was called iris-block, narrow-angle, congestive, acute, or uncompensated glaucoma, and (2) open-angle glaucoma, which is also called simple glaucoma, chronic glaucoma, glaucoma simplex, compensated glaucoma, or wide-angle glau-

coma. Secondary glaucoma is caused by some antecedent or concomitant ocular disease.

In angle-closure glaucoma an anatomic abnormality is present in which the iris root is displaced forward so that the entrance to the chamber angle is narrow. If the iris root mechanically closes the angle so that aqueous humor is not excreted through the trabecular meshwork, the intraocular pressure increases. Angle-closure glaucoma is thus present only when the angle is closed and aqueous humor cannot escape from the eye. Following a prolonged or repeated attack, adhesions form between the iris and the cornea, called peripheral anterior synechiae, and the pressure remains constantly elevated. Many eyes subject to angle-closure glaucoma may be recognized by the shallow anterior chamber, with the iris-lens diaphragm having a convex shape closely paralleling the convexity of the posterior cornea. A history of periods of foggy or hazy vision, occasionally with rainbows around lights and sometimes with headache, may be obtained. Anything that will dilate the pupil, such as prolonged darkness, emotional upset, and mydriatic drops, may cause an attack.

Open-angle glaucoma arises because an abnormality in the trabecular meshwork interferes with the exit of aqueous humor from the anterior chamber. The aqueous humor has access to the angle at all times, and there is no mechanical obstruction between the aqueous humor and the trabecular apparatus.

Secondary glaucoma (p. 316) arises from a number of causes that have only increased ocular pressure as their common denominator. In some diseases, for example, congenital glaucoma, the increased intraocular pressure dominates the clinical picture, whereas in others attention is focused upon the primary disease.

Symptoms

The symptoms of glaucoma arise from two sources: (1) the increased intraocular pressure and (2) the interference with optic nerve function. If the pressure increases slowly, symptoms from increased pressure may be absent or minimal. If there is a sudden increase in pressure, there may be severe, prostrating pain, often unilateral, which may be confused with migraine, internal carotid artery aneurysm, and similar causes of hemicrania. A subepithelial edema of the cornea may occur, with foggy and blurred vision and rainbows around lights, or iridescent vision. Interference with optic nerve function causes subtle defects, often unappreciated by the patient until they are far advanced. In the early stages the range of the peripheral vision (the peripheral isopters) is not affected, and the changes can be demonstrated only by careful measurement of visual function in the area surrounding the point of fixation. Measurement of the visual fields by confrontation is of little diagnostic value, although late in the course of the disease the visual field may be markedly constricted.

The symptoms of angle-closure glaucoma are mainly related to a sudden increase in intraocular pressure. Following movies, emotional upset, and similar factors that cause pupillary dilation, there is a rapid increase in intraocular pressure with halos around lights, pain or discomfort in the eye, and perhaps ciliary injection and lacrimation. Early attacks are often spontaneously relieved by the pupillary constriction that occurs as the patient enters a brightly illuminated area or goes to sleep.

The symptoms of open-angle glaucoma are often mild or absent. Usually the intraocular pressure increases very slowly, and although it may reach high levels, corneal edema and pain do not occur. Cupping of the optic nerve is common, but the patient remains unaware of the field defect until late in the disease.

Diagnostic methods

Three factors must be present to permit the unequivocal diagnosis of glaucoma: (1) increased intraocular pressure, (2) optic nerve atrophy and excavation, and (3) typical visual field defects. Clinically it is desirable to diagnose and treat the disease prior to the development of irreversible organic changes, and the diagnosis is often based upon abnormalities in intraocular pressure and the rate of outflow of aqueous humor from the eye. The increased intraocular pressure is measured by tonometry. The increased intraocular pressure is almost always due to an impairment in the outflow of aqueous humor, and this is evaluated by means of tonography. A number of methods, called provocative tests, are used to distinguish normal from abnormal eyes by inducing an increase in the intraocular pressure under controlled conditions. The configuration of the anterior chamber angle is studied by means of a prism or contact lens combined with a microscope. This examination, called gonioscopy, is used to distinguish angle-closure glaucoma from open-angle glaucoma. The changes of the optic disk are evaluated by means of the ophthalmoscope. The visual field changes are measured by perimetry, using the tangent screen, with particular study of the area surrounding the fixation point.

Tonometry. Intraocular pressure is mea-

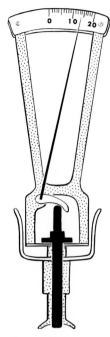

Fig. 19-1. Schiøtz tonometer in which the plunger, in black, measures the ease of indentation of the cornea.

sured by means of a tonometer. There are two main types: the indentation tonometer or Schiøtz (Fig. 19-1) and the applanation tonometer—the applanation tonometer of Goldmann is the one most often used. The cornea must first be anesthetized by the instillation of a local anesthetic such as tetracaine. The indentation tonometer does not measure the intraocular pressure directly but rather measures the ease with which the globe is indented by the plunger of the instrument. A soft eye is easily indented and a low pressure reading is obtained, whereas a hard eye is indented with greater difficulty and a higher pressure reading is obtained. The amount of indentation has been calibrated in enucleated eyes in millimeters of mercury pressure.

The applanation tonometer is used in conjunction with a biomicroscope, and the force required to flatten a segment of the cornea that is 3.06 mm. in diameter is determined. This method is influenced by fewer extraneous factors than indentation tonometry, but it requires greater experience and more costly equipment.

The mean normal intraocular pressure by Schiøtz tonometry is 16.1 mm. Hg, with a standard deviation of ± 2.8 mm. With applanation tonometry, the mean normal is 15.4 mm. Hg, with a standard deviation of ± 2.5 mm. The difference is attributed to the patient being in the upright position with applanation tonometry.

Tonography. Massaging the eyes causes an increased outflow of aqueous humor through the trabecular apparatus, which lowers the intraocular pressure. In most glaucomatous eyes there is an impairment in this outflow so that massage expresses less aqueous humor. Tonography measures the rate at which the intraocular pressure decreases when the eye is compressed by means of an indentation tonometer resting upon it. The weight of the tonometer resting upon the eye expresses aqueous humor through the outflow channels, causing an increase in the amount of indentation by the plunger of the instrument. Inasmuch as the tonometer has been calibrated by determination of the volume of the indentation, the difference between the volume at the beginning and at the end of the test is equal to the amount of aqueous humor expressed from the eye while the tonometer rested upon it. Clinically, tonography is carried out by allowing an electronic tonometer to rest upon the eye for 4 to 5 minutes while recording the pressure response on a galvanometer. The results are expressed as the coefficient of outflow facility, the microliters of aqueous humor expressed from the eye per minute per mm. Hg of intraocular pressure.

Tonography constitutes an unusually valuable method for the diagnosis of and the evaluation of therapy of the glaucomas. Considerable experience is required by the operator before consistently reproducible results are obtained, and frequently the patient must be examined more than once before an adequate record is produced.

The mean normal value of the coefficient of outflow is 0.28, with a standard deviation of ± 0.05. Values of less than 0.18 occur in less than 2.5% of the normal population. The ratio

$$\frac{\text{Intraocular pressure}}{\text{Coefficient facility outflow}}$$

is of unusual value in the diagnosis of glaucoma. A value greater than 100 occurs in 74% of glaucoma patients and in 2.5% of the normal population, whereas a value greater than 138 occurs in 51% of glaucoma patients and in 0.15% of patients with normal eyes.

Provocative tests. The intraocular pressure varies slightly with respiration, heartbeat, and activity. During the day there may be variations in pressure of 4 or 5 mm. Hg in healthy persons and more than 10 mm. Hg in glaucoma patients. Inasmuch as the ocular tension in an individual with glaucoma may be normal when he is examined, a number of tests have been developed to induce an increase in the intraocular pressure to distinguish the normal from the glaucoma population.

These tests are by no means foolproof, and even known glaucoma patients with optic atrophy may react negatively. Such tests are indicated in patients with (1) an intraocular pressure of 21 mm. Hg or more, (2) a coefficient of outflow of less than 0.18, (3) a ratio of intraocular pressure/coefficient facility outflow greater than 100, (4) a shallow anterior chamber, (5) optic nerve changes suggestive of glaucoma, and (6) visual field changes suggestive of glaucoma. Provocative tests permit an earlier diagnosis of glaucoma than is possible if one waits for unequivocal signs of organic change in the eyes.

Water-drinking test. The water-drinking test is probably the most common test for the diagnosis of open-angle glaucoma. The patient is instructed not to use ocular medications for 48 hours prior to the test. The intraocular pressure is measured preferably in the morning while the patient is fasting. The patient then drinks 1 liter of water within 2 to 4 minutes, and tonometry is carried out at 30 and 45 minutes. An increase of intraocular pressure of more than 8 mm. Hg indicates glaucoma. The test is far more reliable if tonography is carried out 45 minutes after the ingestion of water. Some 94% of glaucoma patients will have a ratio of intraocular pressure/coefficient facility outflow of more than 100.

Pupillary dilation. In angle-closure glaucoma, provocative testing is carried out by combining dilation of the pupil with gonioscopy. Angle-closure glaucoma can be diagnosed only when the combination of elevated intraocular pressure and closure of the angle occurs. Inasmuch as dilation of the pupil may induce an acute increase in intraocular pressure, the test is performed cautiously on only one eye at a time, and the pupil is constricted before the patient is released. The pupillary dilation is usually brought about by instillation of an easily neutralized mydriatic such as 5% eucatropine. Placing the patient in a dark room for 60 minutes is a physiologic method of inducing pupillary dilation. Open-angle glaucoma as well as angle-closure glaucoma may respond to pupillary dilation with an increase in intraocular pressure, but such tests are more often positive in angle-closure glaucoma. An increase in intraocular pressure of 8 mm. Hg or more is generally considered pathognomonic. Tonography indicates a decrease in the coefficient of outflow of 25 to 30%. The angle must be observed with the gonioscope to be closed at the time the intraocular pressure is increased in order to be certain that the abnormality is angle-closure glaucoma.

Corticosteroid instillation. Nearly 100% of patients with open-angle glaucoma develop a decreased coefficient of outflow and an increased intraocular pressure following the ocular instillation of 0.1% betamethasone four times daily for 3 weeks. Some 35 to 40% of angle-closure and secondary glaucomas respond similarly. Continued increased intraocular pressure may cause visual field defects and optic atrophy. Every patient who shows a ratio of intraocular pressure/coefficient facility outflow of greater than 100 responds to topical betamethasone. Additionally, every patient with proved glaucoma has offspring who respond to topical corticosteroids with decreased outflow and increased pressure. The parents of patients with proved glaucoma respond to the instillation of betamethasone.

It is evident that topical betamethasone is not only a potent tool for inducing impairment of aqueous outflow but also for the study of the genetic constitution of glaucoma populations. It is postulated that the open-angle glaucoma patient is a homozygote for the abnormal gene, and thus has a gene structure for glaucoma of $g \times g$. If the homozygote mates with another individual with glaucoma, then theoretically all of the offspring are abnormal and respond to corticosteroid administration with a pathologic increase in ocular pressure. The various possibilities are indicated in Table 19-1.

The instillation of corticosteroids pro-vides a valuable method for studying not only glaucoma but also the genetics of a gene controlling an enzyme in the trabecular meshwork. However, the increased intraocular pressure may cause permanent damage to the optic nerve with permanent field defects. Additionally, topical corticosteroids cause lens opacities and decrease local tissue immunity, and such provocative testing and genetic studies must be carried out under controlled conditions with patient understanding of the nature of the study.

Ophthalmoscopy. The examination of the ocular fundus in glaucoma is directed particularly to the appearance of the optic disk. The nerve fibers at the optic disk receive their blood supply from small branches of the arterial circle of Haller-Zinn derived mainly from the posterior ciliary arteries. The blood pressure in this arterial circle is lower than that of the central retinal artery, and the terminal branches of the arterial circle are subject to the intraocular pressure. Thus, when the intraocular pressure is increased, the blood vessels of the disk are much more vulnerable to compression or diversion of blood than the remainder of the blood vessels of the eye. This region is liable, therefore, to selective damage of the nerve fibers of the optic disk, causing optic atrophy.

In the early stages of the disease there may be no change, but as the disease progresses, pathologic excavation (cup-

Table 19-1. Corticosteroid responsiveness for offspring of various phenotypes*

Phenotypes of parents	Number of offspring	< 20 mm. Hg	20 to 31 mm. Hg	> 31 mm. Hg
nn × *nn*	21	95%	5%	0%
nn × *ng*	42	48%	52%	0%
ng × *ng*	25	20%	56%	24%
gg × *gg*	12	0%	0%	100%
Volunteers	100	70%	26%	4%

*From Becker, B.: In Becker, B., and Drews, R. C., editors: Current concepts in ophthalmology, St. Louis, 1967, The C. V. Mosby Co.

ping) and atrophy of the disk occur (Fig. 19-2). Excavation is first noted as an increase in diameter of the normal physiologic cup followed by loss of the rim of nerve tissue between the cup and the temporal margin of the optic nerve. The cupping is evident as a displacement of small blood vessels as they cross the edge of the optic disk. As the cup enlarges, the retinal vessels on the surface of the optic disk are displaced nasally and either run across the floor of the cup or disappear under its nasal edge. With cupping, atrophy of the nerve develops, and the disk becomes pale and gray-white in color.

Perimetry. The measurement of the visual field is the main method of assessing damage to the optic nerve in glaucoma. It

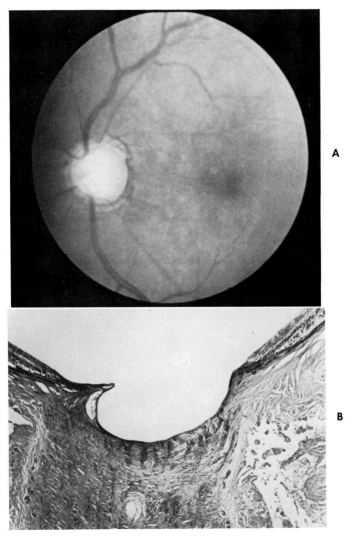

Fig. 19-2. A, Optic atrophy with glaucomatous cupping. Blood vessels are displaced nasally, and no blood vessels can be seen at the temporal portion of the disk. The disk is much whiter than normal. **B,** Advanced cupping, the "bean pot" excavation.

is of particular value in the initial diagnosis and in evaluating progression of the disease and the effectiveness of treatment. The field defect is often proportionate to the amount of optic nerve atrophy present, and a skilled examiner may be able to anticipate the type of perimetric changes present by the ophthalmoscopic appearance of the optic disk. However, the optic disk may have a false appearance of pinkness because of nuclear sclerosis of the lens, and perimetry should not be neglected because of normal-appearing disks. The visual field defect in glaucoma is often transient in the early stages and occurs only when the intraocular pressure is elevated, or it may be induced by an anoxia. As optic nerve damage progresses, the defect becomes permanent.

The nasal visual field is most susceptible to change in glaucoma. It corresponds to axons entering the temporal side of the optic nerve from the temporal periphery. These fibers arc above and below the large mass of fibers from the fovea centralis and do not cross the horizontal midline (Fig. 19-3). With increased pressure, a group of axons arising from an arc-shaped area of the retina lose their function, causing a typical arcuate island of blindness called an arcuate scotoma. The fibers in the temporal periphery are also involved and cause a depression in the peripheral nasal field called Rönne's nasal step. The field defects in glaucoma are usually best demonstrated on a tangent screen using small, white test objects. The macular fibers are resistant to increased pressure or have a less vulnerable blood supply so that central visual acuity is preserved until late.

Gonioscopy. The angle of the anterior chamber cannot be seen by direct inspection because the overlying sclera and the

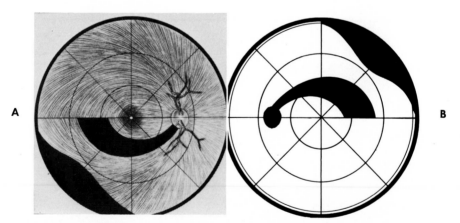

Fig. 19-3. A, Diagram showing the course of the retinal nerve fibers to the optic disk. Fibers temporal to the disk follow an arching course (arcuate) above and below the fovea centralis and do not cross the 180° retinal meridian (horizontal raphe). Fibers arising nasal to the optic disk follow a relatively straight course and cross the horizontal nasal meridian. Arcuate fibers in the blackened area extending from the horizontal raphe to the disk (Bjerrum's area) are particularly vulnerable to increased intraocular pressure and cause the field defect shown in **B.** Involvement of the fibers in the blackened area in the inferior temporal retina causes a depression in the superior nasal peripheral visual field. (Modified from Becker, B., and Shaffer, R. N.: Diagnosis and therapy of the glaucomas, ed. 2, St. Louis, 1965, The C. V. Mosby Co.)

corneoscleral limbus are opaque. It is possible to see this area by means of a contact lens or a prism modified for observation. This method of inspection is of particular diagnostic importance inasmuch as findings in the angle are the basis for distinction between angle-closure glaucoma and open-angle glaucoma. Angle-closure glaucoma cannot be diagnosed definitely unless the angle is observed to be closed when the intraocular pressure is elevated. Gonioscopy has also been used in the development of an effective surgical procedure for congenital glaucoma and in the diagnostic and therapeutic evaluation of many types of secondary glaucoma.

Primary glaucoma
Angle-closure glaucoma

Angle-closure glaucoma is an abnormality in which the intraocular pressure increases because the outflow of aqueous humor from the anterior chamber is mechanically prevented by contact of the iris to the trabecular drainage meshwork and the peripheral cornea. The condition has been designated in the past as narrow-angle, acute congestive, and uncompensated glaucoma. No term is ideal inasmuch as the intraocular pressure is normal when the angle is open, and glaucoma occurs only when a major portion of the angle is closed. If the iris remains in contact with the trabecular meshwork, permanent organic changes occur, and there is an impairment of aqueous outflow. Both eyes are involved, although one eye may present symptoms 2 to 5 years before the fellow eye. There is a familial tendency to shallow anterior chambers.

The disease arises because of an inherited anatomic defect that causes a shallow anterior chamber. The peripheral iris often inserts on the extreme anterior edge of the ciliary body, causing a narrow-angle recess and placing the iris close to the trabecular meshwork. The cornea is often small, and the eye is hyperopic. The lens is closer to the cornea than usual, and with the normal increase in size of the lens with aging, it becomes even closer. The iris appears to bow forward so that it seems to closely parallel the posterior convexity of the cornea. This may be observed by shining a penlight into the anterior chamber from the temporal side of the eye. A shadow, which is not present in the normal eye, is cast on the nasal portion of the relatively convex iris.

Increased intraocular pressure occurs when there is anterior displacement of the peripheral iris. This anterior displacement of the peripheral iris causes it to isolate the trabecular meshwork from the anterior chamber, which prevents the exit of aqueous humor. Two conditions operating singly or together may cause this:

1. A valvelike action of the lens and iris prevents the aqueous humor from flowing freely through the pupil, and there is an accumulation of fluid in the posterior chamber. This pupillary block causes increased pressure in the posterior chamber so that the peripheral iris balloons forward. Since the angle is already a mere slit, the iris isolates the trabecular drainage apparatus from the anterior chamber (Fig. 19-4).

2. Dilation of the pupil causes it to become thicker and crowds into the drainage apparatus, preventing aqueous outflow.

Several stages of angle-closure glaucoma may be recognized:

1. Potential—shallow anterior chamber without symptoms
2. With increased pressure
   a. Intermittent with spontaneous relief
   b. Acute sustained increased pressure
3. Peripheral anterior synechiae formation
   a. Secondary to intermittent or sustained attacks
   b. Chronic without signs of acute increased pressure

Patients who have an anterior chamber with a depth of 2 mm. or less are candidates for the development of angle-closure glaucoma. The shallow anterior chamber may be recognized by the decreased distance between the posterior surface of the cornea and the anterior surface of the iris. Patients with such a mechanism may go for many years without symptoms, and it may be impossible to provoke an increase in intraocular pressure or a decrease in aqueous outflow by means of pupillary dilation. With the gradual increase in size of the lens, however, the margin of safety decreases, and such patients may have the first sustained attack of increased intraocular pressure when they are elderly.

Inasmuch as glaucoma has been defined as increased intraocular pressure combined with characteristic changes of the optic nerve and visual field, it is evident that a shallow anterior chamber does not constitute glaucoma. Many patients with a shallow anterior chamber never develop symptoms of an acute increase in intraocular pressure. Such eyes, however, must be followed with utmost caution if one is to avoid an acute angle-closure episode. Pa-

tients should be warned particularly concerning symptoms of blurry and hazy vision that may be combined with iridescent vision and pain.

Symptoms and signs. Angle-closure glaucoma with increased intraocular pressure occurs in a form in which there is spontaneous relief when the pupil contracts and in a second type in which the pressure remains elevated.

Patients who experience spontaneous relief of increased intraocular pressure are detected on the basis of a shallow anterior chamber (Fig. 19-4) combined with a history of attacks. After a prolonged stay in darkness, such as at a movie, and following emotional upset or other factors that cause pupillary dilation, vision in one eye mainly becomes blurred and foggy. There may be pain in the eye or on the side of the head that can erroneously be attributed to migraine or even to an impending rupture of an intracranial aneurysm. Pupillary constriction with light

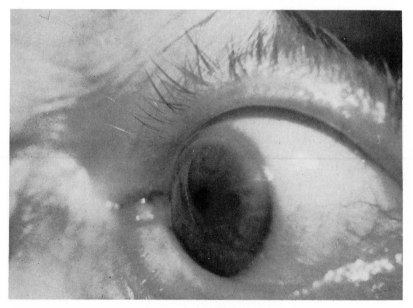

Fig. 19-4. Shallow anterior chamber that may be observed in angle-closure glaucoma. Diagnosis requires that the angle be observed by means of a gonioscope to be closed with the tension elevated.

or with sleep relieves the attack and the symptoms disappear. If the patient is seen during the period of attack, the intraocular pressure may be found to be markedly elevated, but signs of congestion are minimal. These patients may develop peripheral anterior synechiae with a decreased coefficient of outflow from the anterior chamber. Between attacks there are no symptoms, but dilation of the pupil will cause an increase in intraocular pressure of more than 8 mm. Hg or will reduce the coefficient of outflow 25 to 30%. Gonioscopy indicates the angle to be closed when the pressure is elevated.

Patients who have an acute sustained increased intraocular pressure usually have an onset similar to the patients who experience spontaneous relief. The pupil does not constrict, however, the intraocular pressure continues to mount, and the symptoms increase in intensity. A ciliary type of injection is present, and there may be profuse lacrimation. Subepithelial corneal edema becomes marked, and epithelial bullae may form. There is a breakdown of the blood-aqueous barrier with an increase in protein content of the aqueous humor. The blood vessels of the iris stroma become dilated. The pupil is in middilation and does not react to light. Marked systemic symptoms may be present, with nausea, vomiting, and malaise. These symptoms may be aggravated by systemic absorption of anticholinesterase solutions used in the treatment of the angle-closure glaucoma.

As the attack persists, peripheral anterior synechiae form between the root of the iris and the cornea (Fig. 19-5). After several days, these synechiae nearly destroy the function of the drainage meshwork. Adhesions (posterior synechiae) form between the iris and the lens, and if the attack is not relieved, necrosis of the sphincter pupillae muscle results in a permanently semidilated pupil. Fluid vesicles form in the anterior subcapsular region of the lens. If the condition is untreated, there

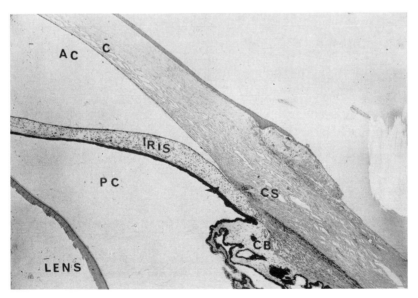

Fig. 19-5. Angle-closure glaucoma with anterior synechiae excluding the anterior chamber, **AC,** from the trabecular area and the canal of Schlemm, **CS.** The posterior chamber, **PC,** is larger than normal. **C,** Cornea. **CB,** Ciliary body. (Hematoxylin and eosin stain; ×38.)

is progressive deterioration of vision with the development of a blind, painful eye. Optic nerve excavation and cupping do not occur until late in the course of the disease.

The development of peripheral anterior synechiae profoundly modifies the disease mechanism in angle-closure glaucoma. Prior to their development, the drainage meshwork of the eye is normal, and the abnormality is limited to the shallow anterior chamber combined with the physiologic iris bombé mechanism. Once peripheral anterior synechiae have developed, the trabecular meshwork is permanently damaged and therefore the glaucoma cannot be cured by eliminating the angle-closure mechanism. These peripheral anterior synechiae develop most commonly during an acute angle-closure attack. In an occasional patient they appear to develop without an acute attack, and it is difficult to determine whether they occur during an intermittent increase in intraocular pressure

or develop because of an additional (and unknown) mechanism.

Diagnosis. The exact diagnosis of angle-closure glaucoma requires that the intraocular pressure of the eye be elevated and a closed angle be demonstrated by gonioscopy. The chief differential points are shown in Table 19-2.

Treatment. Angle-closure glaucoma is essentially a surgical disease. The angle-closure mechanism may be eliminated by providing an opening between the anterior and the posterior chamber. This communication prevents the pressure in the posterior chamber from exceeding that of the anterior chamber and eliminates entirely physiologic iris bombé.

Patients with shallow angles who have never had an attack of angle-closure glaucoma would probably ensure freedom from an attack by an iridectomy. However, inasmuch as it is not known whether they will live long enough to develop an attack, the surgeon and the patient are usually re-

Table 19-2. Differential diagnosis of angle-closure glaucoma

	Angle-closure glaucoma	*Acute iritis*	*Acute conjunctivitis*
Pain	Severe, prostrating	Moderate to severe	Burning, itching
Injection	Ciliary type that is more intense near the corneoscleral limbus and fades toward fornices; not constricted with 1:1,000 epinephrine; vessels do not move with conjunctiva, are violet in color, and individual vessels are not distinguishable		Conjunctival type that is most intense in fornices and fades toward limbus; eye whitened with 1:1,000 epinephrine; vessels superficial, move with conjunctiva, are bright red, and individual vessels evident
Pupil	Semidilated and does not react to light	Miotic, reaction delayed or absent	Normal
Cornea	Steamy and iris details not visible	Usually clear with deposits on posterior surface sometimes visible	Clear and normal
Secretion	Watery	Watery	Stringy pus
Onset	Sudden	Gradual	Gradual
Vision	Markedly reduced	Slightly reduced	Normal
Intraocular pressure	Elevated	Normal or soft	Normal

luctant to undertake intraocular surgery for a disease that is at best potential.

In a patient who is having intermittent symptoms with spontaneous relief, an iridectomy is indicated. A peripheral iridectomy is the operation of choice. This is carried out in the superior temporal quadrant through a small scratch incision. A small opening is made in the iris, and the corneoscleral wound is closed with sutures so as to be watertight. The procedure is relatively simple, and provided the anterior chamber does not remain flat postoperatively, a complication avoided by careful wound closure, the eye tolerates the procedure well.

Angle-closure glaucoma with an acute increase in intraocular pressure presents a difficult problem in management. The type of treatment is often governed by the duration of the attack prior to normalization of the intraocular pressure and whether or not there has been permanent damage to the trabecular meshwork. The intraocular pressure can always be reduced to normal levels by the intravenous infusion of urea or mannitol (p. 107). Once the intraocular pressure is less than 50 mm. Hg, the pupil becomes responsive to miotics, and the attack is usually corrected within several hours. If the pressure remains at a normal level, iridectomy should be done when the signs of ocular congestion have disappeared. It is not customary to operate on both eyes at the same time, but the fellow eye may well be operated upon before the patient is discharged from the hospital.

If following reduction with osmotic agents the pressure again rises despite the use of miotics, in all likelihood the trabecular meshwork has been damaged. These eyes respond poorly to a peripheral iridectomy solely, and it is better to carry out a filtering procedure. Inasmuch as these eyes have been congested, the blood vessels are dilated and bleeding is common.

In eyes in which angle-closure glaucoma has been neglected and that have become blind and painful, enucleation is probably the procedure of choice. Such eyes do not respond well to filtering operations, and it is unwise to subject patients to intraocular surgery to salvage a blind eye.

Open-angle glaucoma

Open-angle glaucoma (simple glaucoma, glaucoma simplex, compensated glaucoma, chronic glaucoma, or chronic simple glaucoma) is that type of primary glaucoma in which there is a pathologic increase in the intraocular pressure in the absence of an obstruction between the trabecular meshwork and the anterior chamber (Fig. 19-6). The increased intraocular pressure leads to a characteristic excavation of the optic disk and typical defects of the visual field. Open-angle glaucoma is the chief cause of blindness of the adult in the United States. It appears to arise because of an abnormality involving the trabecular meshwork that causes an interference of the flow of aqueous humor between the anterior chamber and the canal of Schlemm. There are all degrees of severity, and unquestionably many individuals have mild instances of the disease without knowing it.

Symptoms and signs. Open-angle glaucoma tends to manifest itself usually after the age of 50 years. There is no particular sexual predisposition. As indicated (p. 306), corticosteroid administration suggests that the allele involved in open-angle glaucoma occurs in about one third of all persons. Open-angle glaucoma may occur in myopic as well as hyperoptic eyes, but it is more frequent in hyperopia. External examination of the eye does not indicate an abnormality such as that which may be recognized in angle-closure glaucoma.

Open-angle glaucoma is characterized by an almost complete absence of symptoms and a chronic, insidious course. Halos around lights and blurring of vision do not occur unless there has been a sudden in-

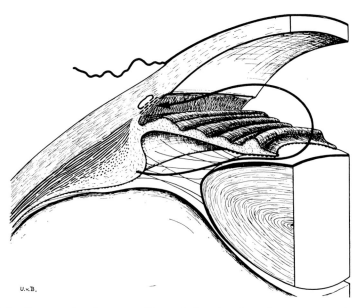

Fig. 19-6. Open-angle glaucoma. The anterior chamber always communicates with the trabecular area.

crease in ocular tension, and many patients never experience iridescent vision. The central visual acuity remains good until very late in the course of the disease. Routine measurement of central vision is of no value as a screening test. As the disease progresses, there is loss of accommodation for near work, so that a premature presbyopia or a more rapid than normal decrease in accommodative power occurs. Additionally, there may be a fairly rapid increase in hyperopia. An early symptom is defective dark adaptation, often manifested by slow recovery of vision in night driving when oncoming headlights disturb adaptation.

Diagnosis. The diagnosis of open-angle glaucoma depends upon demonstration of an increased intraocular pressure combined with characteristic changes in the visual field and optic nerve. The increased intraocular pressure precedes the optic nerve and visual field changes by many years, and it is highly desirable that the abnormality be diagnosed before they occur.

Gonioscopy indicates that the aqueous humor has access to the trabecular meshwork at times when the intraocular pressure is elevated.

Medical treatment. The treatment of open-angle glaucoma is mainly medical in contrast to the treatment of the angle-closure type, which can be cured surgically. Open-angle glaucoma is treated medically unless the pressure cannot be controlled, as indicated by persistently elevated intraocular pressure, by progression of the optic nerve atrophy, or by visual field defects despite apparent normalization of tension. Pilocarpine is the traditional medication and is used in a concentration of 0.5 to 4%. It is desirable to begin therapy with the smallest possible concentration that will maintain normal pressure and prevent progression of the field defect. The concentration is increased gradually as the disease becomes refractory to the effects of the pilocarpine. Pilocarpine is used because it facilitates the aqueous outflow in open-angle glaucoma. It is also used in the management of angle-closure glaucoma, but because of its miotic effect on the pupil.

Treatment with pilocarpine is often combined with topical instillation of anticholinesterase compounds (p. 97) and epinephrine salts. Eserine and the alkyl phosphates, mainly echothiophate iodide, are currently the anticholinesterase agents used. The alkyl phosphates must not be used in angle-closure glaucoma because edema of the ciliary body can aggravate the closure mechanism. Epinephrine salts are used in a 2% concentration and improve aqueous outflow. Epinephrine compounds are moderately irritating to the eye and may cause a melanin pigmentation of the conjunctiva.

Carbonic anhydrase inhibitors are used to reduce the secretion of aqueous humor by the ciliary processes. Acetazolamide is the usual drug used. The drug is effective 2 hours after administration, with its effect lasting for 6 hours. It must be administered every 6 hours to be continuously effective. If side effects prevent use of acetazolamide or if it does not appear effective, other carbonic anhydrase compounds may be substituted.

Frequent examination is necessary to be certain that the glaucoma is controlled. Tonography, ophthalmoscopy, and perimetry are indicated to determine that the pressure is not intermittently elevated and the eyes gradually deteriorating.

Surgical treatment. If the intraocular pressure can be maintained at a normal level by means of drugs, and if there is no progress in the severity of the glaucoma, as judged by the ophthalmoscopic appearance of the optic nerve disk and by careful charting of the central visual fields, medical treatment of open-angle glaucoma is indicated. If the intraocular pressure cannot be controlled medically or if there is progress in the visual field defects or in the degree of optic atrophy, surgery is indicated. In patients who do not use their medication because of defective intelligence or unreliability, surgery is indicated.

If pressure can be maintained at normal levels by medical methods, surgery should not be done. Surgical procedures are particularly likely to be ineffective in Negroes, who tend to develop cicatricial changes that prevent adequate filtering procedures.

The main surgical procedure in open-angle glaucoma is a filtering operation, of which there are many variations. All are based on providing an opening between the anterior chamber and the subconjunctival space through which aqueous humor will flow. The opening may be made by means of a trephine that is 1 or 2 mm. in diameter. Alternatively, an incision may be made into the anterior chamber, and the anterior or posterior lip may be removed so that the wound edges are not adjacent and will not be closed by cicatrix. Cauterization by heat of the scleral wound edges

Causes of secondary glaucoma

  I. Uveitis and postinflammatory glaucoma
     A. Pupillary occlusion
 II. Heterochromia of iris with uveitis
III. Postoperative glaucoma
     A. Pupillary block in aphakic glaucoma
 IV. Phacolytic glaucoma
     A. Swelling of lens
     B. Subluxation of lens
     C. Hypermaturity of lens
     D. Rupture of lens capsule
  V. Epithelial downgrowth
 VI. Glaucoma capsulare
VII. Glaucoma secondary to hemorrhage
VIII. Glaucoma and venous closure
     A. Extraocular
     B. Central
 IX. Traumatic glaucoma
  X. Essential progressive atrophy of iris
 XI. Rubeosis iridis
XII. Thyrotropic exophthalmos
XIII. Intraocular tumors
XIV. Congenital glaucoma

also prevents the wound from closing. The scleral openings into the anterior chamber may be combined with a complete or peripheral iridectomy or with inclusion of a portion of the iris in the scleral wound.

Secondary glaucoma

Secondary glaucoma is an abnormality in which the intraocular pressure is increased to a level incompatible with continued normal function of the eye. The disease may be unilateral or both eyes may be involved, but usually to a different extent. Secondary glaucomas arise from a large number of inflammations, degenerations, trauma, and new growths within the eye.

Special types

Iridocyclitis may cause a secondary glaucoma through obstruction of the trabecular meshwork by inflammatory cells and debris.

Heterochromic iridocyclitis is a nongranulomatous chronic anterior uveitis associated with a secondary glaucoma and a posterior subcapsular cataract. Both the glaucoma and the cataract with which the uveitis is associated may be aggravated by corticosteroids used locally in the treatment of the uveitis. Iridocyclitis may cause a depigmentation of the iris, and some believe that a heterochromic iridocyclitis does not constitute a distinct clinical entity. Glaucoma cyclitic crisis is an acute inflammation of the uveal tract in which the signs of an acute increase in intraocular pressure predominate. There is corneal edema with blurring of vision and marked decrease in the coefficient of outflow. The disease is distinguished from angle-closure glaucoma in that the angle is open. The inflammation may be confined to the trabecular meshwork with minimal inflammatory signs.

Contusion of the eye results in a marked immediate increase in intraocular pressure that persists for 30 to 45 minutes. If hemor-

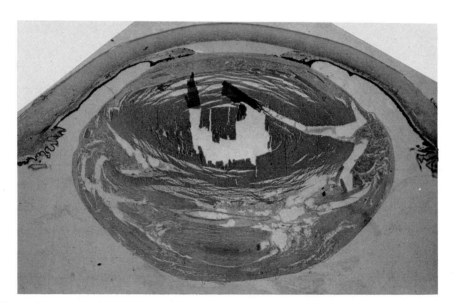

Fig. 19-7. Secondary glaucoma due to swelling of the lens. The anterior chamber has been entirely occluded. There are posterior synechiae binding the pupillary margin to the anterior lens capsule. The increased volume of the posterior chamber has pressed the iris against the trabecular meshwork and the cornea through almost its entire extent.

rhage follows contusion, a secondary glaucoma may ensue. It arises from blockage of the trabecular meshwork with erythrocytes and probably subsequent damage to the trabecular meshwork by hemosiderin.

Subluxation of the lens (Fig. 19-7) may produce a secondary glaucoma, the causes of which are unknown. The mechanism is evident if the lens is trapped in the anterior chamber but not if the intact lens is in the vitreous body. Intumescence, or acute hydration of an immature cataract, may cause glaucoma by blocking the angle. The lens protein may cause a uveitis with secondary glaucoma comparable to that occurring in other types of iridocyclitis. The lens protein is released either through injury of the capsule or in hypermaturity of a cataract. Intraocular tumors initially cause a hypotony. As they increase in size, the coefficient of outflow is reduced, and glaucoma occurs.

Vascularization of the iris as occurs in diabetes or following a central vein closure may cause a neovascularization of the trabecular meshwork and marked increase in intraocular pressure. The downgrowth of epithelium into the anterior chamber from the conjunctiva following surgery or injury may cause a glaucoma that is extremely resistant to therapy.

Pigmentary glaucoma is a variant of primary open-angle glaucoma in which there is a deposition of pigment (Krukenberg's spindle) on the corneal endothelium. There is a deposition of pigment in the trabecular area and on the lens and zonule. Myopic men are often affected.

Exfoliation of the lens capsule occurs in two conditions. True exfoliation occurs in glassblowers' cataract in which the iris absorbs infrared energy and transmits it to the lens capsule, causing a splitting of the zonular lamella. Pseudoexfoliation is an unusual abnormality in which the lens capsule, mainly in a zone between the pupillary area and the equator, is involved, with a deposition of a flaky translucent material. Patients with this condition have a slightly higher incidence of glaucoma than the normal population, but the significance is not known.

Congenital glaucoma

Congenital glaucoma is a secondary type of glaucoma due to a developmental anomaly in the angle of the anterior chamber. This defect interferes with the drainage of the aqueous humor, causing an increase in intraocular pressure, which in turn causes stretching of the elastic coats of the eye with marked enlargement of the globe (total staphyloma). The globe in man is subject to this stretching only until about the age of 3 years. Glaucoma occurring after this age does not cause enlargement of the globe and follows a course similar to adult glaucoma.

True congenital glaucoma is transmitted as an autosomal recessive characteristic. Males are affected twice as often as females. Cardiac, auditory, and cerebral defects may also be present. Signs of infantile glaucoma may be present and even far advanced at birth, or become apparent before the child has reached the age of 3 months. The earliest symptoms are tearing of the eyes, blepharospasm, and sensitivity of the eyes to light. Examination indicates a subepithelial corneal edema that obscures the pattern of the iris. The increase in intraocular pressure causes a stretching of the external coats of the eye, with marked enlargement of the globe (total staphyloma, Fig. 19-8). This is usually evident as an increase in diameter of the cornea from less than 10.5 to 12 mm. or more. There are tears in Descemet's membrane that appear as glassy lines on the back surface of the cornea. The anterior chamber is deeper than normal.

Congenital glaucoma arises from a congenital defect in which there is failure of cleavage of the peripheral iris from the cornea to form the anterior chamber. There is hypoplasia of the scleral spur, and the

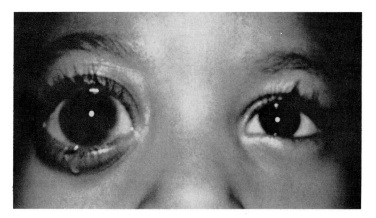

Fig. 19-8. Marked enlargement of the globe in congenital glaucoma.

trabecular meshwork inserts into the anterior portion of the ciliary body. The iris inserts abnormally far forward, often into the trabecular meshwork itself. Gonioscopy indicates the abnormality.

Congenital glaucoma may be recognized by the tearing, photophobia, and blepharospasm. Congenital dacryostenosis also causes tearing but no apparent discomfort. The subepithelial corneal edema causes a characteristic ground-glass appearance. Preferably the disease is recognized before dilation of the globe. Any infant with a cornea more than 10.5 mm. in diameter should be studied.

Accurate measurement of the intraocular pressure must be made with the infant deeply anesthetized. Fluothane markedly reduces the intraocular pressure and should not be used. Superficial planes of anesthesia lead to inaccurate pressure readings and faulty evaluation.

The treatment of congenital glaucoma is primarily surgical by means of the goniotomy procedure in which an incision is made into the region of the trabecular meshwork under direct visual control, using a gonioscope. This procedure may be combined with puncture opening (goniopuncture) between the trabecular area and the subconjunctival space. Surgery may

Patients must be followed carefully posthave to be repeated.

operatively to be certain the glaucoma is controlled. Intraocular pressure must be measured with deep anesthesia.

Chapter 20

The extraocular muscles

A normal pair of eyes is so aligned that an object in space is imaged simultaneously on the fovea centralis of each eye. Thus the eyes are parallel in all directions of gaze, except when they converge on a nearby object. In some 1 to 2% of all children the visual axes of each eye are not so related and the condition of strabismus (squint, walleyes, or cross-eyes) is present.

There are two closely interrelated mechanisms involved in ocular alignment: (1) those related to image formation and perception and (2) those involved in moving the eyes. An abnormality in either mechanism may lead to strabismus.

Definition of the various terms used in describing motor-sensory relationships in the eye may prevent misunderstanding.

Terminology

Strabismus (heterotropia, squint, walleyes, or cross-eyes) is that condition in which an object in space is not imaged simultaneously on the fovea centralis of each eye. It may be divided into paralytic (noncomitant), in which one or more muscles or their nervous connections are impaired, and comitant, in which there is no muscle weakness. Esotropia refers to inward deviation, exotropia to outward deviation. Hypertropia refers to upward deviation; thus the correct usage would be a right hypertropia rather than a left hypotropia. Squint is intermittent or periodic when there are periods when the eyes are parallel and constant when they are never parallel. It is alternating when each eye, first one and then the other, fixates while the fellow eye deviates. A squint is monocular when the same eye always deviates and the fellow eye always fixates. An accommodative squint is one in which the degree of crossing varies with the amount of accommodation present. A congenital strabismus is one present at birth. A sensory strabismus is one in which some abnormality in image formation causes the deviation.

Heterophoria is that condition in which there is a latent tendency for one eye to deviate so as not to look at the same object. This tendency, however, is counteracted by fusion (see below); therefore a heterophoria can be diagnosed only by interrupting fusion. Esophoria refers to the tendency for inward deviation, exophoria to outward deviation, and hyperphoria to upward deviation. Orthophoria is that condition in which there is no deviation of the eye when fusion is interrupted.

Fusion is the condition in which the retinal images from each eye are perceived as a single object. There are three grades of fusion:

Grade 1, simultaneous macular perception (normal correspondence): This is the ability of the brain to receive and appreciate images from the fovea of each eye simultaneously.
Grade 2, fusion with amplitude: This is the ability to blend the images from the two foveas into a single perception. The fusion

Strabismus

I. Comitant (nonparalytic)
  A. Motor anomaly predominantly
    1. Accommodative—vergence movements
    2. Fusional—vergence movements
    3. Convergence—divergence balance
    4. Mixtures of above
  B. Sensory anomaly predominantly
    1. Anatomic malposition of eyes
    2. Interference with image formation
      a. Anisometropia
      b. Irregularities and opacities of media
      c. Disorders of retinal receptors or in transmission
II. Noncomitant (paralytic)
  A. Muscle abnormalities
    1. Congenital, thyroid disease, injury
  B. Nuclei or nerve abnormalities
    1. Congenital, acquired
III. Supranuclear
  A. Conjugate deviation
    1. Paretic
    2. Spastic
  B. Comitant (by definition)
    1. Convergence excess or insufficiency
    2. Divergence excess or insufficiency
    3. Combinations of convergence-divergence anomalies

is maintained by vergence while the images are being moved.

Grade 3, stereopsis: This is the blending of slightly dissimilar images from the two eyes with the perception of depth and solidity.

Fusion-free position is a term applied when an eye is covered or vision is otherwise interrupted or eliminated so as to eliminate fusion.

Binocular rotations of the eyes in opposite directions are called *vergences*. They involve areas in the midbody plane concerned with convergence or divergence (p. 87). The two main mechanisms involved relate to accommodation and convergence. In accommodation, objects remain focused on the retina because of the change in re-fractive power of the lens in response to contraction of the ciliary muscle. The eyes turn inward mainly because of contraction of the medial rectus muscle and relaxation of the lateral rectus muscle. With accommodation, there is an associated balance between convergence and divergence movements so that the fovea of each eye remains directed at an object of regard irrespective of its distance (within limits) from the eye.

Tonic or *initial convergence* is the term applied to the impulse required to give tone to all of the muscles so that the eyes are directed approximately straight ahead. In deep anesthesia or in death when all innervational impulse to the ocular muscles is lost, the eyes are in the anatomic position of rest in which they are divergent. In the waking state and when ocular muscles are actively tonic, the eyes are in the physiologic position of rest because of tonic vergence. In infancy and childhood this position is convergent, while in the adult this position is divergent.

Accommodative vergence is the mechanism by which an object is maintained with a clear image upon the retina, combined with a convergence necessary to maintain the optic axes of each eye directed to the object.

Fusional vergence is the term applied to the fine movements occurring in the eyes when an object is imaged on slightly different parts of the fovea centralis, these movements bringing about the cerebral superimposition of the images. Additionally, there are reflexes that cause the eyes to converge when there is an awareness of nearness, whether this is brought about by sound or by retinal impulses that do not impress themselves upon the cortex.

Physiologic fixation is the faculty of causing the image of an object, to which attention is directed, to fall on the fovea and to be maintained there for a period.

Monocular rotations of the eye are called *ductions*. Binocular rotations of the eye are called *versions* when they are to the right or to the left or up or down. They are called *vergences* when they involve a point in the midbody plane in which convergence or divergence is involved. It will be recalled that ductions and versions involve saccadic eye movements, whereas the vergence movements involve a different mechanism (p. 89).

Visual and oculomotor development

At birth the central visual acuity is approximately 20/700 as measured by opticokinetic nystagmus induced by a rotating drum. There is no central fixation, and the eyes appear to move randomly. Several weeks after birth the eyes will turn toward a light, and by the age of 3 months an infant will fix both eyes on a light and attempt to grasp it. There is a gradual increase in the central visual acuity, so that by the age of 1 year it is approximately 20/200; by the second year, 20/70; and at the end of the third year, about 20/20. Failure to use the eye interferes with the normal development of central visual acuity—this may cause arrest of visual development at the level attained at the time the interference occurred, a functional amblyopia.

At birth the movement of the two eyes does not appear to be coordinated. The eyes may, for a few seconds at a time, seem to turn in different directions. During the first 3 months of life there may be crossing of the eyes, but there are also periods when the two eyes are relatively parallel and appear to be directed simultaneously to the same object. At the age of 3 months the eyes are parallel most of the time, and after the age of 6 months there is normally no deviation from parallelism. Binocular vision appears to be present, but the degree cannot be learned.

From birth until puberty the eyes tend to turn inward when the tone of each ocular muscle is the same (the physiologic position of rest). This inward tendency is called tonic convergence. After puberty there is a tendency for the eyes to turn outward in the physiologic position of rest. Any interference with the normal binocular development of the eyes accentuates this normal tonic convergence, and an inward deviation may occur (sensory esotropia). After puberty there is less tonic convergence, and an exotropia (sensory exotropia) may occur when there is interference with binocular use of the eyes.

For the visual axes to be directed simultaneously to a single object in space, it is evident that the eyes must be placed relatively straight ahead in the head, a condition that occurs only in man and in the higher primates. If the eyes are widely separated, as occurs in Crouzon's disease (p. 193), the visual axes cannot be directed toward the same object, and a heterotropia occurs. This is also likely if one eye is displaced more anterior than the other.

If there is marked interference with the image formation in both eyes, a pendular type of nystagmus occurs (p. 423). There is a failure of development of central neuromuscular controls, and visual acuity remains depressed, with nystagmus dominating the clinical appearance so that a deviation from parallelism is not prominent. If the interference with image formation or perception occurs predominantly in one eye, as in a marked refractive error of one eye or a disease affecting image formation, normal visual development is limited to the fellow eyes. If the neuromuscular mechanisms are superbly adjusted, the eyes may remain parallel. If, however, there is a lack of the stimuli required for parallel adjustment of the eyes, an esotropia may occur. An exotropia occurs if the defective vision develops after the age of 10 years.

Diagnostic measures

The large variety of tests available to study abnormalities of the ocular muscles may be confusing. Worse, they may lead to the erroneous conclusion that diagnosis and treatment should be delayed until the patient is old enough to cooperate in subjective testing, thus permitting the development of poor vision from disuse (functional amblyopia) or other sensory abnormalities. Examination and treatment are indicated in any infant in whom an ocular deviation persists beyond the age of 6 months. In older children, skilled examination is indicated as soon as it is evident that a deviation is present. Emphasis is based upon two major areas: (1) the ocular deviation and (2) the visual (sensory) status.

The presence or absence of an ocular deviation is determined by the alternate cover test (Figs. 20-1 and 20-2). The patient's attention is directed to a fixation target such as a light or small picture, and one eye is covered for about 10 seconds. This eye is then uncovered, and the fellow eye is immediately covered. Attention is directed to the movement made by the covered eye as it is uncovered. If it does not move, orthophoria is probably present, and the eyes are parallel. If the eye

moves as it is uncovered, either a phoria or a tropia is present. If the eye has been rotated inward while under the cover and turns out to fix when it is uncovered, either an esophoria or an esotropia is present. If the eye is turned outward under the cover, it will move inward when the cover is removed, and an exophoria or an exotropia is present.

To distinguish between a phoria and a tropia, the cover-uncover test is used. This test is of more than theoretic importance inasmuch as binocular vision is present if there is only a phoria, whereas if a tropia is present, the individual is either seeing double or is suppressing the image from one eye. The cover-uncover test is performed by directing the patient's attention to a light, covering one eye for about 20 seconds and then uncovering it so that both eyes are uncovered. Attention is directed to movements of the uncovered eye when the fellow eye is occluded and then to movements of both eyes as the cover is removed (Fig. 20-2).

The degree of deviation is often esti-

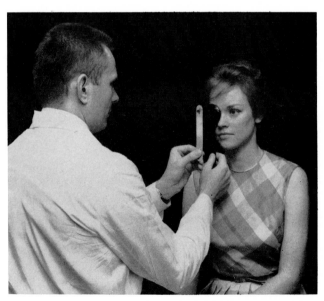

Fig. 20-1. Cover test to determine if the eyes are parallel. A small picture is being used for fixation to stimulate accommodation.

mated by observing the reflection of light from the cornea of the deviating eye. The cornea has a radius of 5 to 6 mm., and each millimeter of displacement of the reflex is equal to about 6° of strabismus. The reflection may be misleading because the visual axis may not pass through the center of the pupil, and a simulated small squint may result.

Noncomitant strabismus (paralytic)

Paralytic strabismus is deviation of the eye from parallelism resulting from weakness (paresis) or paralysis of an ocular muscle. It is characterized by a limitation of movement in the field of action of the paralyzed muscle so that the angle of deviation is greatest in this field. There is less or no deviation in uninvolved fields of action. The deviation is greater when the paralyzed eye is used for fixation than when the normal eye is used. When the normal eye fixes, the paralyzed eye is in the position of primary deviation. When the involved eye fixes, the normal eye deviates in the position of secondary deviation. The secondary deviation is greater than the primary deviation because of the

simultaneous innervational impulse to ocular muscles concerned with the same direction of gaze (Hering's law of equal innervation). Thus, when the involved eye is used for fixation, a greater innervational impulse is required to maintain this fixation, and this greater impulse causes excess deviation or overaction of the muscles of the normal eye.

If the patient has binocular vision, a paralytic strabismus will cause diplopia, which is most marked in the field of action of the involved muscle. Diplopia does not occur in the absence of binocular vision and thus is not found in congenital conditions. The image of the deviating eye is always opposite to the direction of the deviation. To minimize diplopia due to paralysis of a vertical muscle, the head may be tilted toward a shoulder, partially rotated, and the chin elevated or depressed (ocular torticollis). Except with involvement of the superior oblique muscles, the head is tilted toward the shoulder on the affected side and the head slightly rotated in this direction. With superior oblique muscle paralysis, the head is tilted and slightly rotated to the sound side. The chin

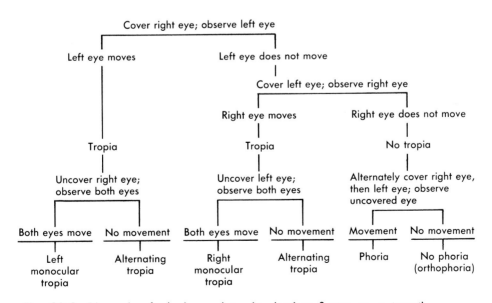

Fig. 20-2. Diagnosis of phorias and tropias (patient fixates on a target).

is elevated in palsies of the elevator muscles and depressed in palsies of the ocular depressor muscles.

The diagnosis of the specific muscle involved in a paralytic strabismus may be difficult. The history may indicate the cause to be head injury, tumor, aneurysm, thyroid oculopathy, etc. The onset of multiple sclerosis (p. 426) may be associated with muscle palsy, and myasthenia gravis (p. 456) may be limited to ocular muscles. Basically the cause is either muscular or nervous and occurs in either the orbit or in the cranial cavity. It may be hereditary, congenital, developmental, traumatic, inflammatory, toxic, metabolic, or neoplastic.

Supranuclear deviations occur because of abnormalities present in the frontal and occipital cortex that are connected by projection fibers with supranuclear centers through the medial longitudinal fasciculus (p. 55). Supranuclear deviations always are bilateral, and diplopia does not occur. Volitional ocular movements are involved, such as eyes up or down or right or left.

Comitant strabismus (nonparalytic)

In comitant strabismus there is no muscle weakness; therefore the angle of deviation is the same in all fields of gaze. Early in the development of the deviation there may be double vision, but this may be quickly eliminated so that the image originating in the deviating eye is suppressed.

Comitant esotropia

The two main types of comitant esotropia (Fig. 20-3) are accommodative and nonaccommodative. There are, in addition, mixtures of these forms.

Accommodative esotropia. Accommodative esotropia occurs because of an anomaly in the accommodative-covergence/accommodation ratio (AC/A ratio), which occurs spontaneously or because of hyperopia. The abnormality has its onset after the age of 1 year, with the usual age of onset between 2 and 3 years. The onset is abrupt in a child who has previously had straight eyes. The deviation is brought about by an attempt to visualize objects clearly, and the amount of crossing varies markedly from time to time. There is often a family history of ocular deviation. The esotropia is often intermittent initially and then develops into a constant type. It is aggravated by fatigue.

Symptoms are ordinarily not conspicuous, although it is evident that diplopia is possible, but the image from the deviating eye is easily suppressed.

Examination may indicate an inward deviation of the eye, and this may be demonstrated with the alternate cover and cover-uncover test. Fixation of a point of light may not stimulate accommodation adequately to demonstrate an intermittent deviation. However, fixation of a small picture requiring accommodation to see will cause deviation. The deviation is frequently greater for near than for distance. A hyperopia of more than 2 diopters may be present, but marked hyperopia is not essential for accommodative esotropia to occur. The deviation is decreased by correction of the hyperopia or by the use of convex lenses

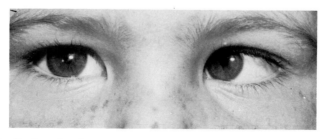

Fig. 20-3. Comitant esotropia.

Comitant esotropia

I. Accommodative
   A. Onset after 1 year (average, 2½ years)
   B. Familial
   C. Abnormal accommodative-convergence accommodation ratio (AC/A)
   D. Sensory mechanisms often normal
   E. Ocular deviation
      1. Greater for near than far
      2. Initially intermittent but tending to become constant
      3. Decreased by convex lenses (which decrease accommodation)
   F. Treatment: decrease accommodative stimulus
      1. Full hyperopic correction
      2. Bifocal lenses
      3. Miotics
II. Nonaccommodative—excessive muscle tone (tonic convergence)
   A. Congenital
      1. Onset at birth
      2. Familial
      3. Abnormal sensory mechanisms common
         a. Strabismic amblyopia
         b. Abnormal retinal correspondence
         c. Defective fusion mechanism
      4. Ocular deviation
         a. Nearly equal for near and far
         b. Does not vary with accommodation
      5. Treatment
         a. Exclude neurologic and ocular disease
         b. Prevent abnormal sensory mechanism
            (1) Mainly patching of eye with better vision
            (2) Pleoptics
         c. Surgery
   B. Sensory interference
      1. Onset after disease or injury
      2. Possibly hereditary eye disease
      3. Defective vision in one or both eyes
         a. Marked anisometropia
         b. Corneal opacity   d. Retinal disease
         c. Cataract   e. Optic nerve or tract disease
      4. Ocular deviation
         a. Equal for near and far
         b. Monocular fixation using eye with better vision
      5. Treatment
         a. Lenses if anisometropic
            (contact lenses, if necessary, as in monocular aphakia)
         b. Cosmetic surgery to straighten eyes
         c. Correction of condition causing defective vision, if possible
   C. Acquired
      1. Onset following neglected accommodative esotropia
      2. Abnormal sensory mechanisms common
      3. Ocular deviation
         a. Equal for near and far
         b. Monocular fixation
         c. Tends to increase initially; exotropia common with aging
      4. Treatment
         a. Prevent neglect of accommodative esotropia
         b. Surgery
   D. Mixed accommodative and nonaccommodative types

for near. Anticholinesterase drugs instilled in each eye decrease the angle of squint by markedly stimulating ciliary body contraction so that additional accommodation is not possible. If the squint becomes constant, functional amblyopia or abnormal retinal correspondence may occur.

Treatment is indicated as soon as the condition is recognized, and it is directed to decreasing the amount of accommodation required. This is done by correcting the full hyperopic error as found by examination with accommodation suspended by means of a cycloplegic drug. If the eyes with correcting lenses are parallel for distance and esotropic for near, it may be desirable to prescribe bifocal lenses to decrease the accommodative stimulus required for near work.

Anticholinesterase drugs may be substituted for, or combined with, lenses. Usually 0.125% echothiophate (Phospholine I) combined with 10% phenylephrine is used. Phenylephrine (a sympathomimetic amine) prevents the development of cysts of the pigmented epithelium of the iris that may become so large as to interfere with vision. As children become older, the convexity of the lenses is decreased, provided the eyes remain parallel. Ultimately the lenses may be discarded unless there is marked astigmatism.

Orthoptic training (p. 332) is of value in teaching the child to maintain parallelism without lenses. It involves teaching the youngster to recognize the diplopia that occurs with the excessive accommodation, which causes the esotropia. This is not always an easy task inasmuch as a child may suppress the image of the deviating eye when he attempts to see clearly by stimulating accommodation. A pure accommodative squint does not require surgery. Accommodative anomalies may be associated with nonaccommodative esotropias, and the surgery must be directed to the nonaccommodative portion of the strabismus.

Nonaccommodative esotropia. Nonaccommodative esotropia involves a variety of mechanisms. In the majority of patients there is no obvious abnormality of ocular image formation or perception. No anatomic factor can be demonstrated. The deviation is usually present at birth or appears shortly thereafter. There is frequently a familial history of squint. The deviation is usually quite large, and it tends to be present for both near and distance. There may be a short period in which there is alternate fixation, but there is a marked tendency for the deviation to become monocular with overaction of a medial rectus muscle and commonly the associated inferior oblique muscles. The angle of deviation tends to remain relatively constant and is not modified by corrective lenses or by anticholinesterase agents. The development of amblyopia and abnormal retinal correspondence is common. The children often have a defective fusion mechanism that cannot be corrected.

When the condition is present at birth, often there is cross-fixation, with the infant using the left eye in looking to the right and the right eye in looking to the left. This fixation encourages equal use of the eyes and combats the development of abnormal sensory mechanisms.

The treatment must be started early, certainly by the sixth month of age. It is important (1) to evaluate the neurologic status of the child to exclude cerebral palsy in which esotropia tends to decrease with passing years and (2) to exclude a visual defect arising either from a marked difference in refraction between the two eyes (anisometropia) or a defect such as cataract or retinal disease that interferes with image formation on the retina. Spontaneous improvement does not occur. Recently, surgery has been recommended in infancy, although the benefits are balanced by the difficulty in making an exact diagnosis. In those cases in which functional amblyopia has developed, the abnormality is treated by occlusion of the habitually fixing eye to force use of the nonfixing eye. This is frequently followed by conversion of a strabismus from a monocular to an alternating type, a condition that may disturb parents who believe that the crossing involved only one eye.

Sensory interference. Children born with an abnormality of the image-forming mechanism of the eyes may also develop an excessive tonic convergence type of defect. This resembles nonaccommodative congenital esotropia in its onset at birth, and a marked deviation for both near and far is present. However, there may not be a family history. The deviation tends to be monocular from the beginning, with the child using the better eye. It is important to distinguish a sensory disturbance from the congenital and acquired types of esotropia. If the individual cannot develop central vision because of a cataract or a retinal disorder, it is important that he not be treated for amblyopia (p. 330).

If a cataract or retinal disease is present, the only treatment of value is cosmetic surgery. Inasmuch as there is no likelihood of providing binocular vision, this may well be delayed to just before the child enters school. These patients tend to become exotropic in later life, and surgery to make the eyes parallel in childhood may accelerate the development of exotropia.

Acquired nonaccommodative esotropia. The acquired type most commonly follows a neglected accommodative esotropia. In this instance a monocular deviation tends to develop, with an excessive tonic convergence and functional amblyopia. The treatment must be directed toward correction of the accommodative factor and correction of the amblyopia. Often surgery is indicated to correct the nonaccommodative portion of the esotropia.

Comitant exotropia

Comitant exotropia (Fig. 20-4) may be divided into accommodative and nonac-

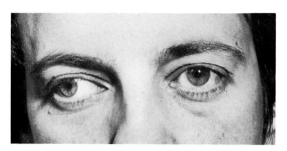

Fig. 20-4. Comitant exotropia.

commodative types. In general, exotropia tends to develop at a later period in life than esotropia, and the development of functional amblyopia is much less common. Abnormalities in image formation and in perception, which give rise to an esotropia when occurring before the age of 10 years, for the most part result in an exotropia when occurring after this age. Functional amblyopia occurring because of esotropia is a common cause of sensory exotropia. Unfortunately, as the eyes pass from esotropia to exotropia, there is a phase in which they are parallel, which leads the naive to believe that the esotropia has been corrected. The eye continues to diverge, with the ultimate development of a constant exotropia that often recurs following surgery.

Accommodative exotropia. Accommodative exotropia is a relatively uncommon disorder and arises because of uncorrected myopia, which decreases the need for accommodation for near work. Inasmuch as most infants are hyperopic at birth, the condition occurs later in life after central visual acuity has developed, and sensory anomalies are uncommon. It may occur in myopic adolescents who prefer poor vision to wearing glasses. There may be a family history of myopia. Symptoms are minimal. The blurred vision arising from myopia prevents appreciation of the diplopia. Examination reveals an intermittent outward deviation of the eyes, which becomes constant if the condition is neglected. The wearing of concave lenses to correct the myopia is all that is required. Youthful individuals often prefer contact lenses.

Nonaccommodative exotropia. Nonaccommodative exotropia may occur in Crouzon's disease in which the eyes are widely separated (p. 193) and in alternating exotropia-exophoria. In Crouzon's disease and in other abnormalities in which the eyes are widely separated, an exotropia is common. It occurs because of mechanical inability of the eyes to converge adequately and provides a mechanism for preventing symptomatic diplopia by keeping the image from each eye widely separated.

Alternating exophoria-exotropia. This is the common type of exotropia. It is usually intermittent and may have its onset between the ages of 6 months and 8 years. There is often a familial history. Its occurrence in infancy may not be noted because the deviation is more marked for distance than for near and is often intermittent. The exotropia may become marked with fatigue or visual inattention, and patients may voluntarily bring their eyes to parallelism.

Examination indicates an exophoria

Comitant exotropia

I. Accommodative
  A. Onset after 5 years
  B. Familial
  C. Uncorrected myopia present
  D. Sensory mechanisms normal
  E. Ocular deviation
    1. Greater for far than near
    2. Initially intermittent but tending to become constant
  F. Treatment: stimulate accommodation by correcting myopia with lenses
II. Nonaccommodative—excessive muscle tone (tonic divergence)
  A. Congenital
    1. Onset with craniostenosis with eyes widely separated
    2. Seldom familial
    3. Sensory mechanisms often normal
    4. Ocular deviation
      a. Nearly equal for near and far
    5. Treatment
      a. Correct craniostenosis
      b. Surgery
  B. Alternating exophoria-exotropia
    1. Onset 6 months to 8 years
    2. Familial
    3. Sensory mechanisms normal
    4. Ocular deviation
      a. Greater for far than near
      b. Aggravated by fatigue, visual inattentiveness
      c. Usually intermittent but becoming constant
    5. Treatment: surgery
  C. Acquired
    1. Onset after 12 years
    2. Deteriorated esotropia or alternating exotropia-exophoria
    3. Sensory abnormalities common
    4. Ocular deviation
      a. Equal for near and far
      b. Poor convergence
      c. Often monocular fixation
    5. Treatment: surgery

much more marked for distance than for near. Convergence is usually adequate. By covering one eye for several minutes, the exophoria may be converted to an exotropia that has the same angle of deviation as the exophoria. The deviation is not influenced by glasses or by local medications. Visual acuity is usually good, and binocular vision is present. The individual suppresses when the eyes deviate, and he is unaware of diplopia.

Treatment is solely surgical and is usually directed to recession of the lateral rectus muscles if fusion is good. Usually a large recession must be performed on each eye, and as much correction is required for an exophoria as an exotropia. Inasmuch as the deviation is intermittent, many patients do not wish surgery, and in time the condition deteriorates with the deviation constant for far and near.

Acquired comitant exotropia. Acquired comitant exotropia occurs because of defective vision developing in one eye or because of a deteriorated exophoria.

Deteriorated exophoria-exotropia. These patients initially have an alternating exophoria-exotropia that is either untreated or neglected. The onset is delayed until the age of 10 to 12 years. Prior to that age, an intermittent alternating exophoria-exotropia is present. The deviation subtly becomes constant, initially for distance and then for near. The exotropia may become marked for both near and far, and attention may not be directed to the deviation until it is marked for near. Central visual acuity is good, but often fusion is poor, and abnormal retinal correspondence may be present. The deviation may be monocular. Convergence is impaired.

Treatment is solely surgical. For the most part, monocular surgery is done with recession of the lateral rectus muscle and resection of the medial rectus muscle. Surgical results are inconsistent, and undercorrections and overcorrections are frequent.

A and V syndromes

A and V syndromes are terms applied to ocular deviations in which the angle of the deviation is more marked on looking upward or downward. In the A type of deviation the visual axes are closer to each other in upward gaze. In the V type of deviation the visual axes are closer together in downward gaze. Thus an A esotropia is greater looking upward than downward, and a V esotropia is greater looking downward than upward. An A exotropia is greater looking downward than upward, and a V exotropia is greater looking upward than downward.

The cause of the abnormality is debated. In V types of esotropia and exotropia there is often, but not always, overaction of both inferior oblique muscles. In A types of deviation there may be overaction of the superior oblique muscles. The overaction of the inferior oblique muscle is noted by having the patient look at the right or left and observing the upward deviation of the adducting eye. Overaction of the superior oblique muscle is noted by observing the downward deviation of the adducting eye in lateral gaze. However, A and V patterns occur without anomalies of the oblique muscles, and physiologically the visual axes tend to converge in downward gaze so that V patterns may be regarded as due to overaction of the medial rectus muscles.

The topic is of more than theoretic interest inasmuch as a frequency as high as 50% has been estimated. Surgery is directed to the muscles believed implicated. In V-pattern anomalies with overaction of the inferior oblique muscles, these muscles are weakened. This may be combined or followed by recession or resection of the lateral rectus and medial rectus muscles. To enhance the effect of these procedures, the new insertions of the horizontal muscles are often displaced upward or downward. The medial rectus muscles are always displaced toward the apex of the A or V, thus upward in A patterns and downward in V patterns. The lateral rectus muscles are displaced away from the apex, irrespective of whether a horizontal recession or resection is done.

Pseudostrabismus

Pseudostrabismus is a condition in which the eyes appear to be crossed although they are in fact perfectly aligned. The appearance arises because of an extra fold of skin at the inner canthus of each eye (epicanthus), because of a broad flat nose, because the eyes are unusually close together, or because of an oval palpebral fissure as occurs in Orientals. Each of these conditions conceals some of the white sclera at the medial side of the eye and gives rise to an appearance that the eyes are turning inward. The alternate cover test indicates that the eyes are parallel and the sole treatment is reassurance of the parents. As the child's face grows, the appearance of strabismus disappears.

Treatment

The treatment of comitant strabismus is directed (1) toward development of normal central visual acuity and fusion with cerebral superimposition of retinal images resulting in depth perception and (2) toward correction of the deviation of the eyes.

Vision in strabismus may be reduced because of defects in image formation that cannot be corrected, such as opacities of the ocular media and retinal or optic nerve defects. More commonly vision is reduced because of the development of amblyopia.

Functional amblyopia. Functional amblyopia is the condition in which there is poor vision in an eye that appears to have no organic disease. Amblyopia may be divided into functional and organic, in which there are retinal, choroidal, or optic nerve lesions. An organic amblyopia may have an associated functional amblyopia superimposed because of inhibition occurring when the blurred image of the dis-

eased eye is superimposed on the clear image of the unaffected fellow eye. Amblyopia is generally diagnosed as present when the best corrected visual acuity in one eye is two or more lines poorer than in the fellow eye as measured on the Snellen chart (see Fig. 6-1). Functional amblyopia usually arises from failure to use the eye during the first few years of life. Central visual acuity is usually arrested at the level of development attained when interference with visual development occurred. The common types of functional amblyopia are strabismic, occurring because one eye constantly deviates, and anisometropic, in which there is a significant (usually more than 2 diopters) difference in refractive error of the two eyes. Usually functional amblyopia may be considered as arising because of inhibition of the false image arising in a deviating eye or because of the blurred image in an eye with a large refractive error.

Examination of the amblyopic eye indicates no decrease of visual acuity in decreased illumination, while an eye with evident organic disease may show a marked decrease. Visual acuity is better when letters are viewed singly than when viewed in a series, an effect that arises because of crowding of details when more than one letter is viewed. The amblyopic eye is also less sensitive than normal in detecting flickering of a light and in following a fast-moving target.

Examination with a special ophthalmoscope (the Visuscope), which projects a minute target on the fundus, may indicate that the fovea centralis is not used for fixation by the amblyopic eye but rather an area adjacent to the fovea centralis. In this case the condition of eccentric fixation is said to be present, and the retinal area selected for fixation varies widely. Severe eccentric fixation is evident if an eye remains deviated when the fellow eye is covered. The prognosis for visual improvement is much poorer when amblyopia is

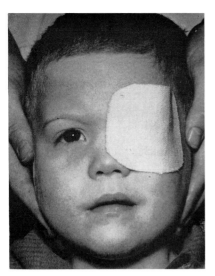

Fig. 20-5. Occlusion of the eye with better vision for treatment of amblyopia.

associated with eccentric fixation, and in general, visual acuity is also poorer than when central fixation is present.

Treatment must be directed toward improvement of vision in the amblyopic eye. This is usually done by excluding the better eye from use by patching it. (Fig. 20-5.) For the most part, the patching must be carried out continuously if it is to be effective. Usually patching must be initiated before the age of 7 years, and it is continued until there is no further improvement in vision. Patching is usually carried out for at least 3 months before it is concluded that there will be no improvement in vision.

When amblyopia is combined with eccentric fixation, the initial step is to induce normal central fixation. Initially the amblyopic eye is patched for 5 weeks and the patient then tested with the Visuscope for central fixation. If central fixation is present, the good eye is continuously patched as described previously. If central fixation is not present, the good eye is patched and the amblyopic eye covered with a red filter until fixation becomes central. Patching of the good eye continues until maximal improvement of visual acuity is attained. If central fixation is not attained, pleoptics (p. 332) is the technique of choice.

Suppression. Suppression is the condition in which the image arising on the retina of one eye is not perceived. Rifle shooters, microscopists, and others using a single eye may without conscious effort intermittently suppress the image from the nonsighting eye. In strabismus the image falling on a peripheral portion of the retina of the deviating eye may be ignored so as to avoid double vision. It not infrequently constitutes a valuable mechanism for avoiding diplopia. Central visual acuity may be good in each eye separately, but the image of the eye that is not being used is suppressed. Sometimes vision is reduced to pretreatment levels following the treatment of functional amblyopia because of suppression. This suppression may take weeks to correct, but invariably vision returns to the level achieved during therapy.

Retinal correspondence. Stimulation of the retina provides not only a sensation of light but also *retinal direction*—the direction from which the light is coming. For each point on the retina of one eye, there is a point on the retina of the fellow eye that has the same visual direction. Corresponding points are thus points on the two retinas that have the same relative directional value in space. If a retinal image falls on points on each retina that do not correspond, two separate images are perceived. If the separation is extremely small, the two objects are fused with the perception of depth, or stereopsis.

In anomalous or *abnormal retinal correspondence* a condition has developed in which corresponding points on the two retinas do not have the same relative direction in space. It may be defined as a condition in which (1) the foveas of the two eyes have different directional values or (2) the fovea of one eye is aligned with an extrafoveal region of the fellow eye. It should be emphasized that abnormal retinal correspondence involves directional values solely and may sometimes be associated with normal vision.

The angle formed by the visual lines of each eye is the angle of the abnormality. If this angle is equal to the angle of a strabismus, the abnormal retinal correspondence is said to be harmonious. Essentially, the visual line of one eye and a line of direction of the fellow eye have developed the same visual direction. If the angle of the abnormality is less than the angle of a strabismus, the abnormal retinal correspondence is called subharmonious or disharmonious.

Therapeutic techniques. To correct abnormalities of image formation and perception, pleoptics and orthoptics have been employed.

Pleoptics. In recent years there has been much attention directed toward the improvement of vision by means of reestablishment of foveal fixation. The equipment is expensive, the treatment sessions are frequent, and some believe simple patching (p. 330) is as effective. The key instrument in pleoptics is the Visuscope, which enables the examiner to find what area of the retina is being used for fixation. Two main methods are used to force fixation. In one the eccentric retinal area used for fixation is dazzled by means of a bright light and the fovea centralis stimulated with different targets. In the second a circular light dazzles the area surrounding the fovea centralis causing an annular after-image (ring scotoma). The patient then places the ring around smaller and smaller targets until ultimately the area of eccentric fixation is not used and the patient learns the visual direction of the true fovea.

Orthoptics. Orthoptic technicians participate in the diagnosis and medical correction of sensory and motor anomalies of the eyes. In the United States they are college-trained individuals with specialization in orthoptics followed by certification by the American Orthoptic Council. Almost universally, orthoptic technicians are sponsored by physicians or universities. Their diagnostic studies consist of the steps that have been mentioned: (1) detection of a deviation, (2) measurement of the deviation by objective and subjective tests, and (3) study of the sensory and motor cooperation between the two eyes. Therapy is carried out to correct amblyopia, AC/A abnormalities, and to improve fusional abilities.

Correction of deviation. Correction of deviation is attained by several methods. In accommodative types of strabismus, correction of the abnormal accommodative-convergence ratio by lenses or anticholinesterase drugs may be all that is required. In many phorias, prisms incorporated into the lenses will be helpful. In some patients the stimulation of their latent fusion may bring about parallelism. In many patients surgery is required.

Surgery is indicated when maximal improvement has been attained by medical methods and a significant manifest deviation is still present. Most instances of strabismus with a small angle in which each fovea centralis is not being used do not require surgery but do require continued care. The accommodative portion of any strabismus should be managed with lenses and not surgery. Surgery usually does not permit patients with comitant strabismus to discard their spectacles that are required to correct astigmatism and accommodative defects or to support the prisms needed to neutralize small residual deviations.

Choice of surgical procedure. Selection of the proper surgical procedure in cases of strabismus involves considerable judgment. In general, it is undesirable to weaken a normally acting muscle; it is more desirable to strengthen an underacting muscle. When vision is equal in the

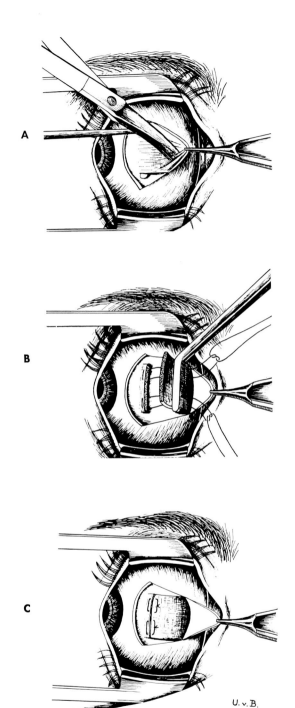

Fig. 20-6. Resection of a medial rectus muscle. **A,** The muscle is isolated. **B,** It is severed from its insertion, and sutures are passed through the muscle at the point of resection. **C,** The shortened muscle is attached to the insertion.

two eyes, it is desirable to perform symmetric surgery, normally carrying out the same surgical procedure in each eye rather than limiting the surgical correction to one eye. Usually the better the fusion, the less surgery is required to achieve a cosmetic and functional result. When vision is markedly decreased in one eye, however, it is impossible to achieve a functional result because surgery will not restore vision to the eye.

In comitant esotropia in which vision is approximately equal in the two eyes and in which correspondence is normal, the usual procedure is bilateral resection of the lateral rectus muscles. In the event that this is inadequate to correct the strabismus, then after a 6-month period a recession may be performed on the medial rectus muscle (Fig. 20-6). If this is unsuccessful, a further recession may be performed on the medial rectus muscle of the opposite eye.

In patients with comitant esotropia in which one eye is markedly amblyopic, the best results are probably achieved by resecting the lateral rectus muscle and recessing the medial rectus muscle in the amblyopic eye (Fig. 20-7). If this is not adequate to achieve parallelism, a similar procedure may be carried out in the opposite eye.

In alternating exotropia, each lateral rectus muscle is recessed if the divergence is mainly for distance and the eyes are parallel for near, provided vision and fusion are good. If the exotropia is monocular, the deviation the same for near and far, and fusion poor, the initial procedure is recession of the lateral rectus muscle and resection of the medial rectus muscle in one eye.

The management of overcorrection is a difficult problem. Often it occurs because of a superimposed A or V abnormality, abnormal retinal correspondence, or surgery in an accommodative type strabismus. When an overcorrection occurs, it is better to op-

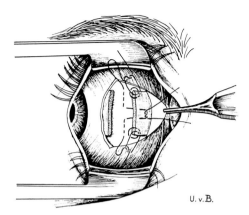

U. v. B.

Fig. 20-7. Recession of the medial rectus muscle. The muscle is severed close to its insertion and reattached to the sclera posterior to the original insertion.

erate on a previously operated muscle rather than on a muscle that has not had surgery. Many instances of overcorrection follow recession of one or both of the medial rectus muscles for esotropia. In such instances, it is necessary to inspect the point of attachment of the weaker muscle that is usually found to be somewhat farther back on the globe than it was believed to have been placed during operation. The muscle is usually reattached to its original insertion. Usually there is never again a conversion to the previous deviation with such a reattachment, and the overcorrection tends to persist.

The surgeon's aim is to perform the minimal procedure that will correct the squint. However, in many patients a series of operations must be done. This does not indicate that the initial procedure was unsuccessful or that more should have been done at the first procedure; moreover, the correction of a horizontal or vertical deviation may reveal anomalies that could not be diagnosed prior to the time of surgery. Usually at least 6 months should elapse between procedures to permit the correction to stabilize.

Chapter 21

Injuries of the eye

Prompt and appropriate care of common eye injuries may prevent much visual disability and in some instances major corrective surgery. Often eye injuries are associated with severe bodily injury demanding immediate attention, and there is failure to recognize and to ' treat the ocular involvement as early as desirable. Conversely, shock must be treated promptly, and appropriate protection against infection must be provided.

Vision is measured, if possible, before the eyes or eyelids are manipulated. Many persons have never known that their vision was defective in one eye until there was occasion to test each eye separately after an injury. If there is no record of visual acuity immediately prior to treatment, the physician may be accused unjustly of causing a defect that, in fact, existed many years prior to the injury. It is not necessary to use a vision testing chart—a newspaper or a telephone book will give some evidence of how much vision is present.

Corneal foreign bodies

Foreign bodies on the surface of the cornea constitute about 25% of all ocular injuries. A history of the injury and the likely character of the foreign body are of assistance in its detection and removal.

The symptoms vary from little or no discomfort to serve pain. Usually there is a sensation of a foreign body that the patient localizes, inaccurately, to the outer portion of the upper lid. This may be associated with tearing and photophobia. There may be an associated ciliary injection.

The foreign body may be seen by careful inspection of the cornea, preferably aided by magnification with a loupe or a magnifying glass. Sterile 2% fluorescein solution instilled into the eye will stain the cornea in the area of the foreign body and accurately demarcate it. Aqueous Mercurochrome may also be used as a vital stain, but it is less effective than fluorescein. Foreign bodies in the cornea should be removed entirely to permit epithelization and to relieve pain. Topical anesthesia must be used to prevent lid closure during removal.

An attempt should be made to remove the foreign body by means of irrigation· A bulb-type syringe or a hypodermic syringe fitted with a sterile needle is used with sterile saline solution as the irrigating fluid. Foreign bodies that are not hot when they strike the eye usually may be removed by directing a stream of fluid against the foreign body so as to float it off the cornea. This is an excellent method for nurses and others to use in removing superficial foreign bodies.

If the foreign body cannot be removed by irrigation, it usually cannot be removed by means of a cotton-tipped applicator, which removes much normal epithelium and is undesirable. Less injury is caused

335

if the foreign body is lifted gently out of the corneal substance by means of a sharp instrument. A sterile spud designed for this purpose, or in an emergency, a 25-gauge to 27-gauge hypodermic needle fitted to a 2 ml. syringe may be used. The instrument is held tangent to the cornea so that the eye will not be penetrated in the event of sudden movement by the patient. The spud is used to elevate the foreign body gently off the cornea. If a ferrous metal has been embedded for several days, a rust ring may remain after the removal of the main portion of the foreign body; this must be removed. If it cannot be removed easily at the first attempt, frequently it can be lifted out entirely 24 hours later when the surrounding corneal tissue has softened.

Following removal of a corneal foreign body, a solution (not ointment) of a sulfonamide such as sulfacetamide or an antibiotic mixture such as neomycin is instilled, and a dressing is applied to the eye. The dressing is used to immobilize the lids and to prevent discomfort arising from the lids blinking over the abraded area. The dressing is not required if it causes discomfort. In the absence of keratitis, local medications to cause pupillary dilation are not used. If marked ciliary congestion and photophobia are present or if the removal of the foreign body has been particularly difficult, a cycloplegic such as 5% homatropine is instilled. Atropine causes a prolonged pupillary dilation and cycloplegia and is usually not indicated. Inasmuch as a foreign body may introduce microorganisms into the cornea, the eye should be inspected for infection each day until the area no longer stains with sterile fluorescein. Foreign bodies that injure only the corneal epithelium do not cause a scar. Scarring follows injuries to Bowman's membrane or to the substantia propria.

Conjunctival foreign bodies

Foreign bodies of the conjunctiva can always be removed with either a spud or a cotton-tipped applicator. Frequently a stream of saline solution directed from a syringe will wash them out of the eye.

Foreign bodies frequently lodge on the upper tarsal conjunctiva at its peripheral margin. The upper lid must be everted (p. 135) to remove them. The operator must be prepared to remove the foreign body when he everts the lid because the foreign body may be dislodged and difficult to locate again if the lid is released.

Intraocular foreign bodies

Foreign bodies may be retained within the eye following injuries in which small particles penetrate the cornea or the sclera. Large foreign bodies cause marked disruption of the globe and so much associated injury that the eye is destroyed and enucleation is required. Foreign bodies composed of vegetable material such as wood or plants may introduce infection that causes a severe purulent panophthalmitis to occur within hours. The majority of intraocular foreign bodies are extremely small and are sterilized by the heat caused by their high velocity. Intraocular foreign bodies mainly consist of small bits of metal, glass, plastics, and similar material. Their nature varies with the types of industry and recreation of the locality.

The diagnosis and treatment depend upon the following:

1. *Size of the foreign body:* A foreign body must have a minimal density and size to be demonstrated by means of roentgenray examination. A number of special techniques have been developed to diagnose and localize foreign bodies by means of roentgen rays. These have been supplemented by devices for locating metal that indicate also whether or not the foreign body is magnetic.

2. *Whether it is magnetic:* Only nickel and iron may be removed by means of a magnet, and for this reason it is helpful to determine whether the tool or other material from which the foreign body originated is magnetic.

3. *Tissue reaction caused by the gradual oxidation of the foreign body within the eye:* Plexiglas and many plastics, stainless steel, glass, and aluminum oxidize very slowly and if retained cause minimal damage to the eye. Often such foreign bodies are not removed. Iron slowly oxidizes within the eye and combines with the protein of the intraocular tissues (siderosis) to form an irreversible ferrous compound that results in gradual loss of vision of the eye. Unlike siderosis, the tissue reaction caused by retention of copper particles, chalcosis, is reversible if the particle is removed. However, copper is much more rapidly injurious to the eye. An intraocular foreign body must always be considered in any patient with uveitis in whom there is a history of injury. Rarely, a foreign body is enmeshed in scar tissue, metallic ions are not released within the eye, and retention of the foreign body causes no symptoms.

4. *Location within the eye:* Foreign bodies in the anterior chamber may be directly observed, although if they are in the chamber angle recess, gonioscopy is required. Metallic foreign bodies within the lens may be tolerated for a long period. If the capsule is markedly injured when the foreign body enters, a cataract forms rapidly. Foreign bodies in the vitreous body and retina are often obscured by hemorrhage but sometimes may be demonstrated by means of ophthalmoscopy, particularly using the indirect ophthalmoscope.

Retained foreign bodies must be suspected in all instances of perforating wounds of the eye. It is customary to make roentgenograms of the orbit in all such injuries to be assured that no foreign body can be demonstrated.

If the point of entry is extremely small, high magnification may be required to see the wound in the cornea or the iris. Minute wounds in the sclera are nearly invisible. Once the presence of a foreign body has been established within the eye, removal is indicated unless the trauma of surgery is more severe than the damage caused by retention of the foreign body. The foreign body is initially localized by means of roentgen rays. Foreign bodies in the posterior ocular segment are removed through the sclera. The corneoscleral limbus approach is used for anterior segment foreign bodies. In removal through the sclera, the foreign body is first localized and the sclera exposed in the quadrant nearest the foreign body. An electronic metal localizer is then used to refine the localization of the foreign body, and a scratch incision is made in the sclera close to it. A suture is placed in the incision but left untied and looped out of the field. A magnet is then applied, and the foreign body is removed. The suture is tied quickly, and the area is surrounded by diathermy to prevent a retinal detachment.

Early removal is important inasmuch as foreign bodies may become enmeshed in fibrin and clot and may be difficult to remove after the lapse of a long period. However, it is probably better to delay treatment until specialized facilities are available than to carry out treatment without the benefit of diagnostic devices.

Lacerations of the lids

Lacerations of the lids are divided into two groups: (1) those that are parallel to the lid margin and hence do not gape and (2) those that are perpendicular to the lid margin and are drawn apart by the pull of the fibers of the orbicularis oculi muscle (Fig. 21-1).

All wounds of the lid must be meticulously cleaned with soap and water, taking care not to irritate the conjunctiva and the cornea. Skin is not excised from the laceration because the excellent blood supply of the lid assures survival, even though it appears markedly contused and damaged.

Lacerations parallel to lid margins require no specialized treatment and are closed with 4-0 or 6-0 black silk sutures. The laceration is parallel to the normal

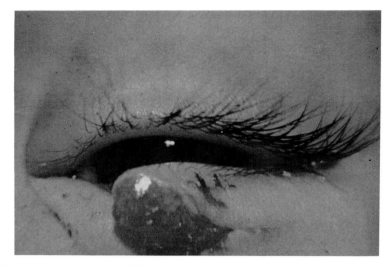

Fig. 21-1. Laceration of the lid margin.

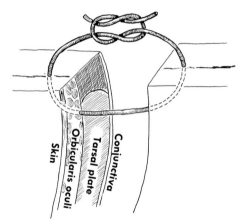

Skin
Orbicularis oculi
Tarsal plate
Conjunctiva

Fig. 21-2. Repair of a laceration of the lid by means of a suture through the gray line. The suture is usually double-armed, and each needle enters the tissue through the laceration and emerges through the gray line. Once the lid margin is approximated without a notch, the skin may be closed with interrupted silk sutures. It is not necessary to close the conjunctiva.

margin, which avulse the canaliculi leading to the tear sac. In those lacerations involving the outer five sixths of the lid margin, the key to successful repair is the placement of the first suture through the gray line of the lid to unite both edges of the laceration with the lid margin in the proper plane (Fig. 21-2). Once the lid margin is closed properly, the remainder of the lid can be closed in layers, using catgut sutures for the tarsus and silk for the skin. Care should be taken that the sutures are not tied on the conjunctival surface where they will irritate the cornea. Unless other injuries are so serious that treatment must be delayed, it is better not to procrastinate, for a delay of even 24 hours may be followed by retraction of the wound edges, and major plastic surgery will be required for repair. If the margins of both the upper and lower lids are involved, a figure-of-eight suture is used in which each lid splints the other.

Laceration of the inner one sixth of the lid in which the canaliculus is torn requires (1) placement of a stent through the canaliculus in the hope that it will be patent, (2) closure of the laceration, and (3) prevention of traction by the mass of orbicularis oculi muscle located lateral to

skin folds, and no conspicuous defect results.

Vertical lacerations are divided into those involving the outer five sixths of the lid (ciliary) margin and those involving the inner one sixth of the lid (lacrimal)

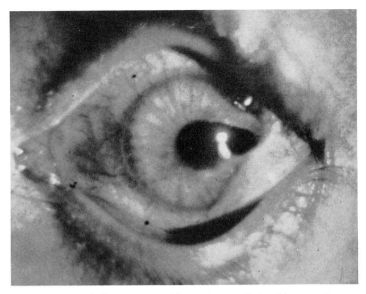

Fig. 21-3. Laceration of the cornea with prolapse of the iris, creating a typical tear-shaped defect of the pupil.

the laceration. Simple closure of the laceration causes a typical notched defect of the lid margin and constant tearing. Even with highly expert repair, it may not be possible to unite the avulsed ends of the canaliculus, and additional surgery is required to correct tearing.

Lacerations of the conjunctiva

Lacerations of the tarsal conjunctiva invariably involve the underlying lid to which the conjunctiva is adherent. The repair of the lid laceration approximates the cut edges of the conjunctiva, for which separate closure is not indicated. Sutures through the tarsal conjunctiva are usually contraindicated because of the damage to the cornea.

Lacerations of the bulbar conjunctiva that do not involve the globe are rarely severe enough to require closure. It is most important, however, that the physician be certain in such injuries that there is not an associated laceration of the sclera. Usually the lacerated conjunctiva is surrounded by an area of subconjunctival hemorrhage,

and the laceration is evident as a white, crescentic area. Fluorescein will stain the margins of the laceration. The eye is uncomfortable, but there is no loss of vision.

Corneal lacerations

Lacerating wounds of the cornea, unless of a puncture type, are followed by prolapse of the iris that closes the wound. A characteristic teardrop distortion of the pupil, which is diagnostic, is present (Fig. 21-3). In severe lacerations there may be frank prolapse of the iris, ciliary body, lens, and vitreous body, causing a completely disorganized globe.

Once the diagnosis of a perforating wound of the globe has been established, no further examination is made until the injury can be corrected surgically. Corneal lacerations are frequently associated with retained intraocular foreign bodies, traumatic cataract, secondary glaucoma, infection, and late complications, so that treatment should be carried out by those able to manage the responsibility of the aftercare. First aid is limited to the diagnosis of the condition. Then both eyes are covered by sterile patches, and the patient is transferred by litter to the place of surgery. A delay of up to 24 hours is not only permissible in the management of these injuries but is also preferable to inexpert examination. In all cases in which the globe has been lacerated, a wide-spectrum antibiotic is administered systemically in large doses. The current choice is a tetracycline in an initial priming dose of 3 Gm. and then 1 or 2 Gm. daily in divided doses. The history of the injury and examination of the eye frequently suggest whether a foreign body is retained.

Local anesthesia may be adequate for repair, but if there has been severe trauma, general anesthesia is preferable. Rapid induction is necessary so that there will be no struggling, which increases the intraocular pressure.

The method of repair depends on whether there has been marked contusion of the wound edges and loss of corneal substance or whether the edges of a laceration are sharply defined. When there has been marked loss of tissue, it may be necessary to draw a conjunctival flap over the wound or to do an immediate corneal transplant. When there is no tissue loss, direct suturing of the cornea is preferred.

The prolapsed iris is grasped with an iris forceps, withdrawn gently a little farther from the wound, and excised. The excision removes enough iris so that its remaining edges will not adhere to the wound. Since the advent of antibiotics there has been some tendency to reposit the iris rather than to excise the prolapse, and thus prevent a glaring cosmetic defect. However, the possibility of introducing infection into an eye and destroying it must be considered, and at present most surgeons tend toward excision.

The placement of appositional sutures in the cornea requires a sharp, fine forceps to grasp the corneal edges. A sharp needle must be used with black silk or catgut sutures. The first corneal suture is placed at the corneoscleral limbus. Other appositional sutures are then placed as needed. The anterior chamber is irrigated before the wound is made completely watertight to prevent pigment debris from adhering to the posterior cornea.

If direct appositional suturing cannot be done because of loss of corneal tissue, the wound is covered with a conjunctival flap. Excision of the prolapsed iris is carried out as described previously, but it is usually delayed until after insertion of sutures so that the globe is not excessively soft during the conjunctival dissection and insertion of sutures. The entire conjunctiva may be circumcised and drawn up purse-string style to cover the entire cornea. Generally, conjunctival flaps have fallen into disfavor because it is impossible to follow the course of wound healing or to inspect the anterior chamber when the cornea is covered with conjunctiva.

If definitive surgery of a corneal laceration cannot be done within 24 hours, the following measures are recommended. The globe is anesthetized using a topical or general anesthesia. The prolapsed iris is excised widely. The cut edges of the cornea are gently stroked into apposition. The eye is then closed gently, and binocular patches are applied. The patient remains in bed for 72 to 96 hours. In many such cases the anterior chamber will re-form, and a useful eye will result.

Corneal lacerations are frequently associated with injuries to the lens causing a cataract. Any rupture in the lens capsule permits aqueous humor to come in contact with the lens cortex and to cause it to become opaque. In corneal lacerations the lens may be lacerated, and at the time of repair of the corneal injury, it is evident that a traumatic cataract is present. The lens should not be removed at the time of repair of the laceration, but cortex in the anterior chamber may be removed by irrigation.

Scleral lacerations

Scleral lacerations often extend to the cornea, and there is prolapse of both the iris and the ciliary body. Involvement of the ciliary body invariably leads to some loss of the vitreous body combined with damage to the zonule of the lens. Such lacerations are much more likely to produce severe damage to the eye than those involving the cornea solely. To repair, the lacerated area is exposed by dissecting the cut edges of the conjunctiva and Tenon's capsule from the scleral laceration. The first suture is placed exactly at the corneoscleral limbus. Prolapsed uveal tissue is then excised, and the laceration is closed with interrupted sutures. The conjunctiva is closed separately.

Sympathetic ophthalmia

Sympathetic ophthalmia is a rare bilateral granulomatous inflammation of the entire uveal tract that follows perforations of the globe. The etiology is unknown, but the disease may constitute an autoimmune reaction to uveal pigment. Most cases develop within 3 months of injury, with extremes of 10 to 14 days and many years. The injured eye (the exciting eye) exhibits a torpid, persistent, granulomatous type of uveitis that is then followed by a similar uveitis in the fellow eye (the sympathizing eye). The inflammation may be suppressed by corticosteroids that may have to be continued for many months or years.

Sympathetic ophthalmia does not occur if the injured eye is removed within 7 to 14 days following the injury. Inasmuch as sympathetic ophthalmia does not occur immediately after an injury, irrespective of the severity of the ocular damage, it is never necessary to enucleate an injured eye as an emergency procedure.

Concussion injuries

Apparently minor blunt trauma to the eye and orbit may result in surprisingly severe injury. Hemorrhage into the lids is in itself usually of little import but may be associated with fractures of the orbital bones. Usually these may be diagnosed by observing the asymmetry of the face and by gently palpating the orbital structures.

A severe subconjunctival hemorrhage and a persistently soft globe following a severe contusion suggest the possibility of a rupture of the posterior sclera. If the hemorrhage involves the entire conjunctiva with bleeding into the lids, there is possibly a fracture of a wall of the orbit.

The cornea may be abraded in contusion injuries, but this is usually not serious and heals quickly. The sphincter pupillae muscle may be ruptured, and if so, the pupil is semidilated and does not react to light or accommodation. In relatively minor contusion injuries there may be minute ruptures of the muscle so that the pupil is no longer round. In more severe injuries the outer edge of the iris may be torn from its insertion to the scleral spur, giving rise to a condition of iridodialysis. This may be so minute as to be visible only with a gonioscope, or it may involve a major portion of the insertion of the iris. An extensive iridodialysis is repaired by drawing the peripheral edge of the iris into a corneoscleral wound. Surgery is usually not indicated unless the iridodialysis is extensive and unless diplopia is present because of the additional pupil.

Contusion of the globe may cause rupture of a portion of the zonule of the lens, causing the lens to become subluxated. Vitreous body bulges into the anterior chamber through the ruptured area. The lens is seldom markedly displaced, and it is rarely necessary to remove it. Curiously, lens subluxation is most common in individuals with syphilis. As years pass, the lens may become opaque. A transient lens opacity may also occur immediately after a blunt injury to the globe.

Glaucoma may develop 10 to 20 years following ocular contusion. The glaucoma resembles open-angle glaucoma except that it is monocular. Gonioscopic examination indicates that a sector of the anterior chamber angle is much deeper than other regions. Often the patient may no longer recall the injury. Blunt contusion of the eye may be the main cause of monocular glaucoma in the adult.

Contusion may cause the release of a large amount of pigment into the anterior chamber, and this may give rise to the appearance of an iritis. There is, however, no tendency toward the formation of keratic precipitates, and posterior synechiae do not form.

Choroidal and retinal hemorrhage, edema, and necrosis following blunt trauma have been discussed earlier (pp. 241 and 273).

Traumatic hyphema

Contusion injuries of the globe frequently are followed by frank bleeding into the anterior chamber. This blood does not clot and, with bed rest, flows to the most dependent portion of the anterior chamber, and a fluid meniscus forms. Frequently the original hyphema, which may be relatively minor, is followed by more severe bleeding 24 to 48 hours following the original injury. A secondary glaucoma may occur immediately or many years later.

The treatment of traumatic hyphema is much debated. If the anterior chamber is not entirely filled with blood, spontaneous recovery will likely take place provided there is no secondary hemorrhage, irrespective of the treatment. Binocular patching, bed rest, and no local medication are often effective. After 96 hours, corticosteroids may be used locally to minimize the traumatic uveitis. If a recurrent hemorrhage occurs that does not fill the anterior chamber, similar treatment is effective.

If the entire anterior chamber is filled with blood and there is no aqueous circulation, the blood should be irrigated from the eye; one of a variety of techniques may be used. It is believed desirable to make

an incision adequate for drainage rather than flushing fluid from a syringe in and out of the anterior chamber. Attempts to remove clots by means of a forceps are contraindicated because of the difficulty in distinguishing between the clots and the iris. Normal saline solution is commonly used for irrigation, although urokinase has been reported to be effective.

Secondary glaucoma developing when the anterior chamber is only partially filled with blood is likely due to vasodilation and is treated by means of systemic acetazolamide. Intravenous urea and mannitol usually do not reduce pressure permanently. Secondary glaucoma developing when the anterior chamber is filled with blood should be managed by irrigation of the blood from the eye. Intraocular pressure is usually reduced with intravenous urea or mannitol initially, and the blood is removed as described previously. General anesthesia is often desirable because of the difficulty in anesthetizing the congested eye.

Fracture-dislocations of orbital bones

Blunt trauma to the orbital region may give rise to fractures and dislocations affecting the bony margins or the walls of the orbit. Many of these injuries are associated with other facial fractures, head injury, and severe lacerations and cannot be treated until shock and life-threatening injuries have been dealt with. It is not necessary to make an emergency decision to remove an injured eye until adequate consultation has been obtained. Roentgenographic views of the skull and the orbit are essential, and laminography may indicate fractures not otherwise evident.

Examination should be particularly directed to asymmetry of the face and to the position of the canthal ligaments. Frequently hemorrhage, lacerations, and serious injury make this unrewarding. Attention should be directed to possible brain injury associated with penetrating wounds of the walls of the orbit. Where the walls communicate with the sinus, penetration causes an emphysema of the tissues that gives rise to a peculiar crepitation on palpation.

Relatively minor trauma to the medial wall of the orbit may fracture the lamina papyracea of the ethmoid bone. This permits air to enter the orbit or the cutaneous tissue of the lid from the sinus. Violent blowing of the nose forces air into the tissues. The condition is self-limited and requires no treatment.

Fractures of the medial margin of the orbit are usually associated with nasal fractures. The lacrimal duct may be sheared off as the bony canal is displaced. Fractures of the inferior orbital margin are often comminuted and associated with lid lacerations. The infraorbital nerve is sheared off in its canal, and there is anesthesia in its area of distribution. The bony fragments may often be placed in a better position, and depressed fractures may be elevated by a forceps introduced through an existing laceration.

Fracture-dislocation of the zygomatic bone and arch occurs commonly. The lateral canthus is depressed, and the prominence of the cheekbone disappears. Relatively minor blows may be a cause. If the arch is fractured, it may be reduced through an incision at the posterior end of the arch and elevation by means of a towel forceps or a periosteal elevator introduced into the temporalis muscle fossa. Much major cosmetic surgery may be avoided if such injuries are corrected within the first 24 hours, the patient's condition permitting.

Fractures of the superior rim of the orbit may involve the trochlea of the superior oblique muscle. This gives rise to the signs of paresis of this muscle, with a diplopia most marked when looking down and particularly when reading. The trochlea tends to reattach itself spontaneously.

Blunt trauma to the orbit may cause a marked increase in intraorbital pressure

that is directed toward the floor of the orbit, causing a blowout fracture. The orbital contents prolapse into the maxillary sinus, and the entire globe may even disappear from sight. The palpebral fissure is narrowed. There is slight enophthalmos and inability to rotate the eye upward. Injection of radiopaque material into the orbit indicates the orbital tissues to be in the sinus. A blowout fracture of the orbit need be repaired only when there is restriction of ocular movement indicating incarceration of orbital tissue in the fracture. The defect may be exposed through a skin incision of the inferior margin of the orbit, and the fracture opening may be bridged with bone or plastic.

Chemical burns

Chemical burns of the conjunctiva and the cornea are best treated by immediate irrigation with water (Fig. 21-4). There should be no delay in seeking the appropriate neutralizing solution (citric or boric acid for alkali burns and sodium bicarbonate for acid burns), but rather the eye should be copiously irrigated with water. In most industries, employees routinely are taught how to do this. The most effective method is plunging the entire face into a container of water and then opening the eyes under water. Immediate dilution is the most important therapy. The fluid used need not be sterile, at body temperature, or even clean, provided the chemical is diluted promptly.

Acid burns are quickly buffered by the tissues, and the immediate injury is usually the full extent of the damage. Alkali burns, however, continue to release hydroxyl ions into the tissue, and the injury is aggravated as time goes by. Meticulous inspection of the conjunctiva is necessary, and all tissue containing alkali is removed. Prolonged irrigation with saline solution is carried out, and as much of the chemical is removed as possible. Irrigation has been carried out for several days with good results. Calcium hydroxide burns may be

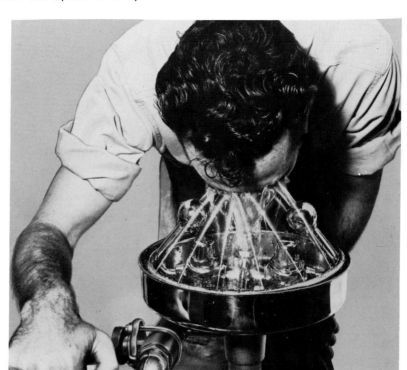

Fig. 21-4. Irrigation of a chemical burn of the eye with an eye-face wash fountain designed for industrial and school use. (Courtesy Haws Drinking Faucet Co., Berkeley, Calif.)

treated by means of chelation of the calcium ion, using ethylenediamine tetraacetic acid. Infection is prevented by the use of systemic and local antibiotics. The pupils are dilated with atropine instilled locally. The systemic use of corticosteroids in high doses following alkali burns appears to limit the amount of scarring. Symblepharon is prevented by the passage of a lubricated probe between the inner surface of the lids and the globe.

Chemical injuries of the eye may cause severe damage, and the prognosis must be guarded until the full extent of the burn is determined.

Thermal burns

Thermal burns of the eyelids usually do not involve the globe since the blinking reflex provides natural protection. Addi-

tionally, tightly closed eyelids usually prevent involvement of the lid margins themselves. Burns of the eyelids require prompt care to prevent severe ectropion. First aid measures consist of application of sterile dressings and systemic control of pain. Definitive treatment should be carried out within 12 hours of the injury. If dirty, the burned area is cleaned gently with sterile saline solution and a sterile, bland soap. Fluid blebs are left intact. The most important step is suturing the upper to the lower lid with 4-0 black silk sutures, or if not available, with other suture material. A mattress suture is placed through the margin of the lower lid and through the margin of the upper lid, care being taken not to penetrate the globe. The sutures bring the two lids together in the closed position, preventing gross contracture and subsequent ectropion formation. Such sutures, if unnecessary, are easily removed. Early skin grafting in severe second- and third-degree burns may speed convalescence and prevent late deformities. Skin for this purpose may be obtained from behind the ear, the inner side of the forearm, or, preferably if uninjured, from the opposite upper lid region.

Radiant energy

Injury to the eye by radiant energy is related to absorption of the energy by the tissues of the eye. Ultraviolet radiation is entirely absorbed by the cornea, and a small band gives rise to an ultraviolet keratitis. Infrared radiation is transmitted by the cornea and lens but comes to focus on the posterior ocular segment, and if the temperature of the tissues is increased enough, it causes a chorioretinitis. Visible light from the laser may be focused on the posterior pole and give rise to choroidal burns because of conversion to heat. Infrared radiation that is absorbed by the iris increases its temperature and that of the adjacent lens, causing an infrared type of cataract.

Electromagnetic energy in the range of radar can cause cataract when focused on the eye for several minutes. The changes are presumably entirely due to increased temperature of the lens and not specifically related to the type of energy. Roentgen rays, gamma rays, and alpha and beta particles may damage any part of the eye. The chief interest arises from their production of radiation cataract through interference with mitoses at the equator of the lens.

For the most part, industrial, warfare, and therapeutic sources of these energies are well known, and appropriate protection measures are undertaken. The majority of injuries are recognized quickly. They may be seen in the following situations: ultraviolet burns of the cornea occurring in arc welding, in mountain climb-

ers and those exposed to snowfields (snow-blindness is ultraviolet keratitis), and in those who expose themselves unwisely to sun lamps. Like sunburn, ultraviolet radiation is cumulative; symptoms arise some time after exposure. A marked foreign body sensation in the eye, lacrimation, and photophobia are present. Symptoms are entirely relieved by a local anesthetic that, however, delays epithelization of the cornea. The condition is entirely self-limited, and treatment is mainly symptomatic: patching and analgesics for discomfort. Healing is usually complete within 12 hours.

Infrared burns of the retina arise mainly in eclipse retinopathy and from various man-made sources of intense energy: the atomic bomb, the laser, and the photocoagulator. The latter two are used therapeutically in the treatment of flat retinal detachments and some retinal tumors. Infrared rays from the laser and the atomic bomb may be reflected from walls or instruments and be brought to a focus at the fovea centralis. They cause minute chorioretinal burns that markedly reduce vision. Inasmuch as the latent period of the blink reflex is 0.1 second, the energy has damaged the eye before one has time to blink.

Cataracts from roentgen rays and beta rays are usually the result of deliberate exposure of the lens to these energy sources in the treatment of the condition that necessitates the risk of cataract. Radiation from the atomic bomb also causes radiation cataracts that are invariably associated with loss of the eyelashes. Radiation cataracts form initially at the posterior pole and have a doughnut shape with a clear center surrounded by opacity. Thereafter, the opacity spreads, as in ordinary posterior subcapsular opacity, and ultimately the lens is entirely opaque. Following initial signs, radiation cataracts do not differ from ordinary senile or other types of lens opacities.

Chapter 22

Optical defects of the eye

A ray of light entering the eye is refracted by the cornea, passes through the anterior chamber, is refracted by the lens, and comes to a focus. The location of this focus within the eye is determined by the total refractive power of the cornea, the lens, the media surrounding them, and the distance separating them. The length of the eye determines whether this focus is in front of the retina as in myopia, upon the retina as in emmetropia, or whether the retina intercepts converging rays before they reach a focus as in hyperopia (Fig. 22-1).

The refractive power of the cornea in individuals with less than 1 diopter of refractive error is about 43 diopters, with extremes of 38 and 47 diopters. (A diopter is a unit of measurement of a lens equal to the reciprocal of the focal distance. Thus, if a lens has a focal distance of 0.2 m., its refractive power is 1/0.2 or 5 diopters. A 5 diopter lens has a focal distance of 1/5 m.) The refractive power of the lens at rest is about 17 diopters, with extremes of 12 and 22 diopters. The total refractive power of the eye is about 58 diopters, with extremes of 53 and 64 diopters. The axial length of the globe varies from 20 to 29 mm., with a mean of 24 mm. Accommodation (p. 86) increases the refractive power of the lens to a maximum of about 33 diopters, an increase of 16 diopters from the refractive power with accommodation suspended.

Refractive errors arise from a disparity between the refractive power of the anterior segment and the length of the globe. Usually there is a remarkable correlation between these two elements, so that long eyes often have less and short eyes have more refractive power so as to minimize any refractive error. It is thus an oversimplification to regard the myopic eye as one that is too long or a hyperopic eye as one that is too short. Instead there has been a failure of correlation between the refractive power of the anterior segment and the length of the globe. For the most part, refractive errors of less than 5 diopters are considered to be biologic variations, and the various components of the refractive system of the anterior segment and the length of the globe follow a binomial distribution. Refractive errors of more than 5 diopters are generally considered to be pathologic and to arise from developmental abnormalities, the origin of which is largely speculative.

Symptoms and signs of refractive error

The cardinal sign of a refractive error is decreased visual acuity, which is entirely corrected by means of lenses. If vision cannot be corrected to normal by means of lenses, the eye must be considered abnormal and an organic cause found to explain the decrease in vision. Decreased vision for distance with normal vision for near is often found in myopia. In hyperopia, vision may be normal or decreased for both

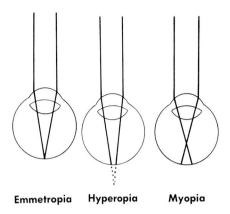

Emmetropia   Hyperopia   Myopia

Fig. 22-1. Major types of refractive error.

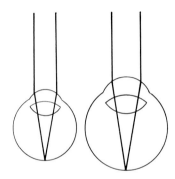

Fig. 22-2. Emmetropia. The refractive power of the anterior segment is so correlated with the length of the eye that parallel rays of light are focused upon the retina. The eye on the left has much less refractive power than the eye on the right, although both are emmetropic. If such a difference were present in the right and in the left eyes, there would be a difference of image size called aniseikonia.

near and far. Inasmuch as hyperopia may be compensated by accommodation, there is often no relationship between vision without lenses and the degree of the hyperopia.

A large variety of symptoms are attributed to errors of refraction. Inasmuch as the eyes play a prominent role in the psychologic development of an individual, these may be difficult to interpret.

There is no relationship between the severity of the symptoms and the degree of the refractive error. Many believe that the minor refractive errors are likely to be more troublesome than those that are marked because the patient exerts greater effort to maintain clear vision than those with marked refractive errors who cannot compensate. Ocular discomfort is a vague symptom referring to nearly any unexplained sensation occurring in or about the eyes. Asthenopia is the term usually used to denote pain or aching around the eyes, conjunctival injection, burning and itchiness of the lids, ready ocular fatigue, and headaches.

Headache is commonly attributed to refractive errors, irrespective of its cause. If it is a significant symptom, it should be related to sustained use of the eyes and should be relieved when the eyes are not used. It is most unlikely that a headache present upon awakening in the morning can be ascribed to excessive use of the eyes the evening before. Additionally, it is important to recognize that symptoms occurring even after prolonged use of the eyes are not necessarily ocular in origin. This is particularly true of those individuals living in unpleasant situations, from which there is no escape, who develop tension headaches that they attribute to the use of the eyes.

Emmetropia

Emmetropia is that optical condition in which parallel rays of light come to a focus on the fovea centralis without accommodation (Fig. 22-2). It is evident that in emmetropia there is an exact correlation between the refractive power of the anterior segment and the axial length of the eye. Clinically, emmetropia virtually never occurs inasmuch as the weight of the upper lid resting upon the eyeball gives rise to a minute amount of astigmatism. An emmetropic eye is defective in decreased illumination in which the increased refractivity of red rays causes an artificial myopia.

Ametropia

Ametropia is that condition in which there is a failure of correlation of the refractive power of the cornea and lens with the length of the globe, that is, a refractive error is present.

Hyperopia. Hyperopia is that refractive condition of the eye in which, with accommodation suspended, parallel rays of light are intercepted by the retina before coming to focus (Fig. 22-3).

The condition arises because of failure of correlation of the refractive power of the anterior segment with the length of the globe. Thus the refractive power of the anterior segment may be too little for the length of the globe, or the globe may be too short for the amount of refractive power present. Accommodation (p. 86) increases the refractive power of the anterior segment and this may compensate for hyperopia in many eyes and provide normal vision. At birth the eyes are hyperopic but not markedly so inasmuch as the small eye is compensated by a relatively flat cornea. With growth of the eye, there is a gradual decrease in hyperopia.

Pathologic degrees of hyperopia may occur with an abnormally small eyeball, which may range in size down to an extreme microphthalmia. A tumor in the ocular muscle cone indenting the retina, edema of the retina, or an intraocular tumor that elevates the retina may cause a hyperopia by displacing the fovea centralis toward the cornea. In such instances the primary disease often causes a concomitant decrease in vision. A decrease of the corneal curvature or the lens curvature or displacement of the lens backward to the vitreous body may reduce the refracting power of the anterior segment and may cause an excessive degree of hyperopia. In aphakia, in which the lens is absent, hyperopia is marked, and additionally, there is loss of accommodation inasmuch as the lens is absent.

The symptoms of hyperopia are (1)

ocular fatigue associated with use of the eyes and (2) poor vision. There is no direct relationship between the symptoms and the degree of accommodation required to neutralize a hyperopia that is present. Since a portion of accommodation must be used to neutralize the refractive error for distance and additional accommodation is required for near work, the symptoms may be more marked for near work than for distance. If the refractive error is neutralized by accommodation,

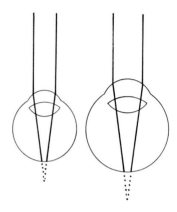

Fig. 22-3. Hyperopia. The refractive power of the eye on the left is less than that on the right. Accommodation may increase the refractive power of the anterior segment in hyperopia so that a distinct image is formed on the retina.

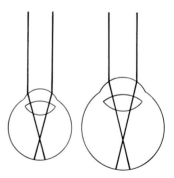

Fig. 22-4. Myopia. The refractive power of the eye on the left is less than that on the right. Accommodation increases the refractive power of the anterior segment and accentuates the refractive error.

vision may be normal. Usually vision for near becomes defective before that for distance.

There are no specific signs of hyperopia. The cornea may appear smaller than normal, and the globe itself may appear small. This should not be confused with the appearance caused by a narrow interpalpebral fissure. Hyperopia that exceeds 5 diopters may be associated with blurring of the disk margin called pseudopapillitis. The disk is not elevated, but the margins appear indistinct and the physiologic cup is absent. This condition is distinguished from early papilledema (p. 283) by the absence of retinal edema, hemorrhages, and the normal caliber and pulsations of the veins. Pseudopapillitis is distinguished from inflammation of the optic nerve at the level of the disk (papillitis, p. 282) by the usually similar involvement of both eyes, the unchanging ophthalmoscopic appearance of the disks, and the normal corrected visual acuity.

Hyperopia is classified as follows:

1. Total hyperopia is the amount of hyperopia present with all accommodation suspended, a condition produced by paralysis of the ciliary muscle by means of a cycloplegic drug (p. 98).
2. Manifest hyperopia is the maximum hyperopia that can be corrected with a convex lens with accommodation active and vision normal.
3. The difference between total and manifest hyperopia is the latent hyperopia.

Inasmuch as hyperopia is associated with an increased accommodation, there may be an increased amount of convergence. This may create an abnormal ratio between accommodation and convergence, giving rise to a convergence excess evident as a tendency for the eyes to deviate inward (esophoria or esotropia, p. 319).

The treatment of hyperopia involves analysis of the interrelation of the symptoms, the visual acuity, and the muscle balance. If visual acuity is good, the muscle balance is normal, and there are no symptoms, correction of the hyperopia is not necessary, irrespective of its severity. Conversely, convex lenses are prescribed when visual acuity is decreased, when a convergence excess is present, or when symptoms arise from the hyperopia.

Myopia. Myopia is that optical condition in which parallel rays of light come to a focus in front of the retina (Fig. 22-4). The condition occurs (1) because the refractive power of the anterior segment is too great for the length of the eye or (2) because the eye is too long for the refractive power present. Inasmuch as the refractive power of the anterior segment is already too great for the length of the globe, accommodation aggravates the defect.

Myopia may be divided into biologic and pathologic types. Biologic myopia, which is by far the most common type, arises because of a failure of correlation of the refractive power of the anterior segment and the length of the globe. These values vary about a mean, and biologic myopia constitutes no greater abnormality than being taller than average or having any other physical measurement that varies from the mean.

Pathologic myopia is a term applied to any myopia that causes degenerative changes in the eye. It is relatively common. In some individuals there is an excessive growth of the eye in all dimensions, a condition known as axial myopia. When the refractive error exceeds 6 diopters, there may be associated choroidal and retinal degenerative changes. Commonly, pathologic myopia tends to increase rapidly during adolescence, and in the past it was called progressive or malignant myopia.

Lenticular myopia is caused by an increase in the refractive power of the crystalline lens that causes an increase in the refractive power of the anterior segment. The increased refractive power occurs in the nucleus of the lens and is known as nuclear sclerosis. Such change occurs at an early stage in the development of senile cataract. Initially, vision may be normal with concave lenses, but ultimately there is a decrease in vision with increasing opacification of the lens. Lenticular myopia is the usual explanation for the elderly who find that they are able to read again without lenses—their distance vision without correction is, of course, poor.

The chief symptom of myopia is a decrease of distance vision. Each myopic eye has a point, a finite distance in front of the eye, which is in conjugate focus with the retina. An object placed here is imaged distinctly on the retina. If there are 4 diopters of myopia, this point is ¼ m. (25 cm.) in front of the eye. An individual with a moderate degree of myopia is thus able to see nearby objects without correction. In more marked degrees of myopia the near point in conjugate focus with the retina is so close to the eye that discomfort results from attempts to do sustained near work at this distance.

The decreased amount of accommodation required for near work in uncorrected myopia may be associated with a decreased amount of convergence, giving rise to a convergence insufficiency with a tendency for the eyes to deviate outward (exophoria, p. 327). In pathologic types the associated retinal and choroidal changes may destroy the fovea centralis and may cause a marked impairment of central vision.

Ophthalmoscopic examination in pathologic myopia may indicate a fluid vitreous body, an abnormal optic disk, and atrophy of the choroid and the retina. A myopic crescent of the optic disk is common. It appears as a white area of sclera adjacent to the temporal side of the optic disk. Sometimes the nasal portion of the disk is obscured by retinal tissue continuing over it. The pigment layer of the retina

may have a decreased amount of pigment so that the choroidal veins are distinctly seen. Atrophy of the choroid permits areas of stark white sclera to be seen. In other areas there may be proliferation of retinal pigment simulating the appearance of chorioretinitis. Atrophy of the choroid involving the region of the fovea centralis causes a loss of central vision. Pigment proliferation in the region of the fovea centralis (Fuchs' spot) occurs between the ages of 30 and 50 years and causes a marked disturbance in central vision. Myopic degeneration of the peripheral retina may lead to the formation of retinal holes and subsequent retinal detachment.

Myopia is neutralized by concave lenses. Lenses should be prescribed for patients dissatisfied with poor central visual acuity. There is no evidence that wearing correcting lenses has any effect on the progression of myopia. A decrease in myopia would necessitate diminution in axial length or refractive power of the eye, and this does not occur.

If a concave lens of greater refractive power than is required to neutralize the myopia is worn, clear vision may be obtained by accommodation. Such individuals may show an apparent decrease in myopia when proper lenses are prescribed. There is no evidence that the use of a bifocal lens has any effect on the progress of the myopia. Inasmuch as biologic myopia is but a variation in growth, nearly any remedy used may be associated with the termination of the growth process, with credit given the therapy. Controlled studies, double-blind techniques, and good experimental design have been lacking in nearly all studies of the treatment of myopia, and numerous remedies have been proposed. When sound experimental studies have been conducted, treatment of myopia has been ineffective.

In pathologic myopia in which the error exceeds 12 to 15 diopters, there is commonly no proportionate increase in vision with an increase in the refractive power of the correcting lens. These patients are sometimes undercorrected in a compromise to achieve the best near and distance vision.

Pathologic myopia is becoming uncommon in the United States. Its treatment is based mainly upon general hygienic measures of adequate nutrition and exercise and avoiding excessive amounts of any one activity, including near work. It is unnecessary that affected children withdraw from school or limit the amount of school work or use textbooks with large type unless defective visual acuity makes this desirable. There is no evidence that faithful wearing of corrective lenses has any effect on the course of myopia. It is not necessary to insist that adolescents wear lenses at all times to correct their myopia.

Astigmatism. Astigmatism is that optical condition in which, with accommodation suspended, the refracting power of the eye is not uniform in all meridians. In such a refracting system the rays of light do not come to focus at a point, but instead are focused at two separate focal lines. Astigmatism is classified as regular and irregular. In regular astigmatism there are two meridians of different refractive power that are at right angles to each other. In irregular astigmatism there are more than two meridians of different refractive power.

Astigmatism usually occurs because of a difference of curvature of the vertical and horizontal meridians of the cornea. This may arise as a biologic variant, from the weight of the upper lid resting upon the eyeball, from surgical incisions into the cornea, from trauma and scarring of the cornea, or from tumors of the lid such as a chalazion (p. 163) pressing upon the globe. An extreme form of curvature astigmatism, frequently irregular, arises in keratoconus (p. 202) in which the cornea becomes cone shaped with the apex of the cone below the center of the cornea. Minor degrees of astigmatism may occur from

variations in the radius of curvature of the lens. This condition is seen in patients who wear contact lenses that neutralize corneal astigmatism and uncover the astigmatism of the lens.

Astigmatism may be myopic, hyperopic, or mixed. In myopic astigmatism, both meridians are in front of the retina. In hyperopic astigmatism, both meridians are intercepted by the retina before reaching a focus. In mixed astigmatism, one meridian is focused in front of the retina, and the opposite meridian would have a focus behind the retina if not intercepted. In simple myopic astigmatism, one focal line is on the retina and the other is in front. In simple hyperopic astigmatism, one focal line is on the retina and the other would be behind it, but it is intercepted by the retina.

The symptoms of astigmatism vary considerably in different individuals. A distinct retinal image cannot be formed. In an attempt to achieve a clear image there may be a constant shifting of accommodation from one focal line to the other. Some believe that small degrees of astigmatism are particularly prone to give rise to the symptoms of ocular discomfort because of this constantly changing accommodation. Small degrees of astigmatism cause no obvious external signs. Marked degrees of astigmatism may cause the optic disk to appear elliptic in shape rather than circular. In irregular astigmatism there may be scars and other abnormalities in the cornea.

Astigmatism is neutralized by cylindric lenses. The amount of astigmatism requiring correction has occasioned debate. Some believe that even minor degrees of astigmatism necessitate correction. If, however, visual acuity is good and there are no symptoms, correction is not indicated. In severe astigmatism, patients may be more comfortable with a correction that does not entirely neutralize the astigmatic error. Irregular astigmatism constitutes a particular problem that must be individualized. Frequently vision is improved if contact lenses are worn. If irregular astigmatism cannot be corrected with contact lenses and if vision is reduced to 20/200 or less, consideration should be given to a corneal transplant to substitute a regular refractive surface.

Presbyopia. We have seen that accommodation (p. 86) increases the refractive power of the anterior segment by causing an increased curvature and thickness of the lens. This change in the shape of the lens occurs because of its inherent elasticity in response to contraction of the ciliary body, which causes relaxation of the zonule (p. 28). The lens becomes less elastic, and there is less accommodation with each year of life. Generally, there are about 14 diopters of accommodation at the age of 10 years, and by the age of 50 years there are only 2 diopters of accommodation. The decrease occurs gradually, but with 2 diopters of accommodation, the near point is ½ m. from the eye, and there is interference with near work.

The optical condition of decreased accommodation is known as presbyopia. The loss of accommodation occurs in all individuals, irrespective of their refractive error. However, a myopic individual may compensate for presbyopia by removing the lens that corrects his distance vision. Presbyopia is aggravated in a hyperopic individual if the lens that corrects the hyperopia is removed.

The chief symptom of presbyopia is inability to see near work distinctly. This is aggravated in dim illumination and with small print. The individual is frequently annoyed at having to place reading matter farther away from his eyes than previously. The necessity to use nearly all accommodation for clear near vision may cause ocular discomfort. There are no external signs of presbyopia except the general appearance indicating the individual to be more than 40 years old.

Presbyopia is treated by means of convex lenses added to the distance correction. The power of the lens required for clear vision for near work varies with an individual's habits, his age, his occupation, the length of his arms, and the distance at which he has become accustomed to do near work. Generally, the weakest possible lenses are prescribed that will permit the individual to carry on his vocation and avocational tasks. Bifocal or trifocal lenses are prescribed not as an aggravating additional burden to the middle-aged, but so that it will not be necessary to wear a separate pair of lenses for near and for far. If an individual requires lenses for distance, he is wise to wear bifocal or trifocal lenses as early as they are indicated. When he does not become accustomed to bifocal lenses relatively early in the development of presbyopia, he frequently suffers insurmountable symptoms in trying to accustom himself to bifocal lenses in later years. If distance lenses are not required, an individual may get along nicely with lenses that correct the presbyopia solely. However, because of the restricted focus of reading lenses, many individuals who do not require a distance correction wear bifocal lenses so that distant objects can be seen without removing the lenses.

Aphakia. Aphakia is the optical condition in which the crystalline lens is not in the visual axis, and rays of light entering the eye are thus refracted solely by the cornea. The most common cause is surgical removal of the lens, but aphakia may arise because of dislocation of the lens out of the pupillary area, as occurs in trauma, Marfan's syndrome, and other diseases (p. 289). Since the lens constitutes a major refracting portion of the eye, its removal causes the eye to become markedly hyperopic with a loss of accommodation.

The chief symptom of aphakia is decreased vision for both far and near. Inasmuch as accommodation is not possible, there are no symptoms of ocular discomfort.

Aphakia may be diagnosed by the loss of the reflected catatropic image from the surface of the lens and by excessive movement of the iris because of loss of support by the anterior lens capsule (iridodonesis).

Aphakia is corrected by means of convex lenses. Inasmuch as accommodation is not possible, an additional convex lens is required for near work. When corrected with ordinary spectacle lenses, the image of the aphakic eye is 25 to 33% larger than the normal eye. If the fellow eye is normal, it is ordinarily not possible for a patient with binocular vision to tolerate this amount of anisometropia because of the difference in size of the retinal images. By means of contact lenses, the difference in image size may be reduced to somewhat less than 10%, which many patients tolerate quite well. Convex lenses are required for near in such eyes corrected for distance with contact lenses.

Anisometropia

Anisometropia is that condition in which there is a difference in the refractive error of the two eyes. Minor differences are nearly universal, but when there is a difference of more than 2 diopters, the difference in image sizes of the two eyes may be the cause of symptoms. Often these patients are asymptomatic until bifocal lenses are prescribed. On turning the eyes downward to use the bifocal segment, the difference in power of the two lenses induces a vertical prism so that the images are on different levels. This may give rise to marked symptoms, but they may be neutralized by prescribing a neutralizing prism in the reading segment or by using separate lenses for near and distance.

Marked anisometropia is a common cause of functional amblyopia (p. 330) because the eye with the lesser refractive error is used by the developing infant.

Failure of central vision to develop leads in turn to strabismus (p. 319). Even when the central visual acuity is normal, binocular vision may fail to develop; then the anisometropia produces no symptoms because the retinal image arising from one eye is suppressed (p. 331).

Aniseikonia

Aniseikonia is that condition in which the size or shape of the retinal images of the two eyes is different. A difference of 0.5 diopter in the refractive error gives rise to a size difference of about 1% in the retinal image. Most patients tolerate a difference up to 5% without symptoms. When the image size difference is greater than 5% because of an anisometropia, it seems likely that many patients suppress the image from one eye and do not have symptoms.

Aniseikonia presents a difficult diagnostic problem when the refractive error of the two eyes is nearly the same and the difference in image size arises because each eye has a different refractive power and length. Special instruments for comparing the sizes of the retinal images are required for diagnosis. The condition is compensated by special lenses with surfaces that yield different size images. Examinations for aniseikonia are carried out at only a few special centers, and although the condition is moderately common, relatively few patients have severe symptoms. Aniseikonia, however, may cause many inexplicable symptoms, and patients present inappropriately severe disability. The physical basis for all symptoms, as with all disorders of binocular vision, is entirely eliminated by covering one eye.

Measurement of the refractive error

The presence or absence of a refractive error may be estimated by a number of methods. Some refractive errors have characteristic symptoms, whereas symptoms of others may be quite misleading. Measurement of near and distance vision may indicate the probable refractive error present. There may be typical ophthalmoscopic signs evident, but the measurement of the severity of ametropia by means of the ophthalmoscopic is quite unreliable.

Visual acuity. Some impression of the degree of ametropia can be learned by measurement of the visual acuity. If vision is 20/20 for distance, the patient is not myopic. If vision is 20/20 for distance and poorer than this for near, the patient is either presbyopic or has a degree of hyperopia that cannot be compensated by accommodation. If vision is less than 20/20 for distance but normal for near, the patient may well be myopic. Patients with hyperopic astigmatism with the cylinder axis at 90° often see the horizontal bars of letters such as E, F, and L more clearly than they do the vertical bars of letters such as N, H, and T. The condition is reversed when the astigmatism is about 180°.

Ophthalmoscopy. The estimation of ametropia by means of the ophthalmoscope may be fairly inaccurate unless the examiner is presbyopic and unable to accommodate. However, in hyperopia the disk may appear smaller than normal, and a pseudopapillitis may occasionally be present. In myopia the disk may appear larger than normal. In pathologic myopia a scleral myopic crescent may be present, there may be attenuation of the pigment epithelium with a prominent choroidal pattern, and there may be areas of pigment proliferation. In marked myopia the fundus can frequently be seen more easily if the patient wears his correcting lens. In astigmatism the optic disk may appear oval rather than round.

• • •

There are two basic methods of measurement of a refractive error: (1) subjective methods and (2) retinoscopy. Frequently the two are combined: the approximate error is estimated by means of retinoscopy and then the results are refined by a subjective method.

Subjective methods. There are many subjective methods for estimating refractive errors, depending in large part upon the patient's response to changes in lenses. When carefully performed by a skilled examiner, these methods may be extremely useful. In the most common type of examination, called fogging, a convex sphere, much in excess of that required for distinct vision, is placed in front of the eyes, and attention is directed to a distant visual acuity chart. Accommodation gradually relaxes to improve vision. The power of the convex lens is then gradually reduced until vision is at about the level of 20/40. The patient's attention may then be directed to an astigmatic dial and the axis of a concave cylinder placed with its axis at right angles to the axis he finds most dark. Subjective testing requires discrimination of moderately small changes in vision by an individual who has moderately rapid reaction times. Subjective techniques are most accurate when the amount of accommodation is limited.

Retinoscopy. Retinoscopy is an objective method of measurement of the refractive error. It is extremely accurate when carried out by a skilled examiner. The basic principle is to substitute lenses in front of the patient's eye so that emerging rays of light from his retina are brought to a focus at the examiner's eye. The light is directed into the patient's eye by means of a mirror or a self-contained light source that has an aperture for observation. Reference is made to the light emerging from the patient's eyes, which is reflected from the retina. If the light rays are diverging as they emerge, they appear to move in the same direction as their apparent origin on the retina. If they focus between the examiner's eye and the patient's eye, they appear to move in the opposite direction from their apparent origin on the retina.

When the emerging rays are brought to a focus at the examiner's eye, there is no movement, and this is the point of reversal. Retinoscopy, or skiascopy, constitutes the single most valuable method of examination for the measurement of ametropia. It is the only method that is of value in children and in individuals with poor discrimination or who respond slowly.

Keratometry. The keratometer is an instrument for measuring the anterior curvature of the cornea. In principle, the size of an image reflected from the cornea is measured. The image is created by an object of known size that is a fixed distance from the cornea. The method was mainly of investigative and academic interest until the increase in popularity of contact lenses. It is now used to select a contact lens of proper curvature.

Cycloplegia. As has been seen, accommodation may cause the refractive power of the eye to vary by as much as 15 diopters between the condition of the eye at rest and when actively accommodated in youth. Paralysis of accommodation by means of drugs (cycloplegia) permits measurement of the refractive error uncomplicated by changes in accommodation. Cycloplegia is indicated in children, in patients with strabismus, when spasm of accommodation is suspected, and in patients with cloudy media in whom retinoscopy through the undilated pupil is not possible.

Inasmuch as adequate ophthalmoscopic examination is not possible through the undilated pupil, many physicians insist that a complete eye examination include pupillary dilation. In many adults, pupillary dilation (mydriasis) is all that is required. In younger individuals, cycloplegia and pupillary dilation are required. The chief precautions are not to dilate the pupil of a patient predisposed to angle-closure glaucoma (Chapter 19) and to constrict the pupils of all adult patients at the conclusion of the examination.

Optical devices

Lenses may provide convex or concave spheres, or cylindric corrections, combined with bifocal and trifocal additions of a variety of sizes and shapes. In addition, prisms may be incorporated into the lenses to compensate muscle imbalance. Lenses may be case-hardened or plastic to resist breaking and may have various metallic salts incorporated in the glass to give color. It should be emphasized that lenses have four functions: (1) to improve vision by neutralizing refractive errors, (2) to relieve symptoms by minimizing the amount of accommodation required, (3) to make the eyes parallel by correcting anomalies of convergence accommodation or by means of correcting prisms, and (4) to protect the eyes.

Lenses do not prevent the progression of refractive errors. Refractive errors are not aggravated by wearing an improper lens or by wearing no lens at all. If an individual is content with blurred vision, he need not be required or urged to wear a correcting lens. However, if a refractive error gives rise to ocular symptoms, aggravates a blepharitis or a chronic conjunctivitis, or causes a disturbance of the ocular muscle balance, it seems ridiculous for a patient to refuse to use the lens that would alleviate the abnormality or to expect the physician to attempt other methods of treatment.

Lenses prescribed to relieve the symptoms arising from excessive amounts of accommodation or required to correct anomalies of the convergence-accommodation ratio may not improve visual acuity. It is important that children with convergence and divergence anomalies arising from accommodative disorders wear lenses to prevent intermittent deviation of one eye, which is often associated with suppression of the image of one eye with resultant interference with binocular function.

Shatter-resistant lenses. Spectacles made of ordinary glass protect the eye significantly. Even greater protection is afforded by shatter-resistant lenses, and they are nearly universally prescribed for children. It is extremely desirable, however, that adults, too, wear such lenses even though not engaged in an occupation having special ocular hazards.

It is evident that it is not possible to make any lens entirely shatter-proof. However, many injuries of the eye may be prevented by a lens that does not shatter when struck. In the main, shatter-resistant lenses are case-hardened by heating followed by cooling or are made of plastic. Plastic lenses scratch easier than case-hardened lenses but are lighter in weight, and many prefer them for this reason. Shatter-resistant lenses come in an industrial thickness and in an ophthalmic thickness. Lenses of industrial thickness in an industrial type of frame are an inexpensive and excellent way of protecting the eyes of children. They should always be worn in industry with ocular hazards. Ophthalmic thickness lenses are suitable for ordinary wear.

Colored lenses. Colored lenses are required in many industries to protect the eye from infrared and ultraviolet radiation. Most such lenses are manufactured by dissolving metallic oxides in glass or plastic so that certain wavelengths of light are absorbed by the lens and others are transmitted. Infrared radiation is usually difficult to protect against, and in this country manufacturing techniques have been developed that minimize exposure to infrared radiation. Ultraviolet radiation may cause a painful superficial keratitis in that the radiation is entirely absorbed by the cornea. Lenses have been specifically designed to protect against ultraviolet radiation, notably in arc welding, and the industrial recommendations should be followed. Lenses designed for industrial protection should not be used in activities other than the industry for which they were prescribed inasmuch as the transmission of light may be markedly reduced with resultant decrease in vision.

The normal, healthy eye does not require a colored lens outdoors. The amount of ultraviolet in sunlight or in artificial light is insufficient to cause any ocular damage under ordinary conditions. Extraordinary conditions include snowfields, deserts, and water where ultraviolet may be reflected into the eyes and cause keratitis. Infrared burns of the eye are possible when viewing an eclipse of the sun where the amount of visible light entering the eye is reduced so that it is possible to focus the sun's rays on the fovea centralis. The direct or reflected beam of a laser or atomic bomb flash may cause a chorioretinal burn at the point of focus.

Colored lenses should never be worn at night inasmuch as they reduce the amount of light entering the eye. Amber and pink lenses may reduce the appreciation of red traffic signals in color-deficient individuals. Deeply tinted lenses may provide considerable comfort to patients with ocular inflammation associated with photophobia, albinism, and conditions in which the pupil is dilated.

Contact lenses. There are essentially two types of contact lenses, corneal and corneoscleral. Corneoscleral lenses are divided into two types: (1) scleral, which have a different radius of the curvature for the cornea and the sclera, and (2) lacrimal lenses, which have a uniform curvature. Corneoscleral contact lenses must be filled with fluid and do not touch the cornea. Corneal contact lenses float on the precorneal tear film of the cornea.

Contact lenses are indicated to improve vision in keratoconus and such conditions as corneal scarring causing irregular astigmatism. Contact lenses are of unusual value in the management of some cases of conjunctival scarring to prevent exposure keratitis, corneal drying, and injury. If there is scarring or irregularity of the cornea, it is desirable to prescribe the scleral type of lenses so as to avoid irritating the cornea with the lens. Additionally, irregularity of the corneal surface may provide inadequate capillarity to maintain corneal lenses in position.

Contact lenses occasionally cause injury to the eye. They separate the corneal epithelium from the atmospheric oxygen necessary for metabolism (p. 68), and after a contact lens has been worn for a period, minute abrasions of the epithelium and subepithelial edema develop. The subepithelial edema is known as Sattler's veil and is identical with the edema observed following sudden increase in intraocular pressure. Infection may be introduced into the cornea by means of a contact lens, and ocular disease may be neglected by patients who believe their symptoms are due to the wearing of contact lenses.

Many athletes and entertainers use contact lenses successfully. The majority of patients, however, wear contact lenses to avoid the use of spectacles, and their successful use depends upon the ratio of the patient's vanity to his tolerance for discomfort.

Contact lenses are contraindicated in patients who have anesthetic corneas; corneal dystrophies, particularly dystrophies involving the endothelium or the epithelium; and glaucoma. Biomicroscopic examination of the cornea should be carried out by one familiar with these conditions prior to the prescription of contact lenses.

The majority of contact lenses are worn by women who wish to discard spectacles. If a useful wearing time is to be obtained, the lenses must be worn nearly daily. It is seldom possible for patients to wear them successfully for infrequent social occasions. Contact lenses are most successfully worn by myopic girls in their late teens who desire clear vision without spectacles. Women in the presbyopic age group often desire them so that it is not necessary to wear reading glasses, but this is seldom successful.

Low vision aids. A number of devices have been designed to permit individuals with poor visual acuity to see more distinctly. All of them magnify and increase the size of the retinal image by bringing the material closer to the eye. The success in wearing such lenses is closely related to the motivation and personality of the patient. Optimistic, self-reliant patients accept optical aids much better than those who are hostile, pessimistic, and inactive. Patients with visual reduction due to vitreous hemorrhage and retinitis proliferans do much more poorly than those with isolated lesions involving the fovea centralis.

A number of different types of lenses are available. A marked increase in the refractive power of the reading portion of a bifocal lens may assist individuals with a relatively good visual acuity. A magnifying lens held in the hand may be helpful, although many patients dislike the inconvenience. Telescopic lenses are theoretically useful but often reduce the peripheral visual field so markedly that patients dislike wearing them. In recent years the use of plastics for lenses permits the manufacture of optical surfaces with a variation in curvature that markedly decreases spheric aberration. Such aspheric lenses are useful to some. In many instances the acceptance of an optical aid appears to depend on the enthusiasm of both the examiner and the patient. Commonly, reading is distinctly difficult inasmuch as one or two letters only may be perceived at one time. The ordinary magnifying lens held by the patient in front of the reading matter is one of the most successful optical aids. Devices for distance are usually not useful, although a small telescope may be helpful in seeing bus signs, street signs, and the like.

Periodic eye examination

Examination of a newborn infant should include inspection of the lids and the external eye. Ophthalmoscopic examination should minimally indicate a red fundus reflex with no opacities of the media. A careful practitioner will view the optic disk and the immediately adjacent area. If the eyes cross after the age of 6 months, a complete eye examination, including cycloplegia and refraction, is indicated.

It is desirable that the vision be measured some time during or before the third year inasmuch as strabismic or anisometropic amblyopia may be corrected at this age. Complete eye examinations are desirable in the first and fourth grades and when the child begins high school and college. More frequent examinations may be necessary if any abnormality is discovered.

Young adults should be examined every 3 or 4 years if correcting lenses are not worn, and at least every 2 years if lenses are worn. After the age of 45 years, examination should be done every 2 years.

An eye examination of a presumably normal individual without specific ocular complaints should include study of the anterior segment of the eye and the lids with a biomicroscope. The ocular fundus should be inspected with the ophthalmoscope. The intraocular pressure should be measured by means of a tonometer. The visual fields should be estimated by confrontation or other screening method or should be measured carefully if the history and examination suggest an abnormality. The muscle balance should be measured for near and far. The central visual acuity should be measured for near and far, and the refractive error should be determined.

Reading defects

A variety of defects in reading are often wrongly attributed to ocular abnormalities, particularly errors of refraction. Individuals with reading problems are characterized by (1) poor word recognition (inability to pronounce words or to identify unfamiliar words); (2) poor comprehension (difficulty in deriving literal and implied meanings, in drawing conclusions, and in following directions); (3) slow reading rate; and (4) difficulty in developing vocabulary.

There are a number of factors that may contribute to or cause reading deficiencies. Since children grow and develop at different rates, not all are ready to begin reading at the same age. Some children may do well at an older age but start slowly. Such a possibility must be considered in evaluating reading skills and reading progress in younger children.

Children with specific reading disability (developmental dyslexia) probably constitute only a small percentage of those with reading difficulties. They do not read despite adequate instruction, proper motivation, a culturally adequate environment, intact senses, normal intelligence, and absence of a gross neurologic defect. This condition is found mostly in boys and may be familial.

Since there are so many causes of reading problems, the diagnosis demands a multidisciplinary approach. Visual, auditory, psychological, neurologic, pediatric, and educational evaluation may be necessary. Defective visual acuity, refractive errors, defective fusion, and muscle imbalance usually have no causative role except insofar as reduced visual acuity makes it difficult for the child to interpret symbols.

It is evident that specific causal factors, if identified, must be treated. Some prob-

---

Contributing factors and causes of reading deficiencies

I. Sociopsychological
   A. Defects in teaching
   B. Deficiencies in cognitive stimulation
   C. Deficiencies in motivation
      1. Associated with social pathology
      2. Associated with psychopathology ("emotional")
II. Psychophysiological
   A. General debility
   B. Sensory defects
   C. Intellectual defects
   D. Brain injury
   E. Specific reading disability (developmental dyslexia)

lems can be handled in the regular classroom. However, many children require the help of the remedial reading specialist for a long period of time. A variety of methods are used in teaching the retarded reader, but no single method can be recognized as the best. Depending upon the child, a variety of methods of sensory stimulation, utilizing visual, auditory and kinesthetic techniques, may be used.

Previously acquired ability to read may be lost because of neurologic defects involving mainly the left (in right-handed persons) angular and supramarginal gyri. This condition may be classed as neurologic dyslexia or acquired dyslexia. The severity and the nature of the defects vary markedly: inability to read letters while retaining the ability to read numbers; the ability to recognize words printed in large type but not small type; and the like. Often the condition is caused by cerebral vascular disease and there is widespread interference with brain function, which complicates exact diagnosis.

Part IV

Systemic diseases and the eye

Chapter 23

Infectious ocular diseases and granulomas

The globe and the ocular adnexa may be involved in inflammation caused by invasion of nearly any infectious agent. In general, if an infecting organism causes skin lesions elsewhere, it may easily involve the skin of the eyelids, often with marked swelling that also involves the conjunctiva. There may be characteristic involvement of the preauricular or submandibular lymph nodes. As we have seen in the section on diseases of the lid (p. 153), the glands associated with hair follicles may become infected and give rise to characteristic lesions. A necrotizing ulcer may occur with tarsal conjunctiva involvement or a superficial abscess with invasion of the bulbar conjunctiva. Introduction of a pathogenic organism into the conjunctival sac can cause a conjunctivitis, often of a typical type. Generally, if organisms affect mucous membranes elsewhere in the body, they will cause a conjunctivitis if introduced in large enough quantities. Additionally, organisms such as the *Streptococcus*, pneumococcus, and *Staphylococcus* can cause conjunctivitis. The epithelium of the cornea acts as a barrier in most infections, although as we have seen (p. 204), abrasion of the corneal epithelium may be followed by ulcers due to bacteria or fungi. The introduction of infectious agents directly into the eye, either by accidental trauma or surgery, not unexpectedly gives rise to immediate inflammation due to multiplication of bacteria or to a response due

to the development of either an antiphylactic type of hypersensitivity or a delayed bacterial type of hypersensitivity. Involvement of the brain and the cranial nerves may give rise to ocular muscle palsies and optic neuritis.

The topic of infectious ocular disease is large, and the discussion here is limited to the more typical ocular manifestations of infection. Additionally, modern therapy has made many infectious diseases a rarity, so rare indeed that they are often not recognized when they do occur. Some of these have been summarized in Table 23-1.

Bacterial infections

Neisseria. The genus *Neisseria* contains two important disease-producing species, the gonococcus and the meningococcus, and several nonpathogenic inhabitants of mucous membrane (*Neisseria catarrhalis, pharyngis,* and *sicca*). Rarely these latter organisms may be a cause of conjunctivitis, but the diseases caused by the gonococcus or the meningococcus are much more important.

Gonococcus. The gonococcus *Neisseria gonorrhoeae* is a gram-negative, nonmotile, nonsporulating diplococcus that may cause inflammation of mucous membranes, particularly of the genital tract. Bacteremia similar to that caused by the meningococcus rarely may follow untreated genitourinary tract infection.

An acute migratory arthritis affecting

Table 23-1. Bacterial disease and the eye

Bacteria	Species or group	Systemic disease	Ocular disease
Bacillus	anthracis	Malignant pustule, hemorrhagic mediastinitis (woolsorters' disease), gastrointestinal inflammation, disseminated disease with meningitis	Necrotic ulcer of lids
Brucella	melitensis (goats), abortus (cattle), suis (pigs), ovis (sheep)	Acute and chronic febrile disease, encephalitis, meningitis	Keratitis (nummular—coins), uveitis (granulomatous), retrobulbar neuritis and papillitis
Corynebacterium	diphtheriae	Fibrinous pseudomembrane upper respiratory tract exotoxin involving myocardium and central nervous system	Membranous conjunctivitis with necrosis, postdiphtheritic paralysis (NVI and accommodation [N III])
	xerose	Nonpathogenic	Found in foamy secretion at inner canthus in elderly
Clostridium	tetani	Tetanus	Miosis, orbicularis oculi spasm
	botulinum	Acute poisoning	Paralysis of intraocular and extraocular muscles
Haemophilus	aegyptius (Koch-Weeks)		Acute catarrhal conjunctivitis
Moraxella	lacunatus and non-liquefaciens		Angular conjunctivitis, indolent corneal ulcer
Bordetella	pertussis	Whooping cough	Lid, orbit, and conjunctival hemorrhage
Neisseria	gonorrhoeae	Mucous membrane inflammation (urethritis)	Purulent conjunctivitis, ophthalmia neonatorum, nongranulomatous iridocyclitis
	meningitidis	Meningitis	Petechiae and ecchymoses during bacteremia, bilateral panophthalmitis
	catarrhalis, pharyngis, and sicca		Conjunctivitis
Mycobacterium	tuberculosis	Nearly any system	Any part of eye involved: lupus vulgaris, phlyctenular disease, uveitis, periphlebitis
	leprae	Lepromatous (cutaneous) Tuberculoid (neural)	Anterior ocular inflammation Rarely anterior ocular inflammation
Pasteurella	tularensis	Generalized febrile illness	Necrotic conjunctival ulcer (Parinaud's syndrome)
	pestis	Severe febrile disease	Severe conjunctival edema
Pneumococci			Hypopyon keratitis, purulent conjunctivitis
Staphylococci			Sty, blepharitis, conjunctivitis
Streptococci	β-hemolytic group A		Pseudomembranous conjunctivitis, keratitis with hypopyon, nongranulomatous uveitis(?)

most commonly the knees, wrists, and ankles is the most common extragenital complication. A catarrhal conjunctivitis may occur. A severe nongranulomatous iridocyclitis (p. 230) may also occur as a metastatic complication. In men, Reiter's disease (urethritis, arthritis, and ocular inflammation, p. 237) as a cause of the symptoms is excluded by demonstration of the gonococcus in the urethral discharge or a rising antibody titer with the gonococcal complement fixation test.

The most serious ocular inflammation caused by the gonococcus is purulent conjunctivitis, which is an important cause of blindness, particularly in the Middle East. The incubation period is 2 to 5 days, with a rapid onset, papillary involvement of the entire conjunctiva, and an initial serous discharge that soon becomes purulent. Chemosis of the bulbar conjunctiva and swelling of the tissues surrounding the eye may be extreme. Corneal ulceration involving the central cornea may lead to panophthalmitis or corneal scarring.

Ophthalmia neonatorum (p. 173) is the term given to any acute conjunctivitis occurring in the first 10 days of life. The most common causes in the United States are *Diplococcus pneumoniae, Neisseria gonorrhoeae,* the *Haemophilus* group, and the virus of inclusion conjunctivitis. The gonococcus has been almost eliminated as a cause of ophthalmia neonatorum in the United States because of the instillation of 1% silver nitrate into the eyes of infants at birth. However, gonococcal inflammation is a common cause of blindness in many medically indigent regions of the world. The disease is so serious that in any conjunctival inflammation of the newborn infant, the gonococcus must be excluded as a cause.

Meningococcus. The meningococcus *(Neisseria meningitidis)* is a gram-negative, nonmotile, nonsporulating microorganism that is often arranged in pairs. They are strictly parasites of man and give rise to a specific infectious disease characterized by invasion through the nasopharynx, bacteremia, and focal involvement, notably of the central nervous system.

Ocular involvement during the stage of bacteremia consists of petechiae and ecchymoses. Intraocular invasion may cause a bilateral panophthalmitis with blindness and eventual phthisis bulbi. A purulent conjunctivitis may develop. Meningeal involvement may cause loss of vision and ocular muscle paralysis. The organism may cause a purulent conjunctivitis in the absence of systemic infection and must be distinguished from the gonococcus.

Mycobacterium. The genus *Mycobacterium* causes a number of chronic infectious granulomas in man and animals. There are a number of nonpathogenic species. The most important human diseases caused by members of the genus are tuberculosis and leprosy.

Tuberculosis. *Mycobacterium tuberculosis* is a nonmotile, encapsulated, rodlike organism that stains with difficulty, but once stained, it resists decolorization with strong mineral acids (acid-fast). Human and bovine varieties are pathogenic for man, whereas the murine and piscine varieties cause tuberculosis in rodents and fish but not in man. The avian (bird) variety rarely causes human disease.

The clinical and pathologic changes of tuberculosis depend upon the tissue involved and the degree of hypersensitivity of the host to the organism. Generally, the initial or primary lesion is an acute process, healing or progressing in a short time, and characterized in the main by an inconspicuous parenchymal lesion and massive tissue necrosis (caseation) of the draining lymph nodes. The postprimary lesion or reinfection occurs in an individual who has developed a hypersensitivity to the bacteria either because of previous infection or immunization with BCG (bacille Calmette Guérin) vaccine. This lesion is more chronic than the primary type and is associated with severe parenchymal involvement with a minor effect on the regional lymph nodes.

As might be anticipated, every portion of the eye and the adnexa may be involved in the tuberculous process. Inasmuch as the causative organism is recovered with difficulty even when tissue is available, diagnosis is frequently based upon the clinical appearance of the lesion and exclusion of other likely causes of the inflammation.

Ocular involvement is uncommon in patients with active pulmonary tuberculosis. Acute miliary tuberculosis may involve any portion of the uveal tract, but the choroid is most commonly affected. Three or four inflammatory nodules may develop rapidly, but they remain inactive, causing minimal cellular reaction.

The skin of the lids may be involved in lupus vulgaris or, more rarely, in other cutaneous manifestations of tuberculosis, each of which may spread to the conjunctiva and the cornea.

Phlyctenular disease involves the conjunctiva and the cornea. In many instances it appears to be a response to sensitivity to tuberculoprotein (tuberculin) and is responsive to local instillation of corticosteroids.

By far the most important ocular involvement is granulomatous inflammation of the uveal tract occurring in an individual hypersensitive to tuberculin. Involvement of the anterior segment causes an insidious low-grade inflammation characterized by the development of mutton-fat keratic precipitates, minute nodules at the pupillary margin (Koeppe nodules), and a tendency to the development of posterior synechiae. Posterior segment involvement causes an exudation of inflammatory cells into the vitreous body with destruction of the overlying retina. A posterior polar cataract (complicated) frequently develops.

Retinal veins are a frequent site of involvement, with development of a periphlebitis with neovascularization and fre-

quently recurrent vitreous hemorrhage (Eales' disease, p. 273). Photocoagulation of the involved area has proved to be an effective means of therapy.

Tuberculous meningitis may involve individuals of any age, but it is usually the result of overwhelming primary infection in childhood. Choroidal tubercles occur, commonly combined with visual loss arising from optic atrophy, caused by adhesive arachnoiditis and internal hydrocephalus.

Treatment of ocular tuberculosis is prolonged chemotherapy, usually with isoniazid and para-aminosalicylic acid. If there is improvement within 3 weeks using these drugs, therapy must be continued uninterruptedly for 12 months. If there is no clinical response within 3 weeks, tuberculosis as an etiologic factor must be questioned. These drugs are commonly combined with local instillation of corticosteroids and atropine to combat inflammation. Desensitization to tuberculin is no longer widely used.

Leprosy. *Mycobacterium leprae* is an acid-fast rod similar to *Mycobacterium tuberculosis*. It causes a chronic infectious disease involving predominantly the skin, the superficial nerves, the pharynx, and the larynx. It occurs as two principal types: (1) the lepromatous (cutaneous) in which there is no body resistance and (2) the tuberculoid (neural) in which there is some body resistance.

Eye involvement occurs commonly in the lepromatous type but rarely in the tuberculoid type, which often tends to localize and not to involve viscera. The eyes are usually involved late in the course of the disease, and there is a marked predilection for the anterior segment, with conjunctivitis, episcleritis, and superficial keratitis. As the disease progresses, the sclera and the cornea are affected, and still later the iris and the ciliary body are affected. The iritis is characterized by small, almost pedunculated nodules (miliary lepromas) on the anterior iris surface. A full-blown granulomatous uveitis ensues. Anterior segment disease is treated with local corticosteroids and atropine.

There may be alopecia of the eyebrows and exposure keratitis because of orbicularis oculi muscle paralysis (keratitis e lagophthalmos, p. 209). Treatment is with sulfones.

Staphylococci. The staphylococci are gram-positive, toxin-producing, nonmotile organisms, typically occurring in irregular clusters. Most pathogenic strains are coagulase positive and may produce a golden pigment, but nonpathogenic variants of *Staphylococcus aureus* may occur.

The skin is the common site of staphylococcic infection, and the majority of deeper infections originate in the skin. This is the common organism found in suppuration of the glands of Zeis or Moll, causing a hordeolum or sty. *Staphylococcus* causes catarrhal conjunctivitis less commonly than do the pneumococcus or *Haemophilus* groups. Staphylococcic infections of the conjunctiva cause typical minute corneal ulcers at the corneoscleral limbus (p. 208).

Streptococci. The streptococci are gram-positive, nonmotile microorganisms that are spherical or oval in shape and tend to grow in chains. Only hemolytic streptococci (beta) are considered pathogenic; the non-hemolytic streptococci are saprophytic. Beta (hemolytic) streptococci have been divided into a number of well-defined serologic groups, the most important in human disease being group A. The manifestations of streptococcic disease vary markedly in different age groups.

Streptococci may cause a pseudomembranous conjunctivitis with a tendency for corneal involvement. Corneal invasion may be associated with hypopyon. These inflammations are readily treated with antibiotics or sulfonamides applied locally. Diagnosis usually is based on culture because chain formation does not commonly occur in ocular infections, and the organism may be confused with staphylococci.

Rheumatic fever (p. 451) rarely causes ocular manifestations. Glomerulonephritis due to streptococci manifests itself in the eye only in the changes of vascular hypertension. Scarlet fever has no ocular signs except the occasional occurrence of ecchymoses and petechiae in severely ill patients after the rash appears on the second day.

Erysipelas is a recurrent, acute, hemolytic streptococcic infection of the skin of the middle-aged and elderly, usually involving the face and head. As a rule, the lesion spreads from a central focus to involve adjacent areas, which become red, glistening, swollen, and sometimes versicolored. The skin of the eyelids may be involved.

Bedsoniae infections

The agents of psittacosis, lymphogranuloma venereum, trachoma, and inclusion conjunctivitis are related, obligate intracellular parasites that are sensitive to antibiotics and occupy a position intermediate between the rickettsiae and the viruses. Those causing *t*rachoma and *i*nclusion *c*onjunctivitis are known as TRIC agents.

Trachoma. Trachoma (p. 174) is a chronic follicular conjunctivitis characteristically involving the upper lid and causing conjunctival and corneal cicatrization with severe visual disability. The disease has been recognized since antiquity and is probably the chief cause of blindness in the world. In the United States it is prevalent mainly in Indians in the Southwest.

Inclusion conjunctivitis. This benign follicular conjunctivitis is caused by the agent that causes a nongonococcal urethritis and cervicitis (p. 175).

In the newborn infant, inclusion conjunctivitis has an incubation period of 5 to 12 days in contrast to gonorrheal ophthalmia, which occurs within 5 days of birth. The onset is acute. A purulent conjunctivitis develops rapidly, with intense infiltration of the conjunctiva and particularly of the lower lid. The infection is not prevented by Credé's prophylaxis.

In the adult the same agent causes an acute follicular conjunctivitis with pre-auricular adenopathy. The follicles, unlike those of trachoma, are more marked in the lower lid and do not contain necrotic material. There is never corneal involvement, and the disease heals spontaneously without residual changes. The genitourinary tract serves as a reservoir for the infection. Oral sulfonamides or broad-spectrum antibiotics are required for healing.

Lymphogranuloma venereum. Lymphogranuloma venereum is a contagious venereal disease manifested by an initial vesicle that bursts, leaving a grayish ulcer and followed by regional lymphadenitis that is frequently suppurative. Mild to severe constitutional signs may be present during the stage of adenitis.

Primary infection of the lid, occurring venereally or through contamination in a laboratory worker, gives rise to an ulcerative lesion of the lid or conjunctiva with preauricular adenopathy (Parinaud's oculoglandular syndrome). There is marked edema of the lids with a characteristic ulcer having clean-cut edges and surrounded by a nonindurated, narrow band of discolored skin.

Hematogenous spread of the disease may cause uveitis, keratouveitis, or sclerokeratitis. A granuloma may occur at the corneoscleral limbus, with an associated keratitis.

The disease may be diagnosed by demonstration of elementary (Donovan) bodies in involved tissue. The Frei skin test is positive 7 to 40 days after infection and remains so thereafter. False positive results are uncommon, but they may be caused by infection with other members of the Bedsoniae group.

Viral infections

Viruses are obligate intracellular parasites that may infect and may cause disease in vertebrates, flowering plants, insects, and bacteria. They vary markedly in the size and complexity of their structure, but they can reproduce only in living cells and depend upon the host cell for a portion of their enzymatic requirements. They may remain latent within a cell without causing any sign until provoked into activity by a physiologic, biochemical, or environmental change.

Viruses cause the same antibody, immunity, and hypersensitivity responses in the infected host as do other infectious agents. Viruses contain a central core of genetic material (nucleic acid) responsible for infectivity and definitive characteristics and an outside coating of protein responsible for antigenic reactivity and involved in the immunity and antibody response of the host. Classification of viruses is not satisfactory and is based on the primary type of host infected, the nucleic acid content (DNA or RNA), the size, the clinical disease, and the common antigens.

The eyes and the surrounding tissues may be affected by nearly any virus, either by direct tissue invasion or by motor or sensory nerve involvement secondary to cerebral infection (Table 23-2). Inasmuch as specific therapy is available for most bacterial diseases, viruses have emerged as a major cause of external inflammatory disease of the eye.

The diagnosis of ocular viral disease is based upon the clinical nature of the disease, laboratory findings, and isolation of the virus. In many instances the ocular involvement is either of minor significance, as in encephalitis, is not recognized, as in measles or mumps, or may dominate the clinical picture, as in herpes simplex keratitis or epidemic keratoconjunctivitis. The recovery of a virus from infected cells by growth in tissue culture or chick allantoic membrane is the only sure way of diagnosing virus disease, but it is usually the most difficult method. Increasing antibody titer to the antigen of a specific virus indicates tissue sensitization to the virus, but

Table 23-2. Virus disease and the eye

Virus	Groups and types	Systemic disease	Ocular disease
Adeno-	Type 3, 4, or 7	Pharyngitis	Conjunctivitis (50%)
	Type 1, 2, or 5	Pharyngitis	None
	Type 8	Children: fever, pharyngitis, gastroenteritis	Conjunctivitis
		Adults: No systemic disease	Epidemic keratoconjunctivitis
Arbor	Equine—various types	Encephalitis	Secondary to cranial nerve involvement
	Yellow fever		
	Dengue		
Chickenpox	1	Chickenpox	Uveitis
		Meningoencephalitis	Cranial nerves
		Zoster	Keratitis, uveitis with invasion of first branch of N V
German measles	1?	German measles, meningo-encephalitis	Congenital defects in embryo: cataract, retinopathy, deafness, heart defects
Herpes simplex	1	Fever sores, stomatitis, Kaposi's eruption	Dendritic keratitis
Measles	1	Measles, meningoencephalitis	Keratitis, uveitis
Molluscum contagiosum	?	Multiple warts	Chronic conjunctivitis
Mumps	1	Parotitis, orchitis, encephalitis	Interstitial keratitis
Newcastle virus of fowl		None	Acute follicular conjunctivitis
Salivary gland	1?	Cytomegalic inclusion disease	Uveitis
Smallpox	1?	Smallpox	Vaccinia of lid, keratitis

in many instances of ocular disease the systemic involvement is so slight that the antibody titer is not affected. Many systemic infections arise from different strains and mutations of virus; therefore specific antigenic tests are difficult to prepare.

In general, those diseases associated with petechial hemorrhage may have associated subconjunctival hemorrhage or ecchymoses of the lids. Widespread systemic infection may be associated with uveal inflammation, which is commonly not diagnosed in light of the grave systemic illness. Conditions characterized by involvement of the skin may affect the lids and, if the lid margin is involved, cause a secondary conjunctivitis or keratitis. Those diseases with

involvement of mucous membranes may affect the conjunctiva or the cornea. If the central nervous system is affected, involvement of the cranial nerves to the eye may give rise to eye signs. Motor nerve involvement causes strabismus. Interference with third cranial nerve fibers to the ciliary muscle causes a loss of accommodation, whereas interruption of fibers to the sphincter pupillae muscle causes pupillary dilation and loss of the direct and consensual light reflexes. The optic nerve may be involved in a neuritis and, less frequently, in a papillitis. Increased intracranial pressure may cause a papilledema.

Adenoviruses. The group of adenoviruses is composed of at least 28 immunologically distinct types of DNA viruses found in man and higher primates. Adenovirus type 8 causes epidemic keratoconjunctivitis in adults, and in children it causes a systemic disease with fever, respiratory or gastrointestinal signs, and a conjunctivitis without corneal opacities. Adenovirus types 3, 4, and 7 prime cause an acute respiratory disease, pharyngoconjunctival fever, and simple follicular conjunctivitis; types 1, 2, 5, and perhaps others cause a febrile pharyngitis.

Pharyngoconjunctival fever. Pharyngoconjunctival fever is an acute sporadic or epidemic disease affecting all age groups but predominantly children. It occurs at all seasons of the year but is more common in summer and is often associated with infection transmitted in swimming pools. The incubation period is 5 to 7 days, and the disease persists 1 to 2 weeks. Clinical manifestations vary markedly in different individuals and epidemics. A usually mild nasopharyngitis is associated with a cervical or a maxillary lymphadenopathy. A fever that may reach 39° C. persists 3 to 14 days. Headache referable to the sinuses, lassitude, malaise, and sometimes gastrointestinal disturbances occur.

The conjunctivitis is acute, sometimes monocular and nonpurulent. Lymph follicle hyperplasia is most marked in the lower cul-de-sac. Congestion is most marked over the palpebral conjunctiva and spares the bulbar conjunctiva. Preauricular adenopathy may be present.

Adenovirus type 3 is most commonly implicated, but types 4 and 7 prime have been found as a cause. The serum of affected patients contains group-specific complement fixation bodies.

Epidemic keratoconjunctivitis. Adenovirus type 8 mainly causes epidemic keratoconjunctivitis in the United States (p. 207). This is an acute infectious corneal disease spread by contaminated eyedrops, eye instruments, or directly by the ocular secretion. In Japan, adenovirus type 8

causes an acute systemic disease in children with a conjunctivitis of varying severity without the production of permanent corneal opacities. The disease is usually associated with fever, malaise, gastrointestinal and upper respiratory symptoms, and a follicular conjunctivitis. Other children exposed to the disease develop the same disease, but exposed adults develop epidemic keratoconjunctivitis.

German measles (rubella). German measles is a mild contagious disease characterized mainly by an evanescent, maculopapular skin eruption beginning on the face and neck, spreading to the trunk and extremities, and fading in 3 days. There may be mild pharyngitis and postauricular adenopathy, sometimes accompanied by slight fever, malaise, lassitude, and myalgia.

Conjunctivitis is common and consists of bilateral bulbar congestion that, unlike measles conjunctivitis, spares the tarsal area. There is no keratitis.

Ophthalmic interest in rubella arises because of the large number of congenital defects occurring in infants whose mothers contract the disease during the first trimester of pregnancy. The incidence of embryopathy may be as high as 90% when infection occurs early in pregnancy. The pigment epithelium of the retina, ciliary body, and iris are severely affected. Because of the role of these tissues in the polarization of the eye, the infection may lead to microphthalmia and cataract formation. Less severe infection causes a discrete pigmentation of the peripheral retina associated with a decreased amplitude of the electroretinogram, poor dark adaptation, and a decreased electro-oculogram. The lens may harbor the virus for as long as 24 months after birth, and cataract surgery carried out during this period may lead to a severe chronic nongranulomatous inflammatory reaction centered around lens remnants. The inflammation involves the uveal tract and is associated with considerable fibroblastic activity that gives rise to overgrowth of the corneal stroma, arising from the site of the corneal incision, and to the formation of an inflammatory membrane. Surgery for rubella cataract should be delayed until children are at least 2 years of age. A sector iridectomy, however, can be done safely at any time and often results in significant visual improvement.

The availability of the vaccine providing complete protection against rubella should result in elimination of periodic epidemics. In the 1963-1964 epidemic it is estimated that over 100,000 affected infants were born between June, 1964, and April, 1965. Nonimmune pregnant women should be protected during the first 4 months of pregnancy by the administration of antirubella gamma globulin, either before contact (in an epidemic area) or early in the incubation period.

Herpesviruses. The herpesvirus group contains three members pathogenic to man: (1) *Herpesvirus varicellae*, which causes chickenpox and zoster; (2) *Herpesvirus hominis*, the virus causing herpes simplex; and (3) *Herpesvirus simiae* (B. virus), which causes a subclinical infection in monkeys but a fatal disease in the accidentally infected human being.

Chickenpox (varicella). Chickenpox is an acute contagious disease characterized by a vesicular exanthem involving predominantly the hands and trunk, developing in crops over a period of 1 to 5 days, and associated with malaise and fever. In adults a varicella pneumonia may develop. Vesicles may occur on the eyelids and rarely on the conjunctiva and the cornea. A very mild iridocyclitis may occur.

Zoster. Zoster is an infectious process of the dorsal root or extramedullary cranial nerve ganglia characterized by a circumscribed vesicular eruption and neuralgic pain in the areas supplied by the sensory nerves extending to the affected ganglia. The causative virus is identical with that causing chickenpox. Varicella may consti-

tute the response to infection in the non-immune host, whereas zoster occurs in the partially immune host. Zoster is most common after the age of 50 years, but occurs also in younger individuals. It may appear in the course of severe and debilitating systemic illness, and patients with lymphosarcoma and reticulum cell sarcoma are particularly susceptible.

Herpes zoster ophthalmicus is an infection with the chickenpox virus of that portion of the gasserian ganglion receiving fibers from the ophthalmic nerve. Most patients are between the ages of 30 and 80 years, the average age being 60 years. The inflammation may constitute the systemic response to infection with varicella in partially immune individuals. With no immunity present, chickenpox occurs.

The disease is ushered in by a severe, unilateral, disabling neuralgia in the region of distribution of the ophthalmic nerve. Several days later there is a vesicular eruption with much swelling and tenderness. The vesicles rupture, leaving hemorrhagic areas that heal in several weeks and leave deep-pitted scars. Pain disappears in about 2 weeks, but in a small percentage of cases a postherpetic neuralgia persists that is resistant to treatment.

The lids may be swollen and tender, but involvement of the globe itself is seen in only about one half of the patients. Ocular involvement is usually heralded by a vesicle on the tip of the nose, an area innervated, as is the cornea, by the nasociliary nerve.

Superficial and deep corneal opacities occur, combined with folds in Descemet's membrane and keratic precipitates due to an anterior uveitis. The disease may persist for weeks and slowly regress, leaving a residue of round corneal infiltrates in the anterior corneal stroma. Secondary glaucoma occurs in about 20% of the patients, and paresis of extraocular muscles occurs in about 10%.

Treatment is often unsatisfactory. Elderly patients should not be exposed to children with chickenpox. Local corticosteroids and atropine appear helpful. In previously healthy individuals, systemic corticosteroids may quickly relieve an attack. In debilitated patients the corticosteroids may cause a fatal dissemination of the virus. The remote possibility that this might occur in an otherwise healthy patient leads many to believe the drug is contraindicated. A large number of nonspecific remedies have been proposed.

Herpes simplex. Two types of infection occur with *Herpesvirus hominis:* (1) primary infection in persons without neutralizing antibodies and (2) recurrent infection (reactivation) in persons with neutralizing antibodies.

Primary infection usually occurs after the age of 6 months, following disappearance of maternal antibodies, and before the age of 5 years, by which time most individuals have been infected. As a rule, there is gingivostomatitis with adenopathy, fever, and malaise. In the majority of cases the primary infection either does not cause clinical signs or is so minor as not to be recalled. If eczema is present, a severe, widespread disease may occur (eczema herpeticum, Kaposi's varicelliform eruption).

After the primary lesion, subsequent disease is entirely local and without systemic signs. Reinfection gives rise to recurrent vesicles on an erythematous base that occur at the same site in each individual. The most frequent manifestation is a fever blister (herpes labialis, herpes facialis, herpes febrilis), which often involves a mucocutaneous junction. Reinfection causes an initial sensation of burning and irritation at the involved site followed by reddish papules that quickly vesiculate. The vesicles quickly become purulent (frequently with localized adenopathy), scale, and heal without a scar.

The eye may be the site of a primary infection in a child. More commonly it is the site of recurrent (reactivation) type of disease. Primary infection of the eye occurs in children and begins as unilateral follicular conjunctivitis with a preauricular adenopathy and malaise. The disease may be confined to the conjunctiva, or the cornea may be involved with superficial punctate erosions or a single vesicle, both types of which develop into a typical dendritic (branching) keratitis (p. 205).

Recurrent disease is triggered by fever, ultraviolet light, mechanical trauma, menstruation, emotional upsets, and allergy. There is an initial foreign body sensation in the eye, and the unfortunate experienced patient usually knows the disease has recurred. Vesicles are present early, but are usually ruptured by the time the patient is seen, and a dendritic pattern can be demonstrated on the cornea with the instillation of 2% sterile fluorescein.

Mumps. Mumps is an acute contagious virus (RNA) systemic disease characterized mainly by a painful enlargement of the salivary glands, most commonly the parotid gland, and, after puberty, by orchitis. Lymphocytic meningitis, pancreatitis, and involvement of other viscera occur rarely.

A transient corneal edema occurs commonly with a decrease in visual acuity. There are no associated ocular inflammatory signs. A uveitis or inflammation of the lacrimal glands may occur. The sole sign of meningeal involvement may be optic neuritis, or there may be widespread ocular signs from cranial nerve involvement.

Measles (rubeola). Measles is a contagious, infectious virus (RNA) disease characterized by prodromal symptoms of fever, cough, conjunctivitis, upper respiratory infection, and Koplik's spots on the buccal mucosa, followed in 3 to 5 days by a maculopapular cutaneous rash. The conjunctivitis is nonpurulent and may be associated with Koplik's spots, particularly on the semilunar fold. The cornea has multiple punctate epithelial erosions, which causes a severe photophobia. The photophobic patient is made more comfortable by either darkness or colored glasses. Local ocular treatment is not indicated in the absence of infection. Permanent corneal scarring does not occur unless there is secondary bacterial infection.

Not infrequently, measles or other acute contagious disease of childhood is the precipitating event in the appearance of strabismus. However, the primary cause of the squint is already present, and the disease seems only to accelerate its appearance or to transform an intermittent type into a continuous type of strabismus.

Vaccination has nearly eliminated measles in the United States. During the period of incubation the administration of gamma globulin may prevent or modify the disease in the nonimmune individual.

Molluscum contagiosum. Molluscum contagiosa is a viral tumor characterized by the development of multiple discrete nodules in the epidermal layer of the skin. The nodules are usually pearly white and painless, with umbilication at the top in which a small white cone can be seen. Man is the only host of the virus; children are attacked most frequently, and the lesion is prevalent in some areas. The nodules occur frequently on the skin of the eyelids and on the lid margins. If on the lid margin, virus material may be released into the conjunctival sac and cause conjunctivitis or keratitis. Excision of the nodule is the treatment of choice.

Vaccinia and variola keratitis (p. 206). Accidental inoculation of the eyelids and the cornea from the vaccinia virus occurs rarely. Treatment with IDU locally or vaccinia hyperimmune gamma globulin systemically is of value.

Variola was a common cause of blindness when smallpox was widespread, and blindness still occurs in those areas where the disease is not prevented by vaccination. Gamma globulin in the incubation period may be effective.

Verrucae (warts). Verrucae are contagious viral tumors characterized by the development of one or more cutaneous masses having a cauliflower-like appearance and comprised of a rough surface made up of many fine projections. When located on the lid margin, the lesions mechanically cause a chronic epithelial keratitis. The conjunctivitis is mild and, like the keratitis, nonspecific. Removal of the lid margin nodules is required to heal the keratitis.

Cat-scratch fever. Cat-scratch fever is a systemic infection, possibly of viral origin, characterized by fever, a localized cutaneous lesion, and lymphadenitis. In years past the lesion was attributed to *Leptothrix (Actinomyces)*, a common nonpathogenic organism of the mouth of man and some lower animals, including cats. The cutaneous lesion, resembling a pustular furuncle, occurs in about 50% of the cases, with a regional lymphadenitis that may be suppurative. Often there has been earlier contact with cats. Involvement of the lid gives rise to a monocular conjunctivitis and preauricular adenopathy. Differential diagnosis includes tularemia, tuberculosis, and Parinaud's oculoglandular disease. An intradermal antigen test is helpful in the diagnosis. Treatment is mainly symptomatic. Chlortetracycline is reported to speed recovery.

Poliomyelitis, rabies, and viral encephalitis. The viruses causing these diseases may affect the optic and motor nerves of the eye. Optic neuritis may occur, with direct invasion of the meningeal covering of the nerve, or papilledema may develop when there is increased intracranial pressure. Involvement of the motor nerves can give rise to a complete ophthalmoplegia that involves ocular movement and accommodation and produces pupillary dilation (N III). There may be bizarre types of motor involvement, with paralytic strabismus. All of these changes may occur as a presenting sign of intracranial involvement but more often occur late in the course of the infection.

Infectious mononucleosis. Infectious mononucleosis is a contagious, presumably viral, disease of benign, though frequently protracted, course. It is characterized by lymphadenopathy and is associated with a lymphocytosis with atypical lymphocytes and an abnormally high serum concentration of heterophilic antibodies against sheep erythrocytes. Conjunctivitis with follicles, periorbital edema, nongranulomatous uveitis, and optic neuritis, sometimes with papillitis, retinal edema, and hemorrhages, may occur. In some epidemics, lacrimal gland inflammation (dacryoadenitis) is prominent. It causes a red, painful swelling, with redness of the outer one third of the upper lid with a typically S-shaped curve of the upper lid margin. Involvement of the central nervous system may cause extraocular muscle paralysis, nystagmus, hemianopsia, and disturbances of conjugate movement.

Treatment is nonspecific, and the disease is usually self-limited.

Rickettsial infections

Rickettsiae are microorganisms that, like bacteria, can be observed with the light microscope but that, like viruses, can multiply only within living cells. They occur in various arthropods that transmit the disease to man, and cause an acute febrile illness usually associated with a skin rash. Satisfactory vaccines have been prepared against some of the microorganisms. Delousing with DDT is effective prophylaxis, and the tetracyclines and chloramphenicol are highly effective therapeutically.

The ocular changes occurring in infections with the group have been best described with epidemic louse-borne typhus fever (*Rickettsia prowazeki* transmitted by the human louse, *Pediculus humanus*) and Rocky Mountain spotted fever (*Rickettsia*

ricksettii transmitted by animal ticks). At the time of onset of the disease, conjunctival hyperemia may occur, sometimes with subconjunctival hemorrhages. Marked venous engorgement with edema of the disk and retina may occur during the second and third weeks of the fever. Venous engorgement may be so severe as to lead to retinal hemorrhages that may burst into the vitreous body. Cotton-wool spots and arterial occlusion may be observed.

The diagnosis of rickettsial disease depends upon clinical signs in an area where the diseases are endemic. The Weil-Felix test in rising titer is helpful, except in Q fever where cross-antigens do not occur.

Mycotic infections

Fungi are single-celled organisms characterized by the formation of filaments (hyphae) and the production of spores. They can be identified only by the type and arrangement of their spores. Many fungi grow on ordinary laboratory media, but Sabouraud's media is preferred. Hyphae may occasionally be demonstrated in material crushed on a coverglass. Complement fixation and delayed skin hypersensitivity tests may also be used, but they are subject to the same limitations that arise in distinguishing an active and a previous infection, as is true of infections caused by other microorganisms. Often the diagnostic procedures are carried out inexpertly or so late that the disease is either not recognized or is diagnosed too late for effective therapy. Antifungal agents are of limited effectiveness, and less toxic and more effective therapeutic agents are needed.

Fungi can involve the eye in four main ways: (1) superficially to produce conjunctivitis, keratitis, and lacrimal obstruction; (2) by extension from infection in neighboring skin, nasal sinuses, or the nasopharynx; (3) by direct introduction into the eye during surgery or accidental trauma, particularly with plants, trees, and other organic material; and (4) by hematogenous infection.

Superficial infection. Fungi may be introduced into the cornea (p. 207) by a foreign body or an epithelial abrasion, frequently from a tree branch or other vegetable matter. A fluffy white spot appears on the cornea, which melts into a shallow ulcer with surrounding infiltrate and hypopyon. The inflammatory reaction is initially deceptively mild, and neovascularization does not occur. The inflammation gradually extends to involve the entire cornea, and there is a violent conjunctival inflammation. If treated with corticosteroids, the cornea slowly melts, sloughs, and perforates, with loss of the eye. Early treatment is by means of local nystatin or amphotericin B, unless the causative organism belongs to the sulfonamide or antibiotic-sensitive group. Medical therapy is frequently not effective, and the cornea does not heal until covered with a conjunctival flap.

A fungus conjunctival inflammation usually is diagnosed only when corneal involvement occurs. In tropical areas, *Rhinosporidium* may produce conjunctival polyps. A monocular necrotic lesion of the conjunctiva, associated with preauricular adenopathy, has been associated with *Leptothrix*, a common inhabitant of the mouths of cats. This organism, however, is now classified as bacterium, and the disease produced is most likely an ocular form of cat-scratch fever.

Unilateral, persistent tearing with patent passages characterizes lacrimal infection with fungi. There is an associated red and pouting punctum. Diagnosis is commonly not made until a lacrimal probe grates against concretions of hardened colonies of fungi in the involved canaliculus.

The skin of the eyelids may be involved by any of the fungi that cause a dermatomycosis. Extension of fungus infection into the orbit may cause a cellulitis or, because of involvement of the optic nerve, a retrobulbar neuritis. Some inflammatory granulomas of the orbit may also be due to fungi.

Intraocular infection. Endophthalmitis may occur from introduction of fungi into the eye at the time of surgery or through accidental trauma. Hypopyon and grayish masses develop, and the condition worsens with steroid therapy. Eventually the eye fills with granulomatous tissue.

Hematogenous intraocular infection has been reported with *Mucor* species, aspergillosis, and coccidioidomycosis. *Cryptococcus* has been reported as a cause of cystic retinal disease. *Candida albicans* has been histologically verified as a cause of retinochoroiditis and indirectly associated with posterior uveitis. Generally, hematogenous infection involves the retina, choroid, and sclera, whereas direct inoculation into the eye causes a vitreous granuloma. Ocular and orbital involvement may occur from cerebral involvement.

A review of cases of mucormycosis indicates that typically the patient is a diabetic in acidosis who develops proptosis, lid edema, and total ophthalmoplegia. Coma continues although the acidosis is corrected, and death occurs about a week later. Hyphae are prominent in the choroid plexus.

Protozoan and metazoan infections

The animal kingdom may be divided into two subkingdoms, the protozoan and metazoan. The protozoa are classically divided into amebas, flagellates, ciliates, and sporozoans. Diseases caused by protozoa include amebic dysentery, leishmaniasis, malaria, toxoplasmosis, and trypanosomiasis. The metazoa consist of all multicelled animals whose various types of cells are not in general capable of independent existence or performing all necessary vital functions. The metazoa range in complexity from simply arranged sponges to the highly specialized structure of man. Human infection by metazoa is chiefly by parasitic worms and some members of the phylum Arthropoda that are transmitters of disease. The larvae of flies are parasitic and may multiply in living tissue, causing myiasis. The adult fly is not a parasite.

The eye and adnexa may be affected by direct invasion by either the adult or larval form, by toxins elaborated by worms or released with death, or by impairment of the health of the host. Diagnosis is based upon the recovery of the parasite, its larvae or eggs, skin tests, and other immunologic studies. A systemic eosinophilia is often present.

Protozoan infections

Toxoplasmosis. Toxoplasmosis is an infectious disease caused by an obligate intracellular parasite, *Toxoplasma gondii.* The organism is capable of infecting a wide range of mammals, birds, and reptiles. Transmission occurs readily by feeding the organism, and it has been suggested that nematodes of cats (*Toxocara cati,* p. 379) are infected with *Toxoplasma* organisms and are capable of transmitting the disease. The life cycle of the organism is unknown. The parasite has been found in all parts of the world. Human beings with antibodies have been identified throughout the world, but the frequency of infection varies from 4 to 80% in different population groups.

Two main types of disease occur: (1) congenital and (2) acquired. The congenital disease is characterized by bilateral chorioretinitis, hydrocephalus, convulsions, and other evidence of encephalomyelitis such as cerebral calcifications demonstrated by x-ray examination. It occurs in infants whose mothers have no obvious illness during pregnancy, but who are found to have circulating antibodies when the disease is discovered in the infant. The main involvement is usually in the eyes and central nervous system, and there are wide variations in severity. Some infants mainly demonstrate visceral and muscular involvement. Onset is at or before birth. There is an inflammatory reaction and necrosis in the brain, with either single or multiple lesions. Disseminated organisms may be found, or pseudocysts may be formed that consist of parasites packed within a cell from which the nucleus has been extruded. With healing, calcification develops. There are associated signs of mental retardation, convulsion, hydrocephalus, and other neurologic abnormalities.

The ocular lesion involves mainly the posterior pole of the eye and a characteristic retinitis with secondary involvement of the choroid (p. 272). The fovea is frequently destroyed, with loss of central vision. The lesion is sharply demarcated, with pigmented borders and atrophy of both the retina and the choroid, so that the white sclera is seen. There may be multiple lesions. Usually the vitreous body is clear, and the inflammation appears inactive. Because of the loss of central vision, there may be an associated esotropia, exotropia, or an ocular type of nystagmus. There may be recurrence of ocular inflammation in later life. The mother and the infant usually have a high methylene blue dye test titer. Children of subsequent pregnancies are not affected.

The acquired form varies in severity from a mild febrile disturbance with lymphadenopathy to a severe, often fatal, disease with a maculopapular rash, pneumonitis, hepatitis, myocarditis, and encephalitis with fever and extreme prostration. Several types of involvement have been described: (1) lymphoadenopathic, (2) exanthematous, (3) pneumonic, (4) meningoencephalic, and (5) ocular.

The ocular lesions of acquired toxoplasmosis vary considerably. The most characteristic are multiple, discrete, sharply defined areas of retinal and choroidal necrosis surrounded with proliferated pigment. The most frequent is a local or generalized intraocular inflammation involving either anterior or posterior ocular tissues. Posterior lesions cause many vitreous exudates and veils, whereas anterior lesions cause mutton-fat keratic precipitates, aqueous flare, posterior synechiae, and complicated cataract. The ocular inflammation may occur because of rupture of a pseudocyst and dissemination of the organisms in the course of, or after, healing of the systemic infection.

Diagnosis of the cause of the ocular inflammation is not difficult when systemic infection is present, but it is most difficult after systemic disease has developed. The skin test is often negative and the blood dye test positive in low dilution. Diagnosis frequently depends upon the exclusion of other causes of uveitis.

The treatment of choice is pyrimethamine (Daraprim) and sulfadiazine. Pyrimethamine is effective in therapy as a folic acid inhibitor. To prevent bone marrow depression, folinic acid, which *Toxoplasma* cannot convert to folic acid, should be administered.

Malaria. Malaria is an infectious febrile disease produced by several species of protozoa belonging to the genus *Plasmodium*. It is transmitted only by the bite of the infected anopheles mosquito. The condition is characterized by recurrent fever. The falciparum type may also be associated with cerebral, renal, or gastrointestinal localization of parasites, causing symptoms and signs directed to these areas.

The most common ocular complication of malaria is herpes simplex keratitis (p. 205) that presumably arises because of proliferation of the causative virus in corneal tissue that has reduced immunity because of the fever. Vascular lesions from malaria may be associated with retinal hemorrhages. Decreased vision, with severe, persistent headache that may be associated with vertigo, photophobia, and orbital pain, commonly occurs. Optic neuritis with papillitis followed by optic atrophy may occur. *Plasmodium vivax* infection may be associated with hyperesthesia of various sensory nerves, with neuralgia of the trigeminal nerve being frequent. For the most part, complications have been observed with untreated malaria and disappear with adequate antimalarial therapy.

Metazoan infections

Tapeworm infections. Tapeworm infections (cestodiasis) are of two types: (1) the intestinal form in which the mature worm is attached to the bowel wall and (2) the visceral or somatic form in which the larval form of the parasite is present in various tissues and organs.

The intestinal type may cause no symptoms or solely symptoms of gastrointestinal disturbances. The visceral type follows ingestion of tapeworm eggs that, after hatching in the intestine, penetrate its wall, resulting in the spread of infection by the bloodstream or lymph stream. An exception to this mode of infection occurs with the larvae causing sparganosis, the adult forms of which are parasitic in frogs, snakes, amphibians, and mammals. In the Orient, fresh, split frogs are used as a poultice for sore eyes and wounds, and the larvae are transferred to human tissue. The conjunctiva becomes red, and there is itching, photophobia, blepharospasm, tearing, and edema of the lid. There may be small nodules harboring the parasite beneath the skin of the upper lid, which are more easily removed after encapsulation. Proptosis and muscle paresis suggest orbital invasion.

The two main types of visceral involvement are (1) ecchinococcus or hydatid cysts and (2) cysticercosis.

Echinococcus cysts. Echinococcus cysts are produced by the larvae of *Echinococcus granulosis*, a minute tapeworm of dogs and cats. Ingestion of the eggs by swine, cattle, or man leads to echinococcus cysts of the liver, lungs, kidney, brain, eye, and other organs. The cyst development is slow and presents the symptoms of a slowly developing tumor. The contained fluid is highly irritating, and the cysts should not be evacuated. Orbital cysts, commoner than intraocular cysts, cause a proptosis with related signs. The intraocular cyst appears as a white, pea-sized mass within the vitreous body, or there may be a progressive, solid retinal detachment. Surgical excision is the only effective therapy, and care must be taken not to rupture the cyst and release toxic fluid.

Cysticercosis. Cysticercosis is infection with the cyst stage of the bladder worm *(Cysticercus cellulosae)*, the pork tapeworm *(Taenia solium)*, or rarely the beef tapeworm *(Taenia saginata)*. It occurs because of ingestion of eggs of the parasite, and autoinfection may occur in a human being harboring the adult parasite in the intestine. The subcutaneous tissues, muscles, brain, eye, heart, and lung are invaded in that order of frequency. Tissue reaction is minimal until the larva dies, when there is a local inflammatory reaction and capsule formation. Increase in size of the cyst in the brain causes the signs and symptoms of an expanding tumor. In the eye the bladder worm is a translucent oval body 6 to 18 mm. in length, without capsule, in which the head of the larva may be seen as a white spot. It may occur in the choroid, causing a retinal detachment, float free in the vitreous body or anterior chamber, or be found beneath the conjunctiva or in the orbit. Removal is the sole therapy, but rupture of the cyst is followed by a violent inflammation.

Nematodes (roundworms). There are an estimated 500,000 species of nematodes that may become parasitic in virtually all arthropods, mollusks, plants, and vertebrates. Typically, they are elongated, cylindric worms that taper more or less at their head and tail ends and have a complete digestive tract and usually different sexes. They vary from minute filiform objects to 1.5 mm. in length. Most human infections are acquired by ingestion of the eggs, but hookworm and *Strongyloides* larvae actively invade the skin.

Ocular involvement occurs with the invasion of the eye by the larva of nematodes parasitic in lower animals, most commonly the roundworms of the dog and cat.

Filariasis. The filariae are slender, threadlike worms that have a tendency to inhabit a particular part of the human body. The female worms of those producing disease in man produce embryos, microfilariae, that live in the blood or skin from whence bloodsucking arthopods, their intermediate hosts, remove them to spread infection.

Onchocerca volvulus. Ocular onchocerciasis, also called "river-blindness," is a chronic filarial infection that occurs endemically in Mexico, Guatemala, Venezuela, and Central Africa. The infection is transmitted from person to person by bites of infected black flies of the genus *Simulium*. Infected larva are injected into the skin or subcutaneous tissue and give rise to nodules (cercoma) of pathognomonic appearance.

The microfilariae of *Onchocerca* swarm in the bulbar conjunctiva and may be seen as squirming, yellowish threads in the aqueous humor. A superficial punctate corneal inflammation occurs initially, followed by deep opacities without vascularization, until they are so numerous as to cause epithelial degeneration. Inflammation of the iris is common, and generalized atrophy of the pigmented epithelium gives a spongy appearance to the iris. The lens is not invaded, but complicated cataract may follow uveal inflammation. There is a circumscribed degeneration of the posterior fundus similar to that seen in choroidal sclerosis. There is irregular deposition of pigment, perivascular sheathing, and an associated optic atrophy. The nature of the posterior segment lesion is quite variable; it is infrequently seen in areas where there is adequate dietary vitamin A. A gross inflammatory lesion due to death of the microfilaria is also seen.

Ocular treatment is largely symptomatic. Surgical excision of nodules is most important. Diethylcarbamazine (Hetrazan) is effective against the microfilaria but not the adult worm. Death of many microfilariae may lead to endophthalmitis. Suramin (Bayer 205) kills the adult worm, but it is very toxic.

Loa loa. *Loa loa* (African eye worm) is a threadlike worm 3 to 5 cm. in length that lives in the subcutaneous tissue of man, travels from place to place beneath the skin, and causes a creeping itch sensation. The disease is seen in the west and central parts of Africa. The worm is responsive to warmth, and in persons sitting before a fire, the worms move to the warm face and eyes.

The adult worm appears like a piece of surgical catgut beneath the conjunctiva or swimming in the anterior chamber. There is local irritation, congestion, and lacrimation, which disappears quickly when the worm moves to deeper tissues. The worm may be removed after first capturing it with a ligature to prevent its escape. A topical anesthetic relieves symptoms.

Calabar swellings are painless, edematous subcutaneous nodules arising as an allergic reaction to metabolic products of the worm or from injured or dead worms. They tend to occur on removal to a cold climate. Systemic antihistamines give relief.

The microfilariae that do not cause ocular disease and some adult worms are destroyed by diethylcarbamazine, which may have to be administered repeatedly.

Bancroft's filariasis. This disease is produced by *Wuchereria bancrofti,* a typical filarial worm that resides in lymph vessels and produces the lymph blockage known as elephantiasis. Physical signs arise from inflammatory reactions due to allergy to the worm and from obstruction of lymph vessels. Rarely the lids or intraocular structures may be involved. Diethylcarbamazine is the drug of choice.

Ascaris lumbricoides. *Ascaris lumbri-* *coides* is the giant intestinal roundworm that affects children predominantly. There is no intermediate host, and infection occurs because of ingestion of eggs. The eggs hatch in the bowel, and the migrating larvae may be the cause of pneumonia, encephalitis, or meningitis. During this phase the larvae may cause intraocular inflammation, varying in severity from iridocyclitis to endophthalmitis. Ascaris larvae in the lungs break through the pulmonary capillaries to enter the air alveoli and then the upper respiratory tract, where they are swallowed and complete their development as mature worms in the intestinal tract.

In the bowel the worm may be asymptomatic or cause intestinal disorders varying in severity from mild colic to obstruction and perforation. Sensitization to the worms or their products may cause allergic manifestations, mainly asthma or urticaria.

The ocular inflammation of the larval migration is nonspecific, but it may be suspected because of the violent ocular tissue reaction combined with an eosinophilia. The eyes that have been enucleated present the pathologic appearance of either Coats' disease or endophthalmitis. The larvae are found in histologic sections.

Visceral larva migrans. This term is applied to the invasion of nematode larvae in tissues other than the skin. The roundworm of the dog and, less frequently, the roundworm of the cat (*Toxocara canis* or *cati*) are common offenders, and the term is also applied to human ascaris larval migration as described previously.

Children particularly become infected by eating embryonated eggs that hatch in the bowel and then migrate throughout the body via the bloodstream and lymphatics. The adult worm of nonhuman types cannot develop in the bowel, but the larva gives rise to hepatic, pulmonary, cerebral, and ocular signs. The children have fever, anorexia, chronic cough, vague pains, persistent eosinophilia, and hepatomegaly.

The ocular lesion may cause a severe granulomatous tissue reaction leading to enucleation of the eye because of the clinical signs of a retinoblastoma. A more subtle reaction involves the posterior pole, with a slight inflammatory reaction combined with hemorrhage and a translucent elevation.

Diagnosis is difficult, but close contact with dogs and cats is usually found. Skin testing antigens are not fully standardized.

Treatment is supportive and symptomatic. Corticosteroids may minimize allergic reactions, and antibiotics may be useful in decreasing secondary bacterial infection. Animal pets should be dewormed.

Trichinosis. Trichinosis is an infestation of striated muscle by the larva of the nematode *Trichinella spiralis*, which infects a wide group of animals of which swine are the chief human reservoir.

The encysted larvae are ingested in undercooked pork and develop in the intestine into sexually mature adults. Eggs develop and hatch in the female, which releases about 1,500 larvae over a 6-week period. The larvae enter the general circulation about 7 days after an individual has eaten infected meat, and they are widely distributed to all tissues. In severe infestations, there are muscle weakness and pain, remittent fever, and edema that is frequently localized to the orbit, particularly the upper lid. Ocular muscle involvement causes pain on movement. There may be subconjunctival hemorrhage.

Diagnosis is based upon muscle tenderness and associated eosinophilia. When these signs are associated with orbital edema, the diagnosis is most suggestive. The larvae may be found in biopsy specimens 10 days after infection. The intradermal ·skin test becomes positive about the third week after infection.

There is no specific therapy. Steroids and ACTH suppress the acute manifestations of the disease.

Necator americanus. *Necator americanus* (common hookworm) is common in the Southeastern United States. There is no intermediate host. Eggs develop in moist soil into larvae that readily penetrate the skin. The cutaneous invasion produces ground itch or hookworm dermatitis. The larvae ultimately reach the lungs, enter the upper respiratory tract, and are swallowed to develop into the mature worms in the intestinal tract. An anemia develops, with malaise, fever, anorexia, and delayed development. The disease is diagnosed by discovery of ova in the stools. Treatment is with tetrachlorethylene.

The ocular signs are those described in visceral larva migrans. Previously, cases of *Toxocara canis* infection of the eye were considered to be caused by the hookworm. The anemia may be associated with retinal hemorrhage.

Ocular myiasis. The deposition of the eggs of flies in wounds of the conjunctiva, lids, and globe gives rise to conjunctival, palpebral, or intraocular myiasis. The eggs hatch into larvae (maggots), which give rise to varying degrees of inflammation or tissue destruction. Removal of the larvae is required.

Spirochetal infections

Syphilis. Syphilis is a specific infectious disease caused by *Treponema pallidum*, which enters the body by direct transfer. Syphilis acquired after birth requires intimate body contact, commonly coitus, with the infected host. In congenital syphilis the transfer occurs through the placenta of a pregnant syphilitic mother.

The outstanding pathologic lesions are perivascular infiltration and vascular endothelial proliferation with obliterative endarteritis, phlebitis, and lymphangitis. A gumma is a lesion consisting of a necrotic central area surrounded by giant and epithelial cells, with a peripheral zone of small lymphocytes and plasma cells.

Acquired syphilis. Acquired syphilis is divided into primary, secondary, and tertiary stages. The incubation period is 2 to 4 weeks, rarely as long as 90 days. The initial lesion is a chancre, usually on the external genitalia, rarely on the conjunctiva or the eyelids. The chancre appears as a papular swelling that becomes ulcerated at the apex and develops a typical punched-out appearance, with a gray, sloughing center and induration. Preauricular and submaxillary adenopathies are present, depending upon the ocular area involved. The *Treponema* may be demonstrated on dark-field microscopic examination, but serologic reactions are negative. The lesion must be distinguished from a sty, infected chalazion, and the other causes of Parinaud's oculoglandular syndrome.

Six weeks to six months following the chancre, the disease passes into its secondary stage of mucous patches, eruptions, and latent syphilis. A nonspecific catarrhal conjunctivitis is the most common conjunctival involvement, but the conjunctiva is less prone to involvement than other mucous membranes. A lesion resembling annular scleritis or a pseudotrachoma with marked papillary (not follicular) formation involving the upper tarsal conjunctiva with pannus may occur.

The iris and the ciliary body are involved early in the secondary stage and late in the tertiary stage. Syphilitic iridocyclitis is usually (75%) associated with the skin rash and occurs in the fourth to the sixth month after the chancre. A severe granulomatous iridocyclitis that may be bilateral occurs. Broad, flat posterior synechiae occur between the stromal layer of the iris and the lens and not between the pigmented epithelium and the lens as is usual in uveal inflammation. The serologic test is positive, but definite diagnosis is based upon the rapid disappearance of the inflammation with penicillin therapy. Chorioretinitis is rarely caused by acquired syphilis but occurs commonly in the congenital disease.

In the late secondary stage of acquired syphilis, up to 10 years after the original infection, there are inflammatory foci of the choroid occurring in crops and preferentially involving the posterior pole. This is followed by marked pigment proliferation with sheets of glial tissue, resembling the lesion of retinitis pigmentosa. The prognosis with treatment is probably better than in the majority of instances of chorioretinitis.

Retrobulbar neuritis may occur in the secondary stage, and late in this stage papilledema occurs due to basilar meningitis. Syphilitic opticoarachnoiditis, which involves the base of the brain and interferes with the optic chiasm or nerves combined with middle ear disease, causes symptoms suggestive of a suprasellar meningioma, that is, optic atrophy, bitemporal visual field defects, and a normal sella. Surgery to correct the adhesions was fairly common at one time, but medical therapy should now be adequate. Rarely a syphilitic gumma causes papilledema with other signs of brain tumor. Diagnosis may be complicated by a glioma causing positive serologic reactions.

The tertiary stage of syphilis occurs 10 or more years after the chancre, or it may never occur. It is characterized by a small number of organisms, extensive parenchymal destruction, gumma formation, and connective tissue proliferation.

A gumma of the conjunctiva is smooth, firm, pink, and is not unlike an injected pinguecula. On the lid a gumma resembles a persistent, necrotizing chalazion. Involvement of the ciliary body may present clinical signs of a tumor. The iridocyclitis of the tertiary stage is clinically similar to that in the secondary stage.

Tabes dorsalis is a degenerative disease of the central nervous system characterized by signs of involvement of the posterior columns and the cranial nerves. Caucasian male individuals are most commonly affected. Frequently there is no history of chancre or skin changes. The disease progresses slowly for 10 to 20 years. Ataxia is common, as is posterior root pain, "lightning pain," with paroxysmal attacks at night involving the legs, abdomen, arms, and face. There is impairment of deep sensibility and position sense and loss of vibratory sense.

Pupillary signs are unusually important in recognizing continued central nervous system progression because earlier therapy may reverse many serologic tests and reassure the patient. Slight inequality in size of the pupils and a sluggish reaction may be the only signs. Argyll Robertson pupils (p. 220) are diagnostic of tabes dorsalis. In an eye with vision the pupil reacts to accommodation but not to light. The pupils are small and irregular, and atrophy of the iris is common. The small pupil contracts further with eserine but dilates poorly with atropine. The lesion is considered to be in the region of the pretectal synapse. Spirochetes morphologically identical to *Treponema pallidum* may be recovered from the aqueous humor despite apparently adequate therapy.

Primary optic atrophy is the next most common ocular sign of tabes dorsalis. It occurs 10 to 20 years after the chancre. There is early loss of dark adaptation, and there is blue (cyanopia) or red (erythropia) vision. The peripheral visual field contracts. Tubular vision may occur in which the central visual acuity is 20/20, but the patient is unable to move unaided because the visual field is contracted to less than 5°. Tests on the blood and spinal fluid may be positive. An increased spinal fluid colloidal gold curve is important. Special serologic examination such as the fluorescent treponemal antibody absorption test is indicated, particularly in individuals with pupillary signs or optic atrophy who may have had syphilis although they do not remember it, or who give a history of prolonged therapy.

General paresis is a chronic, slowly progressive central nervous system disease, with organic psychosis occurring as the result of inflammation rather than glial tissue proliferation as in tabes dorsalis. There are slurred speech, tremor of the lip, tongue, and eyelids, illegible writing, and pyramidal tract signs. The Babinski reflex is positive, and deep reflexes are hyperactive in contrast to tabes dorsalis in which they are hypoactive. Blood and spinal fluid tests are positive, and there is lymphocytosis with descending colloidal gold curve.

At the present time ocular involvement occurs mainly in patients who have previously had inadequate therapy and in whom there may have been serologic reversal on testing but continuation of activity. Other patients have irreversible serologic tests but have been adequately treated. Treatment with massive doses of penicillin over a period of 14 to 28 days is indicated. This may be followed by improvement in the general paresis, but in tabes dorsalis the lesion only is arrested. Further therapy depends upon clinical rather than laboratory signs. If no progression occurs, the disease is considered arrested, irrespective of the serology.

Syphilis in infants is not always congenital. It may be acquired from kissing, from an infected umbilical cord, or from circumcision instruments. Acquired syphilis in infants follows the same course as in adults. The children are usually robust, and fatal termination is uncommon.

Congenital syphilis. Congenital syphilis is an infectious disease due to *Treponema pallidum*. The infection is acquired in utero and is characterized by massive systemic involvement without the occurrence of a primary lesion.

Symptoms are usually present 2 to 6 weeks after birth, but a fatal pemphigus-like lesion may be present at birth. As a rule, a severe, persistent rhinitis develops, followed in a week by a maculopapular eruption. The infant's general nutrition suffers, and he is thin, snuffling, and irritable. Fissures about the mouth are uncommon but diagnostic.

Late signs of congenital syphilis include Hutchison's triad of (1) second dentition pegged, particularly with the upper central incisors notched and enamel absent from the notched edge, (2) nerve-type deafness occurring about the time of puberty, and (3) interstitial keratitis. Other signs are collapse of the bridge of the nose as an end result of necrosis of the nasal septum from syphilitic rhinitis, splenomegaly, lymphadenopathy involving the epitrochlear nodes, saber tibia, and exostosis of the tibia and the cranial bones.

Syphilitic interstitial keratitis is an infiltrative inflammation of the corneal stroma with an associated anterior uveitis. The disease, which affects boys predominantly (61%), occurs between the ages of 5 and 20 years. It commences with anterior uveitis, often preceded by minor ocular trauma. There are endothelial edema and deep staining with fluorescein. After about 2 or 3 weeks there are acute pain, photophobia, and lacrimation. The cornea is hazy, with circumcorneal injection. All corneal layers are affected, with edema of the epithelium and endothelium and cellular infiltration of the stroma. This stage of the disease is usually short and is followed by a period of vascular inflammation with invasion of the cornea from the periphery. The invading vessels, which appear to be pushing the haze in front of them, ultimately meet at the center of the cornea to form a "salmon patch." As soon as the vessels meet, symptoms and inflammation subside. When healing is complete, faint gray lines of empty blood vessels persist in the cornea. There may be late degenerative changes, with band keratopathy or keratoconus and secondary glaucoma.

The chief differential diagnosis involves the interstitial keratitis of tuberculosis, leprosy, and bacterial hypersensitivity. Cogan's syndrome of interstitial keratitis with nerve deafness (p. 207) is due to vascular inflammation.

A penetrating corneal transplant will in many instances restore useful vision in healed interstitial keratitis.

Leptospirosis. Leptospirosis is an acute systemic disease caused by one of the many strains of an animal spirochete. The clinical manifestations depend more upon the host factors than upon the infecting strain. Individuals who work with pigs or in sewers and slaughterhouses are most commonly affected. There are three main types of infection: (1) Weil's disease, in which there are jaundice, oliguria, circulatory collapse, and a hemorrhagic tendency; (2) pretibial fever (Fort Bragg fever), characterized by signs of an acute infectious disease, followed in 4 or 5 days by elevated, irregularly shaped, erythematous cutaneous lesions on the anterior surface of the legs; and (3) leptospiral meningitis (swineherd's disease), a nonpurulent meningitis occurring in young people during the late summer.

Iridocyclitis of either a granulomatous or a nongranulomatous type may occur. The ocular inflammation may appear 4 to 6 weeks after the acute illness, and the association with the original condition may not be recognized. A relatively benign posterior uveitis, with the formation of membranes attached to the optic disk and extending forward to the vitreous body, occurs less frequently than anterior uveitis. Diagnosis depends upon a history of infection, recovery of the organism from the blood, or a persistently elevated antibody titer of the serum. Treatment of the systemic disease with penicillin and broad-spectrum antibiotics is moderately effective.

Sarcoidosis

Sarcoid is a systemic granulomatous disease of unknown etiology and pathogenesis. The characteristic histologic lesion is an epithelioid cell granuloma, similar to a tubercle without caseation, which either resolves or is converted into avascular, acellular, hyaline fibrous tissue. Frequently the tubercle contains refractile or apparently calcified bodies in its giant cells. Most commonly involved are mediastinal and peripheral lymph nodes, lungs, liver, spleen, skin, eyes, phalangeal bones, and parotid glands.

The disease varies widely in incidence from area to area. It is more common in Negroes in the United States and is more prevalent in both the white and black races in the southeastern states. It is more frequent in women than in men, and the peak incidence in both sexes is around 25 to 30 years.

Clinically the disease is often first detected because of an abnormal chest roentgenogram or symptoms of cough, dyspnea, chest pain, or hemoptysis. The onset may be acute, with erythema nodosum, or febrile, with arthralgia. Ocular involvement, skin changes, peripheral lymphadenopathy, or lassitude, fever, and malaise may usher in the disease.

The laboratory signs may be disproportionally abnormal for the symptoms present. The erythrocyte sedimentation rate may be elevated, and there may be a moderate leukopenia with a slight eosinophilia. Increased serum globulin is associated with a decreased serum albumin. The calcium excretion in the urine is higher than normal and there may be a hypercalcemia. The serum phosphorus and phosphatase levels are normal, and the findings suggest a hypersensitivity to vitamin D.

The tuberculin test and similar types of delayed hypersensitivity are usually negative. The Kveim reaction may be helpful in diagnosis provided the specificity of the test material has been fully validated.

Roentgenograms of the chest may indicate bilateral hilar lymph node enlargement as an initial sign, followed by extensive diffuse pulmonary infiltration in the later stages. Rarely the bones, particularly the phalanges of the hand, may show typical cystlike rarefactions.

Ocular involvement is common but may be so minimal as not to cause symptoms. The skin of the eyelids may be inflamed, particularly in the lupus pernio type of skin sarcoid. The inferior conjunctival fornix may contain minute, translucent, slightly yellow elevations. Excision of a typical nodule followed by serial sectioning and skilled interpretation may be a helpful diagnostic procedure.

Gross enlargement of the lacrimal gland is relatively uncommon, but keratoconjunctivitis sicca (p. 210) occurs fairly frequently. Pseudotumor of the orbit has been described, and meningeal involvement may be associated with motor and sensory changes and optic nerve abnormalities. Hypercalcemia may be associated with typical conjunctival and corneal calcium infiltrates of band keratopathy (p. 201).

Uveitis, either anterior or posterior, constitutes the main ocular involvement of sarcoidosis. Iridocyclitis is associated with mutton-fat keratic precipitates and a tendency to form broad, flat, posterior synechiae. There may be sarcoid granulomas of the iris appearing as small nodules. Posterior uveitis is associated with "snowball" opacities in the vitreous and a tendency to periphlebitis in regions adjacent to a nonspecific chorioretinal inflammatory reaction. Inflammation of the pars plana portion of the ciliary body occurs relatively frequently in uveal involvement due to sarcoid. There are often cells in both the vitreous body and anterior chamber and an associated edema of the macula and optic nerve with decreased central vision.

Chapter 24

Endocrine disease and the eye

Diabetes mellitus

Diabetes mellitus is a complex and widespread disorder of carbohydrate metabolism in which the production of insulin is not adequate, or insulin is not available or is not utilized normally by tissue. The resulting inability of tissue to utilize glucose leads to hyperglycemia, glycosuria, and loss of water. The loss of glucose leads to increased catabolism and decreased synthesis of fat and protein, with weakness and weight loss. If the catabolism of fat is excessive, there is accumulation of ketone bodies in the blood and urine, causing increased urinary excretion of cations, which may lead to acidosis. The water excretion causes polyuria, and the resultant dehydration causes polydypsia and dryness of the skin, with pruritus.

In the majority of instances overt diabetes has its onset in adults, particularly between the ages of 40 and 60 years. In other instances the disease manifests itself in the first two decades of life and is known as growth-onset diabetes.

The angiopathy and neuropathy that occur commonly in overt diabetes are rarely found in prediabetes or chemical diabetes.

Ocular changes in diabetes mellitus

Diabetes mellitus may affect the eyes in a variety of ways.

Variations in refractive error. Hyperglycemia may be associated with or followed by increased refractive power of the lens, resulting in a change in the refractive error in the direction of myopia. After the blood sugar has been normal for several days, the refractive power of the lens decreases, and the change is in the direction of hyperopia. The exact mechanism of the change is not known, but it is assumed that during hyperglycemia there is an increased glucose content of the lens cortex with imbibition of water, causing increased thickness of the lens and increased refractive power.

The central visual acuity parallels the change in refraction. Vision may be corrected to normal with lenses. Refraction during hyperglycemia varies, often quite markedly, from that during an interval of normal blood sugar. Paralysis of accommodation by means of a cycloplegic drug does not affect the refractive error. Diagnosis is not difficult in a known diabetic, but the variation in refraction and central visual acuity may be the first indication of the metabolic disease.

A similar change in refractive power may be produced in nondiabetic individuals by some drugs, particularly members of the sulfonamide group. An absolute change in the total refractive power of the eye, as occurs in diabetes, should be differentiated from that occurring with sustained accommodation, which is neutralized with a cycloplegic drug.

Subjective visual symptoms. Patients with diabetes mellitus without organic changes in the eyes may complain of photopsia, not unlike that observed in migraine, or diplopia during periods of hypoglycemia. Presumably these symptoms are of cerebral origin and are abolished by elevating the blood sugar.

Intraocular pressure. The blood volume of the eye is sensitive to the plasma bicarbonate level. A low intraocular pressure is associated with diabetic acidosis, and the hypotension may be augmented by the concurrent dehydration.

Glaucoma in diabetes is a complication of neovascularization of the iris (rubeosis of the iris). It seems likely that wide-angle glaucoma occurs far more frequently in diabetics than in the normal population. Glaucoma is found in the homozygous state and is transmitted as a recessive trait.

Rubeosis of the iris. Rubeosis of the iris is a vascular proliferation of the iris vessels that becomes evident either near the pupillary margin or in the anterior chamber angle. The glaucoma that occurs is resistant to both medical and surgical treatment.

Hydrops of the iris. The pigmented epithelium of the iris is the site of glycogen deposition that appears more marked in the diabetic than in the normal individual (Fig. 24-1). On section, the cells are vacuolated and thickened. Clinically the condition may be suspected by observing the release of pigment into the anterior chamber with dilation of the pupil, or with iridectomy in diabetics. Presumably, release of the pigment is responsible for the microscopic accumulation of pigment on the corneal endothelium.

Cornea. Wrinkles in Descemet's membrane occur at an earlier age and more frequently in diabetics (8 to 33%) than in normal individuals (8%). They are visible with the slit lamp as fine, shining, gray, linear streaks. They are bilateral, and are not as gross as those seen in inflammation, hypotony, and following ocular trauma.

Conjunctiva. It is debatable whether vascular changes characteristic of diabetes occur other than in the ocular fundi. Ditzel reported increased tortuosity, constriction, blood sludging, and edema in prediabetics,

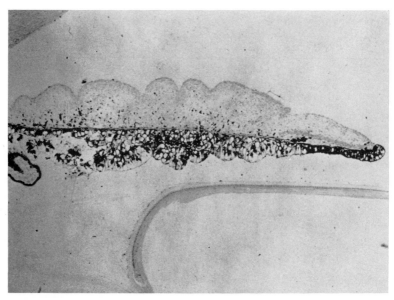

Fig. 24-1. Hydrops of the iris. The cystlike openings contain glycogen. (Courtesy Dr. Bertha A. Klien, Chicago, Ill.)

and he expressed the opinion that the microangiopathy preceded overt diabetes. Because of the exposed position of the conjunctiva, many vascular changes probably occur here because of infection or irritation, but these changes are degenerative rather than specific for diabetes mellitus.

Diabetic cataract. Diabetic cataract is a rare, specific clinical entity occurring in growth-onset diabetes that has been present for 10 to 20 years. Cataract occurring in adult diabetes is indistinguishable from the senile type. The lens opacity develops rapidly and interferes with vision soon after its onset. Both eyes are involved, often simultaneously.

Typically the opacity consists of small, flaky opacities (snowflakes) and water clefts located in the anterior or the posterior cortex immediately beneath the lens capsule. Progression is stopped by adequate control of the diabetes with restoration of normal blood sugar levels. In persistent hyperglycemia a complete (mature) lens opacity may form within 48 hours, but progress is usually more gradual.

The visual results of surgery for diabetic cataract are often disappointing. The patient is often less than 25 years of age, and if extracapsular lens extraction is performed, there may be a violent intraocular inflammation postoperatively. Intracapsular cataract extraction, which requires rupture of the lens zonule with alpha chymotryp-

---

Ocular signs of diabetes mellitus

I. Visual acuity
  A. Transient variations in refraction
  B. Photopsia and diplopia in cerebral hypoglycemia
  C. Decreased accommodation
  D. Depressed in cataract, vitreous hemorrhage, foveal involvement in retinopathy
  E. Diplopia in ophthalmoplegia
II. Intraocular pressure
  A. Decreased in acidosis
  B. Increased in rubeosis of iris
III. Conjunctiva
  A. Sludging of blood, tortuous, constricted blood vessels
IV. Cornea
  A. Wrinkling of Descemet's membrane
V. Iris
  A. Hydrops of pigmented epithelium (glycogen storage)
  B. Rubeosis
VI. Lens
  A. Variation in refractive power (hyperglycemia)
  B. "Sugar" cataract (growth-onset diabetes)
VII. Ocular fundi
  A. Microaneurysms
  B. Deep and superficial hemorrhages
    1. Vitreous hemorrhage
  C. Deposits
  D. Venous dilation (phlebopathy)
  E. Retinitis proliferans
    1. With glial proliferation
    2. Without glial proliferation (rete mirabile)
  F. Macular pigmentation
  G. Lipemia retinalis in ketosis
VIII. Oculomotor nerves
  A. Neuropathy with muscle paralysis (pupil frequently spared in N III involvement)

sin, may yield an excellent anterior segment, but the procedure may be associated with a poor visual result because of diabetic retinopathy.

"Sugar" cataract. Considerable attention has been devoted to "sugar" cataract in experimental animals. The condition may be produced by high blood levels of glucose, xylose, galactose, and ribose. The mechanism of development is not fully known, but it involves a decreased amino acid content of the lens, decreased activity of the phosphogluconate pathway, increased sugar alcohols, and increased hydration of the lens.

Neuropathy. Involvement of the third or the sixth cranial nerve occurs relatively rarely in diabetes. Characteristically a middle-aged to elderly individual with mild overt diabetes or chemical diabetes is afflicted. The onset is sudden and is accompanied frequently by a homolateral headache of an intensity severe enough to lead one to suspect intracranial aneurysm. There may be a history of previous Bell's palsy or similar neural disease. Neuropathy involving other areas may or may not be present. Signs of meningeal irritation do not occur. If the third cranial nerve is involved, the pupil will most likely be spared (in 17 of 24 cases), in contrast to frequent pupillary paralysis, which occurs in cerebral tumors and aneurysms. The abnormality disappears spontaneously within several weeks if the diabetes is of short duration, or it persists up to 6 months if the diabetes has been present for a long time, particularly if poorly controlled.

Unilateral frontal headache and oculomotor paralysis are characteristic of aneurysm of the intracranial portion of the carotid artery (p. 415). The sparing of the pupil, the laboratory signs of diabetes, normal spinal fluid, and absence of meningeal irritation suggest that the disease is due to diabetes.

Other causes of ophthalmoplegia besides intracranial aneurysms include tumors (roentgenographic changes), leukemia (blood count), ophthalmoplegic migraine (history), head trauma, demyelinating disease (painless onset), myasthenia gravis (painless onset), and cerebrovascular disease.

Ocular fundi: retinopathy. Retinopathy is the most important ocular manifestation of diabetes. The introduction of insulin in 1921 followed by the sulfonamides in 1937 and the antibiotics thereafter prevented premature death of the diabetic from coma or infection. Since then, the renal, ocular, and cardiovascular complications have emerged as the chief problem of the disease. Only senile cataract and glaucoma cause more adult blindness than diabetic retinopathy.

Diabetic retinopathy is a specific abnormality caused by diabetes; it does not occur because of concurrent atherosclerosis or hypertensive cardiovascular disease. The incidence of retinopathy generally parallels the duration of the disease and the adequacy of control but not its severity. In unusual individuals, ocular and renal changes characteristic of diabetes may occur before the onset of overt diabetes. The degree and rapidity of involvement of the two eyes may be unequal, and even in the same eye one area may progress while another recedes.

The retinopathy involves mainly the posterior pole of the eye between the superior and inferior vessels but may involve any part of the fundus. In most instances there is no interference with central visual acuity and color vision. There is no relationship between the severity of the retinopathy and the loss of vision. If the fovea centralis is not affected, there is excellent vision with advanced retinopathy, whereas a single lesion involving the fovea centralis may reduce vision to 20/200. The abnormality is limited to the retinal blood vessels; the choroid apparently does not participate.

The main features of diabetic retinopathy are the following: (1) microaneurysms, (2) deep and superficial retinal hemorrhage, (3) deposits, (4) venous dilation, and (5) proliferative retinopathy with glial proliferation or without glial proliferation (rete).

Microaneurysms. Microaneurysms of the retina are considered the most characteristic ocular lesion of diabetes, but they also occur in retinal vein closure, Coats' disease, glaucoma, and a large variety of systemic diseases (hypertension, pernicious anemia,

pulseless disease, and many others). However, in no other disease do as many microaneurysms occur as in diabetes (Fig. 24-2). Those associated with diseases other than diabetes are located on the arterial rather than on the venous side of capillary circulation and in the periphery rather than at the posterior pole. The microaneurysms occur exclusively in the retina and do not occur in tissues other than the retina.

Microscopically, microaneurysms con-

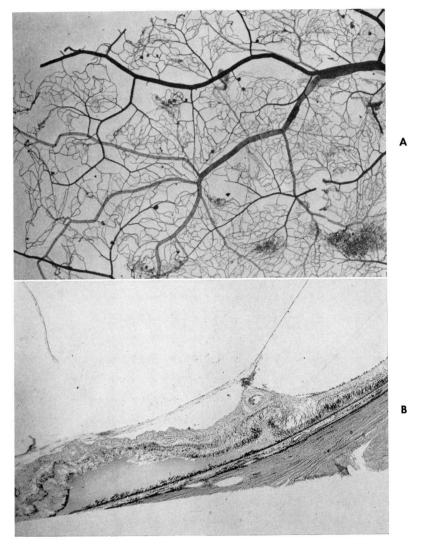

Fig. 24-2. A, Flat preparation of the retina showing microaneurysms in diabetes mellitus.
B, Proliferative retinopathy.

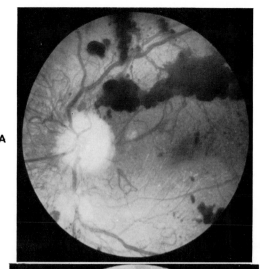

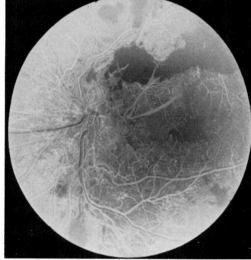

Fig. 24-3. A, Fundus in diabetic retinopathy showing venous dilation, blotlike preretinal hemorrhages, and intraretinal neovascularization nasal to the disk. **B,** Following injection of fluorescein into the brachial vein, more extensive neovascularization and many microaneurysms are evident.

sist of minute spherical or ovoid distentions ranging from 20 to 200μ in size, located on the venous side of the capillary network at the level of the inner nuclear layer. The resolving power of the direct ophthalmoscope is approximately 70 to 80μ. Thus the majority of retinal microaneurysms are not seen with the ophthalmoscope. This is particularly appreciated when the fundus is viewed after intravenous injection of fluorescein (Fig. 24-3) or is seen histologically after trypsin digestion of the retina.

Ophthalmoscopically, microaneurysms appear as minute, deep, round, red bodies, not unlike hemorrhages. They may be distinguished from deep small hemorrhages by their unchanging appearance and their location far from blood vessels.

Retinal hemorrhages. Retinal hemorrhages in diabetes do not differ from those seen in other conditions. Small, round hemorrhages are located in the inner nuclear layer of the retina, the cells of which are arranged so compactly that the hemorrhage cannot spread. Most hemorrhages are larger than aneurysms and tend to disappear.

Flame-shaped hemorrhages located in the innermost layers of the retina commonly reflect the distribution of the nerve fiber layer. Similar hemorrhages are seen in hypertension, blood dyscrasias, papilledema, and central vein obstruction.

Preretinal hemorrhages are held adjacent to the retina by its internal limiting membrane and have a "blot" appearance. Many show a fluid level with bed rest. Trauma and subarachnoid and subdural hemorrhage may produce a similar type of bleeding. There is a tendency for preretinal hemorrhages to burst into the vitreous body, where they cause immediate obscuration of vision.

Vitreous hemorrhage is often absorbed quickly in young individuals, but after repeated episodes or in elderly patients the blood may persist indefinitely. The hemorrhage may produce a black ophthalmoscopic reflex or cause all fundus details to be blurred. As the blood absorbs, large vitreous floaters are observed. Persistence of the blood often leads to proliferative retinopathy and glaucoma.

Deposits. The deposits of diabetes consist of multiple small, glistening, yellow-white areas that gradually coalesce and become larger and confluent. They have a hard, waxy appearance, often more yellowish than those occurring in arteriolar sclerosis. Classically they are areas of ischemia infiltrated with lipids, as occurs in infarcted areas elsewhere in the nervous system. Fluorescein angiography indicates that there is increased capillary permeability surrounding the deposits.

Venous dilation. Venous dilation occurs some time prior to, or in the course of, retinopathy. All of the retinal veins or only a branch become engorged, and the ophthalmoscopic picture suggests an impending central vein closure. However, the veins pulsate normally. Growth-onset diabetes is practically the sole disease found in central vein obstruction in patients 25 years of age or younger.

Proliferative retinopathy. Proliferative retinopathy is a term applied to fibrous vascular proliferation that is associated with retinal detachment. Frequently the retina can be observed with difficulty through the blood-tinged vitreous body, but the uneven pattern and the dark blue blood in both arteries and veins suggest the retinal detachment. Gross strands of whitish tissue with entwined blood vessels enter the vitreous body, and there may be large areas of exudate and many blot-like hemorrhages.

Two types of proliferative retinopathy may be seen:

1. In the most common type there is severe vitreous hemorrhage followed by fibrovascular proliferation. The blood vessels are large, tortuous, and surrounded by glial tissue. The retinitis proliferans is commonly followed by retinal detachment, secondary glaucoma, and severe degenerative changes of the eye.

2. In the more uncommon type there is a delicate growth of lacelike vessels (rete mirabile) that seem to float gracefully in the vitreous body. These vessels usually arise from arterioles near the equator but may arise from those on the surface of the optic disk. Bends and kinks in these vessels suggest microaneurysms. Ultimately the vessels burst and cause vitreous hemorrhage, followed by fibrovascular proliferation.

There are other changes in addition to those discussed that are associated with diabetes and, although less frequently seen, deserve attention.

Pigmentation of the macular area. Pigmentation of the macular area has been described but not fully accepted as a sign of long-term diabetes. A yellowish tinge of the posterior pole of the fundus (xanthosis fundi diabetica) has also been described but occurs uncommonly.

Lipemia retinalis. Lipemia retinalis (Fig. 24-4) is an uncommon abnormality of the ocular fundus arising when the triglyceride concentration of the blood exceeds 2,000 mg./100 ml. and is combined with low-density lipoproteins. Ophthalmoscopically the normal color and size contrast between the arteries and the veins of the fundus are lost, and the vessels become engorged until they stand out like neoprene casts in bold relief. If the triglyceride concentration exceeds 3 or 4%, the color of the blood column changes from salmon pink to a yellow-white-cream color. The choroid appears pinkish rather than red. Vision is not affected, and there are no ocular symptoms.

The condition occurs most commonly in diabetic acidosis, usually in growth-onset diabetes. It may occur also in familial and secondary hyperlipidemia.

Recognition of the ophthalmoscopic picture may establish a presumptive diagnosis of diabetic coma. More frequently a milky, opalescent serum is noted in blood removed for laboratory testing, and the fundi are then studied.

Associated renal changes. Growth-onset diabetes commonly terminates in the fifth

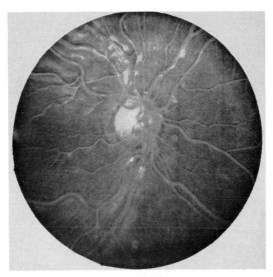

Fig. 24-4. Lipemia retinalis. (From Anderson, W. B., Sr.: Amer. J. Ophthal. **45**:23, 1958.)

decade of life with renal failure. The fundi of many of these patients show an unusual combination of diabetic retinopathy with superimposed changes of severe vascular hypertension (p. 403). There may be papilledema, diabetic deposits, cotton-wool spots of hypertension, angiospasm, hemorrhages, and microaneurysms.

Renal biopsy with study by means of light and electron microscopy indicates that in every case of diabetic retinopathy there are typical diabetic changes in the kidney. Electron microscopy shows specific marked infolding and thickening of the glomerular basement membranes. Intercapillary glomerulosclerosis is a less specific lesion, but it is likely to occur in every instance of diabetic retinopathy—in all probability it precedes the ocular lesion. However, it is of patchy distribution. Not all renal biopsy specimens are taken from an area of involvement, and unless serial sections are made of kidneys removed postmortem, the lesion may be missed.

Etiology. The cause of diabetic retinopathy is unknown. Microaneurysms have been produced experimentally thus far mainly in aged dogs that have been dia-

betic for long periods. There seems to be little doubt that there is marked thickening of basement membranes throughout the body, but why this should be reflected mainly in the eye and the kidney is not known. It has been postulated that the microaneurysms occur because of the following: (1) kinking caused by mesodermal bridgelike interconnections between retinal capillaries; (2) selective interference with contractile cells in the walls of retinal vessels (mural cells), resulting in interference with hydrostatic control of retinal vessels; (3) alterations of serum lipids, mucopolysaccharides, or other compcunds that are deposited in the basement membrane of blood vessels; (4) an autoimmunity to insulin that is bound in the capillary basement membrane and prevents insulin from reaching cells supplied by these cells; (5) a specific retinal tissue enzyme defect unrelated to vascular supply; and (6) abnormality of the secretion of the adrenal or the pituitary gland.

Treatment. The treatment of diabetic retinopathy is not satisfactory. Good control of diabetes apparently minimizes the amount or delays the onset of retinopathy, but seemingly it has little or no effect on the established condition. None of the many drugs proposed for the treatment of retinopathy has been of value when subjected to rigorous double-blind studies.

In recent years attention has focused on the role of the adrenal and the pituitary glands in this disease. Poulsen described complete disappearance of retinopathy in a woman with postpartum hypopituitarism. This report was followed by hypophysectomy for the treatment of diabetic retinopathy and more recently by hypophyseal stalk section, which causes less severe endocrine effects. In general, the procedure appears to accelerate the absorption of vitreous blood, often within several days, and to retard the tempo of a rapidly developing retinopathy, but usually the disease continues. Patients with long-standing retinal degeneration, retinal detachment, macular disease, or fibrovascular proliferation have lost the neuronal requirements for vision, and no therapy can restore vision. Patients selected for hypophysectomy should have in one eye at least a salvageable macula and no proliferative retinopathy. Renal function should be relatively normal, without azotemia, anemia, or hypertension. There should be no arteriosclerotic heart disease, and preferably the diabetes should be of the growth-onset type of less than 25 years in duration. Inasmuch as hypophysectomy causes a far more severe endocrine defect than does diabetes mellitus, patients must be emotionally stable and willing to risk a more severe disease for possible arrest of the retinopathy.

Destruction of areas of retinal neovascularization by means of photocoagulation appears to be of value in some instances of diabetic retinopathy. Patients are usually treated because of recurrent hemorrhage from localized areas of neovascularization. Often large areas of the retina are photocoagulated in a series of operations. Because of the many variables in the progression of retinopathy in different people, it has never been possible to establish an adequate protocol to demonstrate unequivocally the value of the procedure. However, the procedure appears to have merit in patients with bleeding arising from neovascularization distant from the optic disk.

All therapeutic studies are complicated by the tendency for retinopathy to wax and wane and, sometimes, for lesions to increase in one area of the retina and to regress in another. Results must be evaluated by means of careful ophthalmoscopic observation of the ocular fundi combined with accurate diagnosis and, when possible, photographs.

Thyroid gland

The thyroid gland consists of two lateral lobes connected by a medial isthmus. It is located on the ventral surface of the trachea in the midregion of the neck.

The thyroid gland synthesizes, stores, and secretes two hormones: (1) thyroxin, which constitutes about 80% of the total, and (2) triiodothyronine, which constitutes the remainder. The effect of thyroxin appears 2 or 3 days after administration and persists for several days. Triiodothyronine is effective within 6 hours of administration and disappears within 36 hours. These thyroid hormones are stored in the colloid of the thyroid gland as thyroglobulin. They are measured in the butanol-extractable iodine (BEI), and normally they vary between 3.0 and 7.0 μg/100 ml. of blood. Usually the values are within 0.5 μg of the protein-bound iodine.

The thyroid gland is under the control of the thyroid-stimulating hormone (TSH) of the anterior pituitary gland, which in turn is under at least partial control of the hypothalamus. The rate of secretion of TSH varies inversely with the concentration of thyroid hormones in the plasma. Thus, when the thyroid hormones are decreased in the plasma, the amount of TSH increases and stimulates the thyroid gland to increased production of its hormones. When the level of the thyroid hormones increases, the thyroid-stimulating hormone is suppressed.

The release of the thyroid hormones peaks about 2 to 3 hours following the administration of TSH (which is thus short-acting). The long-acting thyroid stimulator (LATS), an IgG immunoglobulin, causes release of thyroid hormones that reach their maximum 10 to 12 hours after its administration. LATS may well be an antibody to some thyroid antigen, but its mechanism of action is not known. It does not seem to be present in individuals who do not have a thyroid abnormality.

The pituitary secretion contains an exophthalmos-producing substance that is normally bound by an alpha 1 and alpha 2 globulin, the exophthalmos-inhibiting factor of the serum. It is postulated that the binding sites on the alpha 1 and alpha 2 globulin may become saturated with growth or luteinizing hormone or other fraction permitting the exophthalmos-producing substance to be active. It is possible that the pituitary gland may produce too much exophthalmos-producing substance for the serum to block, which results in exophthalmos. Most workers believe that the exophthalmos-producing substance is separate from the thyroid-stimulating hormone, but its nature is unknown.

The serum titer of LATS is more likely to be increased in patients with exophthalmos associated with either active or effectively treated thyrotoxicosis than in comparable patients without exophthalmos. Additionally, thyroid antibodies are more common in patients with exophthalmos. However, the titer of LATS and thyroid autoantibodies do not parallel each other, and one may be absent and the other present in high concentration in patients that present apparently similar types of thyroid disease and ocular signs. Thus the two antibodies appear to affect the thyroid by different mechanisms.

Hyperthyroidism

Hyperthyroidism is a systemic abnormality arising from an excessive concentration of thyroid hormones in the blood, usually endogenous in origin. This causes widespread neuromuscular changes and increased tissue metabolism. In some patients a wide variety of ocular signs may occur, but the systemic disease appears to be the same with or without eye changes. Hyperthyroidism with eye signs is known as endocrine exophthalmos, exophthalmic ophthalmoplegia, hyperophthalmia with Graves' disease, and thyrotoxic or thyrotropic exophthalmos.

The onset of the systemic disease is usually insidious, with fatigue, tachycardia, and weight loss despite an increased appe-tite. There may be a fine tremor of the fingers and tongue, heat intolerance, and excessive sweating. The systolic blood pressure is increased, and the pulse pressure is widened. Congestive heart failure may occur in older patients. Muscle weakness may be marked, and true myasthenia gravis may occur.

The basal metabolic rate is increased, and there are an increased uptake of radioactive iodine by the thyroid gland and increased iodine clearance. The protein-bound iodine and butanol-extractable iodine are increased. Serum cholesterol is decreased. The administration of 150 μg of triiodothyronine daily for 1 week does not suppress the radioactive iodine uptake of the thyroid gland.

Ocular signs. In somewhat more than half of the patients with hyperthyroidism, eye signs appear sometime in the course of the disease. These may be unilateral or bilateral and mild or severe. They may precede frank hyperthyroidism or may occur long after the thyroid abnormality has been ameliorated. The severity of ocular signs does not parallel any currently recognized manifestation of the disease or any abnormality of the thyroid, pituitary, or other endocrine glands. The ocular changes involve retraction of the eyelids and the development of exophthalmos. In some patients, paresis of ocular muscles occurs, usually in association with signs of congestion of the orbital contents. Rarely, there is interference with function of the optic nerve. In the most severe instances of exophthalmos the globe is not protected by the eyelids, and an exposure keratitis occurs (keratitis e lagophthalmos, p. 209), which can lead to a destructive infection of the eye.

In considering the possible causes of the ocular signs, most attention has been directed to the sympathetic nervous system and the increased volume of orbital contents. Sympathetic overactivity and contraction of the smooth muscles of the orbit

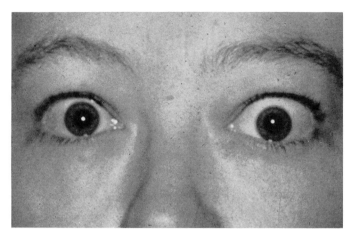

Fig. 24-5. Lid retraction without clinical hyperthyroidism.

Ocular signs of thyroid dysfunction

I. Exophthalmos
   A. Bilateral* or unilateral*
      1. Lid retraction exaggerates or simulates appearance
   B. Compressible
      1. Common type in thyrotoxicosis
   C. Solid (noncompressible)
      1. Common type following medical or surgical ablation of thyroid
II. Eyelids
   A. Lid retraction (Dalrymple)*
      1. Increased by attentive gaze (Kocher) or by conjunctival instillation of epinephrine; decreased by adrenergic blockade (guanethidine locally or block of superior cervical ganglion); forehead does not wrinkle on upward gaze (Joffrey)
   B. Lid lag (von Graefe)
      1. Upper lid delays before following globe in downward gaze
      2. Common in thyrotoxicosis
   C. Infrequent blinking (Stellwag)
   D. Miscellaneous
      1. Globe lags behind upper eyelid on upward gaze (Means)
      2. Lower did lags behind globe on upward gaze (Griffith)
      3. Increased pigmentation of skin (Jellinek)
III. Orbital congestion*
   A. May be associated with fullness of eyelids (Enroth) and prevent eversion of upper eyelid (Gifford)
IV. Extraocular muscles
   A. Contracture of ocular muscle usually
      1. Inferior rectus preventing upward gaze
      2. Most common following thyroid ablation
   B. Weakness of convergence (Mobius)
V. Optic nerve
   A. Most common following thyroid ablation
   B. Papillitis or retrobulbar neuritis
   C. Papilledema
      1. Neuroretinal edema

---

*May occur at any stage of thyroid dysfunction.

have been considered an important cause inasmuch as stimulation of the cervical sympathetic nerve in dogs causes marked exophthalmos and lid retraction. The smooth muscle in the orbit of man is too scanty to produce an exophthalmos when stimulated. Lid retraction in hyperthyroidism does not parallel the increase in thyroxin that potentiates the action of epinephrine. However, the sympathetic nervous system may contribute to upper lid retraction and the lid lag in downward gaze, but it is not considered to play a primary role in the pathogenesis of exophthalmos.

A number of changes occur to increase the volume of the orbital contents in Graves' disease. So few orbits have been studied pathologically and so little is known about the early changes that evidence is inadequate for concluding whether the process is the same in all patients. The ocular muscles may increase three to six times in mass, and there is a marked edema, giving them a pale, swollen, pink appearance. In time there is a fibrous tissue replacement of muscle cells. There are increased mast cells in the orbit and the appearance of an acid mucopolysaccharide.

The orbital fat becomes edematous and increases in weight. It has been suggested that the acid mucopolysaccharide is responsible for marked water binding within the orbit and resultant exophthalmos.

Exophthalmos. In experimental animals, exophthalmos has not been produced by the administration of the thyroid or pituitary hormones (corticotropin, ACTH, gonadotropin, growth hormone, and prolactin). The thyroid-stimulating hormone (TSH) has been implicated, but it is considered at present more likely that an exophthalmos-producing substance of the pituitary gland is responsible. Thyroid-stimulating hormone has been excluded as a cause inasmuch as there is a high level of circulating TSH in primary myxedema and there is lack of correlation in thyroidism between exophthalmos and the level of TSH.

As a rule, the term "exophthalmos" relates to any abnormal prominence of the eyeballs (Fig. 24-6), whereas the term "ocular proptosis" is used to describe a unilateral prominence. Both eyes are usually involved in thyroid disease, although one orbit may be more markedly involved than the other. The asymmetric involvement of

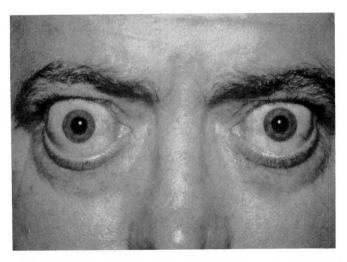

Fig. 24-6. Extreme exophthalmos that developed gradually without signs of orbital congestion.

the orbits is the basis of theories attributing the changes of hyperthyroidism to a local orbital abnormality. Others believe it merely reflects a difference in end-organ sensitivity.

The initial ocular change of hyperthyroidism is usually retraction of the upper lid. The sclera in the 12 o'clock meridian is exposed, and there is widening of the palpebral fissure, with a wide-eyed, staring appearance. Rarely, the sclera is exposed in the 6 o'clock meridian without exophthalmos. There is often a lid lag, which is failure of the upper lid to follow the globe in downward gaze. There is a gradual or sudden increase in prominence of the eyes associated with increased sensitivity to light, increased conjunctival irritation, and sometimes mild conjunctival hyperemia. Extreme degrees of exophthalmos may develop without other signs if hyperthyroidism increases slowly.

Orbital congestion. Signs of marked orbital congestion may develop quickly (Fig. 24-7). The lids become puffy and full. The conjunctiva becomes chemotic and injected. The conjunctival vessels may be so congested as to lead to a diagnosis of conjunctivitis or the suspicion of a carotid fistula.

Chemosis of the palpebral conjunctiva may be marked, and the closed lids may not entirely cover the globe. Edema of the conjunctiva may be so marked as to evert the lower lid, and tearing becomes a prominent symptom. Orbital congestion may occur without increased prominence of the globes, but more often there is a rapid increase in exophthalmos during this period. If the cornea is not protected by the lids, a keratitis e lagophthalmos may develop, causing rapid loss of vision and loss of the eye from infection if not treated.

Ocular muscle palsy. An ocular muscle contracture may develop at any time in the course of thyroid disease. Severe congestion of the orbit may limit ocular movement mechanically. If there is interference with Bell's phenomenon, in which the cornea is usually rotated upward and outward with lid closure, the cornea may be exposed. A weakness of convergence arises from mechanical inefficiency of the medial rectus muscles in rotating the exophthalmic globes inward.

Muscular contracture may develop in hyperthyroidism in the absence of exophthalmos, but more commonly it arises after adequate and appropriate treatment of

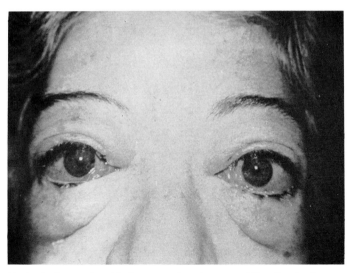

Fig. 24-7. Marked signs of orbital congestion in a rapidly developing exophthalmos.

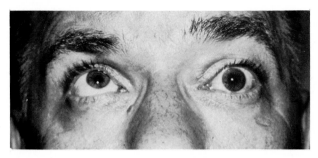

Fig. 24-8. Inability to turn eye upward developing after therapy for hyperthyroidism. The condition arises from a contracture of the inferior rectus muscle that prevents the normal elevators from rotating the eye upward. The contracture may develop without exophthalmos. Myasthenia gravis associated with thyroid disease may cause an isolated muscle paresis.

moderately severe exophthalmos. The vertical muscles are involved, and most commonly there is inability to elevate one or both eyes upward, combined with a vertical diplopia (Fig. 24-8). If the eye commonly used for fixing develops paretic muscles, there may be a marked secondary deviation of the fellow eye. The contracture prevents the unaffected muscles from elevating or depressing the eye. Thus, if the inferior rectus is involved, the superior rectus muscle cannot elevate the globe, and there appears to be weakness of the superior rectus. However, original treatment must be directed to the inferior rectus muscle.

Optic nerve involvement. In occasional individuals, mainly men about 60 years of age, there is involvement of the optic nerve in which papilledema, papillitis, or retrobulbar neuritis may develop. There are associated visual field changes characteristic of the involvement: enlargement of the blind spot, central scotomas, and perhaps peripheral field constriction. Vision is markedly reduced in papillitis and in retrobulbar neuritis.

Patients who develop such optic nerve complications usually have restriction of ocular movements and varying degrees of exophthalmos. Optic neuropathy, like other ocular involvements of hyperthyroidism, may develop long after the original disease

has been corrected. Large amounts of corticosteroids are used in therapy. Treatment must be continued for long periods; usually the corticosteroid dosage may be titrated against the response of the visual acuity.

Medical treatment. The medical treatment of endocrine exophthalmos is neither scientific nor satisfactory. Usually correction of the hyperthyroidism eliminates lid retraction and the exophthalmos appears to regress, although it may well increase 1 or 2 mm. With disappearance of lid retraction, the eyes appear less prominent despite the increased exophthalmos. If ocular signs are marked, it is generally agreed that antithyroid drugs or radioactive iodine should be used in small, fractionated doses and that euthyroid and hypothyroid conditions should be avoided. Even though ocular signs of hyperthyroidism are present, antithyroid drugs should not be administered if the basal metabolic rate is normal.

Medical treatment of established exophthalmos is difficult. Prevention of orbital congestion by sleeping with the head on pillows may be helpful. Methyl cellulose eyedrops may give comfort. Desiccated thyroid is used in large doses if hypothyroidism is present. Corticosteroids in large doses systemically may be helpful.

Surgical treatment. Loss of vision in thy-

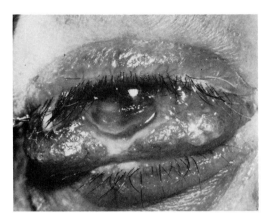

Fig. 24-9. Keratitis e lagophthalmos developing after amelioration of hyperthyroidism.

roid disease occurs either because of keratitis e lagophthalmos (Fig. 24-9) or optic neuritis. Inflammation of the cornea usually requires surgery, while the optic neuritis responds to systemic corticosteroids. In severe orbital congestion with exposure of the cornea, orbital decompression is the treatment of choice. The decompression may be carried out through the lateral wall, or the orbital roof may be removed by means of a transcranial approach. Roentgen radiation of the pituitary gland is often followed by regression of the exophthalmos. Hypophyseal stalk section or hypophysectomy has been reported to be followed by decrease in exophthalmos.

Cosmetic improvement of exophthalmos persisting after correction of the hyperthyroidism is not fully satisfactory. If the exophthalmos developed gradually and congestion is not present, a lateral blepharoplasty narrows the palpebral fissure and improves the cosmetic appearance. Retraction of the upper lid persisting after correction of the hyperthyroidism is corrected by an incision through Müller's smooth muscle of the lid. The procedure is easily accomplished by incising the conjunctiva immediately adjacent to the tarsus. The underlying Müller's muscle is also incised, and the upper lid falls about 2 mm.

Correction of the residual muscle weakness is frequently disappointing. The paresis arises because of a fibrous replacement of muscle tissue with contracture of the muscle. This procedure must be delayed until spontaneous improvement is unlikely, usually a year or more after the onset of the muscle weakness. The contracted muscle is usually recessed.

Parathyroid gland

The parathyroid glands are two pairs of minute structures in close relationship to the dorsal surface of the thyroid gland on either side of the midline. Their function is mainly to control reabsorption of phosphorus from the renal tubule. Excessive parathyroid hormone causes a decreased reabsorption and a decreased serum inorganic phosphorus. This produces a relative undersaturation of extracellular fluids with calcium phosphate and an increase in serum calcium. There is then an increased excretion of urinary calcium.

Hyperparathyroidism

Primary hyperparathyroidism occurs mainly in functioning adenomas of the parathyroid gland. It may follow hyperplasia and carcinoma of the gland. The chief laboratory signs of the disease are increased serum and urinary calcium and decreased serum phosphorus. If calcium is mobilized from the bones, as occurs when dietary calcium is inadequate, the serum alkaline phosphatase is elevated.

The chief clinical signs result from hypercalcemia, hypercalcinuria, and bone disease. The hypercalcemia causes anorexia, weakness, dysphagia, nausea, vomiting, constipation, and muscle hypotonicity. Hypercalcinuria may cause nephrolithiasis or nephrocalcinosis. The bone disease is osteitis fibrosa cystica.

The hypercalcemia may affect the conjunctiva or the cornea, causing a deposition of calcium crystals (p. 201). In the cornea there are subepithelial deposits, usually most marked near the corneoscleral limbus in the palpebral fissure (band keratopathy). The conjunctiva is injected particularly in the palpebral fissure, and glasslike, glistening crystals may be seen with the biomicroscope. The deposits disappear when the blood calcium becomes normal.

Hypoparathyroidism

Decreased secretion of the parathyroid hormone results in a lowered serum calcium, increased serum phosphorus, and a decreased urinary excretion of both calcium and phosphorus. Serum alkaline phosphatase is either normal or decreased. A decreased serum calcium gives rise to a clinical picture dominated by manifestations of tetany and neuromuscular hyperexcitability. In milder cases there is numbness and tingling of the extremities or in the area around the lips. Hoarseness may occur. In more severe cases carpopedal spasm and laryngeal stridor are seen. Generalized convulsions are common. Latent tetany is elicited by Chvostek's sign, in which tapping the finger over the facial nerve causes twitching of the muscles of the mouth and, in severe cases, of the nose and eyelids. Trousseau's sign consists of carpal spasm, with evocation of the so-called obstetric hand that follows nerve ischemia when the arm is constricted by a sphygmomanometer cuff.

Cataracts develop in hypoparathyroidism when the blood calcium falls to a level at which neuromuscular hyperexcitability is observed. Lens changes are bilateral and involve predominantly the subcapsular area of the cortical portion of the lens. The nucleus is usually spared. As lens damage progresses, it may become involved with small, discrete, punctate opacities and crystals of different shapes and colors. Similar opacities may be found in myotonic dystrophy, cretinism, and mongolism.

Papilledema and increased intracranial pressure may occur in hypoparathyroidism. Care must be taken to distinguish brain tumor from hypoparathyroidism with convulsive seizures and papilledema.

Acute hypoparathyroidism responds to parathyroid extract, but refractoriness to the hormone develops rapidly. In chronic hypoparathyroidism, good response follows the use of adequate amounts of vitamin D or dihydrotachysterol (AT-10) and calcium salts. A diet low in phosphorus is important. Aluminum hydroxide given orally will combine with dietary phosphorus to facilitate absorption of calcium. Prompt and early treatment of hypoparathyroidism will prevent cataract formation. Therapy does not bring about regression of cataractous changes once they have formed, although the cataract may be arrested.

Pseudohypoparathyroidism. Pseudohypoparathyroidism is a disorder characterized by failure of response to the normally produced parathyroid hormone, presumably because of a renal end-organ defect. The average age of onset is 8½ years, and the disease usually manifests itself before the age of 20 years. It occurs more frequently in girls than boys.

Clinically, pseudohypoparathyroidism is similar to hypoparathyroidism, but in addition, extraskeletal ossification, calcification, and bony dysplasia are present. The patient is usually short in stature, of stocky build, and has a round face. The metacarpals are shortened. Mental retardation is common. Cataract formation occurs slightly less commonly than in primary hypoparathyroidism.

Pituitary gland

Tumors of the pituitary gland may give rise to a wide variety of endocrine abnormalities together with the chiasmal syndrome (p. 413) in which there is optic atrophy combined with bitemporal hemianopsia due to interference with the decussating visual fibers in the optic chiasm.

Chapter 25

Cardiovascular disease

Using the ophthalmoscope, the careful observer may see and recognize subtle defects of the small retinal arteries and veins, the sole portion of the body's vasculature available for direct visual inspection. However, the ophthalmoscope is not a substitute for the sphygmomanometer, clinical examination, or laboratory data—accurate diagnosis necessitates appraisal of all possible information and not solely an ophthalmoscopic examination. Repeated observation of both eyes over a period of time is frequently necessary before the nature of the retinal abnormality is evident. In addition, the retinal vasculature is a frequent site of a variety of local diseases causing abnormalities, and meaningful ophthalmoscopic study necessitates differentiation between local or focal changes involving a limited portion of the blood vessels and diffuse or generalized changes that arise from systemic disease. Details of the ophthalmoscopic examination are described on pp. 139 and 250.

Arteriosclerosis

Arteriosclerosis is a nonspecific, broadly inclusive term referring to all varieties of processes in which hardening and thickening of the arterial coat have occurred. The three conditions generally included in the term "arteriosclerosis" are Mönckeberg's medial sclerosis, atherosclerosis, and diffuse arteriolar sclerosis. Mönckeberg's medial sclerosis affects medium-sized arteries, particularly in the extremities; there is never

ocular involvement. Atherosclerosis affects large and medium-sized arteries—the central retinal artery and its branches immediately adjacent to the optic disk may be involved. Diffuse arteriolar sclerosis may involve all arterioles in the body in a similar manner. It occurs solely as a result of vascular hypertension.

Retinal vein obstruction from any cause gives rise to changes in adjacent arterioles identical with those occurring in involutionary sclerosis and arteriolar sclerosis. It is postulated that the venous stasis gives rise to a local toxin affecting the arterial wall. The ophthalmoscopic appearance may be distinguished from the changes of arteriolar sclerosis by the presence of adjacent vein disease and the focal localization of the arterial changes.

Atherosclerosis

Atherosclerosis is a vascular abnormality characterized by focal necrosis and thickening of the intima, with intimal and sub-intimal lipid deposition associated with hyperplastic and degenerative changes in the wall of the artery, particularly of the internal elastic lamina. The disease may affect arteries of all diameters, but it has a predilection for the aorta and tends to involve arteries to the heart, brain, and extremities. The condition is absent in puberty, but thereafter its extent and severity increase with advancing years. Atheromas are clinically silent unless there is frank obstruction or localized decrease in blood

401

supply to a region. The lesions may be multiple but are distinctly localized in distribution, so that presence of atheromas in one vessel does not indicate a similar involvement in another vessel. The cause of atheromas is not known, but they are associated with vascular hypertension, emotional stress, turbulence eddies within blood vessels, increased plasma lipids, heredity, and numerous other factors.

Atherosclerosis of retinal vessels. Atherosclerosis may manifest itself in the eye mainly by involvement of the central retinal artery within the optic nerve or in its branches immediately adjacent to the optic disk.

Atheroma formation in the central retinal artery within the optic nerve may cause contraction of the artery and displacement of the retinal arterioles toward the disk. As the bifurcations of retinal vessels are drawn onto the disk, more blood vessels cross the disk margins, the retinal vessels become straighter, and the bifurcations occur at more acute angles. Reduction in the lumen of the central retinal artery by such an atheroma causes diminution in blood flow and narrowing of the caliber of the arterial tree.

Atheromas occurring in branches of the central artery near the optic disk cause subtle changes. Localized indentations in the wall of the artery result in reduction in caliber of the lumen due to projection of an atheromatous plaque into the lumen. Fibrosis may result in a whitish or opaque area in the wall of the involved blood vessel.

Occlusion. Atherosclerosis in the eye, as elsewhere in the body, may give rise to obstruction of the central retinal artery or vein. If the central retinal artery (p. 258) is occluded, a pale coagulation necrosis rapidly involves the inner layers of the retina. The fovea, in which the inner layers are lacking and which receives its nutrition from the choroid, is not involved, and here a cherry red spot is visible. The

entire arterial tree becomes markedly attenuated. Branch occlusion causes a pale coagulation necrosis of the inner layers of the retina in the region of distribution of the involved vessel, the caliber of which is markedly attenuated. A scotoma with very sharp margins corresponding to the involved area can be demonstrated in the visual field.

Dislodgment of a thrombus from an atheromatous plaque in the aorta or heart may produce a shower of small lipid fragments that appear as minute, glistening intra-arterial dots.

Inasmuch as arteries and veins within the eye are bound together at points of crossings, within a common adventitial sheath, atheromatous plaque formation in the artery may impinge on the lumen of the vein, giving rise to central retinal vein occlusion or closure of its immediate tributaries. Retinal vein occlusion is most common at the level of the lamina cribrosa, where obstruction is further favored by the abrupt right-angle turn of the blood vessels on the surface of the disk. The likelihood of venous closure is enhanced by the presence of glaucoma since the increased intraocular pressure favors stagnation of blood and thrombus formation. Atheromatous disease is inferred when involvement within the optic nerve causes sudden loss of vision. The lesion cannot be seen with the ophthalmoscope.

Involutionary sclerosis

Abnormalities of the retinal blood vessels are not uncommon in aged persons but occasionally occur in presenile individuals who do not and have not had vascular hypertension. The outstanding ophthalmoscopic characteristic of involutionary sclerosis is localized involvement of blood vessels, with much of the retinal vasculature appearing normal. There is loss of brilliant light reflexes from the retinal surface, and a coarser texture is reflected from the retina. The light reflex from the convex surface of arterioles is of diminished intensity and more diffuse than is normal. There may be generalized widening of the arteriovenous crossing, but this is far less marked than the crossing changes in arteriolar sclerosis. Very slight reduction in the caliber of arteries may be noted. Associated with the vascular changes are degenerative changes such as colloid excrescences on the lamina vitrea and atrophic changes in the choroid about the optic disk, in the macular region, and in the periphery of the retina.

These changes of involutionary sclerosis occur with aging and do not necessarily parallel any arteriosclerotic process elsewhere in the body. They may be minimal and accompany systemic signs of aging. Their cause is not known, but in all probability they are the consequence of arteriolar fibrosis and loss of elasticity of the affected tissues.

Arteriolar sclerosis

Arteriolar sclerosis is the anatomic reflection of a prolonged, significant increase in blood pressure that results in thickening of the walls and narrowing of the lumen of arterioles in response to the stress and strain of the vascular hypertension. The vascular involvement is generalized, and thus all arterioles throughout the body are affected to a similar degree, in contrast to the spotty, plaquelike involvement of atherosclerosis.

Two types of change may occur in arteriolar sclerosis:

1. Replacement fibrosis may develop in slowly increasing, moderately severe hypertension, associated chiefly with elevation of the systolic blood pressure in the range of 170 to 200 mm. Hg, with the diastolic pressure usually less than 100 mm. Hg. There is increased collagen and elastic tissue in all layers of the blood vessel, with eventual complete loss of cellular detail.

2. Hyperplastic thickening and fibrinoid necrosis are acute, severe reactions to sudden marked elevation of the blood pressure in which the systolic blood pressure exceeds 200 mm. Hg and the diastolic blood pressure exceeds 120 mm. Hg. The marked, diffuse thickening of arteriolar walls, if severe, may lead to necrosis. Hyperplastic thickening and fibrinoid necrosis occur only in vessels containing muscle fibers. Vessels that are the site of involutionary sclerosis or prior replacement fibrosis are not in-

Table 25-1. Ophthalmoscopic signs of arteriolar sclerosis

Replacement fibrosis: diastolic blood pressure usually less than 100 mm. Hg	Fibrinoid necrosis: diastolic blood pressure usually greater than 120 mm. Hg
Attenuation of arterioles	Severe attenuation of arterioles
Changes in vascular light reflex	Edema of retina
Widening	Fluffy cotton-wool exudates
Copper-wire arteries	Hemorrhage
Silver-wire arteries	Papilledema
Irregularities of caliber	Ophthalmoscopic changes of replacement fibrosis
Arteriovenous crossing changes	may precede above signs or remain after
Concealment	condition is corrected
Depression or elevation	
Deviation	
Stenosis	
Hard, shiny exudates	
Hemorrhage	
Sheathing	
Tortuosity	

volved. These changes appear to protect the arterioles from the effects of severe hypertension, and they may explain the infrequency of hyperplastic thickening and fibrinoid necrosis in the age group in which involutionary sclerosis is seen.

Replacement fibrosis and fibrinoid necrosis cause two main groups of ophthalmoscopic changes (Table 25-1). If ophthalmoscopy in a patient with vascular hypertension indicates no arteriolar sclerosis, then the hypertension either is not severe or is of recent onset. If the changes of replacement fibrosis are present, the disease is of long standing and has affected arterioles throughout the body similarly. If the ophthalmoscopic changes are those of hyperplastic thickening and fibrinoid necrosis, the hypertension is very severe, is often of recent onset, and may be associated with renal insufficiency, encephalopathy, and impairment of cardiac function.

Attenuation of arterioles. Attenuation of the arterioles as a sign of hypertension is by far the most difficult ophthalmoscopic finding to interpret. Both generalized and local constriction may be observed, but only the generalized attenuation appears to result from vascular spasm. Attenuation is best appreciated by observation of arterioles beyond their second bifurcation, where they seem to become thin red threads that disappear from view at the equator. The change is observed ophthalmoscopically, uncomplicated by preceding vascular disease, in eclampsia, or in other types of severe vascular hypertension occurring in youthful individuals who have not developed replacement fibrosis.

Changes in light reflex. The walls of retinal arterioles are so thin that the blood column is viewed ophthalmoscopically through a nearly transparent convex wall. The central light reflex arises from the medial coat. With replacement fibrosis, the blood vessel wall becomes less transparent, and the thickening of the medial coat is reflected in changes in the light re-

flex. The changes in light reflex seen in benign hypertension are similar to the changes in involutional sclerosis except for their occurrence in younger individuals.

The major changes in light reflex are as follows:

1. *Widening of the light reflex:* The earliest sign of arteriolar sclerosis is widening of the central light reflex from arterioles. Instead of a bright central line, it becomes broader and softer with less distinct borders.

2. *Copper-wire arteries:* As the reflex broadens, it eventually occupies most of the width of the blood vessel. Early ophthalmologists, using reflected light having less intensity than the modern direct ophthalmoscope affords, described the burnished, metallic reflections as copper-wire arteries.

3. *Silver-wire arteries:* As replacement fibrosis continues, the vessel wall obscures the blood column, and the arteriole appears as a whitish tube containing a red fluid. There is not the white, threadlike appearance of the artery that follows occlusion of the central retinal artery.

4. *Irregularities in caliber:* Widening of the light reflex does not occur uniformly. Initially there are areas of normal width combined with areas of decreased width. This has been interpreted as a sign of focal vasospasm, but unlike generalized vasospasm, it does not disappear with correction of the hypertension.

Arteriovenous crossing changes. Thickening of the wall of an arteriole at the point where it crosses over or under a vein may produce a variety of changes. The earliest and most subtle is loss of translucency of the arteriole so that the vein can no longer be seen beneath the vessel. The formation of atheromatous plaques near the optic disk may cause sheathing of the adjacent arteriovenous crossing, and this region should be excluded in the evaluation of arteriolar sclerosis. Generalized variations in arteriovenous crossing changes are observed solely in arteriolar sclerosis and serve to differentiate the retinal vascular changes of involutionary sclerosis. Occasionally there may be a focal arteriovenous crossing change in involutionary sclerosis. The generalized arteriovenous crossing changes in arteriolar sclerosis are the following:

1. *Concealment:* The loss of transparency of the wall of the retinal arteriole due to thickening of its wall may conceal the underlying vein. The venous blood column may terminate abruptly on either side of the crossing. Alternatively, there may be a tapering type of concealment, with the vein fading on either side of the crossing. The concealment appears to cause a narrowing of the vein commonly described as "nicking" (Fig. 25-1). In all likelihood the venous lumen is not narrowed.

2. *Depression or elevation:* A vein may be deflected deep into the retina or may hump abruptly over the artery (Fig. 25-2). Presumably the thickening of the wall of the arterioles causes displacement of the vein.

3. *Deviation:* Displacement of a vein at the point of crossing is characterized by an abrupt turn in the course of the vein just as it reaches the artery (Fig. 25-3). At a similar distance beyond the artery it again assumes the same direction as prior to the crossing. This gives the vein an S-shape bend. Presumably the lower pressure in the vein compared to the artery permits it to be deflected from its course or compressed with greater ease.

4. *Stenosis:* Because of compression or constriction at the arteriovenous crossing, the vein distal to the crossing becomes dilated and swollen (Fig. 25-4). The crossing is concealed, and thereafter the vein has a normal diameter.

Hard, shiny exudates. The hard, shiny exudates that develop in areas of chronic retinal ischemia are histologically lipid-laden macrophages. These exudates are observed mainly at the posterior pole, vary

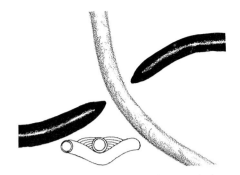

Fig. 25-1. Tapering concealment of the vein appearing as "nicking."

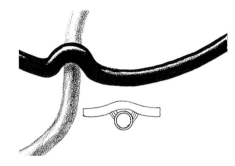

Fig. 25-2. Elevation of vein over artery.

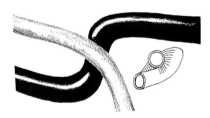

Fig. 25-3. Deviation of vein out of its path.

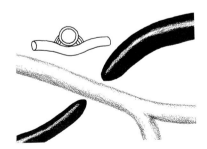

Fig. 25-4. Compression of vein at arteriovenous crossing causing stenosis of distal vein.

in number from a few to 50 or more, and are scattered throughout the inner layers of the retina. In the course of resolution of cotton-wool deposits, shiny, hard exudates may be formed that disappear within a year. Most hard exudates, however, develop gradually. They cause no visual disturbance.

Hemorrhages. Hemorrhages in arteriolar sclerosis are usually superficial and minute. In all probability they are due to minute venous occlusions secondary to closure of small veins.

Sheathing. Sheathing may occur as a result either of arteriolar sclerosis or because of an atheromatous plaque involving an artery adjacent to the optic disk. Normally arterioles near the disk are sheathed with glial tissue. In arteriolar sclerosis, white parallel lines appear at arteriovenous crossings and encase the arteriole, giving rise to the appearance of a white, fibrous-looking cord.

Tortuosity. In fibrous replacement the arterioles increase in length and diameter, with resultant increased tortuosity. This may also be a congenital condition, and its occurrence in hypertension can be evaluated solely by repeated observation.

Cotton-wool spots. Cotton-wool spots are a characteristic change in hypertension when the diastolic blood pressure exceeds 120 mm. Hg. They are located in the nerve fiber layer of the retina at the posterior pole, number usually less than 10, and are about one third of the disk diameter in size. They result presumably from an ischemic infarct of the retina due to occlusion of an arteriole. The occlusion is thought to be caused by fibrinoid arteriolar necrosis or severe spasm giving rise to abnormal endothelial permeability. Similar cotton-wool spots may also be seen in collagen diseases and in a number of other diseases not necessarily associated with vascular hypertension but in which there is generalized endothelial damage. Cotton-wool spots are described histologically as

microinfarcts containing cytoid bodies, which are considered to originate from terminal bulbous swelling of nerve fibers.

Papilledema. The development of hypertensive encephalopathy is associated with the development of papilledema. As in papilledema from brain tumor or other intracranial masses, there is initial congestion of the optic disk with obliteration of the physiologic optic cup. Blurring of the upper and lower nasal margins follows, accompanied by venous dilatation. The veins do not pulsate. Early in the course there are edema and swelling of the retina, which has a wet, watery appearance with many highlights. With increasing venous dilatation, superficial flame-shaped hemorrhages occur. Central visual acuity remains good, but the blind spots are enlarged, as demonstrated by testing on the tangent screen (p. 148). If the primary hypertension is corrected, the ophthalmoscopic changes may disappear without residue.

Choroidal changes. The vasculature of the choroid cannot be seen distinctly with the ophthalmoscope, but vascular changes of the choroid parallel those elsewhere in the body and the eye. Atherosclerosis of choroidal vessels is common, but the rich anastomoses prevent ischemia. Choroidal vessels show an early involutionary sclerosis, which precedes that of the retinal arterioles. In severe hypertension the arterioles may show fibrinoid necrosis, and it has been suggested that this choroidal change plays a role in the retinal lesion of severe hypertension.

Grading of hypertension

The grading of the ocular changes secondary to vascular hypertension has resulted in considerable confusion in the literature and among practitioners. Fundamentally, any grading system is only a form of medical shorthand to be used to summarize the changes observed and to permit grouping of patients with similar disease. Unless all physicians participating in the care of a patient agree upon the same method, the classification of disease findings will confuse, rather than clarify, the diagnosis. It is probably far more instructive to describe and to interpret the changes seen ophthalmoscopically than to use a grading method. It must be emphasized that the ocular changes in hypertension are a result of the increased blood pressure, and one cannot determine the cause of the hypertension by means of the ophthalmoscope.

Atherosclerotic changes may occur in hypertensive vascular disease, but the elevated blood pressure is only one of many factors involved in the pathogenesis. These changes are also seen in normotensive individuals, and it seems quite possible that the majority of adults in the United States have atheromatous plaques somewhere in their arterial system. Observation of their occurrence in the retinal vasculature reflects this process, but because of the spotty distribution of atheromas, it permits no conclusions as to other vessels involved.

Arterial occlusion and venous occlusion are the most conspicuous retinal vascular signs of atherosclerosis. More common is a grayish white opacification involving the wall of an arteriole near the optic disk. It should be distinguished from the bright, shiny, yellowish orange plaque seen with a cholesterol embolus. Retraction of the central retinal artery into the optic nerve requires skilled serial ophthalmoscopic observation.

The ophthalmoscopic changes are similar in involutionary sclerosis and in replacement fibrosis caused by mild or early essential hypertension. Most instances of treated vascular hypertension fall into this category, and arteriolar attenuation and changes in the light reflex are the main changes. Generalized changes in arteriovenous crossings do not occur.

In all likelihood if the observer had no clues to the age of the patient being examined, he could not, by means of the ophthalmoscope, distinguish between involutionary sclerosis and the replacement fibrosis of mild hypertension. However, hypertensive changes occur in a younger age group, and there is a tendency to more generalized arteriolar involvement than is seen in involutionary sclerosis. Involutionary sclerosis is commonly associated with excrescences of the lamina vitrea (drusen) and retinal atrophic changes.

In sustained, untreated, or prolonged vascular hypertension, changes in arteriovenous crossings occur. The arteriolar attenuation and changes in the light reflexes are conspicuous. The hypertension is likely to be less responsive to therapy than when there are no arteriovenous crossing changes. Late in the course of the disease, hard, shiny exudates may develop, and there may be scattered hemorrhages. Hard exudates do not indicate angiospasm or suggest that the hypertension is entering an accelerated phase, as does the occurrence of even one cotton-wool spot.

In some patients the hypertension gradually progresses and enters an accelerated phase. Usually the diastolic pressure exceeds 120 mm. Hg. The replacement fibrosis that has occurred prevents extreme arteriolar attenuation. The developing retinal edema tends to accentuate the irregularities in caliber and arteriovenous crossing changes. It is readily evident that hypertension was present prior to the malignant phase.

In hypertension with a diastolic pressure of more than 120 mm. Hg the outstanding retinal signs are cotton-wool spots, edema of the retina, and ultimately papilledema with venous stasis and hemorrhage. There may be extreme attenuation of the arterioles, particularly if they have not been involved in arteriolar sclerosis. The retinal changes of severe hypertension may occur with dramatic rapidity. In true eclampsia the ophthalmoscopic appearance may change from one of severe, generalized arteriolar attenuation to papilledema, cotton-wool spots, and retinal edema in less than 12 hours.

Keith-Wagener-Barker grouping. This classification relates solely to a grouping of the retinal changes associated with vascular hypertension. It loses its value when applied to other vascular diseases. Inasmuch as hypertension causes generalized, diffuse changes, one should not use the classification for focal changes or for changes secondary to retinal inflammation with venous stasis. Both eyes should have similar changes; involvement of one eye suggests impaired internal carotid circulation on the side of the normal eye (p. 420). Glaucoma tends to minimize the ophthalmoscopic changes of vascular hypertension.

Group I. The light reflex from arterioles is brightened, and there is an increased luster with a burnished copper-wire or polished silver-wire appearance. There is moderate arteriolar attenuation often combined with focal constriction. No marked changes are seen in arteriovenous crossings, although there may be widening with increased translucency of the arteriole, making the underlying vein nearly invisible. Such patients have an essential benign hypertension with adequate cardiac and renal function; the heart size and the electrocardiogram are usually normal. The majority of cases of hypertension fall into this group. The vascular changes of the fundi are virtually identical with those occurring in involutionary sclerosis without hypertension. The ophthalmoscopic changes will probably not progress with adequate treatment of the hypertensive disease.

Group II. The light reflex has a quite definite burnished copper-wire or polished silver-wire luster. Arteriovenous crossing changes may be quite marked and include all the various abnormalities. The arterioles are about half the size of normal, and there are areas of localized constriction. Hard, shiny deposits as well as minute linear hemorrhages may develop late in the course of the disease. These patients have a more sustained hypertension with higher diastolic pressure than those in Group I. Their cardiac and renal functions tend to be normal, but cardiomegaly may develop with corresponding changes in the electrocardiogram. Angina pectoris and proteinuria may also be present.

Group III. Marked attenuation of the arterioles occurs. The retina appears wet and edematous. One or more cotton-wool spots and hemorrhages are present. The significant change is the cotton-wool spot. These patients have a diastolic blood pressure of more than 120 mm. Hg. Depending upon the cause of hypertension, there may be cardiac symptoms, changes in the electrocardiogram, and renal changes of proteinuria and insufficiency.

Group IV. The patients in Group IV have all of the ophthalmoscopic signs of those in Group III, in addition to papilledema. The degree of papilledema may vary from blurring of the disk margins to complete obliteration of the disk structure. Cardiac and renal functions may be seriously impaired. Papilledema and cotton-wool spots may disappear shortly before death.

• • •

A number of systemic abnormalities cause the angiospastic retinopathy of Groups III and IV, and with their correction the ophthalmoscopic appearance of the fundus may be restored to normal. However, if the condition has persisted for some time and if considerable fibrinoid necrosis has occurred, after the blood pressure has been restored to normal, the fundus will resemble that seen in Group II. The originators of this classification did not describe hard, shiny deposits as occurring in Group II. A serious error is introduced if such deposits are the basis for classifying the fundus disease as Group III.

Eclampsia, pheochromocytoma, and renal disease

The retinal manifestation of these diseases is entirely related to the vascular hypertension they produce. In years past the term "renal retinopathy" was used by ophthalmologists to describe the hypertensive fundus changes that occurred with chronic renal disease. Many internists disliked the term because of the implication that the fundus changes reflected a specific renal abnormality rather than the hypertension. The fundi show advanced arteriolar sclerosis. Superimposed upon these changes there is the gradual development of cotton-wool deposits and hemorrhages. The combination suggests a severe hypertensive vascular disease that has been present for a long period.

In true eclampsia the hypertensive vascular changes occur in a fundus that has not previously been the site of vascular change. The rapid onset of a severe hypertension gives rise to a generalized arteriolar spasm. Cotton-wool exudates occur with much retinal edema, giving it a wet, edematous, "shot-silk" appearance. The hemodynamic disturbances may be so severe that a bilateral retinal detachment occurs without holes in the retina. Once the hypertension is corrected, the fundi rapidly revert to normal.

Pheochromocytoma and unilateral renal disease cause hypertension with the fundus changes of severe hypertension without antecedent vascular disease. Usually the hypertension develops more slowly than that seen in eclampsia, and there is less edema in the retina. If the condition is corrected early in the course of the hypertension, the fundus reverts to normal. If the condition has persisted for some time prior to correction of the hypertension, the hemorrhages and deposits disappear, but there tends to be persistent arteriolar constriction and variation in caliber. The ophthalmoscopic picture is not unlike that seen in elderly individuals with treated hypertension.

Chapter 26

The central nervous system and the eye

A wide variety of diseases of the central nervous system may be associated with either involvement of the eye or its adnexa or may give rise to ocular symptoms. Some signs require most elaborate instrumentation and study to demonstrate, whereas others are evident with minimal examination. Even the most cursory physical examination should indicate the absence of papilledema (optic atrophy is more difficult to evaluate), normal ocular movements, and pupils equal in size that react directly to light. If central vision is normal in each eye, an optic neuritis is unlikely; simple testing of the visual fields by confrontation is helpful in excluding abnormalities of the visual pathways.

Optic nerve

Disorders of the optic nerve are discussed in Chapter 17. Optic atrophy may be complete or partial, and it may arise from disease within the eye such as glaucoma or ganglion cell degeneration or from disease in the course of the optic nerve or tract. If optic atrophy is preceded by papilledema or inflammation, it is called secondary; if not, it is called primary.

Optic neuritis or papillitis is nearly always unilateral and is associated with marked reduction of central visual acuity. Papilledema is generally bilateral, is associated with good vision early in its course, is never present when the lamina cribrosa is clearly visible, and is usually associated with disappearance of spontaneous or induced retinal vein pulsation.

Visual pathways

The anatomy of the visual pathways is discussed in the section on anatomy (p. 58). Visual field testing is discussed in the section on examination (p. 147). Lesions in the retina and in the optic nerve anterior to the decussation of nasal retinal fibers in the optic chiasm cause a visual field defect in one eye only. A lesion at the chiasm involves decussating nasal fibers and causes blindness in the temporal one half of each visual field, a bitemporal hemianopsia. Lesions posterior to the chiasm involve the nasal retinal fibers of one eye and the temporal retinal fibers of the fellow eye. The visual field defect is bilateral and involves the right or the left half of the visual field. A right homonymous hemianopsia indicates that the nasal fibers of the right eye and the temporal fibers of the left eye are involved posterior to the chiasm. After synapse in the lateral geniculate body, visual fibers from each eye are exactly superimposed; therefore a visual field defect arising from disease in these fibers is exactly the same, or congruous, in each eye.

Pupils

Disorders involving the pupil are discussed in Chapter 13. The pupils are normally round, approximately equal, and both constrict when the retina of one eye is stimulated with light. Adhesion of the iris to the cornea or the lens, atrophy, or surgical excision of a portion of the pupillary margin gives rise to a pupil that is not round.

Tabes dorsalis may be associated with Argyll Robertson pupils, which are miotic, irregular, and fail to constrict with light but do constrict with accommodation. Adie's syndrome is an abnormality involving postganglionic fibers of the ciliary ganglion in which the pupillary constriction is absent or delayed. Horner's syndrome arises from interruption of the sympathetic nerve fibers to the dilatator iridis. The pupil is miotic and does not dilate when cocaine is instilled into the eye; there is an associated ptosis and failure of sweating on the involved side.

Unilateral pupillary dilation associated with head injury usually indicates a skull fracture on the side of dilation. Head injury with bilateral dilated pupils usually occurs in deeply comatose persons and has a poor prognosis. Rupture of an intracranial aneurysm may cause unilateral mydriasis. Oculomotor nerve involvement in diabetes mellitus is usually without pupillary involvement. Myasthenia gravis never involves the smooth muscle of the iris.

Motor nerves

The motor nerves to the eye may be involved in a variety of abnormalities resulting from trauma, hemorrhage, cerebral edema, inflammation, neoplasm, aneurysms, or demyelination.

Oculomotor nerve. Total paralysis of the oculomotor nerve causes ptosis of the upper lid and paralysis of the superior rectus, medial rectus, inferior rectus, and inferior oblique muscles. The pupil is dilated, reacts slightly, if at all, to light and accommodation, and there is loss of accommodation (internal ophthalmoplegia).

When the unimpaired fellow eye fixes, the paralyzed eye is turned outward by the action of the lateral rectus muscle (N VI). The pupil is often not affected in medical diseases involving the oculomotor nerve (such as diabetes mellitus and multiple sclerosis) but is affected in surgical disease (such as tumors and aneurysms).

Nuclear lesions tend not to involve the pupil or the ciliary muscle. Tumors in the midbrain or the pineal body produce Parinaud's syndrome, in which there is supranuclear conjugate palsy of vertical gaze (inability to elevate or to depress the eyes upon command). Often there are dilated pupils, which are unresponsive to light.

Involvement of the fibers of the oculomotor nerve passing through the red nucleus causes Benedikt's syndrome, in which there is homolateral oculomotor paralysis and contralateral intention tremor. There may be an associated contralateral hemianesthesia. Involvement of fibers near the ventral surface of the brain in the cerebral peduncle interrupts pyramidal fibers and causes Weber's syndrome, with homolateral oculomotor paralysis, contralateral hemiplegia, and paralysis of the tongue and lower part of the face.

Interruption of the oculomotor nerve in the cavernous sinus is likely to be associated with involvement of the fourth and sixth cranial nerves. Involvement in the superior orbital fissure may also involve sympathetic nerve fibers, so that pupillary dilation is not marked.

The third cranial nerve is particularly likely to be involved in tuberculosis or syphilitic meningitis and in herpes zoster. The nerve is frequently spared in purulent meningitis, which is more likely to involve the sixth cranial nerve. All of the ocular nerves are involved in cavernous sinus thrombosis, with the motor involvement likely to precede pupillary involvement. The syndrome of the superior orbital fissure involves all of the motor and sensory nerves of the eye, including the sympathetic nerves. It may be produced by suppuration in the sphenoidal sinus, skull fracture, hemorrhage, or tumor.

Following paralysis of the third cranial nerve, aberrant regeneration of the nerve fibers may give rise to a pseudo–von Graefe phenomenon in which the fibers originally going to the inferior rectus muscle are distributed to the levator muscle. Thus, when an attempt is made to look downward, the inferior rectus muscle is ineffective, but the lid rises. Misdirection of the fibers to the medial rectus muscle so that they extend into the innervation of the sphincter pupillae muscle causes constriction of the pupil on attempts to rotate the eye medially. If nerve fibers destined for the superior rectus muscle abnormally regenerate into the levator palpebrae superioris muscle, attempts to elevate the eye are associated with abnormal elevation of the lid. With closure of the lids as in sleep, an abnormal Bell's phenomenon occurs in which the upper lid elevates rather than closes.

Trochlear nerve. Paralysis of the fourth cranial nerve is particularly evident in looking downward to read, which causes a marked diplopia. Trochlear palsies are particularly likely to be associated with head tilting. The involved eye is higher than the fellow eye, and the head is tilted to the sound side.

Abducens nerve. Paralysis of the sixth cranial nerve results in esotropia with inability to rotate the eye laterally beyond the midline. The long intracranial course of this nerve and its angulation over the sphenoidal bone make it vulnerable in skull fractures, increased intracranial pressure, and purulent meningitis.

Gradenigo's syndrome is due to an osteitis of the petrous tip of the pyramidal bone and follows mastoid and middle ear infections on the homolateral side. It is associated with sixth cranial nerve paralysis, pain on the same side of the face

from fifth cranial nerve involvement, and deafness. Acoustic neuromas are associated with deafness, sixth cranial nerve involvement, facial paralysis due to seventh cranial nerve involvement, and papilledema.

Space-occupying intracranial lesions

A brain tumor, abscess, aneurysm, or hemorrhage may cause many of the same symptoms and signs. The symptoms may be divided into (1) general, arising mainly from increased intracranial pressure, and (2) focal, arising from irritation or damage to a specific part of the brain.

General symptoms. The general symptoms of increased intracranial pressure are diffuse headaches, which are intensified by increased intraventricular pressure brought about by coughing, sneezing, or defecating. Typically the headache is relieved by vomiting, which occurs without nausea. Late in the course there occur slowed pulse (vagus effect), lowered pulse pressure, and increased respiratory rate. There is a clouding of consciousness that varies from somnolence to deep coma, a delirium, or an organic psychosis.

The outstanding ocular sign of increased intracranial pressure is bilateral papilledema. In the absence of ocular or orbital disease, its occurrence suggests brain tumor (or a tumor equivalent) to be the most likely cause. However, many brain tumors do not cause papilledema or are diagnosed before it develops, so that its absence does not exclude tumor. Other ocular signs of increased intracranial pressure occur relatively late. The sixth cranial nerve is involved because of its long intracranial course, but involvement is not of localizing value. A unilateral dilated pupil is suggestive of an ipsilateral supratentorial space-occupying lesion. Initially the pupillary response to light and convergence is normal, but it is lost later in the disease.

Focal symptoms. Focal symptoms may

be divided into those arising from (1) a supratentorial location and (2) those arising from an infratentorial location. The supratentorial group includes the cerebral hemispheres with their frontal, temporal, parietal, and occipital lobes; the pituitary gland, chiasm, and surrounding area; the anterior and middle fossa; and the diencephalon, including the third ventricle. The infratentorial group includes the cerebellopontine angle, the cerebellar hemispheres and vermis, the pons, and the medulla oblongata. Tumors in the mesencephalon may expand in a supratentorial or an infratentorial direction.

Supratentorial tumors. The ocular symptoms of supratentorial tumors differ widely. Visual field defects occur commonly, as do optic atrophy and papilledema. Involvement of ocular movements is not as common as with infratentorial tumors.

Chiasmal syndrome. Interference with the decussating axons arising from the nasal one half of each retina gives rise to a bitemporal hemianopsia combined with optic atrophy. The hemianopsia is often more advanced in one eye than the other. When caused by a pituitary lesion impinging on the chiasm from below, the field defect begins in the superior temporal fields and progresses inferiorly (Fig. 26-1).

A large variety of lesions may give rise to the chiasmal syndrome: tumors and inflammation of the chiasm, pituitary tumors, aneurysms, basal meningitis, injuries, and abnormalities of the structures surrounding the dorsum sellae.

Pituitary adenomas. Pituitary adenomas are of three types:

1. The chromophobe adenoma is the most common type and the most likely to produce ocular signs. Systemic signs are those of hypopituitarism: impotence or amenorrhea with loss of libido, a decreased basal metabolic rate with obesity, a soft, silky skin, and in men, a scanty beard. Bitemporal hemianopsia is the characteristic ocular sign of chiasmal involvement.

2. The acidophilic adenoma causes acromegaly in adults and giantism in children. It is far less likely to produce ocular signs than the chromophobe type, and ocular involvement is not severe. However, treatment by means of radiation should not be delayed because of the absence of ocular signs.

3. Basophilic adenoma causes hypersecretion of the adrenal cortex with development of Cushing's syndrome.

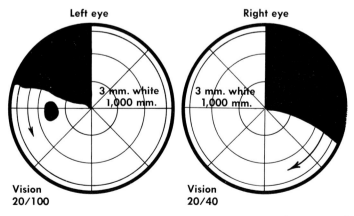

Fig. 26-1. Early field defect in the chiasmal syndrome that begins in the superior temporal field and progresses inferiorly. (Modified from Harrington, D. O.: The visual fields, ed. 2, St. Louis, 1964, The C. V. Mosby Co.)

The ocular signs of adenoma always follow typical ballooning and uniform enlargement of the sella, thinning of the floor, and erosion of the clinoid processes. Suprasellar tumors that cause chiasmal signs give rise to ocular changes prior to roentgenographic changes.

Involvement of the optic chiasm causes a decrease in vision, subjectively noted as cloudy or foggy and not related to a visual field disturbance. Only later does the bitemporal hemianopsia give rise to complaints. The field defect initially involves the superior temporal quadrant and then spreads to the inferior quadrant.

Development of optic atrophy lags behind the field defect. Usually there is a marked difference in the degree of atrophy of the two eyes.

Extreme expansion of the adenoma outside the sella may lead to invasion of the cavernous sinus, causing involvement of cranial nerves III, IV, and VI. Most commonly such expansion follows adrenalectomy in Cushing's syndrome.

Craniopharyngiomas. Craniopharyngiomas originate from epithelial remnants of Rathke's pouch and may be primarily intrasellar (rare) or suprasellar. Although considered more likely to occur in children, adults are equally susceptible.

In children the tumor invades the third ventricle early and causes internal hydrocephalus with papilledema. In adolescents, decreased anterior pituitary secretion may cause dystrophia adiposogenitalis (Fröhlich), cachexia (Simmond), or dwarfism (Lorain). Hypothalamic involvement may cause diabetes insipidus, lethargy, and hyperthermia. In adults, visual disturbances without papilledema occur early. An associated hypopituitarism results in impotence or amenorrhea with loss of libido, obesity, fine, silky skin with loss of body hair, and decreased beard growth in men. Involvement of the hypothalamus causes diabetes insipidus, lethargy, and hyperthermia.

Visual field involvement is typically asymmetric with a tendency to initial involvement of the temporal fields but with defects tending to be far advanced in one eye before involvement of the fellow eye. Because of the cystic nature of the tumor, there may be fluctuation in the visual field even without treatment. Suprasellar calcification demonstrated roentgenographically is helpful in diagnosis. Typically the roentgenographic changes occur after the visual changes.

Frontal lobe tumors. Frontal lobe tumors may reach a huge size or may cause increased intracranial pressure without localizing signs. Mental symptoms frequently dominate the clinical picture with the development of a striking change in character—apathy, euphoria, and a peculiar, silly jocularity (moria). Involvement of Broca's area causes a motor aphasia, whereas involvement of the anterior angular gyrus may cause focal epilepsy. The Foster Kennedy syndrome of ipsilateral optic atrophy and contralateral papilledema is of uncommon occurrence.

Temporal lobe tumors. Temporal lobe tumors cause uncinate fits with unpleasant olfactory or gustatory hallucinations. There may be psychomotor epilepsy or paroxysmal visual hallucinations. The visual hallucinations are typically of the formed type. Involvement of the optic tract causes a homonymous hemianopsia, which is incongruous, that is, of a different extent or intensity in the two eyes. A homonymous superior quadrantanopsia, indicating involvement of Meyer's loop, is much less common but is pathognomonic of temporal lobe involvement.

Parietal lobe tumors. Parietal lobe tumors involve the posterior central gyrus with disturbance of position sense, two-point discrimination, and stereognosis on the contralateral side. Disturbances in reading (dyslexia, alexia) and writing (agraphia) may occur. Late in the course a homonymous hemianopsia may develop.

Inferior homonymous quadrantanopsia is considered pathognomonic of parietal lobe involvement.

Occipital lobe tumors. Occipital lobe tumors manifest themselves almost solely by ocular signs. Tumors elsewhere in the brain may easily injure the posterior cerebral artery and cause occipital lobe ocular signs. A homonymous hemianopsia exactly similar (congruous) in the two eyes is the characteristic sign of occipital lobe involvement. Visual hallucinations are typically of the unformed type and occur rarely. Increased intracranial pressure occurs early in the course of the disease and progresses rapidly, and severe, acute papilledema is common.

Midbrain tumors. Pineal tumors and tumors of the midbrain give rise to Parinaud's syndrome, in which there is a conjugate paralysis of the vertical gaze. There may be associated pupillary signs similar to those of Argyll Robertson, except that the pupils are not miotic or irregular, and there may be involvement of the third and fourth cranial nerves. The name should be distinguished from Parinaud's oculoglandular disease consisting of a conjunctival granuloma with preauricular adenopathy.

Infratentorial tumors. Infratentorial tumors cannot involve the visual pathways, and disturbance in motility is their chief ocular manifestation. They tend to produce embarrassed intracranial circulation earlier than supratentorial tumors.

Cerebellar tumors. Cerebellar tumors cause ataxia, asynergy, dysmetria, and weakness. Ataxia and asynergy are demonstrated by the knee-to-heel test and in testing for diadochokinesis. Dysmetria is demonstrated in the finger-to-finger test. Weakness occurs on the opposite side. There is a distinct tendency to fall toward the side of the lesion.

The earliest ocular sign is jerk nystagmus, which is usually horizontal and accentuated on turning of the eyes from the primary position. Vertical nystagmus may arise from lesions in the vermis and is prominent on upward gaze. Papilledema occurs early and may be the initial sign of disease. Other ocular signs are secondary to increased intracranial pressure. A rare type of cerebellar lesion is the hemangioma of von Hippel's disease, which is associated with peripheral retinal tumors.

Cerebellopontine angle tumors. Cerebellopontine angle tumors are mainly acoustic neuromas causing cerebellar signs, with lesions of the fifth, sixth, seventh, and eighth cranial nerves. Impairment of hearing occurs initially, followed by cerebellar signs with nystagmus and then cranial nerve involvement. The facial nerve is frequently impaired, initially with a tic and later with blepharospasm. Involvement of the fifth cranial nerve causes corneal anesthesia. Increased intracranial pressure occurs late.

Pons and medulla. Tumors of the pons and the medulla are prone to cause disturbance of the abducens nucleus or a disturbance of horizontal conjugate gaze. Horizontal jerk nystagmus occurs occasionally, combined with vertical nystagmus. It is usually absent with the eyes in the primary position and becomes more marked as the eyes are turned toward the side of the lesion. Rarely there are palsies of the third cranial nerve. Corneal anesthesia from trigeminal nerve involvement is common. Increased intracranial pressure does not occur.

Cerebral aneurysms

Infraclinoid aneurysms. Dilation of the internal carotid artery within the cavernous sinus occurs most commonly in women during or after the fifth decade of life. The artery gives off no major branches in this location, and atheromatous plaque formation is common. The cavernous sinus contains the motor nerves to the eye and the ophthalmic and maxillary divisions of the trigeminal nerve. An expanding aneurysm thus gives rise to an ophthalmoplegia of all motor nerves and pain and paresthesia in the face. In infraclinoid aneurysms, unlike supraclinoid aneurysms, corneal and facial sensitivity is reduced.

The most conspicuous sign is an insidious, slowly progressive ophthalmoplegia, with all muscles of the eye involved. The pupil does not constrict with light but may not be dilated because of involvement of sympathetic nerve fibers on the surface of the artery. Pain is a relatively minor symptom. There is pain or paresthesia of the face, the side of the head, about the eye, or along the nose on the same side. Corneal anesthesia usually occurs and is usually associated with anesthesia of the face.

The gradual onset is suggestive of tumor, and arteriography is often necessary for exact diagnosis. Large infraclinoid aneurysms are probably reinforced by the walls of the cavernous sinus and do not rupture. Although it is likely that most spontaneous arteriovenous fistulas represent rupture of an aneurysm, usually they are so small prior to rupture that they do not cause signs of an aneurysm.

If untreated, infraclinoid aneurysms follow one of two patterns. Complete thrombosis of the aneurysm may occur, with spontaneous cure, leaving a residual loss of ocular motility. The artery may expand anteriorly within the cavernous sinus, causing erosion of the optic foramen and the superior orbital fissure, with compression and atrophy of the optic nerve and a proptosis. The development of proptosis is frequently concealed by blepharoptosis. Venous drainage of the orbit is not involved, and there is no chemosis or congestion of bulbar vessels. Posterior expansion may involve the petrous portion of the temporal bone and the acoustic nerve, causing ipsilateral deafness. The treatment of choice is ligation of

the internal carotid artery, provided arteriography indicates adequate filling of the middle and anterior cerebral arteries on the side of the aneurysm from the contralateral carotid artery and provided there is no untoward effect from digital compression of the common carotid artery for 15 minutes. Patients selected for ligation should be under the age of 60 years and should have severe pain, failing vision, or exophthalmos.

Carotid-cavernous fistula. The rupture of an infraclinoid aneurysm shunts blood from the carotid artery into the cavernous sinus, creating an arteriovenous fistula. The arterial blood passes into channels draining the cavernous sinus, and congestion of the superior ophthalmic vein draining the orbit causes visual loss, diplopia, headache, and pain.

Carotid-cavernous fistulas are traumatic (75%) or spontaneous. The traumatic fistula follows skull fracture, particularly basilotemporal fracture. A latent period may occur before the onset of symptoms. Spontaneous fistulas occur most commonly in middle-aged women, presumably from rupture of aneurysms so small that they did not cause symptoms prior to rupture.

The outstanding sign is unilateral proptosis, which may pulsate. A bruit synchronous with the pulse is present and can be heard by the patient as a rushing, roaring sound. The increased venous pressure with stasis causes chemosis, conjunctival injection, lid swelling, dilated retinal veins, and hemorrhages. The sixth cranial nerve may be involved or, less commonly, the third, fourth, or seventh. Visual failure is common from impairment of arterial and venous retinal circulation. Secondary glaucoma may not be diagnosed but may be the chief cause of visual loss.

The ideal treatment is early ligation of the internal carotid artery in the neck combined with simultaneous intracranial

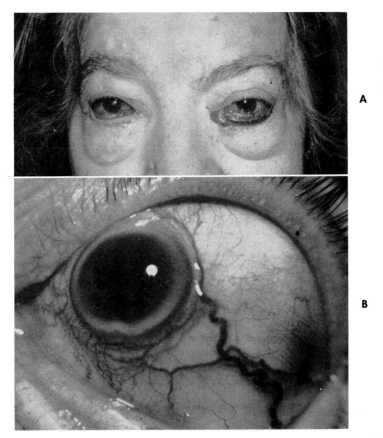

Fig. 26-2. A, Cavernous sinus fistula. **B,** Marked conjunctival vessel dilation with cavernous sinus fistula.

clipping of the internal carotid artery and the ophthalmic artery. The anastomoses between the external carotid artery and the ophthalmic artery will maintain vision in about 75% of patients in whom the ophthalmic artery is clipped. The recommendations described for infraclinoid aneurysms must be followed. Procrastination in favorable patients leads to irreversible tissue changes that cannot be corrected.

Supraclinoid aneurysms. Supraclinoid aneurysms usually arise at the bifurcation of the internal carotid artery into the middle and anterior cerebral arteries or at the junction of the internal carotid artery with the posterior communicating artery. Congenital berry aneurysms are common in

this region, but the majority of patients are middle-aged or older. Women are involved most frequently, and hypertension is present in many patients.

Symptoms occur suddenly, with severe unilateral headache and pain about the face and eye. Pain in the medial canthal region is particularly characteristic. The pain arises from meningeal irritation and not from direct involvement of the trigeminal nerve as occurs in infraclinoid aneurysms. Simultaneously with the headache, or within 72 hours, an oculomotor paralysis develops, with ptosis, exotropia, pupillary dilation, and failure of accommodation.

The prognosis for life is poorer with

supraclinoid aneurysms than with infra-clinoid aneurysms. Death occurs from subarachnoid hemorrhage or from bleeding into the brain. Untreated patients may experience no further episodes, presumably due to intravascular clotting, or may have recurrent attacks. Recovery with regeneration of the oculomotor nerve is seldom complete. A pseudo–von Graefe phenomenon is frequently present (p. 412), and pupillary abnormalities are observed. There may be loss of pupillary constriction, with stimulation of the retina with light and constriction with convergence. The pupil may be widely dilated with no reaction to light or accommodation.

Aneurysms of the middle and anterior cerebral arteries. Aneurysms of the middle and anterior cerebral arteries are particularly prone to cause defects in the visual fields. Optic atrophy is usually present. The visual field changes are bilateral and tend to be variable. An anterior cerebral artery aneurysm may cause a bitemporal hemianopsia, which begins in the inferior temporal quadrant rather than in the superior temporal quadrant, as in early pituitary adenoma. With aneurysm of the middle cerebral artery, there may be loss of vision in one eye, with a hemianopsia in the fellow eye. Subarachnoid hemorrhage is common.

Basilar aneurysms. Congenital berry aneurysms may arise at the anterior end of the basilar artery where it divides into the posterior cerebral arteries or at the posterior end where the vertebral arteries join to form the basilar arteries. The basilar artery is also the most common artery in the body to be affected with atherosclerosis.

The symptoms of basilar-vertebral aneurysms are variable and not characteristic. Dizziness, diplopia, and blurring of vision are the most common symptoms. There may be involvement of motor or sensory nerves on the brain stem, occipital

headache, deafness, memory impairment, and coma. Not infrequently diagnosis is not made until autopsy.

Subarachnoid hemorrhage. The chief causes of spontaneous bleeding into the space between the arachnoid and the pia mater are (1) vascular hypertension, (2) ruptured supraclinoid aneurysms, and (3) angiomas or arteriovenous malformations. Less common causes include blood dyscrasias, necrosis of metastatic or glial brain tumors, and spinal varices.

Subarachnoid hemorrhage is characterized by a sudden, violent head pain of shocking severity followed by photophobia and stiffness of the legs. Unconsciousness persisting a few hours to days may follow. Later there may be rigidity of the neck and spine. Lumbar puncture, in which only a few drops of fluid should be removed, indicates fresh blood. Bilateral carotid arteriography is indicated to determine whether the circle of Willis is normal and to determine the adequacy of blood supply from the contralateral side.

The ocular signs are mainly those described for unruptured supraclinoid aneurysms. In addition, there may be sudden loss of vision, papilledema, and exophthalmos. An uncommon but pathognomonic ocular sign is subhyaloid hemorrhage, which is located at the posterior pole adjacent to the optic disk and develops a fluid level with rest.

Treatment must be individualized. Hypothermia is not universally recommended, but it decreases the metabolic requirements of the brain and prevents cerebral edema. Surgical treatment should be carried out immediately in patients who are conscious or semiconscious, provided the collateral circulation is adequate. If the patient is in poor condition, surgery may be done 5 to 8 days later when the condition has improved or stabilized. Gradual occlusion of the common carotid artery in the neck is moderately effective in subarachnoid hemorrhage arising from ruptured aneurysms of the internal carotid or posterior communicating artery. The treatment of choice is exposure of the aneurysm and either clipping it, coating it with plastic, or inducing intravascular thrombosis by means of an electric current or an animal hair placed in the arterial wall.

Migraine

Migraine is a special type of headache characterized by recurrent, violent, usually unilateral head pain. It is preceded by an aura, usually of a scintillating scotoma, which may be most evident in an area of homonymous hemianopsia. There are nausea, vomiting, and photophobia followed by exhaustion and sleep. Women are affected more commonly than men. There is often a familial history. Onset is usually before the age of 20 years. In the stage of aura a vasoconstrictor such as ergot will prevent the cerebrovascular dilation that causes the headache. Once the headache is established, treatment is seldom effective.

In rare cases there develops a third cranial nerve paralysis with exotropia, ptosis, and pupillary dilation as the headache is receding. The headache persists for several hours or days and then clears without residue. In some individuals, however, the oculomotor paresis becomes permanent. It is debated whether such a paresis constitutes a true entity of ophthalmoplegic migraine or whether it reflects bleeding of a supraclinoid aneurysm.

On the basis of age of onset, history of migraine, and ophthalmoplegia developing as the headache recedes, it seems likely that ophthalmoplegic migraine is a definite disease.

Methysergide, a compound used in treatment of migraine, may cause a retroperitoneal fibrosis with ureteral obstruction, hydronephrosis, and vascular hypertension together with mediastinal fibrosis and sclerosing cholangitis. Associated with these signs may be bilateral pseudotumor of the orbit. This group of signs may also be unrelated to ingestion of the drug.

Diabetes mellitus neuropathy

Diabetes mellitus (p. 385) in rare instances is complicated by a neuropathy involving the cranial motor nerves. There is a severe unilateral headache usually followed by an abducens weakness. More rarely there is an oculomotor nerve palsy that does not involve the pupil in 75% of the instances. Diabetes mellitus neuropathy is distinguished from supraclinoid aneurysms usually by involvement of the abducens nerve, which is never involved individually in an aneurysm. The sparing of the sphincter pupillae muscle aids in the diagnosis of diabetes. Generally, if the pupil is not involved, the cause is medical, whereas if it is involved, the cause is an aneurysm or tumor.

Carotid-vertebral-basilar arterial occlusive disease

Occlusion of major cerebrovascular vessels ranks only after heart disease and cancer as a cause of death in the United States. About 40% of all cerebrovascular accidents are due to occlusive disease within the extracranial portions of the carotid and the vertebral-basilar system that are accessible to surgical approach. The chief cause of obstruction is atherosclerosis. Occasional instances are due to severe angulation, with kinking of arteries or occlusive disease from inflammation of the aortic arch or the subclavian artery.

Incomplete occlusion of the carotid and the vertebral-basilar system is characterized by episodes of focal cerebral ischemia that appear suddenly, last a few minutes, and disappear without residue. These attacks have the same clinical pattern, occur with increasing frequency, and about 50% of the patients will have a serious stroke in an average of 3 years. Of the remainder, one half will continue to have attacks, and the others will recover without further trouble.

Sudden complete occlusion causes loss of consciousness with contralateral motor and sensory defects known as a "stroke." Complete occlusion occurring over a long period may be completely compensated by collateral circulation, and the symptoms resemble those of the preceding insufficiency.

The symptoms of insufficiency are dependent upon the production of a temporary hypoxia in terminal portions of the cerebrovascular tree. Fig. 26-3 shows the wide variety of ophthalmic and neurologic symptoms arising from insufficiency. It is probable that less than 20% have the blood vessel distribution classically depicted in the circle of Willis. Transient ocular signs and symptoms occur in 80 to 90% of patients with carotid or vertebral-basilar insufficiency.

Carotid artery. The internal carotid arterial system or its branches (ophthalmic, anterior choroidal, anterior cerebral, and middle cerebral arteries) supply the frontal and parietal lobes, part of the temporal lobe, the corpus striatum, and the internal capsule. Occlusive disease is associated with contralateral impairment of motor or sensory function of the hand, arm, leg, or lower face. Insufficiency involving the left middle cerebral artery causes aphasia in right-handed persons. Unconsciousness simulating syncope occurs when an anterior cerebral artery is compromised.

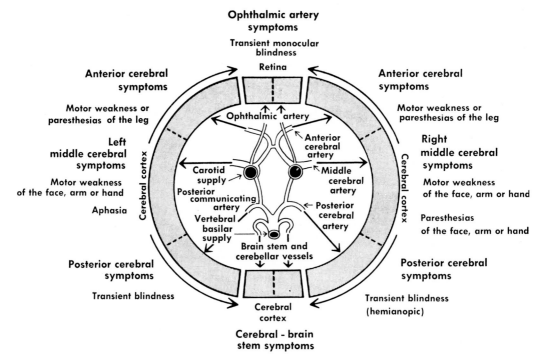

Fig. 26-3. Transient symptoms of cerebral vascular insufficiency. The carotid and vertebral-basilar systems are indicated centrally. The gray band represents the terminal areas of supply of these two systems. Hypoxia may occur at any position on this gray band as a result of decreased blood flow to that area. The wide variety of ophthalmologic and neurologic symptoms that may result is indicated. (From Hoyt, W. F.: Arch. Ophthal. **62:** 260, 1959.)

The chief ocular symptom of carotid insufficiency is transient loss of vision in one eye, called amaurosis fugax. It consists of sudden contraction of the visual field of one eye, varying from hemianopsia to loss of light perception. The pupillary light reflex is absent. The retinal arteries are markedly attenuated during an attack. Vision gradually returns after a few seconds or as long as 10 minutes. Permanent visual loss does not occur. Amaurosis fugax may also occur in migraine, impending central artery closure, and temporal arteritis.

Repeated attacks of amaurosis fugax may give rise to an ophthalmoscopic picture of cotton-wool patches in one eye, probably due to small infarcts secondary to vascular insufficiency. In patients with hypertension the occluded carotid artery may protect the retinal vasculature from the signs of arteriolar sclerosis or even hemorrhages and papilledema.

In both carotid and vertebral-basilar system insufficiency there may be showers of cholesterol emboli. These are observed near or at the bifurcation of retinal arterioles and appear as bright, yellowish orange plaques. With massage upon the globe, they tumble to the periphery.

Rarely in carotid insufficiency, venous stasis is seen on the same side as the diseased artery, with dilation of retinal veins, sludging of venous blood, microaneurysms, and small hemorrhages. If only the diseased eye were examined without regard to the nearly normal fellow eye, the abnormality could be mistaken for the retinopathy of diabetes, impending central vein occlusion, or pulseless disease.

Pulsation in the affected internal carotid artery may be diminished or absent. Palpation through the oropharynx is more reliable than through the neck. Even with complete occlusion of the internal carotid artery, there may be normal pulsation of the common or external carotid artery.

Auscultation of the neck and the mediastinum may reveal a bruit best heard over the bifurcation of the internal and external carotid arteries. The bruit of occlusive disease of the vertebral arteries is best heard over the supraclavicular area and is sometimes accentuated by turning the head to the opposite side.

Compression of the carotid artery may produce syncope suggesting an insufficiency of the vascular supply of the contralateral anterior cerebral artery. In vertebral-basilar artery insufficiency there may be syncope or convulsive movements. Compression is not recommended and has been known to produce permanent complete occlusion.

Angiography will demonstrate the site and extent of the occlusion but carries the risk of permanent complications. It is reserved preferably for the differential diagnosis of "stroke" or tumor in patients whose symptoms have appeared recently and in patients without brain infarcts who are good candidates for surgery.

Measurement of the pressure in the ophthalmic arteries with the ophthalmodynamometer has its greatest application in carotid artery insufficiency. The majority of patients have a 15 to 25% reduction in the diastolic pressure of the ophthalmic artery on the side of the occlusive disease. In about one fourth of the patients with proved disease, the pressure is the same or higher on the involved side. The test is not difficult to perform, but there are a number of limitations.

Vertebral-basilar system. The vertebral-basilar arterial system supplies the brain stem, cerebellum, occipital lobe, and a portion of the temporal lobe. The system arises from the two vertebral arteries, which are the first branches of the subclavian arteries. The vertebral arteries traverse the neck in the vertebral canals of the cervical vertebrae and unite within the cranium to form the basilar artery. The basilar artery supplies branches to the brain stem, the cerebellum, and the posterior cerebral artery supplies branches to the occipital lobe. It connects with the carotid circulation by means of the posterior communicating arteries.

Intermittent insufficiency of the vertebral-basilar arteries causes periodic transient episodes of cerebral ischemia with complicated and widespread neurologic signs. Involvement tends to be bilateral when the basilar artery is involved and unilateral when one vertebral artery is the site of the occlusion.

Involvement of the cochlear-vestibular system causes vertigo, nausea, and a staggering gait. Auditory system symptoms include partial deafness and unilateral tinnitus. There may be paresthesia, hemiplegia, or hemiparesis. Headache, dysarthria, dysphagia, and hiccupping occur.

Ocular symptoms are noted in numerous patients for many months prior to the occurrence of complete occlusion. There may be blurred vision, diplopia, transient homonymous hemianopsia, and scintillating scotomas. Blurring is usually bilateral, and the individual is occasionally blind momentarily. There are no ocular signs, and the condition is not discovered unless examination is made at the time of an attack.

Complete thrombosis causes a congruous homonymous hemianopsia and motor involvement of the eyes. There may be paresis of conjugate gaze, with a conjugate deviation to one side. Internuclear ophthalmoplegia occurs that is identical with that seen in multiple sclerosis. Horizontal or rotatory nystagmus is frequent. Horner's syndrome is occasionally present.

Treatment must be individualized. Surgery may be indicated in patients who have symptoms of recent onset that arise from an accessible artery and who do not have brain infarction or widespread atherosclerotic disease. In other patients with insufficiency, anticoagulation is the therapy of choice. Once a cerebral infarct has occurred, it seems unlikely that anticoagulation will do more than minimize the possibility of further occlusive episodes.

Aortic arch syndrome. Aortic arch syndrome is a chronic disorder arising from obstruction of the subclavian and the carotid arteries (Fig. 26-4). It includes pulseless disease, reversed coarctation of the aorta, and the subclavian steal syndrome. Symptoms arise from insufficiency of the cerebral blood supply and are similar to those described in carotid and vertebral-basilar insufficiency.

Pulseless disease is a giant cell arteritis of the aorta of unknown etiology involving mainly young Japanese females. It is associated with retinal neovascularization, venous engorgement, microaneurysms, and arterial and venous occlusions. The radial pulse is absent. There may be widespread ischemic changes involving the head and the upper extremities. Similar signs occur in an older age group apparently due to atheromatous obstruction near the origin of the subclavian and the carotid arteries.

Reversed coarctation of the aorta occurs in aortic arch occlusion and is a pattern of collateral circulation in which blood reaches the head, neck, and upper extremities through the intercostal, scapular, axillary, posterior and inferior thyroid, inferior epigastric, and internal mammary arteries.

The subclavian steal syndrome arises in stenosis or occlusion of the first portion of the subclavian artery. Blood flows up the contralateral vertebral artery and down the opposite vertebral artery to supply the subclavian artery distal to the area of occlusion. Symptoms arise from cerebral ischemia in the area of distribution of the vertebral-basilar system. A bruit in the subclavicular area and reduction of pulse and blood pressure in the ipsilateral arm suggest the diagnosis.

Brachial-basilar insufficiency arises in patients with occlusive disease of the

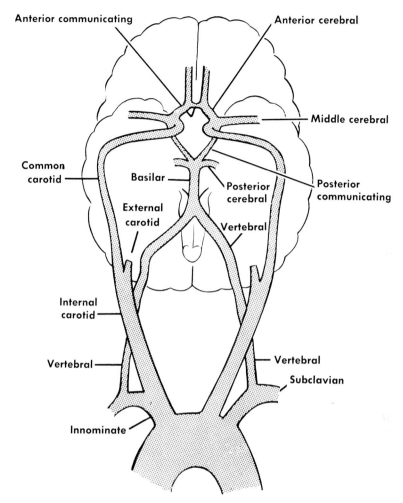

Fig. 26-4. Schematic representation of the primary cerebral arteries. Probably not more than 20% of persons possess the anatomic configuration illustrated in the circle of Willis. (From Callow, A. D.: New Eng. J. Med. **270:**547, 1964.)

proximal segment of the subclavian artery who develop transient ischemic vertebral-basilar symptoms when the arm is exercised. The symptoms arise as in the subclavian steal syndrome from retrograde blood flow through the ipsilateral vertebral artery.

Nystagmus

Nystagmus is an involuntary (usually, see following discussion), more or less rhythmic, back-and-forth movement of the eyes. It is usually easily detected by simple observation of the eyes but when minimal may be detected during ophthalmoscopy, the magnification of the fundus multiplying the movement.

Nystagmus is divided on the basis of its rhythm into pendular and jerk types. When pendular, the rhythm of the movements is regular. In jerk nystagmus there is a slow movement in one direction followed by a quick recovery movement in the opposite direction.

Pendular nystagmus. Pendular nystagmus is characterized by an amplitude of excursion that is approximately equal in the two directions. It is usually associated with loss of central vision involving both eyes. Most commonly it is seen in ocular disease in which central vision either fails to develop or is lost before the age of 2 years. It is seen in bilateral chorioretinitis destroying the macula, in aniridia, in total color blindness, in albinism, in congenital cataract, and in corneal scarring. It does not occur in complete blindness or if there has been several months of macular vision prior to the onset of defective vision.

Spasmus nutans occurs in children less than 2 years of age and is associated with head nodding. It is the most common cause of unilateral nystagmus in children. It has been attributed to poor illumination, but the cause is unknown. It invariably disappears. Miner's nystagmus is a fine, rapid, pendular nystagmus attributed to poor illumination in coal mines; it is not seen in the United States. Voluntary nystagmus is a rare type of pendular nystagmus that occurs in those able to bring about a rapid oscillation of their eyes, usually by extreme convergence. It is of no clinical significance but is an acquired talent, like wiggling one's ears.

Jerk nystagmus. Jerk nystagmus has a slow component in one direction and a rapid corrective movement in the opposite direction. Reference is made to the direction of the rapid component. Two major types of jerk nystagmus are seen: one involves the fixation apparatus or the neuromuscular mechanisms of the eye, and the other arises from the labyrinths or their central connections.

Opticokinetic nystagmus arises from looking at constantly moving objects such as telephone poles from a moving automobile or train. The slow component arises from fixation of the moving object and requires mediation through the striate cortex of the occipital lobe. The fast corrective component is presumably mediated through the higher cortical centers, possibly the opticomotor area of the frontal area. Inasmuch as the subject cannot voluntarily inhibit the eye movements, opticokinetic nystagmus has been widely used in the objective study of vision, particularly in infants and children. Clinically it is studied by having the subject look at a rotating drum or television screen on which there are a series of moving figures or moving alternate white and black lines. More simply, a 20-inch by 2-inch strip of alternating red and white squares, each 2 inches wide, may be used. In homonymous hemianopsia due to parietal lobe lesions, bringing targets from the blind to the seeing side does not elicit nystagmus. Opticokinetic nystagmus may be elicited in temporal lobe and occipital lobe lesions.

Latent nystagmus is an uncommon type of horizontal jerk nystagmus elicited by covering one eye or making the brightness or clarity of retinal images unequal in the two eyes. The slow component is in the direction of the covered eye, with the rapid corrective component in the direction of the open eye. With both eyes open, such patients may have normal vision, but when either eye is covered, vision in the open eye is 20/200 or less. There is no treatment.

End-position nystagmus is seen when the eyes are turned into an extreme position of gaze. It is horizontal or vertical. The slow component is toward the central primary position, and the fast corrective component is toward the extreme position of gaze. This may occur in normal persons who are debilitated or fatigued. It is marked in palsies of conjugate gaze. It may be caused by lesions of the subcortical centers for conjugate gaze.

Congenital nystagmus is a poorly defined abnormality that is usually of the jerk variety. It is first noted in the early months of life. It may be inherited and associated with other ocular defects. The head may be turned to place the eyes in a position of least nystagmus. The condition persists through life.

Vestibular nystagmus. Vestibular nystagmus is a reflex response arising from asymmetric stimulation of the semicircular canals or their central pathways. There are three semicircular canals in each labyrinth: horizontal, superior, and vertical. The otoliths of the inner ear function in controlling body musculature and in maintaining a conjugate deviation of the eyes with changes in position of the head, so that the eyes tend to maintain a primary position in reference to the ground. The major action is evident in torsion of the eyes. The function of the semicircular canals arises in acceleration or deceleration of the body, in which the tendency is for the eyes to oppose a change of position when the body is rotated. The slow component of the nystagmus is in the direction of the displacement of endolymph in the semicircular canals, which causes deviation of the eyes to the opposite side. Thus, if the body is rapidly rotated to the right, the nystagmus during rotation has its slow component to the left. When rotation stops, the slow component is to the right.

Vestibular nystagmus can be conveniently studied by rotation of the body or caloric irrigation of the external auditory canal, which sets up convection currents. Most attention is directed to study of the horizontal canals that involve mainly the medial and lateral rectus muscles. Stimulation of the vertical canals causes vertical and torsional nystagmus, making complicated analysis necessary.

Vestibular nystagmus occurs in diseases of the end-organ, its nuclei, or its central nervous system connections. Peripheral disease may be associated with vertigo, tinnitus, and deafness. The onset is abrupt. The nystagmus is horizontal and rotary and tends to decrease in the course of the disease. The common diseases causing peripheral involvement are labyrinthitis and Meniere's disease.

Involvement of the vestibular nuclei and the central nervous system connections causes a static or increasing nystagmus. Spontaneous vertical nystagmus is virtually always of central origin; spontaneous rotary nystagmus suggests involvement of vestibular nuclei. Both types may be triggered by administration of barbiturates. Nystagmus may occur in multiple sclerosis, encephalitis, vascular disease (particularly occlusion of the posteroinferior cerebellar artery), and cerebellar and cerebellopontine lesions. The latter are likely to produce nystagmus that varies with the position of the head. The fast component is toward the side of the lesion.

Abnormal eye movements

Abnormal eye movements may be rhythmic, as in nystagmus, or irregular and chaotic, as in opsoclonus, ocular dysmetria, ocular flutter, lightening eye movements, and ocular bobbing.

The movements in opsoclonus are in all directions, irregular, hyperkinetic, and often accompanied by myoclonic jerks of the face and body. The ocular movements are not in unison and may persist in sleep. Opsoclonus is most prominent in cerebellar ataxia and abnormalities involving the brain stem. An unexplained association between occult neoplasms, particularly neuroblastoma, and opsoclonus has been described.

Ocular dysmetria is an overshoot of the eyes on attempts to fixate an object. The amplitude of the overshoot progressively diminishes until steady fixation is achieved. Ocular flutter may occur spontaneously or on fixation, and there are intermittent, rapid, to-and-fro oscillations of the eyes of equal amplitude. Dysmetria and ocular flutter occur mainly in patients with cerebellar disease.

Lightening eye movements (ocular myoclonus) consist of rapid bursts of to-and-fro movements of small conjugate saccades (p. 89). The movements usually follow horizontal gaze toward the more paretic or ataxic side of the body. These movements occur in medial lesions involving the pons or pretectal region. Ocular bobbing occurs only in the vertical plane, and the eyes spontaneously, synchronously, and intermittently dip downward and then return to the primary position. Unlike vertical nystagmus, there is no fast and slow component. It has been described in advanced pontine disease.

Demyelinative disease

Demyelination occurs in a variety of disorders in which there is an initial loss of myelin. The group includes multiple sclerosis, neuromyelitis optica (Devic's disease), subcortical encephalopathy (Schilder's disease), and postinfectious encephalitis. These conditions may all affect vision through involvement of the optic nerve or optic radiation. In addition, they may cause ocular muscle weakness.

Multiple sclerosis. Multiple sclerosis is a chronic remittent disease of the spinal cord and brain. It typically involves the white matter of the brain and is characterized by disseminated areas of demyelination and glial scar formation. It affects mainly young adults and involves both sexes equally. There is a relatively high incidence and death rate in the northern regions of the United States and Canada, and there is a low incidence in the South. The etiology is unknown. Patients have antibodies against measles in their spinal fluid. The average duration of the disease is 27 years, and in the majority of patients there are remissions without permanent neurologic residue.

Retrobulbar neuritis is the initial episode of the disease in 15% of the patients, whereas in another 25%, paresis of an ocular muscle occurs. Of patients hospitalized because of multiple sclerosis, 70% have or have had retrobulbar neuritis. The fully developed disease is characterized by Charcot's triad of nystagmus, scanning speech, and optic atrophy. There is no treatment.

Neuromyelitis optica. Neuromyelitis optica appears to be an acute multiple sclerosis. It is characterized by a bilateral acute optic neuritis with a transverse inflammation of the spinal cord. The disease may occur at any age. There are prodromal signs of headache, sore throat, fever, and malaise. The visual loss occurs rapidly, with blindness or near blindness developing within a few days. Ascending paralysis and sensory disturbances occur within a few weeks before or after blindness. Patients may die within a month, or there may be complete remission with recurrences. There is no treatment.

Schilder's disease. Schilder's disease affects children and adolescents and is characterized by progressive involvement of the brain with loss of vision, spastic paralysis, deafness, mental deterioration, and death in a few months to a year. Papilledema occurs in the majority of patients.

Postinfectious encephalitis. Encephalitis may develop following viral infections such as measles, mumps, varicella, and vaccinia. It most commonly follows measles, and the mortality rate of measles encephalitis is 10%. There may be papilledema, papillitis, or retrobulbar neuritis. Recovery of vision is usual.

Familial autonomic dysfunction (Riley-Day syndrome)

Familial or central autonomic dysfunction is commonly associated with decreased or absent tearing, corneal anesthesia, and outward deviation of the eyes. Most but not all cases occur in children of Jewish extraction, and inheritance is via a simple autosomal recessive.

A wide variety of defects occur: (1) autonomic dysfunction with reduced or absent tears, postural hypotension, cold hands and feet, excessive perspiration, and diminished swallowing reflex is usually present; vascular hypertension and skin blotching with excitement, erratic temperature control, and drooling are frequently present; (2) sensory disturbances with relative indifference to pain, corneal anesthesia, and absent corneal nerves are usually present; dysesthesia and Romberg's sign may occur; (3) motor disturbances are manifested by poor motor coordination and dysarthria and less commonly by decreased deep tendon reflexes; and (4) psychologic disturbances with emotional instability (sullen, uncommunicative), mental retardation, and breath holding in infancy occur. The prognosis for life is diminished; general anesthesia presents unusual risks.

The fungiform and vallate papillae containing taste buds are absent. Intradermal injection of 1:1,000 histamine does not cause the usual flare. Partial parasympathetic denervation is suggested by hypersensitivity of the pupil to 2.5% methacholine (Mecholyl) eyedrops as occurs in Adie's syndrome (p. 221). Tearing is induced by subconjunctival or subcutaneous neostigmine. The ratio of urinary excretion of homovanillic acid to vanillylmandelic acid is increased.

The initial finding may be an absence of tears in an infant who has difficulty swallowing and has a feeding problem. By the age of 2 years the child drools constantly, is undernourished and awkward, and walks on his toes with a stumbling gait. High fever of unexplained origin is common, and convulsions occur in about one half of the patients. There is no specific systemic treatment.

In about one third of the patients the deficient lacrimation is associated with chronic, indolent, corneal ulcers, which cause remarkably little discomfort but reduce vision. Protection of the cornea by two intermarginal lid adhesions is the usual treatment.

Ocular differential diagnosis includes congenital absence of the lacrimal gland and a rare disorder, anhidrotic hereditary ectodermal dysplasia, in each of which the corneal sensitivity is normal. Keratoconjunctivitis sicca occurs in later years and, in addition to punctate or filamentary keratitis, has a stringy, mucoid discharge not present in autonomic dysfunction. Vitamin A deficiency with keratomalacia presents feeding problems, decreased tearing, and corneal ulcers, but the conjunctiva is affected initially and loses its luster, with dry spots appearing in it in contrast to the glistening, normal-appearing conjunctiva in autonomic dysfunction. Neuroparalytic keratitis is usually unilateral, follows trigeminal nerve injury, and has no associated systemic findings.

Chapter 27

Hereditary disorders

The accessibility of the eye to examination and the defective vision and the cosmetic defects produced by relatively minor structural abnormalities have led to the recognition of a large variety of ocular defects transmitted by changes in genetic material. Often the changes in the eye are associated with structural or biochemical defects involving other portions of the body, but in many conditions, such as the corneal dystrophies and some cataracts, systemic abnormalities cannot be detected with present methods.

The genetic composition of each human being is determined by 22 pairs of homologous autosomes together with a pair of sex chromosomes that are similar in the female (XX) and unlike in the male (XY). Each parent contributes an equal number of chromosomes to each individual. The male receives a Y chromosome from his father and an X chromosome from his mother. The female receives an X chromosome from each parent.

Each chromosome is composed of genes, which are the units of inheritance. Each gene is responsible for the synthesis of a specific enzyme. Gene differences result in variations in the quantity or quality of proteins by controlling the synthesis of the enzymes responsible for protein structure. Thus all biochemical processes in the body are under genetic control, and each different biochemical reaction is under the control of a different gene.

Possible mechanisms of the abnormality induced by absence of a gene are demonstrated below:

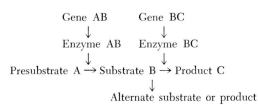

If gene BC is responsible for the enzyme that converts substrate B to product C, then (1) product C will not be formed, as occurs in albinism; (2) there may be an accumulation of substrate B, as occurs in alkaptonuria; (3) there may be an accumulation of presubstrate A, as occurs with glycogen accumulation in von Gierke's disease, a substrate several steps removed from the absent enzyme; or (4) there may be an accumulation of an alternate product or substrate, such as occurs in galactosemia, in which dulcitol appears responsible for the cataract formation.

In addition to these mechanisms, some abnormalities appear to be the result of a genetic defect in the transport of amino acids in renal tubule cells and probably elsewhere in the body. This type of abnormality is distinct from that occurring in alkaptonuria or homocystinuria, in which there is an overflow of a compound that accumulates proximal to an enzyme block.

Each gene has a partner or allele located at the same position (locus) on the corresponding or homologous chromosome contributed by the other parent. When these two allelic genes are similar and determine a similar characteristic, they are homozygous, and when they are different, they are heterozygous.

The occurrence of a genetic defect is determined by the behavior of a pair of allelic genes. If the genetic abnormality requires a double dose of the abnormal gene (the homozygous state), the expression of the abnormality is considered to be recessive. If the condition may be fully expressed by a single dose of the affected gene, the condition is said to be dominant.

Autosomal defects are carried on the nonsex chromosomes, and both males and females are affected and can transmit the abnormality to both sons and daughters. An autosomal dominant condition is one that may be expressed in the heterozygous state. Autosomal dominant conditions are generally less severe than recessive homozygous conditions and in general tend to be structural abnormalities with considerable variation in expression. Often the presence of the abnormal gene cannot be recognized, and some generations are apparently skipped because the carrier of the abnormal gene is clinically normal. When this is the case, the gene is called nonpenetrant. A heterozygous affected individual mated to a normal homozygote will on the average transmit the trait to half of his offspring, both sexes being equally affected. If two individuals are both heterozygous for a dominantly inherited trait, their offspring would be one-fourth homozygous affected, two-fourths heterozygous affected, and one-fourth homozygous normal. The homozygous affected state is frequently lethal, although the heterozygous state may be clinically mild. Autosomal dominant traits are recognized in human pedigrees by transmission from one generation to the next. Except for mutation and illegitimacy, every affected individual has at least one parent with the abnormal gene and may have affected offspring.

Retinoblastoma (p. 274) is an ocular example of an autosomal dominant condition. Most cases are sporadic, but survivors usually transmit the tumor as an autosomal dominant characteristic. Strabismus, some, but not all, congenital cataracts, blepharoptosis, some corneal dystrophies, craniostenosis, and Marfan's syndrome are all transmitted as autosomal dominant traits. Thus only a single dose of the abnormal gene, which may be derived from either parent, is required for clinical expression of the condition.

Autosomal recessive disorders are those conditions that require a double dose of the abnormal gene, such as occur in the homozygous state. In general, the autosomal homozygous affections are more severe than heterozygous affections and often cause inborn errors of metabolism. In the autosomal recessive trait, inheritance is from both parents who are usually normal clinically but are heterozygous for the abnormal gene. Thus, when both parents are heterozygous for a recessive trait, the offspring will be one-fourth homozygous for the abnormal allele, one-fourth normal, and one-half heterozygous for the recessive trait. Since related individuals are more likely to be heterozygous for the same abnormal gene, consanguinity is more likely to produce offspring affected by a recessive disorder.

Complete and circumscript albinism are examples of autosomal recessive expression. (Incomplete albinism may be either recessive or dominant. Albinism involving the eyes solely is a sex-linked recessive disorder.) Infantile amaurotic familial idiocy (Tay-Sachs disease, p. 441) is an autosomal recessive with fatal outcome. Congenital glaucoma (p. 317), galactosemia (p. 437), and the Riley-Day syndrome (p. 426) are examples of autosomal recessive traits.

Defects that are carried on the sex chromosomes may be heterozygous or homozygous in the female and heterozygous in the male. The female, having two X chromosomes and being either heterozygous or homozygous, can demonstrate either recessive or dominant behavior of a trait.

The male has only one X chromosome and thus carries only one half the complement of X-linked genes found in the female. His genotype is therefore referred to as hemizygous, whereas in the female the terms "homozygous" and "heterozygous" usually apply. There can be no father-to-son transmission because the male X chromosome is transmitted only to daughters and not to sons.

On the average, half of the sons of heterozygous females will be normal and half will be affected. An affected male married to a normal female will have daughters who are all carriers and sons who are all normal. Carriers may be clinically abnormal. The carrier daughters will transmit the abnormality to the next generation.

Dominant X-linked traits affect both males and females, who transmit the disorder to their offspring. The heterozygous female with one abnormal X chromosome derived from her father may demonstrate subtle signs of the carrier state and transmit the trait to half of her sons and daughters. The heterozygous male transmits the trait to all of his daughters but to none of his sons.

X-linked dominance occurs in some instances of pigmentary degeneration of the retina. Incontinentia pigmenti appears to be lethal in the homozygous male but nonfatal expressive in the heterozygous female.

In recessive sex-linked traits the heterozygous female frequently shows slight evidence of the carrier state and rarely marked clinical manifestations of the abnormality. In the heterozygous male, however, the deficiency is fully demonstrated. Ocular albinism, choroideremia (p. 267), retinoschisis (p. 265), and color blindness are ocular examples of recessive sex-linked disorders.

Disorders of amino acid metabolism

The major disorders of amino acid metabolism that affect the eye (Table 27-1) involve mainly the metabolism of either tyrosine or methionine. In albinism the biosynthesis of melanin from tyrosine is impaired because of the deficiency of tyrosinase. In alkaptonuria, homogentisic acid produced in the metabolism of phenylalanine and tyrosine accumulates because the enzyme homogentisic acid oxidase is missing. In phenylketonuria (an abnormality associated with minimal ocular signs), plasma phenylalanine increases because L-phenylalanine is not oxidized to tyrosine. In homocystinuria there is a defect in the metabolism of methionine to tyrosine.

Albinism. Albinism is an inherited metabolic defect of the melanocyte in which there is decrease or absence of melanin in the skin, hair, and eyes, resulting in the characteristic fair complexion, blond hair, and impaired vision. Melanocytes are derived from the neural crest and are normally located at the epidermal-dermal junction of the skin, hair bulb, pia-arachnoid, uveal tract, and retinal pigment epithelium. Those melanocytes present in albinism contain nonpigmented melanin granules. The metabolic defect consists of failure of the cells to synthesize tyrosinase, a requirement for the conversion of tyrosine to dopa (3,4-dihydroxyphenylalanine), which, after several more metabolic steps, forms the brown or black insoluble polymer melanin.

All types of albinism, except circumscript cutaneous, affect the eyes. In infants the iris is light gray in color and translucent so that light reflected from the fundus causes a generalized red reflex from the eye. With aging, the iris may become darker in color, but a bright light directed through the sclera indicates that the iris

Table 27-1. Disorders of amino acid metabolism

Disease	Defect	Inheritance	Systemic involvement	Eye involvement	Laboratory findings
Albinism (dopa not converted to melanin)	Absence of tyrosinase (in metabolism of tyrosine to melanin)				
Oculocutaneous		Autosomal recessive or irregular dominant	Diluted pigment of skin and hair	Ocular albinism: translucent iris, prominent choroidal vessels, decreased vision, photophobia, nystagmus	
Ocular		X-linked recessive	None	Ocular albinism	
Cutaneous		Autosomal dominant	Diluted pigment of skin and hair	None	
Chediak-Higashi		Recessive	Diluted pigment of skin and hair	Ocular albinism	Cytoplasmic inclusions in myeloid cells
Alkaptonuria (homogentisic acid excess)	Absence of homogentisic acid oxidase (in metabolism of phenylalanine and tyrosine)	Autosomal recessive	Arthritis (late), pigmentation (ochronosis) of cartilage and connective tissue, heart disease	Ochronosis of sclera and cornea	Homogentisic acid in urine (dark-colored urine)
Homocystinuria (homocysteine not converted to cystationine; homocystine accumulates)	Deficiency of cystathionine synthetase (in metabolism of methionine to cysteine)	Autosomal recessive	Mental retardation, seizures, malar flush, fair skin, thromboembolism	Dislocated lenses, cataract, high myopia	Homocystine in urine
Phenylketonuria (phenylalanine excess)	Absence of phenylalanine hydroxylase (oxidation of L-phenylalanine to tyrosine)	Autosomal recessive	Mental retardation, epilepsy, restlessness, hyperactive tendon reflexes, tremors	Light-colored iris, photophobia	Increased plasma phenylalanine, phenylpyruvic acid in urine

transmits light. Failure of the retinal pigment epithelium (which is present but does not contain melanin) to absorb light results in failure of the fovea centralis to develop. Central visual acuity is reduced. An ocular nystagmus is present. Visual acuity is worse for distance than for near, and often normal schooling is possible although the distance visual acuity is 20/200. Vision tends to improve as patients become older. The decreased vision is associated with a high incidence of strabismus. The outstanding symptom is photophobia with extreme intolerance to light. Ophthalmoscopic examination indicates a bright orange-red reflex with markedly prominent choroidal vessels, which are normally obscured by the retinal pigmented epithelium. The retinal vessels are normal.

A number of ocular defects have been described as occurring in association with albinism, such as hypoplastic iris, heterochromia irides (p. 226), mixed astigmatism (p. 351), and severe myopia (p. 349). Rarely there may be deaf-mutism or mental retardation.

In Caucasian albinos the skin is milk-white, and exposed areas become erythematous and do not tan with exposure to ultraviolet light. The hair is fine in texture, and its color ranges from white to blond. In Negro albinos the skin is copper-red; the hair texture is unchanged, and its color ranges from white to a yellow-brown.

Female carriers of ocular albinism may demonstrate a translucent iris on diaphanoscopy and show brown pigmentation in the equatorial region of the ocular fundus on ophthalmoscopy.

Treatment of albinism is usually directed toward accurate correction of the refractive error and the strabismus if present. The use of a strong reading addition for near work may be helpful. Colored lenses are used to reduce the amount of light entering the eye. Contact lenses with a central clear area surrounded by a pigmented area to simulate the normal pupil and iris

have not been found to improve vision but are helpful in reducing photophobia.

The *Chediak-Higashi syndrome* is a rare autosomal recessive disorder characterized by oculocutaneous albinism, severe pyogenic infections, granulocytopenia, neurologic defects, lymphomatous infiltration, and death before the age of 7 years from infection or hemorrhage. The disease is associated with abnormal giant lysosomes. Abnormal granules are present in myeloid cells, and inclusion bodies occur in cells of both lymphoid and monocytoid origin. The ocular signs and symptoms are those of albinism.

Alkaptonuria and ochronosis. Alkaptonuria is a rare hereditary disorder in which homogentisic acid, produced in the metabolism of phenylalanine and tyrosine, cannot be metabolized further because of the absence of the enzyme homogentisic acid oxidase. Homogentisic acid is a normal intermediate in the metabolism of tyrosine, and the enzyme for its oxidation is normally present in the liver, kidney, and possibly other tissues.

In affected individuals, homogentisic acid is actively excreted by the kidney and appears in the urine (alkaptonuria) in large amounts. It causes the urine to have a dark color or to become dark upon standing, provided the urine is alkaline and large amounts of ascorbic acid are not simultaneously excreted. The substance reduces Benedict's reagent and may give false positive tests for reducing substance in the urine.

Clinically alkaptonuria is characterized by generalized pigmentation of cartilage and other connective tissue (ochronosis), which in turn causes arthritis. The pigmentation is most prominent in the eyes, ears, and nose, and it becomes evident between the ages of 20 and 30 years. The ocular pigmentation arises from deposits of melanin or a melanin-like substance in the collagen bundles of the cornea, sclera, and elastic tissue of the conjunctiva, which de-

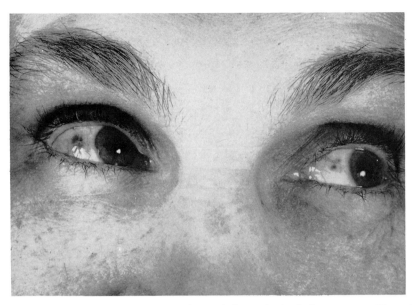

Fig. 27-1. Ochronosis involving the sclera of the palpebral fissure area. (From Hatch, J. L.: Arch. Ophthal. **62:**575, 1959.)

generate. The deposits appear on both globes in the palpebral fissure just in front of the insertions of the horizontal rectus muscle—they are oval in shape and have a slate-gray pigmentation (Fig. 27-1). Biomicroscopy of the cornea reveals tiny, round, golden brown deposits at the level of Bowman's membrane within the palpebral fissure. The concha and the anthelix of the ears have a drab blue-gray color. An associated arthritis commonly involves the spine, shoulders, knees, and hips and may cause the characteristic roentgenographic changes of thinning and calcification of the intervertebral disks and calcification of ear cartilage. There is a tendency for valvular heart disease, calcification of the heart valves, and atherosclerosis, with myocardial infarction a common cause of death.

Differential diagnosis involves pigmentation arising from Atabrine medication, senile hyaline degeneration of the sclera (p. 216), and malignant melanoma of the choroid.

There is no effective treatment.

Phenylketonuria. Phenylketonuria is an abnormality in which there is an absence of phenylalanine hydroxylase in the liver, causing an accumulation of phenylalanine in the plasma and phenylpyruvic acid in the urine. Those afflicted are born with normal neurologic and intellectual capacity but deteriorate progressively during the first 5 or 6 years of life. Phenylpyruvic acid in the urine is demonstrated by an olive-green color when using 5% ferric chloride impregnated on filter paper or testing a wet diaper.

The accumulation of phenylalanine and its metabolites in pigmented cells causes a competitive inhibition of tyrosinase. A defect similar to that in albinism may occur, so that the patient has lightly pigmented hair and skin and blue eyes. Other ocular changes are not specific and are related to the brain damage.

Homocystinuria. Homocystinuria is an autosomal recessive disorder in which patients excrete homocystine in the urine because of a hepatic deficiency of cystathionine synthetase, which functions in the conversion of methionine to cysteine. The disease varies in severity and is important to recognize because of the frequency of fatal thromboembolic accidents.

The main ocular finding is dislocation of both lenses (p. 288), which may cause a secondary glaucoma. A cataract may be present. Peripheral retinal degeneration may be associated with retinal separation (p. 265).

The disease is often recognized in early childhood. Mental retardation is usually, but not invariably, present. There may be convulsions, shuffling gait, and spasticity of the lower extremities. The children have fine, sparse hair, a fair complexion, and often rosy cheeks (malar flush). Some appear to have the same skeletal defects (arachnodactyly, long extremities, malformed thorax, and kyphoscoliosis) as seen in Marfan's syndrome. The platelets are excessively sticky, and death from pulmonary embolism is common. Renal infarction may cause a vascular hypertension, and cerebral infarcts may be the cause of mental retardation.

The cyanide nitroprusside urine color test is used for screening. A positive test indicates the need for amino acid studies to quantitate the urinary abnormality. Early detection is desirable because of the possibility of successful treatment by dietary methods.

Renal tubule transport defects

Cystine storage disease (Lignac-Fanconi) and the oculocerebrorenal syndrome (Lowe) arise from a disturbance in renal function with impaired tubular reabsorption (Table 27-2). This causes an excessive amino acid excretion and gives rise to complex metabolic disturbances often associated with rickets and ocular changes.

Cystine storage disease (Lignac-Fanconi). Cystine storage disease is a rare hereditary metabolic disorder occurring almost exclusively in infants and children. It is characterized by widespread deposition of cystine crystals in the kidneys, liver, spleen, bone marrow, lymph nodes, conjunctiva, and uveal tissues.

The disease begins between the fourth and sixth months of life with failure to grow, repeated emesis, recurrent fever, a severe form of rickets resistant to vitamin D in the usual doses, chronic acidosis, polyuria, and dehydration. An aminoaciduria involves a number of amino acids. There is progressive kidney damage, and chronic glomerulonephritis develops. There may be a terminal vascular hypertension with papilledema and ophthalmoscopic signs of severe vascular hypertension. Death usually ensues from uremia or intercurrent infection.

Crystalline deposits in the conjunctiva and the cornea are pathognomonic of

Table 27-2. Renal tubule transport defects

Disease	Defect	Inheritance	Systemic involvement	Eye involvement	Laboratory findings
Cystine storage disease (Lignac-Fanconi)	Impaired absorption of phosphate by renal tubule	Autosomal recessive	Vitamin D–resistant rickets or osteomalacia, acidosis, polyuria, dehydration	Cystine crystals in conjunctiva and cornea in childhood form	Aminoaciduria, glycosuria, hypophosphatemia, elevated alkaline phosphatase
Oculocerebrorenal syndrome (Lowe)	Not known	X-linked recessive	Rickets, mental retardation	Congenital cataract, congenital glaucoma, keratitis e lagophthalmos	Aminoaciduria

cystine storage disease. Good illumination and magnification are required for their demonstration because of their small size. They appear as tinsel-like, fine refractile crystals or fine white dots uniformly scattered over the entire cornea, predominantly in the anterior stroma (although the corneal bodies appear the same clinically as the conjunctival crystals, they do not have the same x-ray diffraction pattern and may not be cystine). In the conjunctiva the crystals are superficial and tend to aggregate in the walls of blood vessels. Their appearance is so typical that biopsy studies and chemical identification of cystine in the conjunctiva are not necessary for diagnosis. Photophobia is marked, but visual acuity usually seems normal. Ophthalmoscopically there is peripheral patchy depigmentation with pigment clumps that often form small rings. The posterior pole, disk, and blood vessels are normal.

Treatment is directed toward correction of the acidosis and a dietary supplement of phosphate. Improvement in skeletal and biochemical defects occurs with large doses of vitamin D (50,000 to 400,000 I.U. daily). Supplementary calcium may be necessary until the skeleton is normal, but development of hypercalcemia must be prevented. During acidosis, potassium may be depleted and require replacement.

Oculocerebrorenal syndrome (Lowe). Oculocerebrorenal syndrome is a rare sex-linked disorder in which the hemizygote demonstrates mental retardation, a renal defect causing aminoaciduria, and ocular abnormalities (cataract and congenital glaucoma occur). The female carrier has punctate opacities of the lens.

Disorders of carbohydrate metabolism

Diabetes mellitus (p. 385) is clinically the most important abnormality of carbohydrate metabolism, but the nature of the inborn defect is unknown. Galactosemia is an abnormality in which there is failure to

Table 27-3. Disorders of carbohydrate metabolism

Disease	Defect	Inheritance	Systemic involvement	Eye involvement	Laboratory findings
Galactosemia (galactose excess)	Absence of galactose 1-phosphate uridyl transferase	Autosomal recessive	Mental retardation, hepatosplenomegaly, vomiting, and dehydration	Cataracts	Reducing substance in urine (galactose), albuminuria, aminoaciduria, erythrocyte deficiency of galactose 1-phosphate uridyl transferase
Hepatorenal glycogenosis (von Gierke)	Deficiency of glucose 6-phosphatase	Autosomal recessive	Retarded growth, adiposity, hepatomegaly, eruptive xanthomas	Peripheral corneal glycogen deposition	Hypoglycemia, hyperglyceridemia, hypercholesterolemia, acidosis, hyperuricemia
Generalized glycogenosis (Pompe)	Deficiency of alpha glucosidase(?), deficiency of acid maltase(?)	Autosomal recessive(?)	Lethal, anorexia, muscle weakness, tongue enlargement, cardiac and CNS involvement	Clinically negative, but glycogen deposition in eye	Requires muscle biopsy

Table 27-4. Disorders of lipid metabolism in which serum lipids are increased or decreased

Disease	Defect	Inheritance	Systemic involvement	Eye involvement	Laboratory findings
A-beta-lipoproteinemia	Not known (inability to form chylomicrons)	Autosomal recessive	Retarded growth, abdominal distention, steatorrhea, muscle weakness	Pigmentary degeneration of retina, nystagmus	Abnormally shaped erythrocytes (acanthocytes), decreased plasma cholesterol and phospholipids, triglycerides absent
Familial alpha lipoprotein deficiency (Tangier)	Defective synthesis of high-density lipoproteins	Autosomal recessive	Cholesterol deposition in reticuloendothelial system, orange tonsils	Dots in cornea	Low plasma cholesterol and phospholipids, normal triglycerides
Hyperlipoproteinemia Type I (fat-induced hyperchylomicronemia)	Decreased lipoprotein lipase, excessive chylomicrons	Autosomal recessive	Xanthomas, hepatosplenomegaly, episodic abdominal pain, pancreatitis	Lipemia retinalis	Plasma postheparin lipolytic activity (PHLA)
Type II (familial hypercholesterolemia)	Increased beta lipoprotein (low-density protein)	Autosomal dominant or acquired: myxedema, nephrotic syndrome, obstructive hepatic disease	Lethal atherosclerosis, tendon or tuberous xanthomas	Corneal arcus, xanthelasma, lipid keratopathy	Hypercholesterolemia, normal triglycerides and phospholipids
Type III	Increased beta and pre-beta-lipoprotein, carbohydrate induced	Recessive (type II gene + diabetes gene?)	Atherosclerosis, xanthomas, lipids in creases of palms, hepatosplenomegaly, cholelithiasis, cholecystitis	Xanthelasma, corneal arcus	Hypercholesterolemia and hyperlipemia, hyperuricemia
Type IV (familial hyper-pre-beta-lipoproteinemia)	Increased pre-beta-lipoprotein, carbohydrate induced	Recessive: often secondary to diabetes, alcoholism, myxedema, etc.	Same as type III	Same as types I, II, and III	Abnormal glucose tolerance, triglyceridemia, normal cholesterol
Type V (combined hyperchylomicronemia and hyper-pre-beta-lipoproteinemia)	Carbohydrate and fat induced	Gene for types I and IV(?), homozygous type IV(?)	Same as type I	Same as types I, II, and III	High cholesterol and excessive chylomicrons

convert galactose to glucose and lactose. The glycogen storage diseases do not have prominent ocular changes; but in von Gierke's disease, peripheral corneal clouding has been noted, and in Pompe's disease, glycogen is found in retinal ganglion cells, corneal endothelium, pericytes of the retinal capillaries, extraocular muscles, and ciliary muscle.

Galactosemia. Galactosemia is a hereditary abnormality of galactose metabolism in which there is impairment of enzymatic conversion of galactose to glucose. Galactose and glucose combine to form lactose, the main carbohydrate of milk, which is split in the intestine into its two component hexoses. The metabolic block occurs in the enzyme galactose 1-phosphate uridyl transferase responsible for conversion of galactose 1-phosphate to glucose and energy, and there is an accumulation of galactose 1-phosphate, galactose, and dulcitol.

Galactosemia is transmitted as an autosomal recessive. The afflicted children are normal at birth, but soon after they begin to ingest milk they develop feeding problems, with vomiting, diarrhea, and failure to thrive. Bilateral cataracts occur frequently. They appear to be due to the accumulation of dulcitol (a sugar alcohol) and water and not directly to galactose 1-phosphate accumulation. In the early stages there is increased nuclear refractive power (as occurs with senile nuclear sclerosis), and the opacity appears as a

drop of oil in the center of the lens. In other cases a zonular type of opacity develops. If galactose is removed from the diet, cataracts will either not develop or, if present, will not progress.

Systemically there is hepatomegaly with abdominal distention and sometimes with jaundice and ascites. Cirrhosis may develop. Mental retardation is common. Albuminuria and aminoaciduria may be present, and the urine reduces Benedict's solution. It is imperative to identify the reducing substance as galactose.

Diagnosis is based upon the presence of a nonglucose-reducing agent in the urine and the demonstration of the metabolic defect by means of erythrocyte assay for galactose 1-phosphate uridyl transferase. The galactose tolerance test is dangerous and should be avoided.

Treatment involves exclusion of milk and other galactose-containing foods from the diet. If treatment is instituted early, mental retardation, cataract formation, and impairment of hepatic function may be avoided. As the patients grow older, they may tolerate galactose without ill effect.

Disorders of lipid metabolism

The end results of disorders of lipid metabolism are well recognized—an abnormal accumulation of lipids in the plasma or body tissues or both. The underlying defects causing the accumulation are studied with difficulty not only because of the lability of lipid components in blood and

Table 27-5. Disorders of lipid metabolism in which serum lipids are normal

Intracellular accumulation of:	Diseases
Sphingolipids	Sphingolipidosis—Farber's disease, Niemann-Pick disease, Tay-Sachs disease, generalized gangliosidosis, Gaucher's disease, Krabbe's disease, diffuse angiokeratoma, metachromic leukodystrophy
Cholesterol	Cholesterol lipidosis (histiocytosis)—xanthogranuloma (nevoxanthoendothelioma), eosinophilic granuloma, Hand-Schüller-Christian disease, Letterer-Siwe disease
Phytanic acid	Refsum's disease (heredopathia atactica polyneuritiformis)

their intimate relationship to carbohydrate metabolism but also because of the unavailability of analytic tools, mainly ultracentrifugation. The conditions associated with abnormal lipid metabolism may be roughly divided into those in which the plasma lipids are either abnormally elevated or depressed (Table 27-4) and those in which the plasma lipids are normal but there is an intracellular accumulation of sphingolipids, cholesterol, or phytanic acid (Table 27-5).

The major lipids in the plasma are listed in Table 27-4. The fatty acids are derived from adipose tissue triglycerides are not "free" but bound to albumin. The complex releases the fatty acids at sites of utilization. When the amount of fatty acids in the plasma exceeds the capacity of the tissues to utilize them, they are converted by the liver to triglycerides and may give rise to an endogenous hyperlipemia.

Cholesterol and the phospholipids constitute a portion of the alpha and beta lipoprotein molecule and function in transporting triglycerides. Cholesterol is derived from the diet and from intestinal biliary sterols synthesized into cholesterol in the liver. The phospholipids vary only slightly and are present mainly as "biologic detergents" to promote stability at the oil-water interface formed by lipoproteins and plasma.

Glycerides arise either from endogenous synthesis, mainly in the liver, or from dietary fat. Plasma glycerides of endogenous origin are transported predominantly on a very low-density pre-beta-lipoprotein. This is composed predominantly of glycerides (50 to 70%), with a small amount of cholesterol (10 to 25%) and phospholipid (15 to 25%) and a minute amount of protein (2 to 15%). Dietary (exogenous) glycerides are carried on lipid-protein complexes large enough to be seen with the light microscope–chylomicrons. These enter the bloodstream from the intestinal lymphatics through the thoracic duct and are hydrolyzed by the enzyme lipoprotein lipase in adipose tissue, liver, heart, and other organs and the constituent fatty acids resynthesized into triglyceride. The deposition or mobilization of fat is regulated by the presence or absence of food, particularly carbohydrates, and the presence or absence of activities requiring fat for sudden energy.

Beta carotene is converted in the intestine to vitamin A alcohol (retinol) and ester and transported together with other carotenes to the bloodstream in association with chylomicrons. Retinol is transported with a high-density protein in the blood, but the carotenes together with vitamins D, E, and K are found mainly in beta lipoproteins.

The alpha lipoproteins (or high-density proteins) are composed of about 50% protein, 30% phospholipids, 18% cholesterol, and 2% triglycerides. The beta lipoproteins (or low-density proteins) are composed of about 25% protein, 22% phospholipids, 43% cholesterol, and 10% triglycerides. Some 90% of the cholesterol and phospholipid in the plasma are contained in the lipoprotein.

A-beta-lipoproteinemia (acanthocytosis). A-beta-lipoproteinemia is a congenital abnormality in which there is an absence of beta lipoproteins and abolition of virtually all glyceride transport. It is characterized by abnormally shaped erythrocytes (acanthocytes), malabsorption of fat, pigmentary degeneration of the retina leading to blindness, and progressively severe neurologic defects.

The disease is evidenced in infancy by retarded growth, abdominal distention, and steatorrhea. Cholesterol and phospholipids are extremely low and glycerides are absent. In childhood, malabsorption becomes less severe, but muscle weakness, nystagmus, and degeneration of the posterior lateral columns and cerebellar tracts occur. Pigmentary degeneration of the retina (p. 265) is evident at the age of 8 to

10 years. There is no specific treatment and life expectancy is limited.

Familial alpha lipoprotein deficiency (Tangier disease [Tangier Island, Virginia]). Familial high-density lipoprotein deficiency is a genetic disease transmitted as an autosomal recessive and characterized by the deposition of cholesterol esters in reticuloendothelial tissues, particularly the tonsils. The tonsils may be markedly enlarged and of orange color or have stripes of orange alternating with the usual red color. There is an absence of alpha lipoprotein, a low cholesterol and phospholipid concentration in the plasma, but moderately elevated glyceride concentrations. The cornea is diffusely infiltrated with fine dots that are visible only with the biomicroscope. Visual acuity appears not to be affected. Cholesterol is deposited elsewhere in the skin, blood vessels, and reticuloendothelial system.

Hyperlipoproteinemia. It is beyond the scope of this book to discuss the varied manifestations of the hyperlipoproteinemias. For the most part, the ocular involvement, although sometimes of diagnostic significance, is only incidental to the abnormal metabolism and limited life expectancy associated with atherosclerosis.

The major ocular manifestations of hyperlipoproteinemia include lipemia retinalis, corneal arcus, xanthelasma, and ophthalmoscopic signs of atherosclerosis involving the central retinal artery before it bifurcates into arterioles.

Lipemia retinalis (p. 391) occurs because of an excessive number of chylomicrons (dietary lipids) in the plasma. It occurs in a familial form in hyperlipoproteinemia type I and far more commonly in carbohydrate-induced (particularly diabetic ketosis and in pancreatitis and alcoholism) types IV and V. In hyperlipoproteinemia type I there is a decrease of the enzyme lipoprotein lipase manifested by a decrease of plasma postheparin lipolytic activity (PHLA). In types IV and

V, lipemia retinalis is exceptional in the primary type and much more common in secondary types. Usually a triglyceride concentration in excess of 2,000 mg./100 ml. is associated with chylomicrons, giving the appearance of lipemia retinalis.

Corneal arcus (gerontoxon, arcus senilis, embryotoxon, p. 200) is a common deposition of phospholipid and cholesterol in the corneal stroma and anterior sclera. Generally, it appears as a deep, sharply defined, yellowish white ring, frequently incomplete, in the cornea concentric to the corneoscleral limbus (Fig. 27-2). It involves the entire thickness of the cornea but is usually most marked in Descemet's membrane and least marked in the midstroma. The area nearest blood vessels is clear, but when corneal vascularization is present, the opacity affects that area preferentially.

The significance of corneal arcus in lipid metabolism is not established. It is apparently a normal concomitant of the aging process, but this impression should be studied carefully by means of modern lipid chemistry. In individuals under 30 years of age its occurrence suggests an abnormality of lipid metabolism but may be

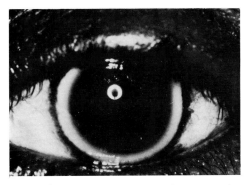

Fig. 27-2. Corneal arcus in Negro patient. Grossly there is a clear interval between the outer periphery of the infiltrate and the corneoscleral limbus. The condition is more common in Negroes.

genetically related to factors other than systemic lipid disease. It occurs commonly in familial hypercholesterolemia (type II) and less frequently in types III, IV, and V.

Xanthelasma (p. 166) is a cutaneous deposition of lipid occurring most commonly in the skin of the lids near the medial canthus. Xanthelasma does not occur with hyperchylomicronemia but is common in other hyperlipoproteinemias, which are often associated with xanthomas of tendons, particularly the Achilles tendon, and tuberous xanthomas over extensor surfaces. These findings are most common in hyperlipoproteinemia types II and III. In types IV and V, eruptive xanthomas are more frequent, but this inflammation is rarely associated with xanthelasma. The relatively frequent occurrence of xanthelasma in patients without demonstrated lipid abnormalities requires additional study.

Atherosclerosis (p. 402) is a vascular abnormality characterized by focal necrosis and thickening of the intima, lipid deposition in the intima and subintima, and hyperplastic and degenerative changes in the muscular coat of the artery, particularly in the internal elastic lamina. Atherosclerosis does not cause symptoms or functional changes unless there is obstruction or a focal decrease in the blood supply to a region, but it is distinctly localized in distribution. Therefore the presence of atherosclerosis in one vessel does not indicate a similar involvement in another vessel.

Sphingolipidosis. The sphingolipids are complex compounds that have ceramide in common. Ceramide consists of a long-chain amino alcohol joined to a fatty acid through an acid-amide linkage. In a variety of hereditary diseases either ceramide or complexes conjugated to it accumulate in the tissues and give rise to visceral, neurologic, and ocular manifestations. These conditions, known collectively as sphingolipidoses, include Farber's disease (unsubstituted ceramide), Niemann-Pick disease (sphingomyelin and cholesterol), Tay-Sachs disease (ganglioside), generalized gangliosidosis, Gaucher's disease (glucocerebroside: ceramide-glucose), Krabbe's disease (ceramide-galactose), diffuse angiokeratoma of Fabry (ceramide-trihexoside), and metachromic leukodystrophy (sulfatide lipidosis).

Farber's disease. Farber's disease is an autosomal recessive abnormality in which there is an accumulation of ceramide in subcutaneous nodules over joints and in nodules in the larynx. The disease begins in the first few months of life. The swelling of the joints of the hands and feet suggests rheumatoid arthritis, and the laryngeal nodules cause a hoarse cry and respiratory difficulties. The macular region may appear gray or cherry red, but there are no visual abnormalities. The infants do poorly and die within 2 years.

Niemann-Pick disease. Niemann-Pick disease is an abnormality in which there is widespread accumulation of lipid, mainly sphingomyelin and cholesterol, in the reticuloendothelial and nervous systems and in the parenchymal cells of many organs. There is patchy destruction of ganglion cells and demyelination of many parts of the nervous system. The involvement of both the nervous and visceral systems is in contrast to Tay-Sachs disease, which involves only the nervous system, and Gaucher's disease, which involves the viscera only in adults.

The condition is probably transmitted as an autosomal recessive and tends to involve children of Jewish parentage. The onset is usually about the sixth month of life, with fatal termination about the third year, although some patients survive until adulthood.

Poor feeding may be the earliest sign, followed by retardation of physical and mental development. Nearly every organ may be infiltrated with lipid, and there is huge enlargement of the liver and spleen with abdominal distention, marked infiltration of lymph nodes and bone marrow, unexplained fever, and yellow-brown pigmentation of the skin. A cherry red spot may develop in one or both eyes, and widespread involvement of the nervous system may cause a variety of sensory, motor, and psychic signs.

Gangliosidosis. Gangliosidosis is a familial disease that involves the central nervous system exclusively in the Tay-Sachs form or the viscera in the generalized type. It is characterized by the accumulation of gangliosides in the tissues. The ganglioside in Tay-Sachs disease is different from that in the generalized type.

Tay-Sachs disease (amaurotic familial idiocy, ganglioside lipidosis) is an autosomal recessive abnormality that has its onset in the first year of life. (Involvements later in life are referred to as [1] late infantile, or Jansky-Bielschowsky disease (onset at the age of 3 or 4 years); [2] juvenile, or Vogt-Spielmeyer disease (onset at the age of 5 to 10 years); and [3] adult, or Kufs' disease. It is not known if ganglioside accumulation occurs in types other than the infantile form or Tay-Sachs disease.) Infants of Jewish parentage are often, but not exclusively, affected.

The disease may have an insidious onset with listlessness, retardation in development, or feeding difficulties. The most common initial symptom is a startled reaction to sound (hyperacusis). Vision is affected early, with inattentiveness, failure to move the eyes, or strabismus. Ophthalmoscopic examination may be normal initially, but soon the macular area shows a whitish area ophthalmoscopically that is approximately 2 disk diameters in size, with a small reddish central area (cherry red spot). Retinal and optic atrophy follow, with eventual blindness. As neurologic involvement progresses, convulsions or a state of decerebrate rigidity may occur.

Death from bulbar involvement usually occurs at about the age of 30 months.

The white spot at the macula is produced by swelling and degeneration of the numerous ganglion cells located there. The cherry red spot arises from the appearance of the choroidal circulation at the fovea centralis where the inner layers of the retina are absent. Changes in the brain include enormously swollen and distorted ganglion cells. Fibers arising from these cells are demyelinated, which also contributes to optic atrophy. Glial cells proliferate and are converted to foam or fat cells.

The neuronal changes are not histologically characteristic, but biochemically there is a large accumulation of ganglioside throughout the nervous system. (Gangliosides also accumulate in the brain in gargoylism. In gargoylism this is considered to be a secondary deposition occurring in degenerated tissue, with the primary abnormality arising in mucopolysaccharide metabolism.)

Children with Tay-Sachs disease do not have fructose 1-phosphate aldolase in their serum. The enzyme is decreased in the serum of their mothers and fathers. The enzyme level is normal in Niemann-Pick disease, Gaucher's disease, Hand-Schüller-Christian disease, and juvenile amaurotic idiocy. Tay-Sachs disease is an autosomal recessive condition that appears in the homozygous state, when each parent contributes an allele to the phenotype.

Generalized gangliosidosis involves viscera as well as nervous tissue. Progressive cerebral degeneration develops early in life and the infants die within 2 years. A cherry red spot has been noted in three of ten cases described.

Gaucher's disease. Gaucher's disease is a rare familial disorder characterized by the accumulation of a lipid, glucocerebroside, in the reticuloendothelial system. It may have its onset at any time of life, the different manifestations depending upon the age of onset. Development of the disease before the age of 6 months leads to widespread neurologic involvement with mental retardation, spasticity, hepatosplenomegaly, and eventual death from intercurrent infection. Development of the condition after the age of 6 months leads to a condition dominated by the effects of an increasing mass of Gaucher's cells in the liver, spleen, lymph nodes, and bone marrow. There are hepatosplenomegaly and lymphadenopathy, bone lesions causing spontaneous fractures, and involvement of the spleen and bone marrow, with resultant pancytopenia often necessitating splenectomy. The skin is pigmented. Ultimately there is interference with blood cell formation and death from intercurrent infection. There is no mental retardation.

The Gaucher cell is typically a large cell in which the cytoplasm has an irregular, streaked appearance resembling wrinkled tissue paper. It stains strongly with periodic acid–Schiff reaction. There is a marked increase in acid phosphatase activity in plasma, tissues, and Gaucher's cells themselves. It is not inhibited by tartrate in contrast to the prostate enzyme. Blood lipids are normal.

Large yellow-brown pingueculas may develop, with their bases at the cornea and extending outward. These occur after childhood, are larger and darker than those occurring spontaneously in middle life, are asymptomatic, and require no treatment. Typical Gaucher's cells have not been described in them.

Krabbe's disease. Krabbe's disease is a familial diffuse sclerosis causing spasticity, dementia, and rigidity. It has its onset in the first 6 months of life and leads to death from emaciation at the age of 1 or 2 years. Blindness due to optic atrophy occurs commonly. Unlike other types of sphingolipidosis, there is no storage of sphingolipids in tissues, but rather an absence or deficiency of sulfur transferase that normally sulfates ceramide-galactose. The globoid cell is characteristic. It resembles a large epitheloid cell and occurs in demyelinated areas.

Diffuse angiokeratoma (Fabry's disease). Diffuse angiokeratoma is a sex-linked hereditary abnormality characterized by the deposition of neutral trihexoside in the endothelium of blood vessels. Its onset is in adolescence. There are burning pain in the extremities, fever, and telangiectasis involving the thighs and genitalia. There are fingerprint lines in the cornea due to epithelial deposition of an abnormal substance. A star-shaped haze of the lens occurs. The veins of the conjunctiva and ocular fundus are abnormally tortuous. The fingerprint lines may occur in the corneas of female carriers.

Metachromic leukodystrophy (sulfatide lipidosis). Metachromic leukodystrophy is an autosomal recessive disorder in which ceramide-galactose accumulates in the nervous system. Typically its onset is in the first 10 years of life. Weakness, ataxia, dysarthria, ocular muscle palsies, and terminally severe mental retardation and spasticity occur. Optic atrophy and blindness eventually develop. Late infantile and adult varieties may occur. Material that stains red with toluidine blue (metachromic) is found in urinary sediment and collects in viscera and ganglion cells, including those of the retina.

Refsum's disease (heredopathia atactica polyneuritiformis). Refsum's disease is a rare autosomal recessive disorder with retinal degeneration, polyneuritis, deafness, ataxia, and other cerebellar signs. Symptoms may arise in childhood, but diagnosis may be delayed until the second or third decade. Retinal pigmentary degeneration and deafness usually precede lower leg weakness, muscular atrophy, drop foot, and loss of deep tendon reflexes. The pupils are miotic and react poorly to light. Nystagmus and cataract may be present. The cerebrospinal fluid protein may be markedly elevated but without an associated pleocytosis. Ataxia, dysarthria, and nystagmus suggest cerebellar involvement. Other common findings include ichthyosis, anosmia, and skeletal abnormalities.

A specific disturbance of lipid metabolism may relate this condition to the sphingolipidoses. Urinary excretion of phytanic acid (3,7,11,15-tetramethyl hexadecanoic acid) causes a thin, fatty layer on its top. Exacerbation with remissions is common. There is no effective treatment.

Disorders of connective tissue

The specialized cells of the eye as well as other parts of the body are supported by connective tissue fibers embedded in a nonstructural matrix. The connective tissue consists of (1) cellular elements, (2) collagenous and elastic fibers, and (3) ground substance.

The cellular elements are derived from mesenchyme and include (1) fibroblasts responsible for the elaboration of the endogenous elements of connective tissue; (2) macrophages, which are histiocytes that function as phagocytes; (3) mast cells, which are implicated in the formation of heparin and possibly of hyaluronic acid, and which are rich in histamine and serotonin; (4) plasma cells, which produce antibodies; and (5) lymphocytes, which carry the genocopy of antigenic determinants that they transmit to immunologically competent cells.

The main fibrous elements of connective tissue are collagen and elastic fibers. Collagen is a fibrous protein of high tensile strength having characteristic striations with regular bands at intervals of 640 Å. It contains two unique amino acids, hydroxyproline and hydroxylysine, and large amounts of proline and glycine.

Elastic fibers are extensible structures that are stained by orcein and digested by elastase. They are found in tissues characterized by extensibility, such as arteries, skin, and some ligaments.

The ground substance (from the German words *grund substanz* meaning fundamental) is the extracellular, extrafibrillar, amorphous matrix of connective tissue. Some components are derived from the fibroblast, such as acid mucoprotein, acid mucopolysaccharide, and soluble or procollagen. In addition, it contains water, molecules such as glucose, cell metabolites, plasma proteins, and similar substances reflecting the passage of metabolites through it between cells.

Pseudoxanthoma elasticum. Pseudoxanthoma elasticum is a hereditary abnormality characterized by changes in the skin, cardiovascular system, and eyes. The basic defect is presumably in the elastic fibers, and widespread systemic changes occur because of involvement of the muscular arteries. The skin of the face, neck, axillary folds, inguinal folds, cubital areas, and periumbilical areas becomes lax and grooved, redundant and relatively inelastic, and resembles coarse-grain Moroccan leather. Involvement of the small muscular arteries may cause hemorrhages in the gastrointestinal tract, which must be distinguished from those occurring with peptic ulcer. Similarly, hemorrhages may occur in the brain, kidney, uterus, bladder, and nose. A severe hypertension that aggravates the hemorrhagic tendency occurs commonly.

The characteristic ocular change is angioid streaks (p. 272), a bizarre network of pigmented lines involving particularly the posterior pole and often associated with hemorrhage and focal chorioretinal atrophy. They arise presumably because of a defect in Bruch's membrane. Ultimately there is involvement of the foveal region, and loss of central vision develops. A disciform degeneration of the macula commonly occurs.

The basic lesion in the skin consists of changes in the deep and middle zones of the corium with the aggregation of a material that stains like elastic fibers. There is no specific treatment for the disease.

Osteogenesis imperfecta. Osteogenesis imperfecta is a hereditary disease that has wide systemic manifestations and an exceedingly large range of clinical severity. It arises from a deficiency in the formation of bone matrix. Characteristically the afflicted adult has short legs as compared with the upper parts of the body. Fractures of the long bones and gross bony deformities are common.

The scleras in patients with osteogenesis imperfecta are vividly blue. The color has been described as robin's egg blue, slate blue, and Wedgewood blue and is apparently caused by thinning of the sclera so that the choroid is seen beneath. Often the corneoscleral limbus is white, resulting in a Saturn ring. Juvenile corneal arcus is common. The eyes are frequently hyperopic, and there may be keratoconus, megalocornea, and maculas of the cornea. The ocular changes resemble those seen in Axenfeld's syndrome (p. 192). The fundamental defect suggests that there is failure of maturation of collagen, which remains in the reticulum fiber stage.

Treatment is symptomatic.

Ehlers-Danlos syndrome. Ehlers-Danlos syndrome is a widespread systemic disorder transmitted by a heterozygous allele. It is characterized clinically by a hyperelastic skin, a defect that permits the afflicted individual to be exhibited as the India rubber man in a sideshow. The skin is fragile and brittle, bruising occurs easily, and pseudotumors commonly occur at pressure points. There is hyperextensibility of the joints with associated flatfoot, clubfoot, and habitual dislocation of the joints. There may be multiple internal abnormalities such as diaphragmatic hernia, spontaneous rupture of the lung, dissecting aneurysm of the aorta, and other congenital defects.

The skin of the eyelids is often involved. Epicanthal folds may be present similar to those seen in mongolism and thalassemia. The eyelids are easily everted. Eso-tropia is common, as are blue scleras, and glaucoma has been recorded. Additionally, there may be ectopia lentis, proliferating retinopathy, hemorrhages into the retina, and detachment of the retina.

The abnormality arises from a lack of normal tensile strength of the collagen fibers, the cause of which is not known.

Marfan's syndrome. Marfan's syndrome is a widespread systemic abnormality basically involving the elastic tissues and transmitted as a dominant trait. The systemic manifestations include aortic dilatation, dissecting aneurysm of the aorta, muscular underdevelopment, femoral and diaphragmatic hernias, and multiple skeletal defects. The extremities are long, and characteristically the pubis to sole measurement is in excess of the pubis to vertex measurement. The arm span is in excess of the height. The more distal bones tend to demonstrate this excessive length, and arachnodactyly (spider fingers) is the result. There is weakness of the joint capsule, with flatfoot, hyperextensibility of the joints, recurrent dislocation of the hip, and kyphoscoliosis. Pigeon breast (pectus excavatum) may occur. Frequently the patient has a long, narrow face and a highly arched palate, and prognathism is present.

There may be widespread ocular changes, with subluxation of the lens being the outstanding change. Characteristic deformities of the chamber angle are present (Fig. 27-3). The lens is usually dislocated upward and inward, and the zonular fibers are drawn taut in the inferior temporal quadrant. Ectopia lentis may be suspected only because of the abnormal mobility of the iris (iridodonesis), which lacks the support of the lens. The lens may be smaller than normal and may be spherical. In some patients, ectopia lentis may be the only stigma of Marfan's syndrome.

Patients with this abnormality tend to be myopic and to develop retinal degeneration with subsequent retinal detach-

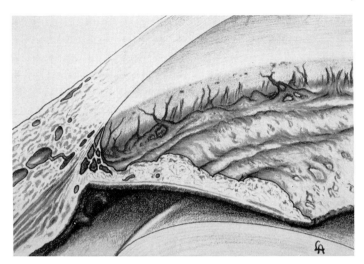

Fig. 27-3. Chamber angle abnormalities in Marfan's syndrome. (From Burian, H. M., von Noorden, G. K., and Ponseti, I. V.: Arch. Ophthal. **64:**671, 1961.)

ment more commonly than normal. The retinal degeneration is apparently related to an elastic fiber defect and not to the myopia. Heterochromia iridis may be present as well as keratoconus, megalocornea, and blue scleras.

In general, surgery is not indicated for the subluxated lens (p. 288). Complications are common, and surgery should be deferred unless necessitated by glaucoma not effectively treated medically.

Mucopolysaccharidoses. Connective tissue contains several distinct acid mucopolysaccharides consisting of repeating and alternating units of hexosamine and hexuronic acid combined with a protein. They are divided into two main groups, nonsulfated and sulfated. There are two nonsulfated mucopolysaccharides, hyaluronic acid and chondroitin. Hyaluronic acids occurs in the vitreous humor, synovial fluid, and umbilical cord. Chondroitin has been isolated only from the cornea. These nonsulfated mucopolysaccharides are apparently not involved in genetic mucopolysaccharidosis, although children with characteristic bone deformities and mental retardation may excrete a modified hyaluronic acid.

Five sulfated mucopolysaccharides have been described: chondroitin sulfate A, B, and C, heparitin sulfate, and keratosulfate. Chondroitin sulfate A and keratosulfate have been found in the cornea and heparitin sulfate solely in the aorta. Chondroitin sulfate A is found also in bone, cartilage, aorta, and ligamentum nuchae. Chondroitin sulfate B has been isolated from skin, tendon, heart valves, aorta, and ligamentum nuchae. Chondroitin sulfate C has been demonstrated in cartilage, umbilical cord, tendon, and nucleus pulposus. Chondroitin sulfate A and C, the major constituents of normal urine, are not apparently involved in genetic mucopolysaccharidoses.

Gargoylism (Fig. 27-4), also known as lipochondrodystrophy or Hurler's disease, is a widespread systemic disorder usually evident within 6 months after birth. It is characterized clinically by skeletal deformities, limitations of joint movements, hernia, hepatosplenomegaly, cardiac abnormalities, deafness, mental retardation, and diffuse corneal clouding. There is urinary excretion of chondroitin B sulfate and heparitin, and presumably the signs arise from accumulation of these mucopolysac-

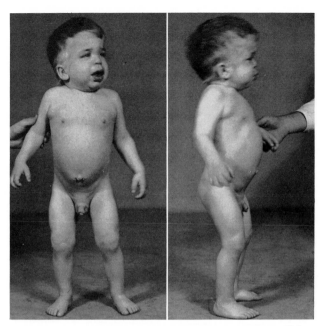

Fig. 27-4. Typical gargoyle appearance. (From Newell, F. W., and Koistenen, A.: Arch. Ophthal. **53**:45, 1955.)

charides in tissues in which they do not normally occur.

The condition is an autosomal recessive. There is no recorded instance of an individual with the disease living to an age to reproduce. Those infants with gargoylism resemble each other far more closely than they do their normal siblings.

Typically the patient has a large and bulging head, the bridge of the nose is flattened and the nostrils are broad, and the posterior pharynx is occluded. The children are mouth breathers and have markedly carious teeth and a fetid breath. The facies are apathetic, the tongue enlarged, and the facial features coarse and ugly. The neck is so short that the head appears to rest directly upon the thorax. Kyphosis is common, as are deformities of the vertebrae. The broad hands have stubby fingers, and on roentgenologic study, the terminal phalangeal bones are found to be hypoplastic. Limitation of extension of the joints is striking. The abdomen is protuberant. Roentgenographic

examination reveals a long and shallow sella turcica.

Clouding of the cornea is quite characteristic. The subepithelial area has the appearance of slightly glazed glass. The central cornea is more cloudy than the periphery, although histologically the periphery seems to be more involved. Not infrequently the initial ocular diagnosis is glaucoma, but the normal tension, absence of tearing, failure of the globe to enlarge, and associated physical changes aid in establishing the correct diagnosis. The main abnormality is in the deep layers of the epithelium (Fig. 27-5). Changes have been described in the endothelium. Rarely, increased intracranial pressure occurs, but associated papilledema is difficult to observe through the cloudy cornea.

The urine of these patients shows marked increase in excretion of chondroitin sulfate B and heparitin sulfate, which is also found in the brain and skin of some of the patients. It is of interest that chondroitin sulfate B normally occurs in all

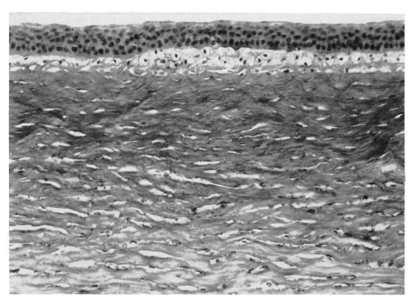

Fig. 27-5. Deposition of mucopolysaccharide in the subepithelial area of the cornea in gargoylism. (Aniline blue–orange fuchsin stain; ×256.) (From Newell, F. W., and Koistenen, A.: Arch. Ophthal. **53:**45, 1955.)

connective tissue except cartilage, bone, and cornea, the tissues that are markedly involved in this disease.

Hunter's syndrome is inherited as an X-linked recessive. Clinically patients resemble those with Hurler's disease, but clinical manifestations are less severe and grossly the corneas are clear, although there may be a slight corneal haze in occasional patients. Patients may survive into adulthood and mental retardation may not occur. Chondroitin sulfate B and heparitin sulfate are excreted in abnormal amounts in the urine, and there may be a greater proportion of heparitin sulfate than in the Hurler type.

Sanfilippo, Podosin, Langer, and Good described an entity characterized by severe mental retardation, but less marked dwarfing, hepatosplenomegaly, and other clinical manifestations than in the Hunter or Hurler syndromes. Corneal involvement is not marked, but retinal pigmentary degeneration occurs. These children excrete abnormal quantities of heparitin sulfate in the urine. Genetic transmission is as an autosomal recessive.

Morquio's syndrome includes a variety of bony disorders described clinically and lacking biochemical confirmation. These patients are markedly dwarfed and later develop characteristic skeletal changes. Clinically they resemble less severe examples of Hurler's disease, but mental retardation is not observed. Transmission is as an autosomal recessive. Diagnosis necessitates the demonstration of excessive urinary excretion of keratosulfate.

Maroteaux, Leveque, and Lamy described a boy with a condition similar to the Hunter disorder in addition to corneal clouding who excreted an excess of chondroitin sulfate B in the urine.

Scheie, Hambrick, and Barnes described an autosomal recessive trait in which patients have severe corneal clouding, moderate dwarfism, and normal intelligence. Two patients were found by Linker to excrete both chondroitin sulfate B and heparitin sulfate in the urine, while McKusick and associates found other patients excreted only chondroitin sulfate B. The clarification of this entity requires further study.

Hereditary corneal dystrophy (macular corneal dystrophy, Groenouw's type II), an autosomal recessive involving the eyes solely, is characterized by slowly progressive visual loss due to the intracellular accumulation of a mucopolysaccharide within keratocytes. There is no abnormal excretion of mucopolysaccharides, and skin fibroblasts do not demonstrate an abnormality of mucopolysaccharides.

Miscellaneous disorders

Hepatolenticular degeneration (Wilson's disease). Hepatolenticular degeneration, or Wilson's disease, is a rare familiar disorder. It is characterized by an abnormality of copper, and perhaps of protein metabolism, and increased tissue and urinary excretion of copper combined with a diminished ceruloplasmin level and increased serum copper.

The disease rarely becomes clinically evident before the eighth year of life, and signs may be delayed until the second or third decade. The cerebral or hepatic signs usually dominate the clinical picture.

Cerebral symptoms involve either (1) classic lenticular degeneration (usually without hepatic signs), with spasticity, rigidity, dysarthria, and dysphagia, or (2) pseudosclerosis (Westphal), with the major symptom being tremor. Symptoms suggesting schizophrenia or other less pronounced behavior or personality abnormality may occur in the absence of motor involvement. Jacksonian epilepsy or hemiplegia may develop, as may a coma that persists for several weeks.

Cirrhosis of the liver may dominate the clinical picture and may occur with minimal neurologic signs. In the mild involvement, symptoms of hepatic dysfunction are uncommon, but retention of Bromsulphalein can be demonstrated. In severe involvement, portal hypertension with esophageal varices and hepatic coma may develop.

Renal function may be affected. There have been reports of aminoaciduria with a predominance of cystine (but without cystine calculi), albuminuria, impaired concentrating capacity, glycosuria, alkaline urine, increased uric acid excretion with low serum uric acid, hyperphosphaturia with low serum phosphate, and osteomalacia.

The Kayser-Fleischer ring of the corneotrabecular region is pathognomonic of the condition. It consists of a brown-green-yellow ring at the corneoscleral limbus, usually first evident above and below and then forming a complete ring. It occurs at the level of Descemet's membrane and, with a gonioscope, can be observed to involve the trabecular area. The ring is present in about 80% of cases. Its absence can be excluded only by biomicroscopic examination of the cornea. The ring is occasionally present when other clinical signs are absent, although an abnormality of copper metabolism can be demonstrated.

Ocular signs other than the Kayser-Fleischer ring include sunflower cataract. This involves the posterior polar area of the lens and is similar to that seen with intraocular retention of a copper foreign body. Night blindness has also been reported, and degenerative changes have been described in the peripheral retina but have not been related to the primary disease.

Treatment is directed toward diminishing the copper in the diet and increasing the copper excretion. Penicillamine chelates copper and increases its excretion. Amelioration of symptoms and signs, including disappearance of the corneal deposits, has been reported. The diagnosis of asymptomatic Wilson's disease is based upon demonstration of low plasma ceruloplasmin and elevated hepatic copper. Early treatment is important to delay or prevent the overt manifestations of the illness.

Amyloidosis. Amyloidosis is a bizarre, nonspecific systemic disorder characterized by the focal or generalized deposition of amyloid, a birefringent, amphorous, fibrillar protein-polysaccharide having a distinctive ultrastructure. Classification is not satisfactory. Amyloidosis may appear spontaneously or in a familial form associated with familial Mediterranean fever (recurring polyserositis). Secondary amyloidosis is related to chronic suppuration, notably tuberculosis, chronic osteomyelitis, and lung abscess, and to bronchiectasis and leprosy. It complicates aging and diseases associated with tissue destruction as occurs in infection, malignant tumors (notably hypernephroma), Hodgkin's disease, rheumatoid arthritis, regional enteritis, chronic ulcerative colitis, chronic pyelonephritis, and paraplegia with suppurating decubitus ulcers. Many instances are associated with multiple myeloma and other tumors.

Ocular symptoms in amyloidosis are due (1) to neuropathy secondary to deposition of the abnormal protein in nerves to the eyes, (2) to vascular fragility and obstruction from amyloid deposition in vessel walls, (3) to functional impairment and structural distortion consequent to the mass effect of amyloid tumor, and (4) to opacification of the vitreous body.

Ocular signs include proptosis, ptosis, thickening of the lids, and hemorrhage into the lids, conjunctiva, sclera, or retina. Ocular palsy and pupillary abnormalities have been reported, as have ocular pain, unexplained blindness, and glaucoma. Vitreous opacities may be pathognomonic of the condition; they appear as veil-like "glass-wool" vitreous opacities. In the absence of an aqueous flare in the anterior chamber, the material is presumably amyloid.

Diagnosis of amyloidosis is best confirmed by biopsy of tissues of the skin, sternal marrow, kidney, or rectal mucosa. The Congo red test is positive less frequently in primary than in secondary amyloidosis.

Secondary amyloidosis is treated by control of the underlying disease, particularly suppuration. The therapy of the primary type is solely symptomatic. Removal of a core of affected vitreous to provide a clear media has recently afforded improvement of vision when the vitreous body was infiltrated.

Chromosome abnormalities. Chromosomal abnormalities in man arise from a variation in their number or an alteration in their structure. In general, chromosomal aberrations are associated with widespread defects involving a number of systems. Adequate diagnosis necessitates chromosomal analysis, which is usually done using skin fibroblasts or peripheral blood.

Numerical variation. Mongolism (p. 295), or Down's syndrome, is the most common cause of mental retardation that can be recognized at birth. The most frequent chromosomal abnormality is trisomy of the G group (chromosomes 21 and 22), resulting in a total of 47 rather than 46 chromosomes. This finding is most common in children of mothers more than 40 years of age. Less frequent and occurring in younger mothers in whom children with Down's syndrome are far less common (14:1) is translocation of chromosome 21 to a nonhomologous chromosome. Rarely there appears to be a normal karotype of 46 chromosomes, but this is presumably due to inability to detect insertion of a G group chromosome into a larger chromosome.

The 13 (13 to 15 group) trisomy syndrome (D-trisomy or Patau syndrome) consists of multiple congenital defects, including harelip, cleft palate, polydactyly, umbilical hernia, and malformations of the heart and central nervous system. Infants seldom live more than a few weeks. Microphthalmia, coloboma of the iris and choroid, and retinal dysplasia are the most frequent ocular findings. Intraocular cartilage has been noted in about half of the cases studied histologically.

Chapter 28

Collagen diseases and muscle disorders

Collagen diseases

The term "collagen disease" was originally introduced to describe a group of maladies characterized by the deposition of fibrinoid material in the ground substance of connective tissue and by widespread inflammation of connective tissue, conspicuously collagen. The fibrinoid material consists of a protein that may be the result of a disturbance in DNA metabolism of mesenchymal cells, as is the case in systemic lupus erythematosus, or may be the product of a hypersensitivity reaction, as is likely in rheumatic fever and polyarteritis.

It has been proposed that the plasma cells initially produce an abnormal gamma globulin, which then causes a diffuse injury to the collagen fibers of connective tissue. The term "dysgammaglobulinemia" has been suggested for the diseases caused by this mechanism. It is likely that there are a variety of causes and that clinical manifestations are governed by the distribution of the changes and their rate of development. Many of the diseases respond favorably to systemic corticosteroids, which has led inaccurately to the designation of "collagen" disease for any disorder of obscure etiology that improves with corticosteroid therapy.

Systemic lupus erythematosus. Systemic lupus erythematosus is a generalized sys-temic disorder that may involve nearly any system and may be associated with severe constitutional signs. Young women are affected predominantly. The disease appears to arise from a hyperreactive immunologic system that causes the synthesis of antibodies to numerous substances, including the patient's own cells. There is marked variation in the major clinical manifestations and their severity. Fever, a rash on the face with a "butterfly" distribution, and an arthralgia may occur. Glomerulonephritis, pericarditis, myocardial and endocardial lesions, or pleurisy may develop. Mental changes, convulsions, and cranial nerves may be involved, with diplopia, nystagmus, and decreased vision. Leukopenia due to a decrease in mononuclear cells is common. Hypergammaglobulinemia is present, and there is an increased fibrinogen and erythrocyte sedimentation rate, false positive tests for syphilis, and positive flocculation tests. An autoantibody, 7S gamma globulin, induces the formation of lupus erythematosus cells, and antinuclear and anticytoplasmic antibodies are present. Lupus erythematosus may simulate almost any clinical disease, and the diagnosis may be neglected because of failure to associate successive involvement of different systems with the same disease.

External involvement of the eye is mainly erythema and puffiness of the eyelids when involved in the "butterfly" rash. The most common ocular sign is cotton-wool deposits (p. 255) of the characteristic type occurring at the posterior pole. The lesions appear during a toxic phase of the disease and disappear with remission. They appear first as soft, white spots that become sharply delineated and gradually disappear over a 1-month to 3-month period. There is no hypertensive vascular disease associated with their appearance. Changes other than cotton-wool deposits have been described rarely: secondary optic atrophy, superficial and deep retinal hemorrhages, and arterial and venous occlusion.

Generalized scleroderma (progressive systemic scleroderma). Generalized scleroderma is a systemic disease of collagen tissue involving adults, with major symptoms that may involve any system. The cutaneous signs are widespread leathery skin, which becomes atrophic and pigmented. The eyelids lose their freedom of movement and then become thin, smooth, and shiny. Cutaneous signs may not occur. Major systemic involvement includes Raynaud's phenomena, dysphagia, pulmonary insufficiency, pulmonary hypertension, cardiac signs, polymyositis, and rheumatoid arthritis. Abnormal gamma globulins are present, with associated reactions similar to those described in systemic lupus erythematosus.

Sjögren's syndrome (p. 452) may occur. An atypical uveitis, with graying of the eyelashes (poliosis), vitiligo, and dysacousia (Vogt-Koyanagi syndrome, p. 241), has been described. Cotton-wool deposits of the retina without vascular hypertension may occur.

Rheumatic fever. Rheumatic fever is an inflammatory disease that occurs following infection with a strain of group A beta hemolytic streptococci. It has major manifestations of carditis, arthritis, chorea, subcutaneous nodules, fever, erythema marginatum, and pulmonary changes. There are numerous laboratory signs of antibodies to streptococcal antigens.

Ocular symptoms are uncommon. Localized, acute, deep choroiditis without involvement of the retina may occur and resolve without residue. The lesions tend to occur in the more severe cases. In bacterial endocarditis complicating rheumatic fever a septic retinitis may occur as the result of an embolus lodging in a retinal artery.

Rheumatoid arthritis. Rheumatoid arthritis is a chronic systemic disease of unknown cause that has a familial tendency with onset between the ages of 25 and 50 years. Women are affected more commonly (75%). The onset is insidious, with pain and swelling in one or more joints, which may become chronic and involve all joints with contraction and deformity. There may be constitutional disturbances such as lymphadenopathy, splenomegaly, fever, tachycardia, leukocytosis, and elevated sedimentation rate. Subcutaneous nodules occur at sites of pressure over bones. They vary in size from 2 to 3 mm. to 3 cm. in diameter. They are composed of a central necrotic area surrounded by a zone of fibroblasts enveloped in a zone of granulation tissue.

The ocular manifestations are due to an inflammatory-exudative alteration in connective tissue elements. Ocular changes are fairly common, so that the possibility of associated rheumatoid arthritis must be considered in every case of nongranulomatous iritis and scleral inflammation.

Iritis may precede or follow the acute disease but usually accompanies it. Most attacks are mild, may involve either eye, and may be recurrent. The severity of the attack varies. It responds quickly to systemic and local corticosteroids. In some patients the inflammation is extremely severe and unresponsive to therapy, with the eye going on to secondary glaucoma and cataract formation.

About 4% of the patients with rheumatoid arthritis develop iritis. In ankylosing spondylitis (p. 236) the incidence is much higher and has been estimated at from 15 to 50%. In Still's disease the incidence is about 15%. Posterior inflammation is uncommon, but bilateral retinal detachment has been described in Still's disease.

Juvenile rheumatoid arthritis (Still's disease). Juvenile rheumatoid arthritis is an uncommon disease identical with the adult form and occurring insidiously about the time of the second dentition. Systemic signs of fever, leukocytosis, splenomegaly, lymphadenopathy, and hepatomegaly are common. Iritis is common and tends to be bilateral and resistant to treatment. Secondary cataract may develop. In 9% of the patients a band-shaped keratopathy develops, with a deposition of calcium in the superficial layers of the cornea. It usually accompanies the iritis. A similar keratopathy occurs in degenerated eyes, in excessive vitamin D intake, and in hypercalcemia.

Scleromalacia perforans. Scleromalacia perforans is a complication of severe progressive rheumatoid arthritis in which rheumatoid nodules develop in the sclera and cause the sclera to gradually melt away (Fig. 28-1). Both eyes are usually involved, although the onset is not simultaneous. Pain is severe, and the eyes often develop a secondary glaucoma. A variety of grafts have been described to repace the sclera: fascia lata, aorta, cadaver sclera, and the like. Treatment is often ineffective.

Rheumatoid nodules in the sclera may also cause a massive granuloma (brawny scleritis or annular scleritis), in which there is massive scar formation, or necroscleritis nodosa, which is limited to small areas of the anterior sclera.

Sjögren's syndrome. Sjögren's syndrome is a chronic systemic disease characterized by the triad of keratoconjunctivitis sicca, xerostomia, and rheumatoid arthritis. The disorder characteristically affects middle-aged women. It is occasionally associated with systemic lupus erythematosus, derma-

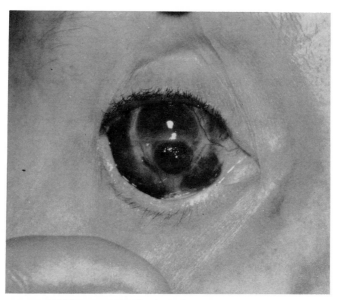

Fig. 28-1. Scleromalacia perforans in rheumatoid arthritis. The iris is prolapsing through a corneal defect, and the choroid is visible through the thinned sclera.

tomyositis, or generalized scleroderma, which replace rheumatoid arthritis in the disorder.

The chief symptoms relate to the eyes. They are dry and burning with moderate photophobia. Dry and hot environments aggravate the symptoms, which are often not immediately diagnosed. Examination rarely indicates a filamentary keratitis with minute horns of epithelium extending forward from the cornea. A foamy xerosis secretion may be present. Large areas of epithelium may be absent, and the conjunctiva and cornea stain with Bengal rose. The Schirmer test (p. 183) indicates less than 5 mm. wetting of the paper strip. The enzyme lysozyme is decreased in the tears early.

Xerostomia is often not recognized by patients, but invariably they are unable to swallow a tablet of medication without drinking water. The arthritis is mild but severe enough frequently to cause the patients to seek relief.

The laboratory signs suggest the disorder. The gamma globulins and the sedimentation rate are elevated. The C reactive protein and similar serologic tests for the rheumatoid factor are positive. Hashimoto's thyroiditis and Sjögren's disease exhibit similar pathologic changes in the thyroid, lacrimal, and salivary glands. Patients with Sjögren's disease develop Hashimoto's thyroiditis in 5% of the instances and positive thyroglobulin titers in some 25% of the instances.

Treatment is often unsatisfactory. Conditions favoring the rapid evaporation of tears should be avoided. The instillation of artificial tears, usually methyl cellulose solution, gives transient relief and is innocuous. Closure of the puncta to conserve remaining tears is usually ineffective, although often not utilized except when involvement is severe.

Dermatomyositis. Dermatomyositis is an acute or chronic disease of middle life characterized by edema, dermatitis, and multiple muscle inflammation. It often follows an infection, and in patients more than 40 years of age may be associated with a neoplasm (20%). A peculiar periorbital edema associated with a reddish brown erythema of the eyelids (heliotrope) may occur. Ophthalmoplegia, nystagmus, and episcleritis have been described. A retinopathy with cotton-wool deposits may be present.

Polyarteritis (periarteritis nodosa). Polyarteritis is a necrotizing angiitis causing a variety of symptoms depending upon the blood vessels involved. Men are involved more frequently (75%), usually between the ages of 20 and 50 years. Constitutional symptoms of fever, weight loss, and arthralgia occur. Presenting symptoms include abdominal pain, renal disease often causing a vascular hypertension when healed, peripheral neuritis, myocardial infarction, pulmonary infiltration, and asthma. Leukocytosis is present, often with a marked eosinophilia, and the sedimentation rate is high. The disease is often fatal, but remissions, and recovery occur. Symptomatic relief follows administration of steroids.

Ophthalmologic findings are common, although frequently the eyes are not examined. Involvement of cerebral vessels may cause subarachnoid hemorrhage, headache, vertigo, and convulsions. There may be involvement of motor nerves of the eye or decreased vision with involvement of the optic tracts or radiation.

Local involvement of ocular vessels has caused conjunctival chemosis and scleral necrosis. Involvement of the pericorneal arcade may be followed by corneal necrosis beginning at the corneoscleral limbus. Involvement of the choroidal vessels in a periarteritis has been found histologically with no history or signs of disturbed function. Choroidopathy has also been observed. Hypertensive retinopathy with papilledema, cotton-wool deposits, and vasospasm may follow renal disease and be in no way different than any other vascular hypertension. Cotton-wool deposits may develop as a toxic sign unrelated to hypertension as in the other collagen diseases.

Temporal arteritis. Temporal arteritis (giant cell arteritis) occurs in patients past 65 years of age and is characterized by malaise, fever, weight loss, and severe headache. The temporal arteries are painful, tender, and prominent, with nodularity and frequently erythema of the overlying skin. Pain on chewing is a common complaint. Other findings include tinnitus, deafness, arthritis, iritis, and spleen and liver enlargement.

In 1 to 4 weeks after the onset of the disease, sudden loss of vision may arise due to closure of the short posterior ciliary arteries supplying the optic nerve. Occlusion of the central retinal artery is less common. There may be branch occlusion of retinal vessels, hemorrhage, exudates, and rarely ocular pain. Often both eyes are affected, the second eye from 1 to 21 days after the first.

Palsies of external ocular muscles especially of the lateral recti muscles, may occur. Loss of vision may occur in some patients without obvious evidence of temporal artery involvement, but biopsy of the vessel may indicate the typical giant cell arteritis.

The diagnosis of temporal arteritis should be considered in all cases of sudden loss of vision, ocular vascular occlusion, and unexplained ophthalmoplegia in the age group past 60 years. The sedimentation rate is elevated during the active disease, and temporal artery biopsy should be performed if the ocular symptoms are associated with an abnormal test. Histologic studies of the involved artery indicate marked reduction of lumen or occlusion of the vessel combined with connective tissue proliferation adjacent to the lumen, with round cells and giant cells

in the region of a ruptured internal elastica.

Once vision is lost it seldom improves, but remarkable recovery has been reported. Corticosteroids should be administered before permanent visual loss has occurred.

Serum sickness. The immunologic mechanism in serum sickness is comparable to that discussed in experimental uveitis (p. 237). A foreign serum is injected, and 7 to 11 days later there is an acute illness with fever, arthralgia, urticaria, lymphadenopathy, abdominal pain, nausea, and vomiting. Cerebral swelling may cause neuritis, asphasia, hemiplegia, and cranial nerve signs. Optic neuritis may occur. The lids are involved in the facial edema, and there may be conjunctival chemosis. Corneal edema has been described. Cotton-wool deposits and retinal and optic nerve edema have occurred. Cataract developed in one case.

Other connective tissue disorders

Connective tissue changes may be involved in a variety of abnormalities in which there are eye signs. Some of these diseases are being discussed here solely for the sake of convenience. They may on occasion present one or more of the signs discussed in collagen diseases, but this appears to be mainly coincidental. Reiter's disease (urethritis, conjunctivitis, uveitis, p. 237) and Behçet's syndrome (aphthous ulcers, uveitis, p. 237) are discussed in the section on uveitis. Cogan's syndrome (p. 207), in which there are interstitial keratitis deafness, and vestibular signs, is described in the diseases of the cornea, although periarteritis nodosa and aortitis have been described as occurring with it. The several aortic arch inflammations that may be variants of polyarteritis are described in the section on central nervous system disease (p. 442). A variety of localized ocular disorders arise because of connective tissue abnormalities but are seldom classed as such: pterygia, pinguecula, corneal dystrophies, and keratoconus.

Erythema multiforme (Stevens-Johnson disease). Erythema multiforme is an acute inflammatory systemic disease that varies in severity from an inconsequential skin or mucous membrane lesion to a severe, sometimes fatal systemic disorder. Ophthalmologists tend to describe the disease with ocular involvement as Stevens-Johnson syndrome (Fig. 28-2), although there is no historical justification. The disease affects all ages. The etiology is unknown, although hypersensitivity to drugs, microorganisms, and foods has been described.

The onset is variable, with mild to severe constitutional symptoms of fever, malaise, myalgia, arthralgia, and those of an upper respiratory infection. Skin and mucous membrane lesions develop 1 to 14 days later, often with systemic reaction. The skin lesions develop symmetrically and in crops and vary considerably in appearance. Vesicles and bullae may develop on preexisting macular papules or wheals. They may be surrounded by varying shades of erythema, called iris, target, or bull's-eye. Ulcerations and scaling take place with healing, leaving pigmented and

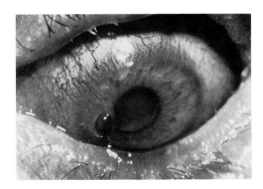

Fig. 28-2. Spontaneous corneal perforation in a 17-year-old male patient who had erythema multiforme when 4 years old. The iris has prolapsed into the corneal opening, and there is ciliary injection and corneal neovascularization.

depigmented areas. The mouth, pharynx, vagina, and rectum may be involved in similar lesions, with erosions and ulcerations. These heal, leaving scarred areas that suggest the diagnosis long after the disease has cleared.

The skin of the eyelids may be involved. A conjunctivitis develops, varying in severity from catarrhal to pseudomembranous. There may be marked swelling of the lids. An acute iritis may occur. In severe cases the cornea may perforate, with loss of the eye. The active inflammation may persist for weeks. Treatment during the acute phase is mainly supportive. Secondary bacterial infection may be combated with antibiotics; corticosteroids may be used.

With healing there are often adhesions between the tarsal and the bulbar conjunctiva (symblepharon). Trichiasis is common. The most marked symptoms arise from keratoconjunctivitis sicca due to scarring of the orifices of the lacrimal glands. The eyes are dry, uncomfortable, injected, and corneal vascularization occurs easily. Infection may occur. Treatment is by means of scleral contact lenses that must be meticulously fitted and adjusted and by transplantation of the parotid duct to provide saliva as a substitute for tears.

Muscle disorders

Myotonic dystrophy. Myotonic dystrophy is an autosomal dominant disorder affecting not only muscular tissue but causing widespread ocular involvement, testicular and ovarian atrophy, endocrine changes, and mental deterioration. There is muscle wasting, often of the extremities, and inability of muscles to relax after voluntary contraction. Cardiac muscle is often involved. Frontal baldness, atrophy of the muscles of mastication, enophthalmos, and ptosis of the upper lid combine to produce a long, expressionless, hawklike face. The onset is often in the third or fourth decade of life, although the myotonia may cause persistent closure of the eyelids after crying in infancy.

Cataract is the most common ocular finding and may precede muscular weakness. The lens opacities may be minute, brilliantly colored specks (iridescent dust) or snowball shaped. They seldom progress enough to cause visual disturbance. Ptosis of the upper lid and weakness of the extraocular muscles are almost constant in later years. Blepharitis (p. 164) and hordeola (p. 162) are common. The pupils are miotic and react sluggishly to light. Macular degeneration has been described recently.

Treatment is symptomatic.

Ataxia-telangiectasia. Ataxia-telangiectasia is a rare autosomal recessive disorder (Louis-Bar) characterized by progressive cerebellar ataxia beginning in infancy, telangiectasis of the conjunctiva, mental and growth retardation, and immunologic incompetence, with absence of Ig A globulin. The dilated blood vessels of the conjunctiva may be confused with the injection of conjunctivitis but is progressive and ultimately appears on the eyelids, ears, and neck and in a butterfly pattern on the face. In addition, there may be nystagmus, absence of opticokinetic nystagmus, and frequent blinking. Inability to look to either side on command leads the child to turn the head first, with the eyes then following.

Myasthenia gravis. Myasthenia gravis is a chronic disease of skeletal muscle characterized by easy fatigability of muscle groups. In approximately 15% of the cases, unilateral or bilateral ptosis and ophthalmoplegia constitute the only evidence of the disease. In an additional 40% of cases, ocular signs are combined with skeletal or oropharyngeal weakness, while in the remainder there are no ocular signs. Women are affected in 75% of the cases, with the age of onset less than 35 years; thereafter there is no sexual predilection. Weakness is often exacerbated in the premenstrual period in young women.

The diagnosis is based upon the history of fluctuations in strength and confirmed by the administration of edrophonium (Tensilon). (Atropine sulfate, 0.4 mg., should be available to counteract cholinergic toxicity.) Edrophonium is administered intravenously in a dosage of 2 to 10 mg.; if myasthenia gravis is present, relief of ptosis, improvement of speech, and generalized muscle strengthening will occur within 30 to 60 seconds and persist 2 to 3 minutes. The extraocular muscles are resistant to cholinergic effects, and ophthalmoplegia may not be grossly responsive, although diplopia may decrease slightly, intraocular pressure may increase, and electromyography of an affected ocular muscle may show increased activity.

Hyperthyroidism occurs in some 3 to 8% of patients with myasthenia gravis and must be excluded. A myasthenia-like syndrome occurs in association with oat cell carcinoma of the lung, presumably on a toxic basis.

The classic treatment for systemic myasthenia gravis is anticholinesterase medication. Ptosis of the upper lid responds well, but the extraocular muscle paresis may be resistant. The instillation of 0.25% eserine solution into the conjunctival cul-de-sac may be helpful.

Chapter 29

Diseases of the blood

Abnormalities of the number or function of normal constituents of the blood may cause marked alterations in the eye. On occasion the changes in the eye may lead to the appropriate tests as in some hemoglobinopathies and macroglobulinemias, whereas in other instances the ocular changes are only incidental to the blood disease. This topic is so encompassing that reference will be made mainly to those diseases in which there are more or less specific ocular changes.

Sickle cell disease

Hemoglobin is a molecule consisting of two pairs of polypeptide chains. There are four normal polypeptide chains, designated as alpha, beta, gamma, and delta. Normal adult hemoglobin (Hgb A) is composed of a pair of alpha polypeptides and a pair of beta polypeptides. There is also a trace of hemoglobin composed of a pair of alpha chains and a pair of delta chains (Hgb A_2). Fetal hemoglobin (Hgb F), which is normally present in fetal life and in decreasing amounts in infancy, contains a pair of alpha chains and a pair of gamma chains. Alteration of a single amino acid in the polypeptide chain gives rise to abnormal hemoglobins. These abnormal hemoglobins are transmitted genetically, and a large number of combinations are possible. The most important variations in causing ocular disorders are those that cause sickling of blood. Hemoglobin S is a hemoglobin in which

the beta polypeptide chain is abnormal because of the substitution of a molecule of valine for glutamic acid. Such hemoglobin undergoes marked distortion when oxygen is deficient. This hemoglobin is insoluble and forms crystals that cause the erythrocytes to take the shape of sickles, crescents, and filaments in venous circulation. In arterial circulation they may revert to normal. Sickle cells have a greater fragility and a life-span of 60 days rather than the normal 120 days.

Sickle cell anemia or homozygous Hgb S disease arises when each parent provides one gene for the abnormal hemoglobin. There is from 70 to 98% Hgb S, and the remainder is Hgb F, normal fetal hemoglobin. In sickle cell trait, or heterozygous Hgb SA disease, one parent provides the gene for sickle cell hemoglobin, and the other provides the gene for normal hemoglobin. Homozygous Hgb C is not a form of sickle cell disease and causes a very mild hemolytic anemia. However, if one parent provides a gene for Hgb C and the other for Hgb S, the resultant Hgb SC provides a combination that leads to a particularly severe retinopathy.

Sickle cell trait involves about 9% of the Negroes in the United States. These patients are frequently asymptomatic, with the major sign being painless hematuria arising from thrombosis and infarction of the kidney papillae. In patients with Hgb S disease, low oxygen tension

457

may lead to infarction of the spleen, brain, and lungs. Symptoms and signs arise from sickling, with a cycle of sickled erythrocytes trapped in capillaries leading to stasis deoxygenation and decreased pH with further sickling, thrombosis, and infarction. The disease becomes manifest as fetal hemoglobin is replaced by hemoglobin S. There are episodic attacks of abdominal or joint pain or aplastic anemia. Patients have increased susceptibility to many infectious agents. Cerebrovascular accidents, aseptic necrosis of bones, ulcers, and hepatic and hemologic disorders occur.

The ocular lesions arise from the intravascular changes either in the conjunctiva or in the retinal vessels. The conjunctival changes are asymptomatic and consist of sausagelike dilation of fine vessels and saccular microaneurysms. They may be seen with the +40 diopter lens of the ophthalmoscope. The most marked changes are retinal. Hemorrhage may occur into the retina, optic disk, or vitreous body. Typically lesions are in the temporal periphery, with proliferative retinopathy combined with aneurysmal vascular dilations, arborizing vascular networks, focal constriction, dilation, sheathing, and obstruction of arterioles and venules (Fig. 29-1). Changes in the contents of vessels cause them to become chalk-white. In addition to the sickle cell retinopathy, angioid streaks (also associated with pseudoxanthoma elasticum and Paget's disease) have been observed (see Figs. 15-13 and 15-14).

Caucasians of Mediterranean ancestry or Negroes who develop angioid streaks, recurrent vitreous hemorrhage (Eales' disease), or a hemorrhagic retinopathy should be tested for a sickling tendency, and if sickling is present, hemoglobin electrophoresis should be done. In patients with sickle cell disease the ocular fundi, particularly the peripheral portions, should be studied through a maximally dilated pupil. Photocoagulation of newly formed blood vessels by means of a xenon arc photocoag-

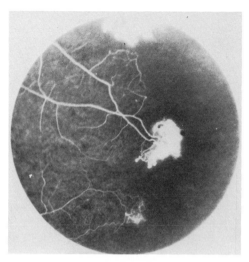

Fig. 29-1. Peripheral neovascularization in the retinal periphery in sickle cell disease following intravenous fluorescein. (Courtesy Retina Service, Wills Eye Hospital, Philadelphia; John Justice, photographer.)

ulator or laser may minimize bleeding into the vitreous.

Thalassemia syndromes

Thalassemia syndromes are hereditary abnormalities of hemoglobin polypeptide chains in which there is a suppression of beta chains and an excess of alpha subunits. In thalassemia major (Cooley's anemia), hemolysis, hypochromic anemia, and iron storage in the spleen and liver dominate the systemic aspects of the condition. The onset is in infancy, and the children have mongoloid facies with prominent epicanthal folds. There may be neovascularization of the peripheral retina as in sickle cell disease. The thalassemia syndromes may be combined with sickle cell hemoglobinopathies.

Polycythemia

In polycythemia there is an abnormal increase in hemoglobin concentration or red blood cell mass. It is divided into primary and secondary. Secondary polycythemia occurs in response to persistent low oxygen tension in mountain dwellers, in patients with chronic lung disease, in Cushing's syndrome, in brain tumor, in hepatocarcinoma, in uterine fibroids, and in renal disease. The brain tumors are usually vascular, in the posterior fossa, and associated with papilledema.

Polycythemia has been reported as associated with conjunctival injection and retinal vein dilation. There may be retinal vein occlusion (p. 260) with visual loss. Ocular abnormalities may disappear with venesection. Papilledema has been reported as a complication of polycythemia without brain tumor. Transient loss of vision may occur. Retinal artery spasm has been reported.

Pernicious anemia

Pernicious anemia is a chronic macrocytic anemia produced by a deficiency of vitamin B_{12} and characterized by anemia, achlorhydria, and degenerative changes in the spinal cord. The disease is often familial, associated with thyroid abnormalities and antibodies against parietal cells of the gastric mucosa. The optic nerve may be involved in retrobulbar neuritis and optic atrophy. Symptoms are referable solely to decreased vision with a central scotoma. In some instances this has been diagnosed as alcohol-tobacco amblyopia. Pipe smoking has been stressed rather than cigarettes. The diagnosis of pernicious anemia may be unusually difficult in patients receiving folic acid in a vitamin preparation inasmuch as folic acid prevents the hematologic but not the neurologic abnormalities of pernicious anemia. The ocular symptoms may improve with vitamin B_{12} therapy. With the development of severe anemia, there may be retinal hemorrhages and soft deposits resembling cotton-wool spots. These may contain cytoid bodies on histologic examination. The retinopathy disappears with correction of the anemia. Orbital hemorrhages have been reported.

Hemorrhage

A rare complication of severe hemorrhage is optic atrophy. The hemorrhage is often spontaneous from bowel lesions rather than traumatic. Immediately or up to several days later there may be loss of vision. The arteries and the veins are small, the retina is pale, and the optic disk may be swollen. Cotton-wool deposits may occur and have been demonstrated to contain cytoid bodies. There may be persistent, complete blindness, or vision may improve to normal. More often the vision is about 20/200, and optic atrophy is present. The arteries remain constricted. Acute blood loss may also cause visual defects from cortical interference, with no fundus changes.

Chronic anemia or an acute anemia may cause a transient loss of vision in one or both eyes. The symptoms are most suggestive of occlusive disease involving the carotid-basilar system.

Leukemia

Leukemia is a disease of unknown cause of the blood-forming tissue characterized by abnormal proliferation of a precursor of one of the types of leukocytes. It may be classified as acute or chronic according to the degree of maturity of cells in the peripheral blood or bone marrow and according to the cell type involved: myelocytic, monocytic, or lymphocytic. Its greatest incidence is before the fifth and after the fiftieth year of life.

The clinical features arise from infiltration of tissues, hemorrhage, and infection. Infiltration commonly involves the liver, spleen, and lymph nodes. Subperiosteal infiltration causes bone pain, and pathologic fractures may occur.

Infiltration and direct extension into the central nervous system may involve cranial nerves with ophthalmoplegia, deafness, or Meniere's syndrome. Leukemic meningitis is common in treated cases, presumably because the chemical antileukemic agents do not cross the blood-brain barrier, so that leukemic cells proliferate in the meninges. Internal hydrocephalus may occur, with headache, nausea, increased cerebrospinal fluid pressure, and papilledema. Hydrocephalus may occur in an infant.

Hemorrhage usually occurs when the platelet count is less that 20,000/mm³. It may involve the mucous membranes, skin, kidney, conjunctiva, orbit, and retina. Subarachnoid hemorrhage may cause death.

Infections are common, particularly infections of the oral cavity, skin, and rectum. Fungi and usually nonvirulent organisms may be involved, possibly because of predisposition secondary to antibiotic and steroid therapy.

The diagnosis is made by hematologic examination. Types of treatment include steroids, antimetabolites, irradiation (with radioactive phosphorus in chronic leukemias), and supportive treatment.

The ocular changes in leukemia arise from infiltration and hemorrhage involving the conjunctiva, sclera, retina, and particularly the choroid. Acute forms of leukemia are far more likely to cause ocular signs than chronic forms, but in both types, changes are likely to be reversible with remission. There is no clinical difference in ocular changes in lymphatic leukemia and in myelogenous leukemia.

The conjunctiva is subtly and frequently involved in acute leukemias, with a slight thickening near the limbus arising from leukemic infiltrates. Infiltrates in the sclera are found on histologic study but do not cause clinical signs. The main ophthalmoscopic signs are the following: (1) change in color of blood column due to anemia or high leukocyte concentration; (2) dilated, tortuous veins of irregular caliber; (3) gray-white lines on either side of a vessel; (4) "hard," yellow-white exudates and occasionally "cotton-wool" patches; and (5) superficial and deep hemorrhages, commonly with a white spot, and leading on occasion to (7) vitreous

hemorrhage. The choroid is often packed with leukemic cells, but visual symptoms are absent.

Leukemic infiltration may give rise to obstruction of lacrimal drainage with the occurrence of a typical dacryocystitis. Intracranial infiltration may cause papilledema and cranial nerve abnormalities. Orbital filtration may cause a severe proptosis.

Neoplasms

Lymphomas, lymphosarcomas, reticulum cell sarcoma, and Hodgkin's disease are closely related neoplasms affecting lymphoid tissue and causing symptoms because of infiltration, compression, or obstruction of vital tissues or organs. The onset is insidious, the course long, and diagnosis is based on the histologic study of involved tissue.

The ocular changes are the following: (1) lid involvement with painless, progressive infiltration; (2) a characteristic subconjunctival tumor with smooth surfaces frequently presenting in the lower cul-de-sac; and (3) orbital or lacrimal gland involvement with proptosis causing diplopia, ocular compression, and the like.

Treatment is individualized as to site of involvement and symptoms and utilizes surgery, irradiation, chemotherapy, and steroids. Commonly the ocular manifestations can be resolved with a dosage of radiation too low to cause cataract.

Paraproteinemias (abnormal globulins)

There are four major groups of immune globulins in adults: (1) Ig G, or γ-G, which contains most antibacterial and antiviral antibodies; (2) Ig A, or γ-A, to which belong diphtheria, tetanus toxin antibodies, typhoid O agglutinins, and paratyphoid B antibodies; (3) Ig M, or γ-M, to which belong isohemagglutinins, Rh antibodies, cold agglutinins, and the rheumatoid factor; and (4) Ig D, or γ-D. It is postulated that proliferation of one clone among immunologically competent cells is responsible for excessive production of a single type of immune globulin giving rise to a variety of disorders.

Multiple myeloma is a neoplasm of plasma cells that elaborate an excess of γ-A of an abnormal type. In cryoglobulinemia, abnormal proteins precipitate when cooled and return to normal at body temperature. Many of the patients have multiple myeloma; others are asymptomatic but have chronic lymphatic leuemia or other disease. In Waldenström's macroglobulinemia, more than 5% of the globulin is of the γ-M type.

In multiple myeloma, ocular signs may be divided into two main groups: (1) those arising from the neoplasm itself such as orbital tumor, compression of cranial nerves within the orbit or head, and papilledema and (2) those arising from blood changes such as retinal hemorrhage and vascular occlusion. Cysts of the pars plana filled with protein, possibly a myeloma globulin, are found in about one third of the eyes removed at autopsy from patients with multiple myeloma.

Diffuse uveal accumulation of leukocytes may occur. Sludging and dilation of conjunctival blood vessels occur in cryoglobulinemia, and the signs may be accentuated by irrigating the conjunctiva with cold water.

Waldenström's macroglobulinemia is associated with a spectacular retinal venous dilation with hemorrhages, cotton-wool deposits, and exudative retinal detachment. These retinal changes may occur in the other paraproteinemias.

Corneal dystrophy has been reported in all types. In multiple myeloma and cryoglobulinemia the deposits are suggestive of cholesterol. The dystrophy has appeared as early as 5 years prior to the onset of the overt systemic disease.

Histiocytosis X

Unlike the abnormalities of lipid metabolism described in Chapter 27, there is no demonstrable metabolic defect in eosin-ophilic granuloma, Hand-Schüller-Christian disease, Letterer-Siwe disease, and juvenile ocular xanthogranuloma (nevoxanthoendothelioma). Lipid, when present, is liberated as part of a local destructive, inflammatory, and probably infectious process.

These conditions are likely different clinical expressions of the same fundamental malady, and signs and symptoms are dependent upon the sites involved and the rapidity of the course. Juvenile ocular xanthogranuloma (nevoxanthoendothelioma) may represent a transitional form between the solely cutaneous involvement of nevoxanthoendothelioma and the systemic involvement of the other conditions. There are many transitional forms between eosinophilic granuloma, Hand-Schüller-Christian disease, and Letterer-Siwe disease, all of which are associated with a diffuse reticuloendothelial hyperplasia.

Different histopathologic pictures may develop simultaneously in the same patient. The characteristic four stages are as follows: (1) a histiocytic proliferative phase with accumulation of eosinophils, (2) vascular granulomatous stage, (3) diffuse xanthomatous phase with abundance of "foam" cells, and (4) fibrous dysplasia stage.

Eosinophilic granuloma. Eosinophilic granuloma is an abnormality localized to bone that may have one, several, or many areas of histiocytic proliferation, with eosinophils. There is no intracellular lipid accumulation. An orbital bone may be involved with a circumscribed osteolytic granuloma demonstrable with roentgen-ray examination.

Hand-Schüller-Christian disease. Hand-Schüller-Christian disease is an idiopathic, nonspecific type of reticuloendothelial and histiocytic proliferation occurring usually before the age of 10 years. It is characterized by the development of multiple lipid granulomas. The classic triad is polyuria, exophthalmos, and skull defects. The polyuria arises from a diabetes insipidus due to a deficiency of antidiuretic hormone secondary to involvement of the tuber cinereum and the hypothalamus. Histiocytic lesions commonly involve the skull, particularly the temporoparietal region, and give rise to otitis media. The skeletal involvement is painless and in the skull gives rise to large, confluent areas with a maplike x-ray appearance. Growth abnormalities are commonly present. Exophthalmos is usually present and arises from orbital accumulation of granulomatous tissue that may be combined with granulomas of orbital bones. Ophthalmoplegia, papilledema, and loss of vision may follow either mechanical displacement or actual infiltration of the skull or orbit.

The skeletal lesions, but not the visceral manifestations, respond to localized roentgen-ray therapy. The polyuria tends to resist treatment, and the occurrence of spontaneous improvement suggests involvement of the adrenal glands, the anterior pituitary gland, or the hypothalamus. Corticosteroids and ACTH have been helpful, as have folic acid antagonists, sometimes in combination with corticosteroids.

Letterer-Siwe disease. Letterer-Siwe disease is a rapidly fatal disease of infancy characterized by fever, osseous lesions, hemorrhage, progressive anemia, and hepatosplenomegaly. Ocular signs may be secondary to skull involvement.

Juvenile ocular xanthogranuloma (nevoxanthoendothelioma). Juvenile ocular xanthogranuloma is an ocular manifestation of what is usually considered a disease solely of the skin. The only evidence of the skin disease is the occurrence of inconspicuous, small, yellow-orange plaques on the head and trunk during the first 5 years of life. The plaques disappear without treatment and, if removed for study, the scar may be infiltrated with a similar plaque. When there is ocular involvement, there may be frank bleeding into the anterior chamber, which may cause secondary glaucoma. Glaucoma with enlargement of the globe may occur without a hyphema. The iris and the ciliary body are infiltrated with histiocytes, which become fused to form giant (Teuton) cells. The skin shows similar histologic changes. The ocular disease is sensitive to small doses of radiation.

Other causes of hyphema such as retinoblastoma, leukemia, injury, and persistent primary vitreous should be excluded. The occurrence of typical skin lesions should distinguish the secondary glaucoma from congenital glaucoma due either to a malformation of the chamber angle or to neurofibromatosis of von Recklinghausen.

Glossary

ablepharon absence of the eyelids.

abnormal retinal correspondence see anomalous retinal correspondence.

accommodation process by which the refractive power of the lens is increased through contraction of the ciliary muscle (N III), causing an increased thickness and curvature of the lens.

accommodative esotropia inward deviation of the eyes characteristically more marked for near than far and increased by ciliary muscle contraction in accommodation.

accommodative exotropia outward deviation of the eyes, usually secondary to uncorrected myopia.

achromatopsia color blindness; often applied to complete color blindness.

after-image visual sensation occurring after the stimulus causing it has ceased.

agnosia inability to recognize objects by sight with ability to recognize by touch; a sign of lesions of the angular gyrus of the parieto-occipital fissure.

agraphia (visual) loss of ability to write.

albinism inherited deficiency of tyrosinase characterized by an absence or decrease of melanin in the skin, hair, and eyes.

alternating cross-eyes deviation of the eyes in which either eye may be used for fixation while the other deviates.

amaurosis nearly obsolete term indicating loss of vision.

amblyopia subnormal visual acuity.

> *ex anopsia* refractive, functional, or strabismic amblyopia now preferred.
>
> *functional* there is inhibition as in refractive or strabismic amblyopia.
>
> *organic* caused by organic disease such as optic atrophy, macular degeneration, or cataract.
>
> *refractive* arises from a refractive error, particularly a marked difference in refraction of the two eyes (anisometropia).
>
> *relative* associated with organic amblyopia upon which is superimposed an inhibition as in strabismic amblyopia.
>
> *strabismic* associated with crossing of the eyes that occurs before the establishment of normal visual acuity in each eye; there appears to be active inhibition of perception of the retinal image transmitted by one eye.

ametropia optical condition in which parallel rays of light do not focus on the retina; a refractive error.

angioid streaks abnormality of the elastic layer of Bruch's membrane giving rise to pigmented striations of the ocular fundus; associated with a variety of systemic diseases such as pseudoxanthoma elasticum, sickle cell disease, and osteitis deformans (Paget's disease) and a variety of generalized diseases affecting the elastic lamina of blood vessels.

angle of anomaly in strabismus, the degree an eye deviates from parallelism.

angle-closure glaucoma ocular abnormality in which the intraocular pressure increases, often quickly, because the anterior aqueous humor is mechanically prevented from reaching the trabecular meshwork.

angstrom (Å) unit of wavelength equal to 10^{-10} (one ten-billionth) meter.

aniridia absence of iris, usually incomplete, with iris root present.

aniseikonia optical condition in which the retinal images in the two eyes are of different sizes.

anisocoria condition in which the pupils of the two eyes are of unequal size.

anisometropia condition in which the refractive errors in the two eyes are different.

ankyloblepharon condition in which the margins of the eyelids are fused together.

anomalous (abnormal) retinal correspondence condition in which corresponding points on the two retinas do not have the same relative direction in space.

> *disharmonious* angle of abnormality is less than the angle of strabismus.
>
> *harmonious* angle of abnormality is the same as the angle of strabismus.

anomalous trichromatism defect of color vision in which there appears to be a deficiency of one of the cone pigments (*see also* deuteranomaly, protanomaly, tritanomaly).

anophthalmos absence of the eye.

aphakia absence of the crystalline lens of the eye.

aqueous flare Tyndall beam observed with a biomicroscope when excessive protein is present in the anterior aqueous humor.

aqueous humor fluid that fills the posterior and anterior chambers.

arcuate scotoma area of blindness in the field of vision of characteristic arc shape caused by interruption of a nerve fiber bundle in the retina; most often seen in glaucoma.

argyria discoloration of the skin or mucous membranes produced by prolonged administration of silver salts with deposition of metallic silver in tissue.

asteroid hyalosis fixed opacities composed of a calcium lipid complex that occur in an otherwise normal vitreous body; there are no symptoms.

asthenopia ill-defined ocular discomfort arising from use of the eyes.

astigmatism optical condition in which the refractive power is not uniform in all meridians; when regular, there are two main meridians of refractive power; when irregular, there are a number of meridians of different power.

avulsion of caruncle term usually applied to a laceration involving inner one sixth (lacrimal portion) of lower eyelid with rupture of the inferior canaliculus.

band keratopathy deposition of calcium in the cornea most marked in horizontal meridian; occurs in degenerating eyes, hypercalcemia, and juvenile arthritis (of Still).

bedewing of cornea subepithelial corneal edema, often associated with sudden prolonged increase in intraocular pressure or wearing of contact lenses for an excessively long period (Sattler's veil).

Bell's palsy peripheral paralysis of the facial nerve (N VII).

Bell's phenomena upward and outward deviation of the eyes occurring with forcible closure of the eyelids or sleep.

Bergmeister's papilla small mass of glial cells that surrounds the hyaloid artery in the center of the optic disk; on occasion it persists and obliterates the physiologic cup of the optic disk.

biomicroscope microscope for examining the eye and consisting essentially of a dissecting microscope combined with a light source that projects a rectangular light beam that can be changed in size and focus.

Bitot's spot highly refractile mass with silver-gray hue and having a foamy surface that appears on the bulbar conjunctiva in vitamin A deficiency.

blepharitis inflammation of the margin of the eyelids; occurs in squamous (seborrheic) and ulcerative forms.

blepharochalasis relaxation of the skin of the eyelid due to atrophy of the elastic tissue; the upper eyelid is commonly involved and a fold of tissue hangs over the lid margin.

blepharophimosis narrowing of the palpebral fissure, often associated with excessive distance between the inner canthi and drooping of the upper eyelid (blepharoptosis).

blepharoplasty plastic surgery of the eyelids.

blepharoptosis drooping of the upper lid due to paralysis of the oculomotor (N III) nerve or the sympathetic nerves or to excessive weight of the upper lids.

blepharospasm tonic spasm of the orbicularis oculi muscle.

blind spot (of Mariotte, of Vito) area of blindness in the visual field marking the site of the optic nerve in the eye where there are no photoreceptors.

blindness inability to see; defined by Internal Revenue Service as reduction of best corrected visual acuity to 20/200 or less in better eye or restriction of the visual field to 20° or less; defined by Social Security Agency as reduction of vision in best corrected eye to 5/200 or less; in industry, reduction of the best corrected visual acuity to less that 20/200.

  color see deuteranopia, protanopia, tritanopia, deuteranomaly, protanomaly, tritanomaly.

  cortical caused by a lesion in the cortical visual center.

  night inefficient dark adaptation so that vision is markedly reduced in reduced illumination.

  snow inability to open eyes to see; secondary to ultraviolet keratitis.

blowout fracture of orbit comminuted fracture of the roof of the maxillary sinus with prolapse of intraorbital contents into the antrum; there is enophthalmos, blepharoptosis, inability to turn the eye upward, and usually infraorbital anesthesia.

blue sclera abnormality in which the sclera is thin and has a blue appearance arising from the underlying pigmented choroid.

Brushfield's spots transient whitish areas in the iris at birth that occur in Mongolian idiocy.

buphthalmos enlargement of the eye usually occurring as a result of congenital glaucoma.

campimeter alternative term for perimeter.

campimetry alternative term for perimetry.

canaliculitis inflammation of the lacrimal canaliculi, often due to fungus infection.

candela unit of luminous intensity; one candela is defined as the luminous intensity of 1/60 of a square centimeter of projected area of a blackbody radiator operating at the temperature of solidification of platinum.

candle power luminous intensity as expressed in candelas.

carotid-cavernous fistula rupture of a carotid aneurysm into the cavernous sinus (infrasellar) that causes an increased venous pressure in the sinus.

cataract any opacity of the lens is a cataract; the opacity arises from either denatured protein or imbibition of fluid by the lens.

central angiospastic retinopathy condition characterized by separation of the neural retina from the pigment epithelium in the macular area by a serous fluid.

centrocecal scotoma area of blindness in the field of vision involving both the fixation point and the blind spot (cecum); characterizes toxic amblyopias.

chalazion chronic lipogranuloma of a meibomian gland.

Charcot's triad nystagmus, intention tremor, and scanning speech, which occur as a late sign in demyelinating disease, particularly multiple sclerosis.

chemosis edema of the conjunctiva.

cherry red spot ophthalmoscopic appearance of the fovea centralis (which contains only the layers of the retina adjacent to the choroid) when surrounded by either edematous or lipid-filled inner layers of the retina, as occurs in occlusion of the central retinal artery, in amaurotic familial idiocy, and in Niemann-Pick disease.

choroideremia sex-linked abnormality characterized by atrophy of the choriocapillaris and degeneration of the retinal pigment epithelium.

choroiditis inflammation of the choroid.

chromatic aberration imperfection of an image produced by variations in the refractability of the various wavelengths of white light.

C.I.E. abbreviation for Commission Internationale de l'Eclairage.

C.I.E. observer hypothetical observer having color-mixture data recommended in 1931 by C.I.E.

circinate retinopathy rare monocular disorder, mainly of elderly women, characterized by a girdlelike zone of small, discrete, coalescing white spots engirdling the macular area.

collyrium eyewash.

coloboma fissure of a part of the eye.

commotio retina traumatic lesion of the posterior pole with edema and hemorrhage following contusion of the anterior ocular segment.

complementary after-image after-image in which the hue is approximately complementary to the hue of the sensation produced by the original stimulus.

complementary chromaticities pairs of different samples of light that produce an achromatic (colorless) stimulus when combined in suitable proportions.

complementary colors pairs of samples of light that have complementary chromaticities; also the proper relative amounts of luminous flux to produce an achromatic (colorless) mixture.

congruous field defects visual field defects that are exactly the same in extent and intensity in both eyes; characterizes lesions in the optic radiation and occipital cortex.

conical cornea keratoconus.

conjugate ocular movements similar ocular movements of both eyes such as eyes right, eyes down, eyes left, eyes up, eyes down.

conjunctivitis inflammation of the conjunctiva.

consensual light reflex constriction of the pupil in the fellow eye when the retina is stimulated by light.

conus of optic disk abnormality in which the choroid and retinal pigment epithelium do not extend to the optic disk, allowing the sclera to be observed ophthalmoscopically at its margin.

corectopia displacement of pupil from its normal position.

corresponding points points on the two retinas that have the same directional value in space.

cover-uncover test alternate covering and uncovering of one eye to distinguish between a phoria and a tropia.

Credé's prophylaxis instillation of 1% silver nitrate in the eyes of a newborn infant to prevent gonococcal conjunctivitis.

crescent, myopic term applied to a conus of the optic disk in myopia.

cryotherapy procedure carried out with a freezing probe.

cyclodialysis surgical procedure for glaucoma to establish a communication between the anterior chamber and the suprachoroidal space.

cyclodiathermy destruction of a portion of the ciliary body by diathermy to reduce the quantity of aqueous humor produced in glaucoma.

cycloplegia paralysis of the ciliary muscle giving rise to paralysis of accommodation.

cycloplegic agent that causes cycloplegia.

cylinder in optics, a lens having no refracting power in one meridian and maximal refracting power at the meridian at right angles to this.

dacryoadenitis inflammation of the lacrimal gland, often chronic and due to a granulomatous disease; acute dacryoadenitis occurs with mumps and infectious mononucleosis.

dacryocystitis inflammation of the lacrimal sac that usually results from interference with lacrimal drainage.

dacryocystorhinostomy surgical procedure in which the mucous membrane of the lacrimal sac is anastomosed with the mucous membrane lining the middle meatus of the nose to establish lacrimal drainage.

dacryostenosis atresia of the lacrimal duct.

dark adaptation biochemical and neurologic process by which the eye becomes more sensitive to light.

dendritic keratitis inflammation of the corneal epithelium by the *Herpes hominis* virus.

denervation supersensitivity sensitivity to neural effector substance that follows postganglionic interruption of the nerve supply of organs innervated by the autonomic nervous system.

descemetocele herniation of the basement membrane of the corneal endothelium.

detachment, retinal separation of the neural retina from the retinal pigment epithelium.

deuteranomaly form of anomalous trichromatism for which there appears to be a deficiency of green-sensitive cones so that there is poor green-purple and red-purple discrimination, green insensitivity, and normal luminosity function.

deuteranopia form of dichromatism in which there are but two cone pigments present and there is complete insensitivity to green.

deviation

   primary ocular deviation seen in paralysis of an ocular muscle when the noninvolved eye is used for fixation.

   secondary ocular deviation seen in paralysis of an ocular muscle when the involved eye is used for fixation.

   supranuclear binocular paralysis of the volitional ocular movements arising because of abnormalities in the frontal or occipital cortex.

dialysis of retina separation at the ora serrata of the neural retina from the retinal pigment epithelium.

diaphanoscopy transillumination of a body cavity; used in ophthalmology to demonstrate the diminution of pigment in the iris in the female carriers of albinism or in the diagnosis of intraocular tumors.

dichromatism abnormality of color vision in which only two of the three cone pigments are present; mixtures of two, rather than the normal three, components are necessary and sufficient to match all colors (protanopes, red absent;

deuteranopes, green absent; tritanopes, blue absent).

diopter unit of measurement of the refractive power of lenses equal to the reciprocal focal length of the lens expressed in meters.

diplopia double vision; simultaneous perception of two grossly dissimilar images.

   crossed double vision in which the image arising from the right is observed to the left of the image arising from the left eye; associated with conditions in which the eyes turn outward.

   uncrossed condition in which the image of the right eye is to the right of the image belonging to the left eye; observed in conditions in which the visual axes of the eye are directed toward each other, as in esotropia.

disciform degeneration of macula secondary type of macular degeneration, often arising from abnormalities in the elastic layer of the lamina vitrea.

disciform detachment of retina term commonly applied to separations of the retina in the macular region arising because blood or serous fluid separates the neural retina from the retinal pigment epithelium.

disciform keratitis stromal type of corneal inflammation, roughly circular in shape, often seen as secondary stromal involvement to herpes simplex keratitis.

disinsertion of retina retinal dialysis at the ora serrata in which the neural retina is separated from the retinal pigment epithelium.

dislocation of lens condition in which the crystalline lens is completely unsupported by the zonular fibers so that the lens is free, either in the vitreous body or the anterior chamber.

Doyne's honeycomb choroiditis noninflammatory condition with excrescences (drusen) of the cuticular layer of the lamina vitrea; fundus appears to be studded with yellowish white dots.

drusen hyaline excrescences of the lamina vitrea.

dry eye keratoconjunctivitis sicca.

ductions ocular movements of one eye only.

dyslexia psychologic abnormality in which despite adequate intelligence, motivation, and, instruction and in the absence of a physical handicap, emotional disturbance, or cultural deprivation an individual fails to master printed and written language.

dysmetria abnormality of ocular movements in which there is a disturbance in the power to control the range of movement.

dystrophy, corneal noninflammatory developmental, nutritional, or metabolic abnormality characterized by the occurrence of opaque material in the central cornea.

   Salzmann's nodular inflammatory opacity of the

cornea associated with bacterial hypersensitivity, particularly to *Mycobacterium tuberculosis*.

eccentric fixation visual abnormality in which a retinal area other than the fovea centralis is used for visual fixation.

ecchymosis extravasation of blood beneath the skin.

ectasia of sclera localized bulging of the sclera lined with uveal tissue; a staphyloma.

ectropion turning outward of the margin of the eyelid occurring in spastic, cicatricial, and paralytic forms.

eikonometer device for measuring the retinal image size in each eye; used in the diagnosis of aniseikonia or a difference in image size of the two eyes, most often arising from a difference in refractive power of the eyes.

electromagnetic spectrum range of radiant energy that has a variable frequency and a constant velocity (energy = Planck's constant × frequency).

electro-oculogram ratio of standing potential between retina and cornea in light and dark adaptation.

electroretinogram action potential that follows stimulation of the retina.

emmetropia refractive condition in which no refractive error is present with accommodation at rest.

emphysema, orbital air in the orbit; generally follows traumatic rupture of a nasal sinus, particularly the lamina papyracea of the ethmoid bone.

endogenous uveitis inflammation of the uveal tract arising from causes within the body in contrast to that introduced from outside the body as in injuries (exogenous).

endophthalmitis purulent inflammation of the intraocular contents.

enophthalmos abnormal recession of the eyeball within the orbit.

entropion inward turning of the eyelid observed in cicatricial, spastic, and paralytic forms.

enucleation removal of the eyeball.

epidemic keratoconjunctivitis inflammation of the cornea and conjunctiva by an adenovirus, often adenovirus type 8.

epiphora tearing in which faulty drainage of tears permits their overflow.

episcleritis localized inflammation of the superficial tissues of the sclera.

epithelial downgrowth epithelialization of the interior of the eye that may follow faulty wound healing of the anterior ocular segment.

erysiphake instrument that uses a vacuum to grasp the lens in cataract extraction.

esodeviation inward deviation of the eye.

esophoria latent inward deviation of the eye in which, with binocular vision suspended, the eyes deviate inward.

esotropia manifest inward deviation that occurs with both eyes open.

essential atrophy of iris rare, progressive unilateral disease of the iris in which there is a patchy loss of all layers of the iris, causing a distorted and migrating pupil and often a secondary increase in intraocular pressure.

evisceration in ophthalmology, the surgical procedure in which the intraocular contents are removed, retaining the cornea (sometimes) and the sclera.

exenteration, orbital removal of all of the orbital tissues, including the eye and its nervous, vascular, and muscular connections.

exfoliation of lens capsule condition in which the anterior lens capsule degenerates and appears to be wiped from the lens by the movement of the iris; true exfoliation follows infrared injury to the lens; pseudoexfoliation is more common; the cause is unknown.

exodeviation turning outward of the eyes.

exophoria latent outward deviation of the eyes in which, with binocular vision suspended, the eyes deviate outward.

exophthalmos abnormal protusion of the eyes.
   endocrine associated with abnormalities of the thyroid gland.
   ophthalmoplegic inability to move the eye because of exophthalmos.
   pulsating associated with a carotid-cavernous fistula.

exotropia outward deviation of the eyes.

eye
   exciting initially injured eye that gives rise to sympathetic ophthalmia in fellow eye, the sympathizing eye.
   fixating in strabismus, the eye directed to the object of regard.
   reduced, schematic simplified eye used in optics.
   squinting deviating eye in strabismus.

field of vision area simultaneously visible to an eye without movement; usually measured by means of an arc (perimeter) located 330 mm. from the eye.

flare, aqueous see aqueous flare.

floater object seen in the field of vision that originates in the vitreous body; the most common floaters are muscae volitantes, minute flecks of protein seen in bright, uniform illumination.

fluorescence reradiation of energy with increase of wavelength by an absorbing substance.

flux short form for radiant flux, or luminous flux, according to context.

focus point of convergence of light rays.

foot-candle unit of illuminance equal to one lumen incident per square foot.

foot-lambert unit of luminance.

fructose 1-aldolase deficiency enzymatic deficiency associated with amaurotic familial idiocy in the homozygote; parents of such children are heterozygotes and have a much less severe enzyme deficiency.

Fuchs' black spot area of proliferation of the retinal pigment layer in the macular region occurring in degenerative myopia.

Fuchs' dystrophy corneal abnormality in which there is initially a degeneration of the endothelium followed sometimes by epithelial changes.

funduscope inasmuch as many organs have a fundus, a more precise term for the instrument used in ophthalmoscopy is ophthalmoscope.

fusion reflex, the stimulus of which is the simultaneous stimulation of the two retinas by two images of an object.

Grade 1, simultaneous macular perception (normal correspondence) ability of the brain to receive and appreciate images from the fovea of each eye simultaneously.

Grade 2, fusion with amplitude blending of the similar images from the two foveas into a single perception.

Grade 3, stereopsis blending of slightly dissimilar images from the two eyes with the perception of depth.

glare sensation produced by brightnesses within the visual field that are sufficiently greater than the luminance to which the eyes are adapted to cause annoyance, discomfort, or loss in visual performance and visibility.

glasses popular name for spectacles or eyeglasses.

goniopuncture surgical procedure for the treatment of congenital glaucoma in which a knife blade is passed through the trabecular area to the subconjunctival space.

gonioscope special instrument for studying the angle of the anterior chamber of the eye.

goniotomy operation for congenital glaucoma in which the trabecular meshwork in the region of Schlemm's canal is incised.

hallucinations perception without external stimulus that may occur in every field of sensation; visual hallucinations are formed when composed of scenes and unformed when composed of sparks, lights, and the like; formed hallucinations characterize temporal lobe disturbances and unformed visual hallucinations characterize occipital lobe disorders, particularly migraine.

Hassall-Henle bodies hyaline deposits of Descemet's membrane that occur as a sign of aging.

heterochromia of iris condition in which the irides of the two eyes are not of uniform color.

heterophoria condition in which there is a latent tendency of the eyes to deviate which is prevented by fusion.

heterotropia condition in which the eyes deviate; a strabismus.

hippus spasmodic dilation and contraction of the pupil independent of stimulation with light.

hole, retinal break in the continuity of the neural retina so that there is a communication between the vitreous cavity and the potential space between the neural retina and the retina pigment epithelium.

Holmgren's color test color vision test utilizing colored yarns.

homonymous in ophthalmology, having the same side of the field of vision; thus a right homonymous hemianopsia is right half-blindness and arises from a defect involving the nasal fibers of the right eye that decussate and the noncrossing fibers of the left eye; the lesion is on the left side, posterior to the optic chiasm.

hordeolum acute inflammation caused by infection of one of the sebaceous glands of Zeis; a sty; the term "internal hordeolum" is sometimes applied to a chalazion.

horopter plane in space that localizes the visual direction of corresponding retinal points.

Hudson-Stähli line pigmented iron line of the cornea.

hydrophthalmos buphthalmos or the distended eye that occurs in infantile glaucoma.

hydrops of iris term applied to the vacuolization of the pigment layer of the iris as occurs when these cells are filled with glycogen in diabetes mellitus.

hyperopia refractive state of the eye in which the parallel rays of light would come to focus behind the retina if not intercepted by it.

absolute cannot be corrected completely by accommodation so that there is indistinct vision both for near and for distance.

axial caused by abnormal shortness of the anteroposterior diameter of the eye.

latent portion of total hypermetropia that cannot be overcome, or the difference between the manifest and total hypermetropia.

manifest amount of hypermetropia indicated by the strongest convex lens a patient will accept while retaining normal visual acuity.

total entire hypermetropia, both latent and manifest.

hyperphoria tendency for the eyes to deviate vertically which is prevented by binocular vision.

hypertelorism excessive width between two organs; in ocular hypertelorism there is increased distance between the eyes that is often associated with mental deficiency and exotropia.

hypertropia deviation of the eyes in which one eye is higher than the other.

hypotony, ocular diminished ocular pressure.

illuminance luminous flux incident per unit area of a surface.

image visual impression of an object formed by a lens or mirror.

   false in diplopia, the image arising in the deviating eye.

   Purkinje's images reflected from the surface of the cornea, the anterior surface of the lens, and the posterior surface of the lens.

   real in optics, the inverted image in which refracted rays pass through the image point.

   true in diplopia, the image received by the nondeviating eye.

   virtual in optics, the erect image in which the refracted rays do not pass through the image point, but appear to come from it.

incongruous field defects visual field defects that are dissimilar in the two eyes; occur in lesions involving that portion of the visual pathways anterior to the lateral geniculate body.

infrared radiation portion of the electromagnetic spectrum that has a wavelength of more than 700 nm. and less than 10,000 nm.

interstitial keratitis inflammation of the corneal stroma with neovascularization, often complicating congenital syphilis.

intrascleral nerve loop condition in which a long posterior ciliary nerve loops in the anterior sclera; gives rise to a minute dark spot of uveal tissue on the sclera.

iridectomy cutting out of a part of the iris.

   peripheral removal of a portion of the peripheral iris.

   sector removal of an entire sector, extending usually from the pupillary margin to the root of the iris.

iridencleisis surgical procedure for glaucoma in which an incision is made at the corneoscleral limbus and the iris is incarcerated in the wound to create a filtering wick between the anterior chamber and subconjunctival space.

iridocapsulotomy surgical procedure in which the iris and adherent lens capsule is incised to create a new pupillary opening; procedure is necessitated by a cataract extraction in which a large amount of lens capsule remains.

iridocyclitis inflammation of the iris and ciliary body.

iridodialysis separation of the base of the iris from the ciliary body; main cause is blunt trauma to the eye.

iridodonesis tremulousness of the iris as occurs following loss of support after lens removal.

iridoplegia paralysis of the sphincter pupillae of the iris.

iris bombé condition in which the pupil is adherent to the lens so that aqueous humor accumulates in the posterior chamber; iris tends to balloon forward peripherally and it may close the angle, causing secondary glaucoma.

iris coloboma defect of the iris that follows iridectomy or occurs as a congenital abnormality.

iritis inflammation of the iris.

irradiance density of radiant flux incident on a surface.

Ishihara color plates device for screening for color discrimination using forms composed of different colored dots.

joule ten million ergs.

Kayser-Fleischer ring golden deposit of copper in the periphery of the cornea observed in hepatolenticular degeneration (Wilson's disease).

keratectomy excision of the cornea.

keratic precipitates clumps of leukocytes adhering to the corneal endothelium in uveal tract inflammation; customarily divided into mutton-fat (macrophages), which occur in granulomatous inflammations, and punctate (lymphocytes), which occur in nongranulomatous inflammations.

keratitis inflammation of the cornea.

keratocele hernia of Descemet's membrane through the cornea; a descemetocele.

keratoconjunctivitis simultaneous inflammation of the cornea and conjunctiva.

keratoconus conical protusion of the cornea.

keratomalacia softening of the cornea, often occurring in severe vitamin A deficiency.

keratome knife with a triangular blade used for corneal incision.

keratometer instrument for measuring the radius of curvature of the cornea.

keratomycosis keratitis due to fungus infection.

keratoplasty transplantation of a portion of the cornea.

   lamellar superficial layers are replaced.

   penetrating entire thickness of a portion of the cornea is replaced.

keratotomy incision of the cornea carried out in years past to limit the spread of an ulcer.

Koeppe nodule accumulation of epithelioid cells at the pupillary margin in granulomatous uveitis.

Krukenberg's spindle accumulation of pigment on

the corneal endothelium in the shape of a vertical spindle that occurs in pigmentary glaucoma.

lagophthalmos condition in which the globe is not entirely covered with the eyelids closed.

lambert unit of luminance.

laser acronym for *l*ight *a*mplification by *s*timulated *e*mission of *r*adiation; the laser produces a nearly monochromatic and coherent beam of radiation.

lens glass or other transparent material used optically to modify the path of light.

> *bifocal* spectacles that contain two foci, usually arranged with the focus for distance above and a smaller segment for near below; such lenses are used in the correction of presbyopia and to relieve excessive accommodation in accommodative strabismus of children.

> *colored* selectively absorb or reflect certain wavelengths of light.

> *contact* worn beneath the lids.

> *crystalline* transparent biconvex tissue located behind the pupil and in front of the vitreous.

> *prism* transparent solid with triangular ends and two converging sides; separates white light into its spectral components and bends rays of light toward its base; used to measure or to correct ocular muscle imbalance.

> *safety* lens resistant to shattering made either of plastic or by means of case-hardening.

lensometer instrument for determining the refractive power of a lens.

lenticonus rare abnormality of the lens characterized by a conical prominence on the anterior or posterior lens surface.

leukoma opacity of the cornea; a less marked opacity is a macula, and the most minor type of opacity is a nebula.

> *adherent* corneal opacity to which the iris is adherent.

light that portion of the electromagnetic spectrum that gives rise to a sensation through stimulation of the retina.

lumen unit of luminous flux equal to the flux in a unit of solid angle (one steradian) from a uniform point source of one candela.

luminance luminous flux per unit solid angle emitted per unit of projected area.

luminosity ratio of lumens per watt of any kind of radiant energy.

luminous emittance density of luminous flux emitted from a surface.

luminous flux rate of flow of luminous energy.

lux unit of illuminance equal to one lumen per square meter.

lysozyme antibacterial enzyme found in tears, leukocytes, egg albumin, and plants; mainly effective against nonpathogenic bacteria.

macula minute corneal opacity.

macula lutea yellow spot; the ill-defined retinal area surrounding the fovea centralis.

megalocornea cornea having a diameter of 12 mm. or more.

microcornea cornea having a diameter of less than 9 mm.

microphakia anomaly in which the crystalline lens is abnormally small.

microphthalmia condition in which the eyeball is abnormally small.

micropsia disturbance of visual perception in which objects appear smaller than their true size.

millimicron unit of wavelength equal to 10^{-9} meter; nanometer now preferred.

miosis condition in which the pupil is constricted.

miotic pertaining to or characterized by constriction of the pupil.

morgagnian cataract hypermature cataract in which the cortex is liquefied, permitting the lens nucleus to float within the capsule.

muscae volitantes flitting flecks darting about in the field of vision caused by opacities in the vitreous humor or erthyrocytes in retinal capillaries.

mydriasis dilation of the pupil.

mydriatic pertaining to mydriasis.

myopia optical condition in which parallel rays of light come to focus in front of the retina.

> *axial* caused by abnormal length of anteroposterior diameter of the eye.

> *degenerative* associated with conus of optic disk and retinal abnormalities.

> *refractive* caused by increased index of refraction of lens as occurs in nuclear sclerosis.

Nagel anomaloscope device for mixing two colors to match a third; used for analysis of color perception.

nanometer (nm.) unit of wavelength equal to 10^{-9} (one one-billionth) meter; formerly called millimicron (mμ).

narrow-angle glaucoma glaucoma arising because apposition of the iris to the peripheral cornea prevents the aqueous humor from draining through the trabecular meshwork.

nebula of cornea minor opacity of the cornea.

neurotrophic keratitis keratitis arising because of anesthesia of the cornea.

nodal points locations in an optical system toward and from which are directed corresponding incident and transmitted rays that make equal angles with the optic axis.

nystagmus oscillatory movement of the eyeballs.

> *end-position* involuntary rhythmic movement of the eyes observed when in extreme positions of gaze.

jerk occurs with a fast and a slow phase.

labyrinthine occurs when the labyrinths are irritated or diseased (synonym, vestibular nystagmus).

miner's nystagmus caused by darkness.

optokinetic occurs in normal individuals when a succession of moving objects traverse the field of vision such as occurs when gazing out of the window of a moving vehicle at a succession of stationary objects (synonym, railroad nystagmus).

pendulous occurs when vision in both eyes has been defective since birth.

rotatory eyeball partially rotates around the visual axis.

ophthalmoplegia paralysis of the ocular muscles.

externa paralysis of the external ocular muscles.

interna paralysis of the muscles of the iris and the ciliary body.

total combination of both intrinsic and extrinsic paralysis.

ophthalmoscope instrument for examining the interior of the eye.

direct provides an upright image of about 15 diameters magnification.

indirect convex lens is held in front of the eye and an inverted image is observed; provides a magnification of about four times but allows examination of a more peripheral portion of the fundus than direct ophthalmoscopy.

optic atrophy atrophy of the optic nerve.

orthophoria tendency for the eyes to be parallel; normal ocular muscle balance.

orthoptics technique of providing correct and efficient visual responses, usually by the form of visual training; these measures include the treatment of functional amblyopia, management of convergence insufficiency, and diagnosis of muscle imbalance and strabismus.

pannus vascularization and connective tissue deposition beneath the epithelium of the cornea.

Panum's area spatial area surrounding the horopter in which objects are viewed with stereopsis; outside this area, diplopia occurs.

papilla small nipplelike eminence.

lacrimal small conical eminence on the upper and lower eyelid at the inner canthus pierced by the lacrimal punctum; particularly evident in the elderly.

optic optic disk (a misnomer in that the disk does not project into the eye).

papilledema passive edema of the optic disk.

papillitis inflammation of the optic disk, or optic neuritis.

perimeter instrument used to measure the visual field.

phakomatoses group of hereditary diseases characterized by the presence of spots, tumors, and cysts in various parts of the body; types recognized as associated with ocular findings are tuberous sclerosis, Lindau–von Hippel disease, von Recklinghausen's disease, Bourneville's disease, and Louis-Bar disease.

photophobia ocular discomfort induced by bright lights.

photopsia subjective sensation of sparks or flashes of light that occur in some pathologic conditions of the optic nerve, the retina, or the brain.

phthisis bulbi degenerative shrinkage of the eyeball.

pinguecula small yellowish white subconjunctival elevation composed of elastic tissue located between the corneoscleral limbus and the canthus.

pits in optic disk coloboma of the optic disk causing poor vision, sometimes associated with central serous chorioretinopathy.

Placido's disk device composed of concentric black and white lines that is reflected onto the anterior surface of the cornea to detect astigmatism.

poliosis condition characterized by the absence of pigment in the hair; poliosis of the eyelashes occurs in sympathetic ophthalmia, syphilis, and Vogt-Koyanagi's bilateral uveitis.

polycoria occurrence of more than one pupil in the iris.

presbyopia refractive condition in which there is a diminished power of accommodation arising from impaired elasticity of the crystalline lens, as occurs with aging.

protanomaly form of anomalous trichromatism for which, in a red-green mixture, more than the normal amount of red is required than for normal observer.

protanope person having protanopia.

protanopia form of dichromatism in which red and bluish green are confused, and relative luminosity of red is much lower than for normal observer.

pseudoisochromatic plate *see* Ishihara color plates.

pterygium abnormality arising basically in the cornea in which a triangular patch of conjunctiva extends into the cornea; apex of the patch points toward the pupil.

ptosis *see* blepharoptosis.

pupil aperture in the iris of the eye for the passage of light.

Adie's abnormality in the reaction of the pupil to light and associated with hypotonic deep reflexes.

Argyll Robertson pupil that does not constrict to light, but constricts to accommodation; pupils are small, unequal in size, and irregular; seen mainly in tabes dorsalis.

cat's-eye pupil with a white reflex when light is directed into it; most commonly associated with retinoblastoma.

pupillary membrane anomaly of the iris, usually minor, in which there is failure of the fetal pupillary membrane to atrophy; often a persistent strand extends between the iris collarette and the anterior lens capsule.

Purkinje shift luminosity curve of dark-adapted individual peaks at 500 nm., whereas the luminosity curve of light-adapted individual peaks at 550 nm.; indicates two types of retinal photoreceptors.

radiance radiant intensity per unit of projected area.

radiant absorptance ratio of absorbed radiant flux to incident flux.

radiant emittance radiant flux emitted per unit area of a source.

radiant energy energy being transferred, unaccompanied by transfer of matter.

radiant flux rate of transfer of radiant energy.

radiant intensity flux radiated per unit solid angle.

radiant power alternative term for radiant flux.

radiant reflectance ratio of reflected radiant flux to incident flux.

red eye lay term applied to any condition with dilation of conjunctival or ciliary blood vessels.

reflex involuntary, invariable, adaptive response to a stimulus.

accommodation constriction of the pupils when the eyes converge for near vision; an associated reaction and not a reflex.

auditory brief closure of the eyelids resulting from a sudden sound.

conjunctival (lid) closure of the eyelids induced by touching the conjunctiva (also called corneal reflex).

consensual light (crossed) constriction of the pupil when the opposite retina is stimulated with light.

cutaneous pupillary (ciliospinal) dilation of the ipsilateral pupil on pinching the skin on one side of the neck.

direct light contraction of the sphincter pupillae induced by stimulation of retina with light (also called pupillary reflex).

eyeball compression (oculocardiac) decrease of heartbeat caused by pressure on the eyeball.

fixation direction of the eye so that an image remains upon the fovea centralis of each eye.

foveolar bright dot of light arising from the foveola when an ophthalmoscope light is directed upon the region of the fovea centralis.

lacrimal secretion of tears induced by irritation of the cornea and conjunctiva.

red red glow of light seen to emerge from the pupil when the interior of the eye is illuminated.

refraction deviation of rays of light when passing from one transparent medium into another of a different density.

retinitis inflammation of the retina.

retinoblastoma common autosomal dominant malignant retinal tumor of infancy.

retinopathy any disease condition of the retina.

retinopexy surgical procedure to correct retinal detachment by means of diathermy.

retinoschisis retinal abnormality in which the neural retina splits at the level of the bipolar layer.

retinoscopy objective method of determining the refraction of the eye by observing the movements of the reflection of light from the eye (skiascopy).

retrobulbar neuritis inflammation of the optic nerve occurring without involvement of the optic disk.

retrolental fibroplasia condition of cicatricial neovascularization of the retina that occurs predominantly in infants who weigh less than 1,500 grams at birth and who require oxygen in an excessively high concentration for a long period.

salmon patch central area of intense vascularization that occurs in interstitial keratitis with the confluence of all blood vessels at the center of the cornea.

Sattler's veil subepithelial corneal edema, particularly that following prolonged wearing of a contact lens.

Schirmer's test test for tear formation in which filter paper is folded over the lid margin and the amount of wetting in 4 minutes is measured in millimeters.

scleritis inflammation of the sclera.

scleromalacia perforans disease condition in which rheumatoid nodules form in the sclera and cause it to become necrotic; there is usually an associated severe rheumatoid arthritis.

sclerosing keratitis inflammation of the cornea in which it becomes white and opaque resembling the sclera.

scotoma area of blindness in the field of vision.

scotopic adaptation adaptation to low levels of luminance at which only rod vision is operative.

serous chorioretinopathy term applied to limited separation of the sensory layer of the retina from the pigment epithelium layer by fluid.

siderosis chronic inflammation of the eye due to a retained iron foreign body within the eye.

slit lamp see biomicroscope.

Snellen letter letter so constructed that at a given distance from the eye it subtends an angle of

5 minutes, with each portion of the letter sub-tending an angle of 1 minute.

squamous blepharitis seborrheic inflammation of the lid margins.

squint cross-eyes (strabismus).

staphyloma ectasia of the wall of the eye that is lined with uveal tract.

Stiles-Crawford effect light passing through the center of the pupil of the eye is more effective in evoking the sensation of brightness than the same amount of light passing through an equal area near the edge of the pupil.

strabismus condition in which the eyes are not simultaneously directed to the same object.

comitant deviation of the eye in which there is no ocular muscle paralysis and the degree of crossing is the same in all directions of gaze.

noncomitant deviation of the eyes from parallelism in which a muscle is paretic or paralytic.

sty purulent inflammation of a gland of Zeis; hordeolum.

subconjunctival hemorrhage bleeding beneath the conjunctiva, often occurring spontaneously.

subhyaloid hemorrhage hemorrhage between the neural retina and the vitreous body; a meniscus level is often present.

subluxation of lens condition of the lens when a portion of the supporting zonule is absent and the lens lacks support in one or more quadrants.

suppression physiologic mental process whereby the retinal image transmitted by one eye is ignored.

symblepharon adhesion between palpebral and bulbar conjunctiva.

sympathetic ophthalmia granulomatous uveitis that follows in the opposite eye when there are penetrating injuries of one eye; the eye secondarily affected is called the sympathizing eye, while the injured eye is called the exciting or activating eye.

syndrome group of symptoms and signs that occur together; disease or definite morbid process having a characteristic sequence of symptoms; may affect the whole body or any of its parts.

A and V cross-eyes in which the eyes are closer together in looking up than down (A) or closer looking down than up (V).

Adie see pupil.

Anton form of anosognosia in which the patient denies his blindness; usually accompanied by confabulation, with the patient claiming to see objects in the blind field.

Bassen-Kornzweig progressive ataxic neuropathy associated with retinal pigmentary degenera-

syndrome—cont'd

tion and a crenated appearance of erythrocytes (A-beta-lipoproteinemia).

Batten-Mayou juvenile form of amaurotic familial idiocy with macular degeneration and optic atrophy.

Behçet recurrent iridocyclitis, aphthous ulcers of the mouth, ulcerations of the genitalia, and in some cases erythema nodosum.

Behr macular degeneration seen in adult life.

Benedikt hemianesthesia and involuntary movements of a choreiform nature in the extremities on the side opposite to the lesion in the medial lemniscus and region of the red nucleus.

Berlin retinal edema following ocular contusion.

Best hereditary type of vitelliruptive macular degeneration characterized by a macular lesion having an ophthalmoscopic appearance of an egg fried "sunny side up" and associated in this stage with good vision; when egg is "scrambled," vision deteriorates.

Bielschowsky-Jansky late form of infantile amaurotic familial idiocy.

Bowen intraepithelial epithelioma; when the eye is involved, it commonly involves the conjunctiva at the corneoscleral junction in chronically irritated eyes.

cavernous sinus thrombosis of the cavernous sinus with third, fourth, and sixth cranial nerve palsy and edema of the face and eyelids and infection.

cerebellopontine angle tumor ataxia, tinnitus, deafness, ipsilateral paralysis of the sixth and seventh cranial nerves, involvement of the fifth cranial nerve, vertigo, and nystagmus.

chiasma optic atrophy and bitemporal hemianopsia.

Coats chronic progressive retinal abnormality characterized by retinal deposits and malformation of retinal blood vessels.

Cogan nonsyphilitic interstitial keratitis with associated nerve deafness.

Collins (Franceschetti) mandibulofacial dysostosis.

crocodile tears spontaneous lacrimation that occurs with the normal salivation of eating; follows facial nerve paralysis and is due to aberrant regenerating nerve fibers so that some destined for the salivary glands go to the lacrimal gland.

Crouzon craniofacial dysostosis with eyes widely separated.

Danlos-Ehlers widespread systemic disorder with overextensibility of joints, hyperelasticity of the skin, fragility of the skin, and pseudotumors following trauma; there may be epi-

syndrome—cont'd

canthal folds, esotropia, blue sclera, glaucoma, ectopic lenses, and proliferating retinopathy.

Devic optic neuroencephalomyelopathy.

Down mongolism.

Duane's retraction narrowing of the palpebral fissure on the side on which the lateral rectus muscle is paralyzed when the patient looks toward the opposite side.

Eales vasculitis of the retinal vessels characterized by inflammation, occlusion, neovascularization, and recurrent retinal hemorrhages, occurring particularly in young men.

familial autonomic dysfunction (Riley-Day) reduced or absent tears, postural hypotension, excessive sweating, corneal anesthesia, exotropia, and absence of taste buds.

Foster Kennedy optic atrophy on the side of the lesion and papilledema on the opposite side that occur in tumors of the frontal lobe of the brain.

Foville paralysis of the limbs on one side of the body and of the face on the opposite side together with loss of power to rotate the eyes to that side.

Fuchs unilateral heterochromia, inflammation of the iris and ciliary body, and secondary cataract.

Gaucher familial disorder characterized by splenomegaly, skin pigmentation, and pigmented pingueculas.

Gradenigo palsy of the lateral rectus muscle (N VI) and severe unilateral headache in suppurative disease of the middle ear.

Grönblad-Strandberg angioid streaks of the fundus and pseudoxanthoma elasticum of the skin.

Hand-Schüller-Christian insidious and progressive abnormality of children characterized by exophthalmos, diabetes insipidus, and softened areas in the bones, particularly in femurs and those of the skull, shoulder, and pelvic girdle.

Harada Vogt-Koyanagi syndrome combined with retinal detachment.

Heerfordt uveitis, fever, and parotid gland swelling; now recognized as a manifestation of sarcoidosis.

hepatolenticular degeneration (Wilson) abnormality of copper metabolism associated with progressive degeneration of the liver and lentate nucleus, mental retardation, and a brownish ring (Kayser-Fleisher) composed of copper at the periphery of the cornea.

Horner sympathetic nerve paralysis with miosis, blepharoptosis, and anhydrosis of face.

Hunter sex-linked form of mucopolysaccharido-

syndrome—cont'd

sis in which the corneas remain clear until the third decade.

Hurler (gargoylism) autosomal recessive mucopolysaccharidosis characterized by dwarfism with short, kyphotic spinal column, short fingers, depression of bridge of the nose, heavy, ugly facies, stiffness of joints, cloudiness of cornea, retinal degeneration, hepatosplenomegaly, and mental retardation.

Hutchinson neuroblastoma with orbital metastasis.

Kufs late juvenile form of cerebromacular degeneration.

Laurence-Moon-Biedl inherited disturbance of the pituitary gland characterized by girdle-type obesity, hypogenitalism, mental retardation, polydactyly, and pigmentary retinal degeneration.

Leber sex-linked form of retrobulbar neuritis occurring about the age of 20 years.

Leterer-Siwe nonfamilial reticuloendotheliosis of early childhood.

Lindau angioma of the central nervous system, particularly in the cerebellum, and associated Lindau–von Hippel disease with angioma of the cerebellum, retina, pancreas, and kidney.

Marcus Gunn jerky movements of the upper eyelid occurring when the jaw moves, often associated with blepharoptosis.

Marfan widespread systemic abnormality involving elastic tissues.

Mikulicz chronic lymphocytic infiltration and enlargement of the lacrimal and salivary glands.

Niemann-Pick heredofamilial lipid disorder.

orbital apex oculomotor paresis and neuralgia resulting from involvement of structures at apex of the orbit by a tumor, often a neoplasm of the nasopharynx.

osteogenesis imperfecta (Van der Hoeve) bone fragility, blue sclera, and deafness.

paratrigeminal (Raeder) rare abnormality due to a lesion of the semilunar ganglion and related sympathetic fibers from the carotid plexus, characterized by trigeminal neuralgia, often followed by sensory loss on the affected side of the face, weakness and atrophy of the muscles of mastication, miosis, and blepharoptosis.

Parinaud conjunctivitis associated with palpable preauricular lymph nodes.

Purtscher traumatic angiopathy of the retina.

Refsum hereditary lipid abnormality with retinal degeneration, polyneuritis, deafness, and cerebellar signs.

Reiter disease of males marked by initial diar-

syndrome—cont'd

rhea and followed by urethritis, conjunctivitis, and migratory polyarthritis.

Riley-Day see familial autonomic dysfunction.

Sjögren keratoconjunctivitis sicca, xerostomia, enlargement of the parotid gland, and polyarthritis.

Stargardt degenerative disease of the macula lutea occurring before puberty.

Stevens-Johnson form of erythema multiforme characterized by consitutional symptoms and marked inflammation and later scarring of the conjunctiva and oral mucosa.

Sturge-Weber-Dimitri nevus flammeus, often associated with glaucoma.

Tay-Sachs infantile amaurotic familial idiocy.

Vogt-Koyanagi bilateral uveitis, poliosis, vitiligo, alopecia, and dysacousia.

Vogt-Spielmeyer juvenile amaurotic familial idiocy.

Weber paralysis of the oculomotor nerve (N III) on the same side as the lesion and spastic hemiplegia on the side opposite the lesion with increased reflexes and loss of superficial reflexes.

synechiae adhesion between the iris and adjacent structures.

anterior synechiae between the iris and the cornea.

peripheral anterior occurs with unrelieved attacks of angle-closure glaucoma when the iris remains in contact with the cornea for a long period; may occur following injury or surgery when the anterior chamber does not form.

posterior adhesion between the iris and the lens as occurs commonly in uveitis.

talbot unit of light equal to one lumen-second.

tangent screen device used in perimetry for the study of the field of vision within 30° of the fixation point; usually made of black felt and testing is carried out 1 or 2 meters from the eye; called tangent because it would be tangent to the arc of a perimeter, placed at 1 or 2 meters from the eye.

tarsorrhaphy operation in which the lids are sutured together as in lagophthalmos.

temporal arteritis giant cell arteritis.

tonography test by means of which the amount of fluid forced from the eye by a constant pressure during a constant period is determined.

tonometer instrument for measuring ocular tension.

applanation instrument used to measure intraocular pressure in which the globe is not indented.

Schiøtz indentation type of instrument.

trachoma cicatrizing conjunctivitis caused by a member of the Bedsoniae group of microorganisms.

TRIC agents acronym derived from *tr*achoma and *i*nclusion *c*onjunctivitis, members of the psittacosis–lymphogranuloma venereum–trachoma *(Chlamydia* or Bedsoniae) group of microorganisms.

trichiasis condition in which there are supernumerary lashes.

tritanopia form of dichromatism in which there are but two cone pigments present and there is a complete insensitivity to blue.

uveitis inflammation of the uveal tract.

vernal conjunctivitis inflammation of the conjunctiva presumably due to allergy and characterized by giant papillary hypertrophy of the conjunctiva.

vision

binocular faculty of using both eyes synchronously, without diplopia.

color ability to distinguish subjectively a large variety of wavelengths of light in the visible spectrum.

photopic vision in bright illumination.

scotopic vision in dim illumination or vision following the biochemical or neurologic changes occurring in dark adaptation.

visual angle angle that an object or detail subtends at the point of observation; usually measured in minutes of arc.

visual field locus of objects or points in space that can be perceived when the head and eyes are kept fixed; the field may be monocular or binocular.

visual line that line which connects a point in space with the fovea centralis.

xanthelasma flat, sharply circumscribed deposits of lipid in the eyelids, sometimes associated with hypercholesterolemia.

yellow spot term applied to macula lutea.

Selected references

The *Archives of Ophthalmology* each month publishes a critical review of the current literature concerning a different topic. Each reviewer has a particular interest in the subject and a new reviewer is selected every 3 years. The monthly schedule is approximately as follows: neuro-ophthalmology—January; eyelids, lacrimal apparatus, and conjunctiva—February; cornea and sclera—March; uvea—April; glaucoma—May; retina and optic nerve—June; optics and visual physiology—July; strabismus—August; orbit—September; pharmacology and toxicology—October; orbit—November; chemistry—December.

The *American Journal of Ophthalmology* publishes some 2,000 abstracts annually and each 10 years a Ten Year Index. This appeared most recently in 1962. A Ten Year Index of the *British Journal of Ophthalmology* was published in 1966, and the most recent index of the American Ophthalmological Society is bound in their 1962 *Transactions*.

The *System of Ophthalmology*, edited by Sir Stewart Duke-Elder (St. Louis, The C. V. Mosby Company) offers a remarkably comprehensive and authoritative review. The following volumes have thus far appeared: vol. 1, *The Eye in Evolution*, 1958; vol. 2, *Anatomy of the Visual System*, 1961; vol. 3, pt. 1, *Embryology*, 1963; vol. 3, pt. 2, *Congenital Deformities*, 1964; vol. 4, *Physiology of the Eye and of Vision*, 1968; vol. 7, *Foundations of Ophthalmol-ogy: Heredity, Pathology, Diagnosis and Therapeutics*, 1962; vol. 8, pt. 1, *Diseases of the Conjunctiva and Associated Diseases of the Corneal Epithelium*, 1965; vol. 8, pt. 2, *Diseases of the Cornea and Sclera, Epibulbar Manifestations of Systemic Disease, Cysts and Tumors*, 1965; vol. 9, *Diseases of the Uveal Tract*, 1966; and vol. 10, *Diseases of the Retina*, 1967.

The monograph published each year by the French Ophthalmological Society surveys one topic in detail and provides an exhaustive review. The *Transactions of the Ophthalmological Society of the United Kingdom* is clinically oriented with considerable emphasis on systemic disease, whereas the *Year Book of Ophthalmology* surveys recent literature and provides interesting comments.

ANATOMY AND EMBRYOLOGY
Anatomy

Cogan, D. G.: Neurology of the ocular muscles, ed. 2, Springfield, Ill., 1956, Charles C Thomas, Publisher.

Fink, W. H.: Surgery of the vertical muscles of the eye, ed. 2, Springfield, Ill., 1962, Charles C Thomas, Publisher.

Jakus, M. A.: Ocular fine structures, Boston, 1964, Little, Brown & Co.

Rohen, J. W., editor: The structure of the eye, Stuttgart, 1965, F. K. Schattauer-Verlag, vol. 2.

Salzmann, M.: The anatomy and histology of the human eyeball in the normal state: its development and senescence, Brown, E. V. L., translator, Chicago, 1912, The University of Chicago Press.

Smelser, G. K., editor: The structure of the eye, New York, 1961, Academic Press, Inc.

Whitnall, S. E.: The anatomy of the human orbit and accessory organs of vision, London, 1921, Oxford University Press.

Wolff, E.: Anatomy of the eye and orbit, ed. 6, revised by Last, R. J., Philadelphia, 1968, W. B. Saunders Co.

Choroid

Feeney, M. L., and Hogan, M. J.: Electron microscopy of the human choroid. I. Cells and supporting structures. II. The choroidal nerves. III. The blood vessels, Amer. J. Ophthal. **51**: 1057, 1072, 1085, 1961.

Friedman, E., and Smith, T. R.: Clinical and pathological study of choroidal lipid globules, Arch. Ophthal. **75**:334, 1966.

Potts, A. M.: Anatomic methods for study of bulbus oculi, Amer. J. Ophthal. **65**:155, 1968.

Ring, H. G., and Fujino, T.: Observations on the anatomy and pathology of the choroidal vasculature, Arch. Ophthal. **78**:431, 1967.

Ciliary body

Fenton, R. H., and Hunter, W. S.: Histopathologic findings in eyes with paralysis of the oculomotor (third) nerve, Arch. Ophthal. **73**: 224, 1965.

Fine, B. S.: Limiting membranes of the sensory retina and pigment epithelium. An electron microscopic study, Arch. Ophthal. **66**:847, 1961.

Fine, B. S., and Zimmerman, L. E.: Müller's cells and the "middle limiting membrane" of the human retina, Invest. Ophthal. **1**:304, 1962.

Fine, B. S., and Zimmerman, L. E.: Light and electron microscopic observations in the ciliary epithelium in man and rhesus monkey, Invest. Ophthal. **2**:105, 1963.

Cornea

Kayes, J., and Holmberg, A.: The fine structure of Bowman's layer and the basement membrane of the corneal epithelium, Amer. J. Ophthal. **50**:1013, 1960.

Teng, C. C.: The fine structure of the corneal epithelium and basement membrane of the rabbit, Amer. J. Ophthal. **51**:278, 1961.

Corneoscleral limbus

Allen, L., Burian, H. M., and Braley, A. E.: The anterior border ring of Schwalbe and the pectinate ligament, Arch. Ophthal. **53**:799, 1955.

Ashton, N.: The exit pathway of aqueous, Trans. Ophthal. Soc. U. K. **80**:397, 1960.

Flocks, M.: The anatomy of the trabecular meshwork as seen in tangential section, Arch. Ophthal. **56**:708, 1956.

Preziosi, V. A.: The periphery of Descemet's membrane, Arch. Ophthal. **80**:197, 1968.

Theobald, G.: II. Further studies on the canal of Schlemm, Amer. J. Ophthal. **39**:65, 1955.

Theobald, G.: The limbal area, Amer. J. Ophthal. **50**:543, 1960.

Zimmerman, L. E., Smelser, G. K., Tormey, J. M., Fine, B. S., Feeney, L., Wissig, S., and Becker, B.: Symposium—Contribution of electron microscopy to the understanding of the production and outflow of aqueous humor, Trans. Amer. Acad. Ophthal. Otolaryng. **70**:737, 1966.

Eyelids

Berke, R. N.: Simplified Blascovic's operation for ptosis, Arch. Ophthal. **48**:460, 1952.

Fox, S. A.: The palpebral fissure, Amer. J. Ophthal. **62**:73, 1966.

Jones, L. T.: The anatomy of the lower eyelid, Amer. J. Ophthal. **49**:29, 1960.

Iris

Eninger, B.: Double innervation of the feline iris dilator, Arch. Ophthal. **77**:541, 1967.

Paulson, G. W., and Kapp, J. P.: Dilation of the pupil in the cat via the oculomotor nerve, Arch. Ophthal. **77**:536, 1967.

Toumis, A. J., and Fine, B. S.: Ultrastructure of the iris: intercellular stromal components, Arch. Ophthal. **62**:974, 1959.

Toumis, A. J., and Fine, B. S.: Ultrastructure of the iris: an electron microscopic study, Amer. J. Ophthal. **48**:397, 1959.

Lens

Wanko, T., and Gavin, M. W.: The fine structure of the lens epithelium, Arch. Ophthal. **60**:686, 1958.

Nerves to the eyes

Carpenter, M. B., and Strominger, N. L.: The medial longitudinal fasciculus and disturbances of conjugate horizontal eye movements in the monkey, J. Comp. Neurol. **125**:41, 1965.

Hayreh, S. S., and Vrabec, F.: The structure of the head of the optic nerve in rhesus monkey, Amer. J. Ophthal. **62**:136, 1966.

Henderson, J. W.: The neuroanatomy of ocular motility and of strabismus. In Haik, G. M., editor: Strabismus, symposium of the New Orleans Academy of Ophthalmology, St. Louis, 1962, The C. V. Mosby Co.

Jampel, R. S., and Bloomgarden, C. I.: Individual extraocular muscle function from faradic stimulation of the oculomotor and trochlear nerves of the macaque, Invest. Ophthal. **2**:265, 1963.

Rucker, C. W., Keefe, W. P., and Kernohan, J. W.: Pathogenesis of paralysis of the third cranial nerve, Trans. Amer. Ophthal. Soc. **57**:87, 1959.

Ocular muscles

Brandt, D. E., and Leeson, C. R.: Structural differences of fast and slow fibers in human extraocular muscle, Amer. J. Ophthal. 62:478, 1966.

Cheng, K., and Breinin, G. M.: Fine structure of nerve endings in extraocular muscle, Arch. Ophthal. 74:882, 1965.

Diefert, S. W.: The demonstration of different types of muscle fibers in human extraocular muscle, Invest. Ophthal. 4:51, 1965.

Jampel, R. S.: The action of the superior oblique muscle. An experimental study in the monkey, Arch. Ophthal. 75:535, 1966.

Leopold, I. H., editor: Symposium on extraocular muscles, Invest. Ophthal. 6:217, 1967.

Miller, J. E.: Cellular organization of rhesus extraocular muscle, Invest. Ophthal. 6:18, 1967.

Optic nerves

Cohen, A. I.: Ultrastructural aspects of human optic nerve, Invest. Ophthal. 6:294, 1967.

Retina

Cogan, D. G.: Retinal architecture and pathophysiology, Amer. J. Ophthal. 54:347, 1962.

Fine, B. S., and Zimmerman, L. E.: Müller's cells and the "middle limiting membrane" of the human retina, Invest. Ophthal. 1:304, 1962.

Friedman, E., and Kuwabara, T.: The retinal pigment epithelium. IV. The damaging effects of radiant energy, Arch. Ophthal. 80:265, 1968.

Friedman, E., and Ts'o, M. O. M.: The retinal pigment epithelium. II. Histologic changes associated with age, Arch. Ophthal. 79:315, 1968.

Polyak, S. L.: The retina, Chicago, 1941, University of Chicago Press.

Polyak, S. L.: The vertebrate visual system, Chicago, 1957, University of Chicago Press.

Straatsma, B. R., Landers, M. B., and Kreiger, A. E.: The ora serrata in the adult human eye, Arch. Ophthal. 80:3, 1968.

Ts'o, M. O. M., and Friedman, E.: The retinal pigment epithelium, Arch. Ophthal. 78:641, 1967.

Ts'o, M. O. M., and Friedman, E.: The retinal pigment epithelium. III. Growth and development, Arch. Ophthal. 80:214, 1968.

Vrabec, F.: The temporal raphe of the human retina, Amer. J. Ophthal. 62:926, 1966.

Vitreous body

Hogan, M. J.: The vitreous: its structure and relation to the ciliary body and retina, Invest. Ophthal. 2:418, 1963.

Zonule

McCulloch, C.: The zonule of Zinn. Its origin, course and insertion, and its relation to neighboring structures, Trans. Amer. Ophthal. Soc. 52:525, 1954.

Pappas, G. D., and Smelser, G. K.: II. Studies on the ciliary epithelium and zonule, Amer. J. Ophthal. 46:299, 1958.

Vail, D.: The zonule of Zinn. The Doyne lecture, Trans. Ophthal. Soc. U. K. 77:441, 1957.

Embryology

Barber, A. N.: Embryology of the human eye, St. Louis, 1955, The C. V. Mosby Co.

Davies, J.: Human developmental anatomy, New York, 1963, The Ronald Press Co.

Espinasse, P. G.: The regeneration of the lens and its initial development, Exper. Eye Res. 1:466, 1962.

Mann, I.: The development of the human eye, ed. 2, London, 1949, British Medical Association.

Papaconstantinou, J.: Molecular basis of lens cell differentiation, Science 156:338, 1967.

Pettit, T. H.: A study of lens regeneration in the rabbit, Invest. Ophthal. 2:243, 1963.

Walls, G. L.: The vertebrate eye and its adaptive radiation, Bloomfield, Hills, Mich., 1942, Cranbrook Press; reissued, New York, 1963, Hafner Publishing Co., Inc.

PHYSIOLOGY OF THE EYE

Adler, F. M.: Physiology of the eye, clinical application, ed. 4, St. Louis, 1965, The C. V. Mosby Co.

Allen, J. H., editor: Strabismus, ophthalmic symposium I, II, St. Louis, 1950, 1958, The C. V. Mosby Co.

Ascher, K. W.: The aqueous veins, Springfield, Ill., 1961, Charles C Thomas, Publisher.

Cogan, D. G.: Neurology of ocular muscles, ed. 2, Springfield, Ill., 1956, Charles C Thomas, Publisher.

Dartnall, H. J. A.: The visual pigments, New York, 1957, John Wiley & Sons, Inc.

Davson, H. M.: Physiology of the ocular and cerebrospinal fluids, London, 1956, J. & R. Churchill, Ltd.

Davson, H. M., editor: The eye: vol. 1, Vegetative physiology and biochemistry; vol. 2, The visual process; vol. 3, Muscular mechanisms; vol. 4, Visual optics and the optical space sense, New York, 1962, Academic Press, Inc.

Gibson, G. G., and Harley, R. D.: Sensorimotor anomalies of the extrinsic ocular muscles, Rochester, Minn., 1962, American Academy of Ophthalmology and Otolaryngology.

Graham, C. H., editor: Vision and visual perception, New York, 1965, John Wiley & Sons, Inc.

Granit, R.: Sensory mechanism of the retina, London, 1947, Oxford University Press.

Haik, G. M., editor: Strabismus, symposium of the New Orleans Academy of Ophthalmology, St. Louis, 1962, The C. V. Mosby Co.

Linksz, A.: Physiology of the eye; vol. 1, Optics; vol. 2, Vision; vol. 3, Physiology, New York, 1962, Grune & Stratton, Inc.

Pirie, A., and Van Heyningen, R.: Biochemistry of the eye, Oxford, 1956, Blackwell Scientific Publications.

Rubin, M. L., and Walls, G. L.: Studies in physiological optics, Springfield, Ill., 1965, Charles C Thomas, Publisher.

Wolken, J. J.: Vision, biophysics and biochemistry of the retinal photoreceptors, Springfield, Ill., 1966, Charles C Thomas, Publisher.

Wright, W. D.: The measurement of colour, ed. 3, Princeton, N. J., 1964, D. Van Nostrand Co., Inc.

Aqueous humor

Becker, B.: Hypothermia and aqueous humor dynamics of the rabbit eye, Trans. Amer. Ophthal. Soc. **58**:337, 1960.

Kinsey, V. E.: Aqueous composition and dynamics in glaucoma. In Newell, F. W., editor: Transactions of Fifth Conference, New York, 1961, Josiah Macy, Jr., Foundation.

Cornea

Kinoshita, J. H.: Some aspects of carbohydrate metabolism of the cornea, Invest. Ophthal. **1**:178, 1962.

Maurice, D. M.: The structure and transparency of the cornea, J. Physiol. **136**:263, 1957.

Extraocular muscular mechanisms

Robinson, D. A.: Eye control in primates, Science **161**:1219, 1968.

Intraocular pressure

Bárány, E.: A mathematical formulation of intraocular pressure as dependent upon secretion, ultrafiltration, bulk-out flow and osmotic reabsorption of fluid, Invest. Ophthal. **2**:485, 1963.

Becker, B., and Shaffer, R. N.: Diagnosis and therapy of the glaucomas, ed. 2, St. Louis, 1965, The C. V. Mosby Co.

Retina—metabolism

Brown, P. K., and Wald, G.: Visual pigments in single rods and cones of the human retina, Science **144**:45, 1964.

Marks, W. B., Dobelle, W. H., and MacNichol, E. F.: Visual pigments of single primate cones, Science **143**:1181, 1964.

Wald, G.: Retinal structure and visual function. In Smelser, G. K., editor: The structure of the eye, New York, 1961, Academic Press, Inc.

Wald, G., Brown, P. K., and Gibbons, I. R.: The problem of visual excitation, J. Opt. Soc. Amer. **53**:20, 1963.

Wolken, J. J.: Structure and molecular organization of retinal photoreceptors, J. Opt. Soc. Amer. **53**:1, 1963.

Tears

François, J., and Rabaey, M.: Agar microelectrophoresis of tears, Amer. J. Ophthal. **50**:793, 1960.

Mishima, S.: Some physiological aspects of the precorneal tear film, Arch. Ophthal. **73**:233, 1965.

Wright, J. C., and Meger, G. E.: A review of the Schirmer test for tear production, Arch. Ophthal. **67**:564, 1962.

Visual mechanisms

Brown, K. T.: The electroretinogram: its components and their origin, Vision Res. **8**:633, 1968.

Committee on Colorimetry, Optical Society of America: The science of color, Washington, D. C., 1963, The Society.

Hubel, D. H.: Integrative processes in the central visual pathways of the cat, J. Opt. Soc. Amer. **53**:58, 1963.

Ikeda, H., and Ripps, H.: The electroretinogram of a cone-monochromat, Arch. Ophthal. **75**:513, 1966.

Kolder, H., and Brecher, G. A.: Fast oscillations of the corneoretinal potential in man, Arch. Ophthal. **75**:232, 1966.

Muntz, W. R. A.: Vision in frogs, Sci. Amer. **210**:111, 1964.

Penn, R.: The mechanism of dark adaptation, Survey Ophthal. **10**:510, 1965.

Rushton, W. A. H.: Organization of the retina. In Creese, R., editor: Recent advances in physiology, ed. 8, Boston, 1963, Little, Brown & Co.

Wald, G.: Molecular basis of visual excitation, Science **162**:230, 1968.

Vitreous body

Balazs, E. A.: Molecular morphology of the vitreous body. In Smelser, G. K., editor: Structure of the eye, New York, 1961, Academic Press, Inc.

Fine, B. S., and Tousimis, S. A.: The structure of the vitreous body and the suspensory ligaments of the lens, Arch. Ophthal. **65**:95, 1961.

Hogan, M. J.: The vitreous: its structure and relation to the ciliary body and retina, Invest. Ophthal. **2**:418, 1963.

Schepens, C. L., editor: Importance of the vitreous body in retina surgery with special emphasis upon reoperations, St. Louis, 1960, The C. V. Mosby Co.

Schwarz, W.: Electron microscopic observations of the human vitreous body. In Smelser, G. K., editor: The structure of the eye, New York, 1961, Academic Press, Inc.

PHARMACOLOGY

Becker, B., and Shaffer, R. N.: Diagnosis and therapy of the glaucomas, ed. 2, St. Louis, 1965, The C. V. Mosby Co.

Ellis, P. P., and Smith, D. L.: Handbook of ocular therapeutics and pharmacology, ed. 2, St. Louis, 1966, The C. V. Mosby Co.

Goodman, L. S., and Gilman, A., editors: The pharmacological basis of therapeutics, New York, 1965, The Macmillan Co.

Grant, W. M.: Toxicology of the eye, Springfield, Ill., 1962, Charles C Thomas, Publisher.

Havener, W. H.: Ocular pharmacology, St. Louis, 1966, The C. V. Mosby Co.

Leopold, I. H.: New dimensions in ocular pharmacology, Amer. J. Ophthal. 62:396, 1966.

Leopold, I. H., editor: Ocular therapy, complications and management, St. Louis, 1966, 1967, 1968, The C. V. Mosby Co., vols. 1, 2, 3.

Potts, A. M.: The effect of drugs upon the eye, Physiol. Pharm. 2:329, 1965.

Antimicrobial therapy

Carter, W., and McCarty, K. S.: Molecular mechanisms of antibiotic therapy, Ann. Intern. Med. 64:1087, 1966.

Kagan, B. M., editor: Antimicrobial therapy, Pediat. Clin. N. Amer. 15:1, 1968.

Records, R. E., and Ellis, P.: The intraocular penetration of ampicillin, methicillin and oxacillin, Amer. J. Ophthal. 64:135, 1967.

Autonomic drugs

Acheson, G. H., editor: Second symposium on catecholamines, Pharmacol. Rev. 18:1, 1966.

Criswick, F. B., and Drance, S. M.: Comparative study of four different epinephrine salts on intraocular pressure, Arch. Ophthal. 75:768, 1966.

Langham, M. E., and Weinstein, G. W.: Horner's syndrome. Ocular hypersensitivity to adrenergic amines, Arch. Ophthal. 78:462, 1967.

Sears, M. L.: The mechanism of action of adrenergic drugs in glaucoma, Invest. Ophthal. 5:115, 1966.

Shaffer, R. N., and Hetherington, J.: Anticholinesterase drugs and cataracts, Amer. J. Ophthal. 62:613, 1966.

Von Euler, U. S., Rosell, S., and Unvas, B., editors: Mechanism of release of biogenic amines, Long Island City, N. Y., 1966, Pergamon Press, Inc.

Carbonic anhydrase inhibitors

Becker, B.: Carbonic anhydrase and the formation of aqueous humor, Amer. J. Ophthal. 47:342, 1959.

Maren, T. H.: Carbonic anhydrase: chemistry, physiology, and inhibition, Physiol. Rev. 47:595, 1967.

Cardiac glycosides

Bonting, S. L., Caravaggion, L. L., and Hawkins, N. M.: Studies on sodium-potassium-activated adenosine-triphosphatase. VI. Its role in cation transport in the lens of cat, calf, and rabbit, Arch. Biochem. 101:47, 1963.

Simon, K. A., and Bonting, S. L.: Possible usefulness of cardiac glycosides in treatment of glaucoma, Arch. Ophthal. 68:277, 1962.

Chloroquine toxicity

Burns, R. P.: Delayed onset of chloroquine retinopathy, New Eng. J. Med. 275:693, 1966.

Carr, R. E., Gouras, P., and Gunkel, R. D.: Chloroquine retinopathy, Arch. Ophthal. 75:171, 1966.

Carr, R. E., Henkind, P., Rothfield, N., and Siegel, I. M.: Ocular toxicity of antimalarial drugs: long-term follow-up, Amer. J. Ophthal. 66:738, 1968.

McClanahan, W. S., Harris, J. E., Knobloch, W. H., Tredici, L. M., and Udasco, R. L.: Ocular manifestations of chronic phenothiazine derivative administration, Arch. Ophthal. 75:319, 1966.

Scherbel, A. L., MacKenzie, A. H., Nousek, J. E., and Atojian, M.: Ocular lesions in rheumatoid arthritis and related disorders with particular reference to retinopathy: study of 741 patients treated with and without chloroquine drugs, New Eng. J. Med. 273:360, 1965.

Complications

Burns, C. A.: Indomethacin, reduced retinal sensitivity, and corneal deposits, Amer. J. Ophthal. 66:825, 1968.

Burns, R. P.: Ocular effects of systemic medication, Northwest Med. 60:1083, 1961.

Carpenter, W. T., Jr.: Precipitous mental deterioration following cycloplegia with 0.2% cyclopentolate HCl, Arch. Ophthal. 78:445, 1967.

Lansche, R. K.: Systemic reactions to topical epinephrine and phenylephrine, Amer. J. Ophthal. 62:95, 1966.

Markman, H. D., Rosenberg, P., and Dettbarn, W. D.: Eyedrops and diarrhea, New Eng. J. Med. 271:197, 1964.

Corticosteroids and ACTH

Gartner, J.: Complications of corticoid hormones, Amer. J. Ophthal. 59:1141, 1965.

Schwartz, B., editor: Corticosteroids and the eye, Int. Ophthal. Clin. 6:753, 1966.

Digitalis

Gibson, H. C., Smith, D. M., and Alpern, M.: Pi (π) specificity in digitoxin toxicity, Arch. Ophthal. 74:154, 1965.

White, P. D.: An important toxic effect of digitalis overdosage on the vision, New Eng. J. Med. 272:904, 1965.

Dyes

Forster, H. W., Jr.: Rose bengal in diagnosis of deficient tear formation, Arch. Ophthal. 45:419, 1951.

Lansche, R. K.: Vital staining in normal eyes and in keratoconjunctivitis sicca, Amer. J. Ophthal. 60:520, 1965.

LaPiana, F. G., and Penner, R.: Anaphylactoid reaction to intravenously administered fluorescein, Arch. Ophthal. 79:161, 1968.

Oral contraceptives

Cole, M.: Strokes in young women using oral contraceptives, Arch. Intern. Med. 120:551, 1967.

Walsh, F. B., Clark, D. B., Thompson, R. S., and Nicholson, D. H.: Oral contraceptives and neuroophthalmologic interest, Arch. Ophthal. 74:628, 1965.

Hyperosmotic agents

Becker, B., Kolker, A. E., and Krupin, T.: Isosorbide, an oral hyperosmotic agent, Arch. Ophthal. 78:147, 1967.

D'Alena, P., and Ferguson, W.: Adverse effects after glycerol orally and mannitol parenterally, Arch. Ophthal. 75:201, 1966.

Galin, M. A., Davidson, R., and Shachter, N.: Ophthalmological use of osmotic therapy, Amer. J. Ophthal. 62:629, 1966.

Quinine

Knox, D. L., Palmer, C. A. L., and English, F.: Iris atrophy after quinine amblyopia, Arch. Ophthal. 76:359, 1966.

HISTORY AND INTERPRETATION

Givner, I.: Ocular sign posts to systemic diagnosis, Amer. J. Ophthal. 60:792, 1965.

Heaton, J. M.: The pain in eyestrain, Amer. J. Ophthal. 62:104, 1966.

Huber, A.: Eye symptoms in brain tumors, St. Louis, 1961, The C. V. Mosby Co.

PHYSICAL EXAMINATION OF THE EYES

Givner, I.: Ocular sign posts to systemic diagnosis, Amer. J. Ophthal. 60:792, 1965.

Goldmann, H.: Biomicroscopy of the eye, Amer. J. Ophthal. 66:789, 1968.

Hales, R. H.: Monocular diplopia, Amer. J. Ophthal. 63:459, 1967.

Rutnin, U.: Fundus appearance in normal eyes. I. The choroid, Amer. J. Ophthal. 64:821, 1967.

Rutnin, U., and Schepens, C. L.: Fundus appearance in normal eyes. II. The standard peripheral fundus and developmental variations, Amer. J. Ophthal. 64:840, 1967; III. Peripheral degenerations, Amer. J. Ophthal. 64:1040, 1968; IV. Retinal breaks and other findings, Amer. J. Ophthal. 64:1063, 1968.

Voipio, H., and Hyvarinen, L.: Objective measurement of visual acuity by arrestovisography, Arch. Ophthal. 75:799, 1966.

FUNCTIONAL EXAMINATION OF THE EYES

François, J., Verriest, G., Matton-Van Leuven, M. T., De Rouck, A., and Manavian, D.: Atypical achromatopia of sex-linked recessive inheritance, Amer. J. Ophthal. 61:1101, 1966.

Krill, A. E., and Newell, F. W.: The diagnosis of ocular conversion reaction involving visual function, Arch. Ophthal. 79:254, 1968.

Leinfelder, P. J.: Ophthalmoscopy: an investigative challenge, Amer. J. Ophthal. 61:1211, 1966.

Linksz, A.: The Farnsworth panel D-15 test, Amer. J. Ophthal. 62:27, 1966.

Wheeler, P. C.: The physician and his blind patient, Missouri Med. p. 265, Apr. 1965.

Zuckerman, J.: Diagnostic examination of the eye, Philadelphia, 1964, J. B. Lippincott Co.

THE EYELIDS

Beard, C.: Ptosis, St. Louis, 1969, The C. V. Mosby Co.

Callahan, A.: Reconstructive surgery of the eyelids and ocular adnexa, Birmingham, Ala., 1966, Aesculapius Publishing Co.

Cole, J. G.: Reconstructive surgery of the ocular adnexa: modifications and selected techniques, Trans. Amer. Ophthal. Soc. 63:454, 1965.

Johnson, C. C.: Epiblepharon, Amer. J. Ophthal. 66:1172, 1968.

Johnson, C. C.: Epicanthus, Amer. J. Ophthal. 66:939, 1969.

Mustardé, J. C.: Repair and reconstruction of the orbital region, Baltimore, 1966, The Williams & Wilkins Co.

Peterson, R. A., Aaberg, T. M., and Smith, T. R.: Solid vs. cystic basal cell epitheliomas of the eyelids, Arch. Ophthal. 79:31, 1968.

Reeh, M. J.: Treatment of lid and epibulbar tumors, Springfield, Ill., 1963, Charles C Thomas, Publisher.

THE CONJUNCTIVA

Boniuk, M., editor: Precancerous and cancerous melanosis in ocular and adnexal tumors, St. Louis, 1964, The C. V. Mosby Co.

Conference on trachoma and allied diseases, Amer. J. Ophthal. 63:1027, 1967 (monograph).

Donaldson, D. D.: Atlas of external diseases of the eye; vol. 1, Congenital anomalies and systemic diseases, St. Louis, 1966, The C. V. Mosby Co.

Reese, A. B.: Tumors of the eye, ed. 2, New York, 1963, Hoeber Medical Division, Harper & Row, Publishers.

THE LACRIMAL APPARATUS

Green, W. R., and Zimmerman, L. E.: Ectopic lacrimal gland tissue, Arch. Ophthal. 78:318, 1967.

Jones, L. T.: The lacrimal secretory system and its treatment, Amer. J. Ophthal. 62:47, 1966.

Lemoine, A. N., Jr.: The lacrimal system, Survey Ophthal. 7:325, 1962.

Reese, A. B.: Tumors of the eye, ed. 2, New York, 1964, Hoeber Medical Division, Harper & Row, Publishers.

Spaeth, E. B.: Dacryocystotomy, dacryocystectomy, dacryocystorhinostomy, Trans. Amer. Acad. Ophthal. Otolaryng. 67:68, 1963.

Viers, E. R.: The lacrimal system, clinical application, New York, 1955, Grune & Stratton, Inc.

Zimmerman, L. E.: New concepts regarding certain orbital and lacrimal gland tumors. In Boniuk, M., editor: Ocular and adnexal tumors, St. Louis, 1964, The C. V. Mosby Co.

THE ORBIT

Anderson, F. M., and Geiger, L.: Craniosynostosis, J. Neurosurg. 22:241, 1965.

Blodi, F. C.: Developmental anomalies of the skull affecting the eye, Arch. Ophthal. 57:593, 1957.

Boniuk, M., editor: Ocular and adnexal tumors, St. Louis, 1964, The C. V. Mosby Co.

Conley, J., editor: Cancer of the head and neck. Papers presented at the International Workshop on Cancer of the Head and Neck, New York, May 10-14, 1965, Washington, D. C., 1967, Butterworth, Inc.

François, J., editor: The tumors of the eye and its adnexa, Basel, 1966, S. Karger, A. G.

Hartmann, E., and Gilles, E.: Roentgenologic diagnosis in ophthalmology, Philadelphia, 1959, J. B. Lippincott Co.

Iliff, C. E., and Ossofsky, H. J.: Tumors of the eye and adnexa in infancy and childhood, Springfield, Ill., 1962, Charles C Thomas, Publisher.

Kennedy, R. E.: The effect of early enucleation on the orbit, Amer. J. Ophthal. 60:277, 1965.

Lemoine, A. N., Jr.: The orbit, Survey Ophthal. 7:443, 1962.

Lombardi, G.: Radiology in neuro-ophthalmology, Baltimore, 1967, The Williams & Wilkins Co.

Porterfield, J. F., and Zimmerman, L. E.: Rhabdomyosarcoma of the orbit, Virchow, Arch. Path. Anat. 335:329, 1962.

Van der Werf, A. J. M.: Craniostenose, Amsterdam, 1966, Scheltema & Holkema.

THE CORNEA

Berliner, M. L.: Biomicroscopy of the eye, New York, 1966, Hafner Publishing Co., Inc.

Brown, S. I., and Grayson, M.: Marginal furrows, Arch. Ophthal. 79:563, 1968.

Brown, S. I., and Kitano, S.: Pathogenesis of the retrolental membrane, Arch. Ophthal. 75:518, 1966.

Burns, R. P.: *Pseudomonas aeruginosa* keratitis: mixed infections of the eye, Amer. J. Ophthal. 67:257, 1969.

Cogan, D. G., and Dickerson, G. R.: Nonsyphilitic interstitial keratitis with vestibulo-auditory symptoms: a case with fatal aortitis, Trans. Amer. Ophthal. Soc. 61:113, 1963.

Detels, R., and Dhir, S. P.: Pterygium: a geographical study, Arch. Ophthal. 78:485, 1967.

DeVoe, A. G.: The management of endothelial dystrophy of the cornea, Amer. J. Ophthal. 61:1084, 1966.

Dohlman, C. H., and Brown, S. I.: Treatment of corneal edema with a buried implant, Trans. Amer. Acad. Ophthal. Otolaryng. 69:267, 1966.

Guerry, D. P.: Observations on Cogan's microcystic dystrophy of the corneal epithelium, Amer. J. Ophthal. 62:65, 1966.

Haik, G. M., Perez, L. F., and Murtagh, J. J.: Changes in the cornea and lens in patients on long-term chlorpromazine therapy, Southern Med. J. 59:839, 1966.

Hogan, M. J., Kimura, S. J., and Thygeson, P.: Pathology of herpes simplex kerato-iritis, Trans. Amer. Ophthal. Soc. 61:74, 1963.

Hughes, W. F.: Treatment of herpes simplex keratitis, Amer. J. Ophthal. 67:313, 1969.

Kaufman, H. E., Robbins, J. E., and Capella, J. A.: The endothelium in normal and abnormal corneas, Trans. Amer. Acad. Ophthal. Otolaryng. 69:931, 1965.

Leigh, A. G.: Corneal transplantation, Oxford, 1966, Blackwell Scientific Publications.

McLarnen, D. S.: Malnutrition and the eye, New York, 1963, Academic Press, Inc.

McLean, J. M.: Oculomycosis, Amer. J. Ophthal. 56:537, 1963.

McPherson, S. D., Jr., and Kiffney, G. T., Jr.:

Some histologic findings in keratoconus, Arch. Ophthal. **79**:669, 1968.

Paton, D., and McLarnen, D. S.: Bitot's spots, Amer. J. Ophthal. **50**:568, 1960.

Spencer, W. H., Ferguson, W. J., Jr., Shaffer, R. N., and Fine, M.: Late degenerative changes in the cornea following breaks in Descemet's membrane, Trans. Amer. Acad. Ophthal. Otolaryng. **70**:973, 1966.

Teng, C. C.: Macular dystrophy of the cornea. A histochemical and electron microscopic study, Amer. J. Ophthal. **62**:436, 1966.

Thomas, C. I., and Parnell, E. W.: Prevention and management of early and late complications of keratoplasty, Amer. J. Ophthal. **60**: 385, 1965.

Thygeson, P.: Further observations on superficial punctate keratitis, Arch. Ophthal. **66**:158, 1961.

THE SCLERA

McCarthy, J. L.: Episcleral nodules and erythema nodosum: report of a case with the pathologic findings, Amer. J. Ophthal. **52**:60, 1961.

Wolter, J. R., and Bentley, M. D.: Scleromalacia perforans and massive granuloma of the sclera: a report of an unusual combination of ocular pathology in rheumatoid arthritis, Amer. J. Ophthal. **51**:71, 1961.

THE PUPIL

Alpern, M., Mason, G. L., and Jordinico, R. E.: Pupil size changes associated with changes in accommodative vergence, Amer. J. Ophthal. **52**:762, 1961.

Giles, C. L., and Henderson, J. W.: Horner's syndrome: an analysis of 216 cases, Amer. J. Ophthal. **46**:289, 1958.

Langham, M. E., and Weinstein, G. W.: Horner's syndrome, Arch. Ophthal. **78**:470, 1967.

Laties, A. M., and Scheie, H. G.: Adie's syndrome. Duration of methacholine sensitivity, Arch. Ophthal. **74**:458, 1965.

Loewenfeld, I. E., and Thompson, H. S.: The tonic pupil: a re-evaluation, Amer. J. Ophthal. **63**:46, 1967.

Lowenstein, O.: The Argyll Robertson pupillary syndrome. II. Mechanism and localization, Amer. J. Ophthal. **42**:105, 1956.

Lowenstein, O., and Loewenfeld, I. E.: Influence of retinal adaptation upon the pupillary reflex to light in normal man. I. Effect of adaptation to bright light on the pupillary threshold, Amer. J. Ophthal. **48**:536, pt. 2, 1959; II. Effect of adaptation to dim illumination upon pupillary reflexes elicited by bright light, Amer. J. Ophthal. **51**:644, 1961.

Lowenstein, O., and Loewenfeld, I. E.: Pupillotonic pseudotubes. Syndrome of Markus-Weil and Reys-Holmes-Adie, Survey Ophthal. **10**: 129, 1965.

Pruett, R. C.: Horner's syndrome following intra-oral trauma, Arch. Ophthal. **78**:420, 1967.

Thompson, H. S.: Afferent pupillary defects. Pupillary findings associated with defects of the afferent arm of the pupillary light reflex arc, Amer. J. Ophthal. **62**:860, 1966.

Walsh, F. B., and Hoyt, W. F.: Clinical neuro-ophthalmology, ed. 3, Baltimore, The Williams & Wilkins Co. (In press.)

THE UVEA

Allen, H. F.: Aseptic technique in ophthalmology, Trans. Amer. Ophthal. Soc. **57**:377, 1959.

Albers, E. C., and Klien, B. A.: Iridoschisis, a clinical and histopathologic study, Amer. J. Ophthal. **46**:794, 1958.

Albert, D. M., Rubenstein, R. A., and Scheie, H. G.: Tumor metastasis to the eye, Amer. J. Ophthal. **63**:723, 727, 1967.

Aronson, S. B., Gamble, C. N., Goodner, E. K., and O'Connor, G. R., editors: Clinical methods in uveitis, St. Louis, 1968, The C. V. Mosby Co.

Ashton, N.: Larval granulomatoses of retina due to Toxocara, Brit. J. Ophthal. **44**:129, 1960.

Blodi, F. C., and Hervouet, F.: Syphilitic chorioretinitis, Arch. Ophthal. **79**:294, 1968.

Denko, C. W., and Von Haam, E.: Reiter's syndrome, J.A.M.A. **186**:632, 1963.

DiGeorge, A. M., and Harley, R. D.: The association of aniridia, Wilms' tumor, and genital abnormalities Arch. Ophthal. **75**:796, 1966.

Feldman, H. A.: Toxoplasmosis, New Eng. J. Med. **279**:1370, 1431, 1968.

Gillespie, F. D.: Aniridia, cerebellar ataxia and oligophrenia in siblings, Arch. Ophthal. **73**: 338, 1965.

Hogan, M. J., Kimura, S. J., and Thygeson, P.: Signs and symptoms of uveitis. I. Anterior uveitis, Amer. J. Ophthal. **47**:155, 1959.

Kaufman, H. E.: The uvea, Arch. Ophthal. **75**: 407, 1966.

Kimura, S. J., Hogan, M. J., O'Connor, G. R., and Epstein, W. V.: Uveitis and joint diseases, Arch. Ophthal. **77**:309, 1967.

Kimura, S. J., Thygeson, P., and Hogan, M. J.: Signs and symptoms of uveitis. II. Classification of the posterior manifestations of uveitis, Amer. J. Ophthal. **47**:171, 1959.

Knox, D. L.: Ischemic ocular inflammation, Amer. J. Ophthal. **60**:995, 1965.

Maumenee, A. E., editor: Symposium—Toxoplasmosis, with special reference to uveitis, Baltimore, 1962, The Williams & Wilkins Co.

McCarty, B., and Lewis, P. M.: Reiter's syndrome, Amer. J. Ophthal. **34**:1008, 1962.

McKusick, V. A., Stauffer, M., Knox, D. L., and Clark, D. B.: Chorioretinopathy with hereditary microcephaly, Arch. Ophthal. **75**:597, 1966.

Monacelli, M., and Nazzaro, P., editors: Behçet's disease, Basel, 1966, S. Karger, A. G.

Norton, E. W. D., and Gutman, F.: Fluorescein angiography and hemangiomas of the choroid, Arch. Ophthal. **78**:121, 1967.

Perkins, E. S.: Uveitis and toxoplasmosis, Boston, 1961, Little, Brown & Co.

Schlaegel, T. F., Weber, J. C., Helveston, E., and Kennery, D.: Presumed histoplasmic choroiditis, Amer. J. Ophthal. **63**:919, 1967.

Schultze, R. R.: Rubeosis iridis, Amer. J. Ophthal. **63**:487, 1967.

Silverstein, A. M.: Effect of x-radiation on development of immunogenic uveitis, Invest. Ophthal. **2**:58, 1963.

Smith, J. L., and Singer, J. A.: Histoplasmosis, Amer. J. Ophthal. **3**:413, 1021, 1964.

Sugar, H. S.: Heterochromia iridis. With special consideration of its relation to cyclitic disease, Amer. J. Ophthal. **60**:1, 1965.

Van Meter, T. E., Knox, D. L., and Maumenee, A. E.: The relation between toxoplasmosis and focal exudative retinochoroiditis, Amer. J. Ophthal. **58**:6, 1964.

Winter, F. C., and Yukins, R. E.: Ocular pathology of Behçet's disease, Amer. J. Ophthal. **62**:267, 1966.

Wirostko, E., and Spalter, H. F.: Lens-induced uveitis, Arch. Ophthal. **78**:1, 1967.

Woods, A. C.: Endogenous inflammations of the uveal tract, Baltimore, 1961, The Williams & Wilkins Co.

THE RETINA
General

Ballantyne, A. J., and Michaelson, I. C.: Textbook of the fundus of the eye, Baltimore, 1962, The Williams & Wilkins Co.

Blodi, F. C., and Allen, L.: Stereoscopic manual of the ocular fundus in local and systemic disease, St. Louis, 1964, The C. V. Mosby Co.

Braley, A. E., editor: The retina, Int. Ophthal. Clin. **2**:3, 1962.

François, J.: Heredity in ophthalmology, St. Louis, 1961, The C. V. Mosby Co.

Meyer-Schwickerath, G.: Light coagulation, Drance, S. M., translator, St. Louis, 1960, The C. V. Mosby Co.

Pischel, D. K., Clark, G., and Cibis, P. A.: Symposium—photocoagulation, Trans. Amer. Acad. Ophthal. **66**:57, 1962.

Reese, A. B.: Tumors of the eye, ed. 2, New York, 1963, Hoeber Medical Division, Harper & Row, Publishers.

Coats's disease

Imre, G.: Coats's disease, Amer. J. Ophthal. **54**:175, 1962.

Wise, G. N., and Horava, A.: Coats's disease, Amer. J. Ophthal. **57**:17, 1963.

Degeneration

Carr, R. E., and Gouras, P.: Oguchi's disease, Arch. Ophthal. **73**:528, 1965.

Hogan, M. J., and Alvarado, J.: Studies on the human macula. IV. Aging changes in Bruch's membrane, Arch. Ophthal. **77**:410, 1967.

Hogan, M. J.: Bruch's membrane and disease of the macula, Trans. Ophthal. Soc. U. K. **87**:113, 1968.

Krachmer, J. H., Smith, J. L., and Tocci, P. M. Laboratory studies in retinitis pigmentosa, Arch. Ophthal. **75**:661, 1966.

Maumenee, A. E.: Fluorescein angiography in the diagnosis and treatment of lesions of the ocular fundus, Trans. Ophthal. Soc. U. K. **87**:529, 1968.

Morgan, W. E., III, and Crawford, J. B.: Retinitis pigmentosa and Coats's disease, Arch. Ophthal. **79**:146, 1968.

O'Malley, P., Allen, R. A., Straatsma, B. R., and O'Malley, C.: Paving stone degeneration of the retina, Arch. Ophthal. **73**:169, 1965.

Hyperplastic vitreous

Acers, T. E., and Coston, T. O.: Persistent hyperplastic primary vitreous: early surgical management, Amer. J. Ophthal. **64**:734, 1967.

Wolter, J. R., and Flaherty, N. W.: Persistent hyperplastic vitreous, Amer. J. Ophthal. **47**:491, 1959.

Inflammation

Elliott, A. J.: Recurrent intraocular hemorrhage in young adults (Eales's disease), Trans. Amer. Ophthal. Soc. **52**:811, 1954.

Ophthalmoscopy

Ashton, N., Dollery, C. T., Henkind, P., Hill, D. W., Paterson, J. W., Ramalho, P. W., and Shakib, M.: Focal retinal ischemia: ophthalmoscopic, circulatory, and ultrastructural changes, Brit. J. Ophthal. **50**:281, 1966.

Christensen, L.: The nature of the cytoid body, Trans. Amer. Ophthal. Soc. **56**:451, 1958.

Hollenhorst, R. W.: Significance of bright plaques in the retinal arterioles, J.A.M.A. **178**:23, 1961.

Hollenhorst, R. W., Lensink, E. R., and Whisnant, J. P.: Experimental embolization of the retinal arterioles, Trans. Amer. Ophthal. Soc. **60**:317, 1962.

Kennedy, J. E., and Wise, G. N.: Clinicopathological correlation of retinal lesions, Arch. Ophthal. **74**:658, 1965.

Klien, B. A.: Comments on the cotton-wool lesion of the retina, Amer. J. Ophthal. **59**:17, 1965.

Smith, R., Ashton, N., and Sanders, A. G.: Symposium—Neovascularization in ocular disease, Trans. Ophthal. Soc. U. K. **71**:125, 1961.

Wise, G. N.: Factors influencing new blood vessel formation, Amer. J. Ophthal. **52**:637, 1961.

Retinal separation

Hagler, W. S., and North, A. W.: Retinal dialyses and retinal detachment, Arch. Ophthal. **79**:376, 1968.

McPherson, A., editor: New and controversial aspects of retinal detachment, New York, 1968, Hoeber Medical Division, Harper & Row, Publishers.

Schepens, C. L., editor: Importance of the vitreous body in retina surgery with special emphasis on reoperations, St. Louis, 1960, The C. V. Mosby Co.

Tassman, W., and Annesley, W., Jr.: Retinal detachment in the retinopathy of prematurity, Arch. Ophthal. **75**:608, 1966.

Retinoschisis

Balian, J. V., and Halls, H. F.: Congenital vascular veils in the vitreous: hereditary retinoschisis, Arch. Ophthal. **63**:92, 1960.

Yanoff, M., Rah, E. H., and Zimmerman, L. E.: Histopathology of juvenile retinoschisis, Arch. Ophthal. **79**:49, 1968.

Retinoblastoma

Ellsworth, R. M.: Treatment of retinoblastoma, Amer. J. Ophthal. **66**:49, 1968.

Howard, G. M., and Ellsworth, R. M.: Differential diagnosis of retinoblastoma. A statistical survey of 500 children, Amer. J. Ophthal. **60**:610, 1965.

Hyman, G. A., Ellsworth, R. M., Feind, C. R., and Tretter, P.: Combination therapy in retinoblastoma, Arch. Ophthal. **80**:744, 1968.

Retrolental fibroplasia

Patz, A.: New role of the ophthalmologist in prevention of retrolental fibroplasia, Arch. Ophthal. **78**:565, 1967.

Patz, A.: Retrolental fibroplasia, Trans. Amer. Ophthal. Soc. **66**:940, 1968.

Reese, A. B., Owens, W. C., Friedenwald, J. S., Silverman, W. A., Kinsey, V. E., Hemphill, F. M., and Patz, A.: Symposium—Retrolental fibroplasia (retinopathy of prematurity), Amer. J. Ophthal. **40**:159, 1955.

Silverman, W. A.: Oxygen therapy and retrolental fibroplasia, Arch. Ophthal. **80**:810, 1968.

Serous retinopathy

Peabody, R. R., Zweng, H. C., and Little, H. L.: Treatment of persistent central serous retinopathy, Arch. Ophthal. **79**:166, 1968.

Spalter, H. F.: Photocoagulation of central serous retinopathy, Arch. Ophthal. **79**:247, 1968.

Vascular occlusion

Dahrling, B. E.: Histopathology of early central retinal artery occlusion, Arch. Ophthal. **73**:506, 1965.

Dryden, R. M.: Central retinal vein occlusions and chronic simple glaucoma, Arch. Ophthal. **73**:659, 1965.

Hardenbergh, F. E.: Idiopathic central artery occlusion. Case report and presentation of a general guide to therapy, Arch. Ophthal. **67**:556, 1962.

Klien, B. A.: Macular and extramacular serous chorioretinopathy: with remarks upon the role of an extrabulbar mechanism in its pathogenesis, Amer. J. Ophthal. **51**:231, 1961.

Smith, J. L.: Central retinal and internal carotid arterial occlusions, Arch. Ophthal. **65**:550, 1961.

THE VITREOUS BODY

Kasner, D., Miller, G. R., Taylor, W. H., Sever, R. J., and Norton, E. W. D.: Surgical treatment of amyloidosis of the vitreous, Trans. Amer. Acad. Ophthal. Otolaryng. **72**:410, 1968.

Kaufman, H. E., and Thomas, L. B.: Vitreous opacities diagnostic of familial primary amyloidosis, New Eng. J. Med. **261**:1267, 1959.

Luxenberg, M., and Sime, D.: Relationship of asteroid hyalosis to diabetes mellitus and plasma lipid levels, Amer. J. Ophthal. **67**:406, 1969.

Paton, D., and Duke, J. R.: Primary familial amyloidosis, Amer. J. Ophthal. **61**:736, 1966.

Schepens, C. L.: Clinical aspects of pathologic changes in the vitreous body, Amer. J. Ophthal. **38**:8, 1954.

Schepens, C. L., editor: Importance of the vitreous body in retina surgery with special emphasis on reoperations, St. Louis, 1960, The C. V. Mosby Co.

Teng, C. C., and Chi, H. H.: Vitreous changes and the mechanisms of retinal detachment, Amer. J. Ophthal. **44**:335, 1957.

Tolentino, F. I., Schepens, C. L., and Freeman, H. M.: Massive preretinal retraction, Arch. Ophthal. **78**:16, 1967.

THE OPTIC NERVE

Carroll, F. D., Henderson, J. W., Zimmerman, L. E., Walsh, F. B., and Rucker, C. W.: Symposium—Disease of the optic nerve, Trans. Amer. Acad. Ophthal. Otolaryng. **56**:7, 1956.

Day, R. M., and Carroll, F. D.: Corticosteroids in the treatment of optic nerve involvement associated with thyroid dysfunction, Arch. Ophthal. **79**:279, 1968.

Dreyfus, P. M.: Blood transketolase levels in

tobacco-alcohol amblyopia, Arch. Ophthal. **74:** 617, 1965.

Forster, H. W., Jr., and Bouzarth, W. F.: Meningioma of the tuberculum sellae as a cause of optic atrophy, Amer. J. Ophthal. **64:**908, 1967.

Hoyt, W. F., and Beeston, D.: The ocular fundus in neurologic disease, St. Louis, 1966, The C. V. Mosby Co.

Hoyt, W. F., and Pont, M. E.: Pseudopapilloedema: anomalous elevation of the optic disc. Pitfalls in diagnosis and management, J.A.M.A. **181:**191, 1962.

Miller, A., Bader, R. A., and Bader, M. E.: The neurologic syndrome due to marked hypercapnia with papilloedema, Amer. J. Med. **33:** 309, 1962.

Miller, G. R., and Smith, J. L.: Ischemic optic neuropathy, Amer. J. Ophthal. **62:**103, 1966.

Pollack, I. P., and Becker, B.: Hyaline bodies (drusen) of the optic nerve, Amer. J. Ophthal. **54:**651, 1962.

Richards, R. D., and Lynn, J. R.: The surgical management of gliomas of the optic nerve, Amer. J. Ophthal. **62:**60, 1966.

Schlossman, A., and Phillips, C. C.: Optic neuritis in relation to demyelinating disease, Amer. J. Ophthal. **37:**487, 1954.

Sugar, H. S.: Congenital pits on the optic disc with acquired macular pathology, Amer. J. Ophthal. **53:**307, 1962.

Taub, R. G., and Rucker, C. W.: The relationship of retrobulbar neuritis to multiple sclerosis, Amer. J. Ophthal. **37:**494, 1954.

Victor, M., and Dreyfus, P. M.: Tobacco-alcohol amblyopia, Arch. Ophthal. **74:**649, 1965.

Walsh, F. B., and Hoyt, W. F.: Clinical neuro-ophthalmology, ed. 3, Baltimore, The Williams & Wilkins Co. (In press.)

Williamson-Noble, F. A.: Physiological cupping, Trans. Ophthal. Soc. U. K. **81:**437, 1961.

THE LENS

Byron, H. M.: Differential diagnosis of the shortened angle, Amer. J. Ophthal. **52:**492, 1961.

Cinotti, A. A., and Patti, J. D.: Lens abnormalities in an aging population of nonglaucomatous patients, Amer. J. Ophthal. **65:**25, 1968.

Cogan, D. G.: Symposium on the lens, Exper. Eye Res. **1:**293, 1962.

Cogan, D. G., and Kuwabara, T.: Pathology of cataracts in mongoloid idiocy: a new concept of the pathogenesis of cataracts of the coronary-cerulean type, Docum. Ophthal. **16:**73, 1962.

Curtin, V. T., Joyce, E. E., and Ballin, N.: Ocular pathology in the oculo-cerebro-renal syndrome of Lowe, Amer. J. Ophthal. **64:**533, 1967.

Donaldson, D. D.: The significance of spotting of the iris in mongoloids, Brushfield's spots, Arch. Ophthal. **65:**26, 1960.

Fasanella, R. M., editor: Modern advances in cataract surgery, Philadelphia, 1963, J. B. Lippincott Co.

Feiler-Ofry, V., Stein, R., and Godel, V.: Marchesani's syndrome and chamber-angle anomalies, Amer. J. Ophthal. **65:**862, 1968.

Fonda, G.: Subnormal vision correction for aphakia, Amer. J. Ophthal. **55:**247, 1963.

François, J.: Syndromes with congenital cataract, Amer. J. Ophthal. **52:**207, 1961.

Girard, L. J.: Aspiration-irrigation of congenital and traumatic cataracts, Arch. Ophthal. **77:**387, 1967.

Greaves, D. P.: Symposium on metabolic diseases of the eye: galactosemia, Proc. Roy. Soc. Med. **56:**24, 1963.

Guerry, D., and Geeraets, W. J.: Complications of anterior chamber lenses, Amer. J. Ophthal. **54:**229, 1962.

Jarrett, W. H., II: Dislocation of the lens, Arch. Ophthal. **78:**289, 1967.

McGavic, J. S.: Weill-Marchesani syndrome, Amer. J. Ophthal. **62:**820, 1966.

Merz, E. H., Tausk, K., and Dukes, E.: Mesoectodermal dysplasia and its variants with particular reference to the Rothmund-Werner syndrome, Amer. J. Ophthal. **55:**488, 1963.

Muller, S. A., and Brunsting, L. A.: Cataracts associated with dermatologic disorders, Arch. Derm. **88:**330, 1963.

Riddell, W. J. B.: Congenital cataract, Trans. Ophthal. Soc. U. K. **82:**761, 1962.

Rosenbaum, L. J., and Podos, S. M.: Traumatic ectopic lentis: some relationships to syphilis and glaucoma, Amer. J. Ophthal. **64:**1095, 1967.

Rosenthal, J. W., and Kloepfer, H. W.: The spherophakia-brachymorphia syndrome, Arch. Ophthal. **55:**28, 1956.

Sand, B. J., and Abraham, S. V.: Anterior lenticonus, Amer. J. Ophthal. **53:**636, 1962.

Symposium on the lens, Invest. Ophthal. **4:**373, 1965.

Tarkkanen, A.: Pseudoexfoliation of the lens capsule: a clinical study of 418 patients with special reference to glaucoma, cataract, and changes of the vitreous, Acta Ophthal. **71:**1, 1962.

Wilson, W. A.: Cataracts and galactose metabolism, Trans. Amer. Ophthal. Soc. **65:**661, 1967.

GLAUCOMA

Armaly, M. F.: The heritable nature of dexamethasone-induced ocular hypertension, Arch. Ophthal. **75:**32, 1966.

Armaly, M. F.: Ocular pressure and visual fields, Arch. Ophthal. **81**:25, 1969.

Becker, B., and Ballin, N.: Glaucoma and corticosteroid provocative testing, Arch. Ophthal. **74**:621, 1965.

Becker, B., and Hahn, K. A.: Topical corticosteroids and heredity in primary open-angle glaucoma, Amer. J. Ophthal. **57**:543, 1964.

Becker, B., Keates, E. U., and Coleman, S. L.: Gamma-globulin in the trabecular meshwork of glaucomatous eyes, Arch. Ophthal. **68**:643, 1962.

Becker, B., and Shaffer, R. N.: Diagnosis and therapy of the glaucomas, ed. 2, St. Louis, 1965, The C. V. Mosby Co.

Bill, A., and Barany, E. H.: Gross facility, facility of conventional routes, and pseudofacility of aqueous humor outflow in the cynomolgus monkey, Arch. Ophthal. **75**:665, 1966.

Blanton, F. M., and Pollack, I. P.: Therapy of open-angle glaucoma, Arch. Ophthal. **75**:763, 1966.

Chandler, P. A., and Grant, M. W.: Lectures on glaucoma, Philadelphia, 1965, Lea & Febiger.

Christensen, L.: Pathogenesis of primary shallow chamber angle-closure glaucoma, Arch. Ophthal. **75**:490, 1966.

Drance, S. M.: Studies in the susceptibility of the eye to raised intraocular pressure, Arch. Ophthal. **68**:478, 1962.

Ernest, J. T., and Potts, A. M.: Pathophysiology of the distal portion of the optic nerve. I. Tissue pressure relationships. II. Vascular relationships, Amer. J. Ophthal. **66**:373, 380, 1968.

Haas, J.: Principles and problems of therapy in congenital glaucoma, Invest. Ophthal. **7**:140, 1968.

Hogan, M. J., editor: Medical and surgical management of glaucoma, Boston, 1963, Little, Brown & Co.

Kirsch, R. E.: A study of provocative tests for angle-closure glaucoma, Arch. Ophthal. **74**:770, 1965.

Kurz, G. H.: Phacolytic glaucoma, Arch. Ophthal. **69**:327, 1963.

Leydhecker, W.: Glaucoma in ophthalmic practice, Boston, 1966, Little, Brown & Co.

Lowe, R. F.: Acute angle-closure glaucoma: the second eye; an analysis of 200 cases, Brit. J. Ophthal. **46**:641, 1962.

Redmond, J. H., and Smith, J. H.: Clinical glaucoma, Philadelphia, 1965, F. A. Davis Co.

Shaffer, R. N.: Genetics and the congenital glaucomas, Amer. J. Ophthal. **60**:981, 1965.

Spivey, B. E., and Armaly, M. F.: Tonographic findings in glaucomatocyclitic crises, Amer. J. Ophthal. **55**:47, 1963.

Thomas, R. P., and Riley, M. W.: Acetazolamide and ocular tension, Amer. J. Ophthal. **60**:241, 1965.

Zimmerman, L. E.: Acute secondary open-angle glaucoma ten years after contusion, Survey Ophthal. **8**:26, 1963.

THE EXTRAOCULAR MUSCLES

Adler, F. H.: Physiology of the eye, ed. 4, St. Louis, 1964, The C. V. Mosby Co.

Allen, J. H., editor: Strabismus ophthalmic symposium I, II, St. Louis, 1950, 1958 (vol. 1 reissued in 1968), The C. V. Mosby Co.

Bedrossian, E. H.: Bilateral superior oblique tenectomy for the A-pattern in strabismus, Arch. Ophthal. **78**:334, 1967.

Breinin, G. M., Chin, N. B., and Ripps, H.: A rationale for therapy of accommodative strabismus, Amer. J. Ophthal. **61**:1030, 1966.

Burian, H. M.: Occlusion amblyopia and the development of eccentric fixation in occluded eyes, Amer. J. Ophthal. **62**:853, 1966.

Burian, H. M.: Pathophysiologic basis of amblyopia and of its treatment, Amer. J. Ophthal. **67**:1, 1969.

Cashell, G. T. W., and Durran, I. M.: Handbook of orthoptic principles, Baltimore, 1967, The Williams & Wilkins Co.

Cogan, D. G.: Neurology of ocular muscles, ed. 2, Springfield, Ill., 1956, Charles C Thomas, Publisher.

Cook, G., and Stark, L.: The human eye-movement mechanism, Arch. Ophthal. **79**:428, 1968.

Dunlap, E. A.: Present status of the A and V syndromes, Amer. J. Ophthal. **52**:396, 1961.

Ernest, J. T., and Costenbader, F. D.: Lateral rectus muscle palsy, Amer. J. Ophthal. **65**:721, 1968.

Gibson, G. G., and Harley, R. D.: Sensorimotor anomalies of the extrinsic ocular muscles, Rochester, Minn., 1961, American Academy of Ophthalmology and Otolaryngology.

Haik, G. M., editor: Strabismus—Symposium of the New Orleans Academy of Ophthalmology, St. Louis, 1962, The C. V. Mosby Co.

Helveston, E. M., and von Noorden, G. K.: Microtropia, Arch. Ophthal. **78**:272, 1967.

Parks, M. M., and Friendly, D. S.: Treatment of eccentric fixation in children under four years of age, Amer. J. Ophthal. **61**:395, 1966.

Pratt-Johnson, J. A., Wee, H. S., and Ellis, S.: Suppression associated with esotropia, Canad. J. Ophthal. **2**:284, 1967.

Reinecke, R. D., and Miller, D.: Strabismus, a programmed text, New York, 1966, Appleton-Century-Crofts.

Scott, A. M.: Extraocular muscles and head tilting, Arch. Ophthal. **78**:397, 1967.

Sloan, L. L., Sears, M. L., and Jablonski, M. D.:

Convergence-accommodation relationships, Arch. Ophthal. 63:111, 1960.

Sugar, H. S.: The extrinsic eye muscles, Rochester, Minn., 1955, American Academy of Ophthalmology and Otolaryngology.

Swan, K. C.: False projection in comitant strabismus. Alleviation by anomalous retinal correspondency, Arch. Ophthal. 73:189, 1965.

Swan, K. C.: Surgery for exotropia: fusional ability and choice of procedure, Amer. J. Ophthal. 50:1158, 1960.

Von Noorden, G. K.: Pathogenesis of eccentric fixation, Amer. J. Ophthal. 61:399, 1966.

Von Noorden, G. K., and Maumenee, A. E.: Atlas of strabismus, St. Louis, 1967, The C. V. Mosby Co.

INJURIES OF THE EYE

Abrahams, I. W., and Dodd, R. W.: Orbital floor fractures: a combined procedure of early surgical management, Arch. Ophthal. 68:159, 1962.

Allen, L., and Webster, H. E.: Modified impression method of artificial eye fitting, Amer. J. Ophthal. 67:189, 329, 1969.

Brown, J. L.: Flash blindness, Amer. J. Ophthal. 60:505, 1965.

Browning, C. W., and Walker, R. V.: The use of alloplastics in 45 cases of orbital floor reconstruction, Amer. J. Ophthal. 60:684, 1965.

Callahan, A.: Surgery of the eye—injuries, Springfield, Ill., 1950, Charles C Thomas, Publisher.

Converse, J. M., and Smith, B.: Symposium—Midfacial fractures: nasoorbital fractures, Trans. Amer. Acad. Ophthal. Otolaryng. 67:622, 1963.

George, C. W., and Slack, W. J.: Corneal and scleral lacerations: a 5-year review, Amer. J. Ophthal. 54:119, 1962.

Gorn, R. A., and Kuwabara, T.: Retinal damage by visible light. A physiologic study, Arch. Ophthal. 77:115, 1967.

Hoefle, F. B.: Initial treatment of eye injuries, Arch. Ophthal. 79:33, 1968.

Marr, W. G., and Marr, E. G.: Some observations on Purtscher's disease: traumatic retinal angiopathy, Amer. J. Ophthal. 54:693, 1962.

Merriam, G. R., Jr., and Focht, E. F.: A clinical and experimental study of the effect of single and divided doses of radiation on cataract production, Trans. Amer. Ophthal. Soc. 60:35, 1962.

New Orleans Academy of Ophthalmology: Industrial and traumatic ophthalmology, St. Louis, 1964, The C. V. Mosby Co.

Paton, D., and Goldberg, M. F.: Injuries to the eye, the lids, and the orbit, Philadelphia, 1968, W. B. Saunders Co.

Spaeth, G. L.: Traumatic hyphema, angle recession, dexamethasone hypertension, and glaucoma, Arch. Ophthal. 78:714, 1967.

Spivey, B. E., Allen, L., and Burns, C. A.: The Iowa enucleation implant, Amer. J. Ophthal. 67:171, 1969.

Stallard, H. B.: Eye surgery, ed. 4, Baltimore, 1965, The Williams & Wilkins Co.

Wolter, J. R.: Coup-contrecoup mechanism of ocular injuries, Amer. J. Ophthal. 56:785, 1963.

OPTICAL DEFECTS OF THE EYE

Benton, C. D., and Welsh, R. C.: Spectacles for aphakia, Springfield, Ill., 1966, Charles C Thomas, Publisher.

Bettman, J. W., Jr., Stern, E. L., Whitsell, L. J., and Gofman, H. F.: Cerebral dominance in developmental dyslexia, Arch. Ophthal. 78:722, 1967.

Duke-Elder, S. W.: The practice of refraction, ed. 7, St. Louis, 1963, The C. V. Mosby Co.

Fonda, G.: Management of the patient with subnormal vision, St. Louis, 1965, The C. V. Mosby Co.

Gettes, B. C.: Practical refraction, New York, 1957, Grune & Stratton, Inc.

Girard, L. J., Soper, J. W., and Sampson, W. G.: Corneal contact lenses, St. Louis, 1964, The C. V. Mosby Co.

Hiatt, R. L., Costenbader, F. D., and Albert, D. G.: Clinical evaluation of congenital myopia, Arch. Ophthal. 74:31, 1965.

Keeney, A. H., and Keeney, V.: Dyslexia, St. Louis, 1968, The C. V. Mosby Co.

Money, J., editor: The disabled reader: education of the dyslexic child, Baltimore, 1966, The Johns Hopkins Press.

Ogle, K.: Optics, ed. 2, Springfield, Ill., 1968, Charles C Thomas, Publisher.

Reinecke, R. D., and Herm, R. J.: Refraction: a programmed text, New York, 1965, Appleton-Century-Crofts.

Rubin, M. L., and Waus, G. L.: Studies in physiological optics, Springfield, Ill., 1965, Charles C Thomas, Publisher.

Sloan, L. L.: Reading aids for the partially sighted, Arch. Ophthal. 80:35, 1968.

Sloan, L. L.: Recommended aids for the partially sighted, New York, 1966, National Society for the Prevention of Blindness, Inc.

Sloane, A. E.: Manual of refraction, Boston, 1961, Little, Brown & Co.

Snydacker, D., and Newell, F. W.: A manual of refraction, ed. 2, Rochester, Minn., 1964, American Academy of Ophthalmology and Otolaryngology.

Woods, A. C.: Report from the Wilmer Institute on the results obtained in the treatment of myopia by visual training, Amer. J. Ophthal. **29:**28, 1946.

INFECTIOUS OCULAR DISEASE AND GRANULOMAS

Beeson, P. B., and McDermott, M., editors: Cecil-Loeb textbook of medicine, ed. 12, Philadelphia, 1967, W. B. Saunders Co.

Blank, H., and Rake, G.: Viral and rickettsial diseases of skin, eye and mucous membranes of man, Boston, 1955, Little, Brown & Co.

Chandler, A. C., and Read, C. P.: Introduction to parasitology, ed. 10, New York, 1961, John Wiley & Sons, Inc.

Dubos, R. J., and Hirsch, J. G.: Bacterial and mycotic infections of man, ed. 4, Philadelphia, 1965, J. B. Lippincott Co.

François, J., and Elewaut-Rysselaere, M.: Les mycoses oculaires, Bull. Soc. Belge Ophtal. **147:**1, 1968.

Horsfall, F. L., Jr., and Tamm, I., editors: Viral and rickettsial infections of man, ed. 4, Philadelphia, 1965, J. B. Lippincott Co.

Scadding, J. G.: Sarcoidosis, London, 1967, Eyre & Spottiswoode (Publishers), Ltd.

Woods, A. C.: Endogenous inflammations of the uveal tract, Baltimore, 1961, The Williams & Wilkins Co.

Bacteria

Capolongo, G.: Some observations on the therapy of diphtheritic eye manifestations with antibiotics, Ann. Ottal. **61:**347, 1957.

Harley, R. D.: Ocular leprosy in Panama, Amer. J. Ophthal. **29:**295, 1946.

Mooney, A. J.: Further observations on the ocular complication of tuberculosis meningitis and their implications, Amer. J. Ophthal. **48:**297, 1959.

Sears, M. L.: Ocular leprosy, Amer. J. Ophthal. **46:**359, 1958.

Simmonds, N. T.: Anthrax of the eyelid, Amer. J. Ophthal. **49:**838, 1960.

Thygeson, P.: The cytology of conjunctival exudates, Amer. J. Ophthal. **29:**1499, 1946.

Fungi

Ferry, A. P.: Cerebral mucormycosis (phycomycosis). Ocular findings and review of literature, Survey Ophthal. **6:**1, 1961.

McLean, J. M.: Oculomycosis, Amer. J. Ophthal. **56:**537, 1963.

Pettit, T. H., Learn, R. N., and Foos, R. Y.: Intraocular coccidioidmycosis, Arch. Ophthal. **77:**655, 1967.

Spaeth, G. L.: Absence of so-called histoplasmic uveitis in 134 cases of proven histoplasmosis, Arch. Ophthal. **77:**41, 1967.

Parasites

Daguid, I. M.: Features of ocular infestation by *Toxocara*, Brit. J. Ophthal. **47:**789, 1961.

Ghosh, M., Levy, P. M., and Leopold, I. H.: Therapy of toxoplasmosis uveitis, Amer. J. Ophthal. **59:**55, 1965.

Heath, C. W., Jr., Alexander, A. D., and Galton, M. M.: Leptospirosis in the United States, New Eng. J. Med. **273:**857, 1965.

Maumenee, A. E., editor: Symposium—Toxoplasmosis, with special reference to uveitis, Baltimore, 1962, The Williams & Wilkins Co.

Rose, L.: Filarial worm in anterior chamber of eye in man, Arch. Ophthal. **75:**13, 1966.

Toussaint, D., and Danis, P.: Retinopathy in generalized *Loa loa* filariasis, Arch. Ophthal. **74:**470, 1965.

Unsworth, A. C., Fox, J. C., Rosenthal, E., and Shelton, P. A.: Larval granulomatosis of the retina due to nematode, Amer. J. Ophthal. **60:**127, 1967.

Von Noorden, G. K., and Buck, A. A.: Ocular onchocerciasis, Arch. Ophthal. **80:**26, 1968.

Wood, R. M., Ellison, A. C., Kelley, K. C., and Kaufman, H. E.: Antibody to *Toxocara canis* in humans, Arch. Ophthal. **73:**482, 1965.

Spirochetes

Harner, R. E., Smith, J. L., and Israel, C. W.: The FTA-ABS test in late syphilis, J.A.M.A. **203:**545, 1968.

Smith, J. L., and Israel, C. W.: Treponemes in aqueous humor in late seronegative syphilis, Trans. Amer. Acad. Ophthal. Otolaryng. **72:**63, 1968.

Viruses

Alfano, J. E.: Ocular aspects of the maternal rubella syndrome, Trans. Amer. Acad. Ophthal. Otolaryng. **69:**235, 1966.

Blodi, F. C.: Ophthalmic zoster in malignant disease, Amer. J. Ophthal. **65:**686, 1968.

Boniuk, M., Phillips, C. A., Hines, M. J., and Friedman, J. B.: Adenovirus infections of the conjunctiva and cornea, Trans. Amer. Acad. Ophthal. Otolaryng. **70:**1016, 1966.

Boniuk, M., and Zimmerman, L. E.: Ocular pathology in the rubella syndrome, Arch. Ophthal. **77:**455, 1967.

Conference on trachoma and allied diseases, Amer. J. Ophthal. **63:**1027, 1967.

Copenhaver, R. M.: Chickenpox with retinopathy, Arch. Ophthal. **75:**199, 1967.

Croffead, G. W., and Harrison, S. W.: Vaccinia conjunctivitis, Amer. J. Ophthal. **53:**531, 1962.

Geltzer, A. I., Guber, D., and Sears, M. L.: Ocular manifestations of the 1964-65 rubella epidemic, Amer. J. Ophthal. **63:**221, 1967.

Hogan, M. J., Kimura, S. J., and Thygeson, P.: Pathology of herpes simplex keratoiritis, Trans. Amer. Ophthal. Soc. **61:**75, 1963.

Jarcho, L. W., Fred, H. L., and Castle, C. H.: Encephalitis and poliomyelitis in the adult due to Coxsackie virus group B, type 5, New Eng. J. Med. **268:**235, 1963.

Kaufman, H. E., Brown, D. C., and Ellison, E. D.: Herpes virus in the lacrimal gland, conjunctiva and cornea of man—a chronic infection, Amer. J. Ophthal. **65:**32, 1968.

Leopold, I. H., and Sery, T. W.: Epidemiology of herpes simplex keratitis, Invest. Ophthal. **2:**498, 1963.

McKee, A. P.: The biology of the herpes simplex virus, Invest. Ophthal. **2:**490, 1963.

Merselis, J. G., Jr., Kaye, D., and Hook, E. W.: Disseminated herpes zoster, Arch. Intern. Med. **113:**679, 1964.

Morax, P. V., Saraux, H., Moday, S., and Coscas, G.: The ocular manifestations of rickettsiosis and of neorickettsiosis, Ann. Oculist. **194:**929, 1961.

Phillips, C. A., Melnick, J. L., Yow, M. D., Bayatpour, M., and Burkhardt, M.: Persistence of virus in infants with congenital rubella and in normal infants with a history of maternal rubella, J.A.M.A. **193:**1027, 1965.

Presley, G. D.: Fundus changes in Rocky Mountain spotted fever, Amer. J. Ophthal. **67:**263, 1969.

Roy, F. H.: Microsurgery of congenital rubella cataract: modification of linear extraction, Amer. J. Ophthal. **65:**81, 1968.

Roy, F. H., Hiatt, R. L., Korones, S. B., and Roane, J.: Ocular manifestations of congenital rubella syndrome, Arch. Ophthal. **75:**601, 1966.

Symposium on trachoma, Invest. Ophthal. **2:**460, 1963.

Yanoff, M., Schaffer, D. B., and Scheie, H. G.: Rubella ocular syndrome. Correlation of clinical, viral, and pathologic studies, Trans. Amer. Acad. Ophthal. Otolaryng. **72:**906, 1968.

Zimmerman, L. E.: Histopathologic basis for ocular manifestations of congenital rubella syndrome, Amer. J. Ophthal. **65:**837, 1968.

ENDOCRINE DISEASE AND THE EYE
Diabetes mellitus
Ocular fundi

Ashton, N.: Diabetic microangiopathy, Advances Ophthal. **8:**1, 1958.

Caird, F. I., Burdette, A. F., and Draper, G. J.: Diabetic retinopathy, Diabetes **17:**121, 1968.

Cogan, D. C., and Kuwabara, T.: Capillary shunts in the pathogenesis of diabetic retinopathy, Diabetes **12:**293, 1963.

Conteras, J. S., Field, R. A., Hall, W. A., and

Sweet, W. H.: Ophthalmological observations in hypophyseal stalk resection, Arch. Ophthal. **67:**428, 1962.

Davis, M. D.: Vitreous contraction in proliferative diabetic retinopathy, Arch. Ophthal. **74:**741, 1965.

Henderson, J. W.: Induced hypopituitarism in the management of diabetic retinopathy, Amer. J. Med. Sci. **250:**220, 1965.

Jain, I. S., and Luthra, C. L.: Diabetic retinopathy, Arch. Ophthal. **78:**198, 1967.

Kimura, S. J., and Caygill, W. M., editors: Vascular complications of diabetes mellitus: with special emphasis on microangiopathy of the eye, St. Louis, 1967, The C. V. Mosby Co.

Meyer-Schwickerath, G. R. E., and Schott, K.: Diabetic retinopathy and photocoagulation, Amer. J. Ophthal. **66:**597, 1968.

Norton, E. W. D., and Gutman, F.: Diabetic retinopathy studied by fluorescein angiography, Ophthalmologica **150:**5, 1965.

Okun, E., and Cibis, P. A.: The role of photocoagulation in the therapy of proliferative diabetic retinopathy, Arch. Ophthal. **75:**337, 1966.

Patz, A., and Maumenee, A. E.: Studies on diabetic retinopathy. I. Retinopathy in a dog with spontaneous diabetes mellitus, Amer. J. Ophthal. **54:**532, 1962.

Poulsen, J. E.: The Houssay phenomenon in man. Recovery from retinopathy in a case of diabetes with Simmonds' disease, Diabetes **2:**7, 1953.

Tolentino, F. I., Lee, P., and Schepens, C. L.: Biomicroscopic study of vitreous cavity in diabetic retinopathy, Arch. Ophthal. **75:**238, 1966.

Yanoff, M.: Ocular pathology of diabetes mellitus, Amer. J. Ophthal. **67:**21, 1969.

Cornea

Henkind, P., and Wise, G. N.: Descemet's wrinkles in diabetes, Amer. J. Ophthal. **52:**371, 1961.

Conjunctiva

Ditzel, J., Beaven, D. W., and Renold, A. E.: Early vascular changes in diabetes mellitus, Metabolism **9:**400, 1960.

Lens

Kinoshita, J. H., Merola, L. O., and Dikmak, E.: Osmotic changes in experimental galactose cataracts, Exp. Eye Res. **1:**405, 1962.

Patterson, J. W., Patterson, M. E., and Bunting, K. W.: Experimental carbohydrate cataracts, Exp. Eye Res. **1:**411, 1962.

Motor nerves

Goldstein, J. E., and Cogan, D. G.: Diabetic ophthalmoplegia with special reference to the pupil, Arch. Ophthal. **64:**592, 1960.

Lincoff, H., and Cogan, D. G.: Unilateral headache and oculomotor paralysis not caused by headache, Arch. Ophthal. **57**:181, 1957.

Rucker, C. W.: Paralysis of the third, fourth and sixth cranial nerves, Amer. J. Ophthal. **46**:789, 1958.

Snydacker, D.: Diabetic neuropathy as a cause of extraocular muscle palsy, Trans. Amer. Acad. Ophthal. Otolaryng. **62**:704, 1958.

Hyperthyroidism

Day, R. M.: Ocular manifestations of thyroid disease, Arch. Ophthal. **64**:324, 1960.

Day, R. M., and Carroll, F. D.: Optic nerve involvement associated with thyroid dysfunction, Trans. Amer. Ophthal. Soc. **59**:220, 1961.

Haddad, H. M.: Tonography and visual fields in endocrine exophthalmos: report on 29 patients, Amer. J. Ophthal. **64**:63, 1967.

Henderson, J. W.: Relief of eyelid retraction, Arch. Ophthal. **74**:205, 1965.

Irvine, W. J., editor: Thyrotoxicosis. Proceedings of an international symposium, Edinburgh, May 1967, Baltimore, 1967, The Williams & Wilkins Co.

Ochi, Y., and DeGroot, L. J.: Long acting thyroid stimulator of Graves's disease, New Eng. J. Med. **278**:718, 1968.

Schultz, R. O., Van Allen, M. W., and Blodi, F. C.: Endocrine ophthalmoplegia, Arch. Ophthal. **63**:217, 1960.

Werner, S. C.: The thyroid, a fundamental and clinical text, New York, 1955, Hoeber Medical Division, Harper & Row, Publishers.

Werner, S. C., Feind, C. R., and Aida, M.: Graves's disease and total thyroidectomy. Progression of severe eye changes and decrease in serum long acting thyroid stimulator after operation, New Eng. J. Med. **276**:132, 1967.

Hyperparathyroidism

Cogan, D. G., Albright, F., and Bartter, F. C.: Hypercalcemia and band keratopathy, Arch. Ophthal. **40**:625, 1948.

Pronove, P., and Bartter, F. C.: Diagnosis of hyperparathyroidism, Metabolism **10**:349, 1961.

Hypoparathyroidism

Hanno, H. A., and Weiss, T. I.: Hypoparathyroidism, pseudohypoparathyroidism and pseudopseudohypoparathyroidism, Arch. Ophthal. **65**:238, 1961.

CARDIOVASCULAR DISEASE

Ashton, N., and Harry, J.: The pathology of cotton-wool spots and cytoid bodies in hypertensive retinopathy and other diseases, Trans. Ophthal. Soc. U. K. **83**:91, 1963.

Ballantyne, A. J., and Michaelson, I. C.: Textbook of the fundus of the eye, Baltimore, 1962, The Williams & Wilkins Co.

Christensen, L.: The nature of the cytoid body, Trans. Amer. Ophthal. Soc. **56**:451, 1958.

Friedenwald, J. S.: Retinal and choroidal arteriosclerosis. In Ridley, F., and Sorsby, A., editors: Modern trends in ophthalmology, New York, 1940, Hoeber Medical Division, Harper & Row, Publishers.

Harry, J., and Ashton, N.: The pathology of hypertensive retinopathy, Trans. Ophthal. Soc. U. K. **88**:71, 1963.

Hill, D. W., and Dollery, C. T.: Calibre changes in retinal arterioles, Trans. Ophthal. Soc. U. K. **83**:61, 1963.

Keith, N. M., Wagener, H. P., and Barker, N. W.: Some different types of essential hypertension: their course and prognosis, Amer. J. Med. Sci. **197**:332, 1939.

McMichael, J., and Dollery, C. T.: Hypertensive retinopathy, Trans. Ophthal. Soc. U. K. **83**:51, 1963.

Moses, C.: Artherosclerosis. Mechanisms or a guide to prevention, Philadelphia, 1963, Lea & Febiger.

Seitz, R.: Retinal vessels, Blodi, F., translator, St. Louis, 1964, The C. V. Mosby Co.

Wise, G. N.: Arteriosclerosis secondary to retinal vein obstruction, Trans. Amer. Ophthal. Soc. **56**:361, 1958.

THE CENTRAL NERVOUS SYSTEM AND THE EYE

Acers, T. E., and Cooper, W. C.: Cortical blindness secondary to bacterial meningitis, Amer. J. Ophthal. **59**:226, 1965.

Acers, T. E., and Tenney, R.: Ocular symptomatology of posterior fossa tumors, Arch. Ophthal. **65**:872, 1968.

Botterell, E. H., Lloyd, L. A., and Hoffman, H. J.: Oculomotor palsy due to supraclinoid internal carotid artery berry aneurysm, Amer. J. Ophthal. **54**:609, 1962.

Breger, B. C., and Leopold, I. H.: Incidence of uveitis in multiple sclerosis, Amer. J. Ophthal. **62**:540, 1966.

Callow, A. D.: Surgical management of varying patterns of vertebral artery and subclavian artery insufficiency, New Eng. J. Med. **270**:546, 1964.

Cheek, C. W., Simon, K. A., and Gay, A. J.: Acquired cranial nerve lesions affecting the ocular system, Amer. J. Ophthal. **59**:13, 1965.

Cogan, D. G.: Neurology of the visual system, Springfield, Ill., 1966, Charles C Thomas, Publisher.

Croll, M.: The ocular manifestations of multiple sclerosis, Amer. J. Ophthal. **60**:822, 1965.

Galin, M. A., Rodriguez-Barrios, R., Pola, R., and McLean, J. M.: Cerebro-vascular insufficiency, Trans. Amer. Acad. Ophthal. Otolaryng. **71:** 119, 1967.

Gills, J. P., Jr., Kapp, J. P., and Odom, G. L.: Benign intracranial hypertension, Arch. Ophthal. **78:**592, 1967.

Glaser, J. S.: Myasthenic pseudo-internuclear ophthalmoplegia, Arch. Ophthal. **75:**363, 1966.

Goldberg, M. F., Payne, J. W., and Brunt, P. W.: Ophthalmologic studies of familial dysautonomia; the Riley-Day syndrome, Arch. Ophthal. **80:**732, 1968.

Green, W. R., Hackett, E. R., and Schlizinger, N. S.: Oculomotor nerve paralysis, Arch. Ophthal. **72:**154, 1964.

Gurdjian, E. S., Hardy, W. G., Lindner, D. W., and Thomas, L. M.: Diagnostic evolution and treatment of occlusive cerebro-vascular disease. Trans. Amer. Acad. Ophthal. Otolaryng. **66:** 149, 1962.

Harley, R. D., Baird, H. W., and Craven, E. M.: Ataxia-telangectasia, Arch. Ophthal. **77:**582, 1967.

Hedges, T. R.: The aortic arch syndrome, Arch. Ophthal. **71:**28, 1964.

Henderson, J. W., and Schneider, R. C.: The ocular findings in carotid fistula in a series of 17 cases, Amer. J. Ophthal. **48:**585, 1959.

Hollenhorst, R. W.: Ocular manifestations of insufficiency or thrombosis of the internal carotid artery, Trans. Amer. Ophthal. Soc. **56:**474, 1958.

Hollenhorst, R. W.: Carotid and vertebral-basilar arterial stenosis· and occlusion; neuro-ophthalmologic considerations, Trans. Amer. Acad. Ophthal. Otolaryng. **66:**166, 1962.

Hoyt, W. F.: Some neuro-ophthalmological considerations in cerebrovascular insufficiency, Arch. Ophthal. **62:**260, 1959.

Hoyt, W. F., and Beeston, D.: The ocular fundus in neurologic disease, St. Louis, 1966, The C. V. Mosby Co.

Huber, A.: Eye symptoms in brain tumors, van Wien, S., translator, St. Louis, 1961, The C. V. Mosby Co.

Kearns, T. P., and Hollenhorst, R. W.: Venous-stasis retinopathy of occlusive disease of the carotid artery, Mayo Clin. Proc. **38:**304, 1963.

Mannick, J. A., Suter, C. G., and Hume, D. H.: The "subclavian steal" syndrome: a further documentation, J.A.M.A. **182:**258, 1962.

Riley, C. M., and Moore, R. H.: Familial dysautonomia differentiated from related disorders: case reports and discussions of current concepts, Pediatrics **37:**435, 1966.

Ross, A. T.: Cranial nerve palsies in diabetes mellitus, Neurology **12:**180, 1962.

Smith, J. L., editor: Neuro-ophthalmology—Symposium of the University of Miami and the Bascom Palmer Eye Institute, St. Louis, 1965, 1967, 1968, The C. V. Mosby Co., vols., 2, 3, 4.

Smith, J. L., Singer, J. A., Moore, M. B., and Yobs, A. R.: Seronegative ocular and neurosyphilis, Amer. J. Ophthal. **59:**753, 1965.

Solomon, G. E., and Chutorian, A. M.: Opsoclonus and occult neuroblastoma, New Eng. J. Med. **279:**475, 1968.

Walsh, F. B.: Visual field defects due to aneurysms at the circle of Willis, Arch. Ophthal. **71:** 15, 1964.

Walsh, F. B., and Hoyt, W. F.: Clinical neuro-ophthalmology, ed. 3, Baltimore, The Williams & Wilkins Co. (In press.)

Williams, D., and Wilson, T. G.: The diagnosis of the major and minor syndromes of basilar insufficiency, Brain **85:**741, 1962.

HEREDITARY DISORDERS

Kertesz, E. D., and Falls, H. F.: Genetic application to pediatric ophthalmology. In Liebman, S. D., and Gellis, S. S., editors: The pediatrician's ophthalmology, St. Louis, 1966, The C. V. Mosby Co.

McKusick, V. A.: Heritable disorders of connective tissue, ed. 3, St. Louis, 1966, The C. V. Mosby Co.

Stanbury, J. B., Wyngaarden, J. B., and Fredrickson, D. S., editors: The metabolic basis of inherited disease, ed. 2, New York, 1966, McGraw-Hill Book Co.

Waardenburg, P. J., Franceschetti, A., and Klien, D.: Genetics and ophthalmology, Springfield, Ill., 1963, Charles C Thomas, Publisher.

Albinism

Fonda, G.: Characteristics and low-vision corrections in albinism. Report of 161 patients, Arch. Ophthal. **68:**754, 1962.

Johnson, D. L., Jacobson, L. W., Toyama, R., and Monahan, R.: Histopathology of eyes in Chédiak-Higashi syndrome, Arch. Ophthal. **75:** 84, 1966.

Kanfer, J. N., Blume, R. S., Yankee, R. A., and Wolff, S. M.: Alteration of sphingolipid metabolism in leukocytes from patients with the Chédiak-Higashi syndrome, New Eng. J. Med. **279:**410, 1968.

Spencer, W. H., and Hogan, M. J.: Ocular manifestations of Chédiak-Higashi syndrome, Amer. J. Ophthal. **50:**1197, 1960.

Alkaptonuria and ochronosis

Brookler, M. I., Martin, W. J., Underdahl, L. O., Worthington, J. W., and Mathiewson, D. R.:

Alkaptonuria and ochronosis: further experiences, Mayo Clin. Proc. **39**:107, 1964.

Hatch, J. L.: Hereditary alkaptonuria with ochronosis, Arch. Ophthal. **62**:575, 1959.

Amyloidosis

Cohen, A. S.: Amyloidosis, New Eng. J. Med. **277**:522, 1967.

Crawford, J. B.: Cotton wool exudates in systemic amyloidosis, Arch. Ophthal. **78**:214, 1967.

Kaufman, H. E.: Primary familial amyloidosis, Arch. Ophthal. **60**:1036, 1958.

Paton, D., and Duke, J. R.: Primary familial amyloidosis, Amer. J. Ophthal. **61**:736, 1966.

Smith, M. E., and Zimmerman, L. E.: Amyloidosis of the eyelid and conjunctiva, Arch. Ophthal. **75**:42, 1966.

Smith, M. E., and Zimmerman, L. E.: Amyloid in corneal dystrophies, Arch. Ophthal. **79**:407, 1968.

Stafford, W. R., and Fine, B. S.: Amyloidosis of the cornea, Arch. Ophthal. **75**:53, 1966.

Wong, V. G., and McFarlin, D. E.: Primary familial amyloidosis, Arch. Ophthal. **78**:208, 1967.

Carbohydrate metabolism

Toussaint, D., and Davis, P.: Ocular histopathology in generalized glycogenosis (Pompe's disease), Arch. Ophthal. **73**:342, 1965.

Chromosomal abnormalities

Ginsberry, J., and Perrin, E. V. D.: Ocular manifestations of 13-15 trisomy, Arch. Ophthal. **74**:487, 1965.

Cystine storage disease

Ben-Ishay, I., Dreyfuss, F., and Ullman, T. D.: Fanconi syndrome with hypouricemia in an adult, Amer. J. Med. **31**:793, 1961.

Cogan, D. G., and Kuwabara, T.: Ocular pathology of cystinosis, Arch. Ophthal. **63**:51, 1960.

Wong, V. G., Lietman, P. S., and Seegmiller, J. E.: Alterations of pigment epithelium in cystinosis, Arch. Ophthal. **77**:361, 1967.

Disorders of lipid metabolism

Abrahamson, I. A., Sr., and Abrahamson, I. A., Jr.: Hypercarotenemia, Arch. Ophthal. **68**:4, 1962.

Anderson, B., Margolis, G., and Lynn, W. S.: Ocular lesions related to disturbances of fat metabolism, Amer. J. Ophthal. **45**:23, 1958.

Avioli, L. V., Lasersohn, J. T., and Lopresti, J. M.: Histiocystosis X (Schüller-Christian disease), Medicine **42**:199, 1963.

Baum, J. L., Tannenbaum, M., and Kolodny, E. H.: Refsum's syndrome with corneal involvement, Amer. J. Ophthal. **60**:699, 1965.

Blodi, F. C., and Yarbrough, J. C.: Ocular manifestations of familial hypercholesterolemia, Trans. Amer. Ophthal. Soc. **60**:304, 1962.

Brady, R. O.: The sphingolipidoses, New Eng. J Med. **275**:312, 1966.

Cogan, D. G., Kuwabara, T., Moser, H., and Hazard, G. W.: Retinopathy in a case of Farber's lipogranulomatosis, Arch. Ophthal. **75**:752, 1966.

Cogan, D. G., and Kuwabara, T.: The sphingolipidoses and the eyes, Arch. Ophthal. **79**:437, 1968.

Frederickson, D. S., Levy, R. I., and Lees, R. S.: Fat transport in lipoproteins—an integrated approach to mechanisms and disorders, New Eng. J. Med. **276**:34, 94, 148, 215, 276, 1967.

Hsia, D. Y., Naylor, J., and Bigler, J. A.: Gaucher's disease: report of two cases in father and son and review of the literature, New Eng. J. Med. **261**:164, 1959.

Jampel, R. S., and Falls, H. F.: Atypical retinitis pigmentosa, acanthrocytosis, and heredodegenerative neuromuscular disease, Arch. Ophthal. **59**:818, 1958.

Macaraeg, P. V. J., Lasagna, L., and Snyder, B.: Arcus not so senilis, Ann. Intern. Med. **68**:345, 1968.

Schneck, L., Volk, B. W., and Saifer, A.: The gangliosidoses, Amer. J. Med. **46**:245, 1969.

Spaeth, G. L., and Frost, P.: Fabry's disease, Arch. Ophthal. **74**:760, 1965.

Thannhauser, S. J.: Lipidoses, diseases of the intracellular lipid metabolism, New York, 1958, Grune & Stratton, Inc.

Volk, B. W., Aronson, S. M., and Saifer, A.: Fructose-1 phosphate aldolase deficiency in Tay-Sachs disease, Amer. J. Med. **36**:481, 1964.

Galactosemia

Cordes, F. C.: Galactosemia cataract: a review, Amer. J. Ophthal. **50**:1151, 1960.

Wilson, W. A.: Failure to produce cataracts in rats with galactosemia diet, Amer. J. Ophthal. **67**:224, 1969.

Hepatolenticular degeneration (Wilson's disease)

Goldberg, M. F., and von Noorden, G. K.: Ophthalmologic findings in Wilson's hepatolenticular degeneration, Arch. Ophthal. **75**:162, 1966.

Goldstein, N. P., Randall, R. V., Gross, J. B., Rosevear, J. W., and McGuckin, W. F.: Treatment of Wilson's disease (hepatolenticular degeneration) with DL-penicillamine, Neurology **12**:231, 1962.

Mitchell, A. M., and Heller, G. L.: Changes in Kayser-Fleischer ring during treatment of hepatolenticular degeneration, Arch. Ophthal. **80**:622, 1968.

Sternlieb, I., and Scheinberg, I. H.: The diagnosis of Wilson's disease in asymptomatic patients, J.A.M.A. **183**:750, 1963.

Histiocytosis

Petersen, R. A., and Kuwabara, T.: Ocular manifestations of familial lymphohistiocytosis, Arch. Ophthal. **79**:413, 1968.

Zimmerman, L. E.: Ocular lesions of juvenile xanthogranuloma, Amer. J. Ophthal. **60**:1011, 1965.

Homocystinuria

Carey, M. C., Donovan, D. F., FitzGerald, O., and McAuley, F. D.: Homocystinuria. I. Clinical and pathological study of nine subjects in six families, Amer. J. Med. **45**:26, 1968.

Chase, H. P., Goodman, S. I., and O'Brien, D.: Treatment of homocystinuria, Arch. Dis. Child. **42**:514, 1967.

Lieberman, T. W., and Podos, S. M.: Homocystinuria. In Becker, B., and Drews, R. C., editors: Current concepts in ophthalmology, St. Louis, 1967, The C. V. Mosby Co.

Presley, G. D., and Sidbury, J. B.: Homocystinuria and ocular defects, Amer. J. Ophthal. **63**:1723, 1967.

Presley, G. D., Stinson, I. N., and Sidbury, J. B.: Homocystinuria: at the North Carolina State School for the Blind, Amer. J. Ophthal. **66**:884, 1968.

Schimke, R. N., McKusick, V. A., Huang, T., and Pollack, A. D.: Homocystinuria, J.A.M.A. **193**:711, 1965.

Mucopolysaccharidoses

McKusick, V. A., Kaplan, D., Wise, D., Hanley, W. B., Suddarth, S. B., Sevick, M. E., and Maumenee, A. E.: The genetic mucopolysaccharidoses, Medicine **44**:445, 1965.

COLLAGEN DISEASES AND MUSCLE DISORDERS

Anderson, B., Sr.: Ocular lesions in relapsing polychondritis and other rheumatoid syndromes, Amer. J. Ophthal. **64**:35, 1967.

Bianchine, J. R., Macaraeg, P. V. J., Lasagna, L., Azarnoff, D. L., Brunk, S. F., Hvidberg, E. F., and Owens, J. A., Jr.: Drugs as etiologic factors in the Stevens-Johnson syndrome, Amer. J. Med. **44**:390, 1968.

Bloch, K. J., Buchanan, W. W., Wohl, M. J., and Bunim, J. J.: Sjögren's syndrome. A clinical, pathological and serological survey of 62 cases, Medicine **44**:187, 1965.

Blodi, F.: Sympathetic ophthalmia as an allergic phenomenon. With a study of the association with phacoanaphylactic uveitis and a report on the pathologic findings in sympathizing eyes,

Trans. Amer. Acad. Ophthal. Otolaryng. **63**:642, 1959.

Boeck, J.: Ocular changes in periarteritis nodosa, Amer. J. Ophthal. **42**:567, 1956.

Burian, H. M., and Burns, C. A.: Electroretinography and dark adaptation in patients with myotonic dystrophy, Amer. J. Ophthal. **61**:1044, 1966.

Burian, H. M., and Burns, C. A.: Ocular changes in myotonic dystrophy, Trans. Amer. Ophthal. Soc. **64**:250, 1966.

Burian, H. M., von Noorden, G. K., and Ponseti, I. V.: Chamber angle anomalies in systemic connective tissue disorders, Trans. Amer. Ophthal. Soc. **58**:301, 1960.

Caughey, J. E., and Myrianthopoulos, N. C.: Dystrophia myotonia and related disorders, Springfield, Ill., 1963, Charles C Thomas, Publisher.

Christensen, L.: The nature of the cytoid body, Trans. Amer. Ophthal. Soc. **56**:451, 1958.

Cogan, D. G.: Myasthenia gravis. A review of the disease and a description of lid twitch as a characteristic sign, Arch. Ophthal. **74**:217, 1965.

Frenkel, M.: Myasthenia gravis: current trends, Amer. J. Ophthal. **61**:522, 1966.

Hogan, M. J., Thygeson, P., and Kimura, S. J.: Uveitis in association with rheumatism, Trans. Amer. Ophthal. Soc. **54**:93, 1956.

Hollenhorst, R. W.: Effect of posture on retinal ischemia from temporal arteritis, Arch. Ophthal. **78**:569, 1967.

Howard, G. M.: The Stevens-Johnson syndrome, Amer. J. Ophthal. **55**:893, 1963.

Manshot, W. A.: The eye in relation to collagen disease, Trans. Ophthal. Soc. U. K. **80**:137, 1960.

Retzlaff, J. A., Kearns, T. P., Howard, Jr., F. M., and Cronin, M. L.: Lancaster red-green test in evaluation of edrophonium effect in myasthenia gravis, Amer. J. Ophthal. **67**:13, 1969.

Wolter, J. R., and Bentley, M. D.: Scleromalacia perforans and massive granuloma of the sclera, Amer. J. Ophthal. **51**:71, 1961.

DISEASES OF THE BLOOD

Alfano, J. E., and Roper, K. L.: Visual disturbances following acute blood loss, Amer. J. Ophthal. **38**:817, 1954.

Allen, R. A., and Straatsma, B. R.: Ocular involvement in leukemia and allied diseases, Arch. Ophthal. **66**:490, 1961.

Aronson, S. B., and Shaw, R.: Corneal crystals in multiple myeloma, Arch. Ophthal. **61**:541, 1959.

Chernoff, A. I.: The human hemoglobins in health

and disease, New Eng. J. Med. **253**:322, 365, 416, 1955.

Ellis, P. P., and Hamilton, H.: Retrobulbar neuritis in pernicious anemia, Amer. J. Ophthal. **49**:95, 1959.

François, J., and Rabaey, M.: Corneal dystrophy and paraproteinemia, Amer. J. Ophthal. **52**:895, 1962.

Funahashi, T., Fink, A., Robinson, M., and Watson, R. J.: Pathology of conjunctival vessels in sickle cell disease, Amer. J. Ophthal. **57**:713, 1964.

Geeraets, W. J., and Guerry, D. III: Angioid streaks and sickle cell disease, Amer. J. Ophthal. **49**:450, 1960.

Goodman, G., von Sallman, L., and Holland, M. G.: Ocular manifestations of sickle-cell disease, Arch. Ophthal. **58**:655, 1957.

Levine, R. A., and Kaplan, A. M.: The ophthalmoscopic findings in C + S disease, Amer. J. Ophthal. **59**:37, 1965.

Lieb, W. A., Geeraets, W. J., and Guerry, D., III: Sickle-cell retinopathy, Acta Ophthal. **58**:1, supp., 1959.

Marks, P. A.: Thallasemia syndromes, New Eng. J. Med. **275**:1363, 1966.

Massa, J. M., De Vloo, N., and Jamotton, L.: Les manifestations oculaires des hemopathies, Bull. Soc. Belg. Ophthal. **142**:1, 1966.

Oglesby, R. B.: Corneal opacities in a patient with cryoglobulinemia with reticulohistiocytosis, Arch. Ophthal. **65**:63, 1961.

Reese, A. B.: Tumors of the eye, ed. 2, New York, 1963, Hoeber Medical Division, Harper & Row, Publishers.

Sanders, T. E., and Podos, S.: Pars plana cysts in multiple myeloma, Trans. Amer. Acad. Ophthal. Otolaryng. **70**:951, 1966.

Welch, R. B., and Goldberg, M. F.: Sickle-cell hemoglobin and its relation to fundus abnormality, Arch. Ophthal **75**:353, 1966.

Index